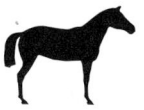

Clinical Examination of Horses

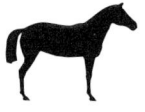

Clinical Examination of Horses

Victor C. Speirs
MVSc, PhD, Dr. med vet Habil, FACVSc, Diplomate ACVS,
Diplomate ECVS, Specialist Equine Surgeon
Melbourne, Australia

Formerly:
Professor, Large Animal Surgery
College of Veterinary Medicine
Auburn University
Alabama

Professor and Head, Equine Surgery
Klinik für Nutztiere und Pferde
Universität Bern, Switzerland

With contributions by:
Robert H. Wrigley
BVSc, MS, DVR, MRCVS, Diplomate ACVR
Associate Professor, Department of Radiological Health Sciences
College of Veterinary Medicine and Biomedical Sciences
Colorado State University
Fort Collins, Colorado

Illustrations by **Gale E. Mueller**

W.B. SAUNDERS COMPANY
A Division of Harcourt Brace & Company
Philadelphia London Toronto Montreal Sydney Tokyo

W.B. SAUNDERS COMPANY
A Division of Harcourt Brace & Company

The Curtis Center
Independence Square West
Philadelphia, Pennsylvania 19106

Library of Congress Catalog Card Number 96-72080.

CLINICAL EXAMINATION OF HORSES   ISBN 0–7216–6506–3

Printed in the United States of America.

Last digit is the print number: 9   8   7   6   5   4   3   2   1

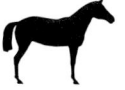

Acknowledgments

I am grateful to the staff of W.B. Saunders for their assistance in getting this text to publication. Special thanks especially to Sandra Valkhoff and Ray Kersey.

Gale Mueller is acknowledged for her artwork, and especially for her patience with the difficulties associated with working with an author who resides on another continent.

Thanks are extended to Dr. Robert Wrigley, who wrote the section on ultrasonography and supplied most of the ultrasonographic figures for the different organ sections.

Thanks are also extended to the following individuals for providing photographs from their personal files:

Dr. A.O. McKinnon

Dr. J.R. Blogg

Dr. S. Church

For assistance with photography: Dr. G.D. Jeffrey and his staff at the Cranbourne Equine Hospital, Drs. J.C. Sewell, G.D. Duncan, R.H. Selth and their staff at the Epsom Veterinary Center, Dr. J.C. van Veenendaal, Dr. R.B. Lavelle, Dr. A.A. MacLean, Dr. A.G. Turner, and Professor V.D. Studdert for permission to photograph within the Veterinary Clinical Center of the University of Melbourne.

Finally, thanks especially to my wife, Kaye, and daughters, Naomi and Camilla, for their endless patience during this most time-consuming undertaking.

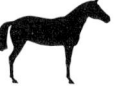

Preface

As the type and complexity of diagnostic aids available to the clinician increase it has become easy to forget that an accurate diagnosis rests basically on a competent clinical examination supplemented with results from selected ancillary aids. The use of specialized diagnostic aids usually requires that the site of disease has been localized by a clinical examination. Therefore, a competent clinical examination, in addition to making a diagnosis possible, will dictate use of appropriate ancillary testing, thereby reducing the unnecessary use of such tests.

A competent clinical examination should be systematic and thorough, an approach that is automatic to a good diagnostician. A systematic approach ensures that all appropriate body regions are examined and it is made easier if protocols for recording the results of the clinical examination are utilized. This author's experience of teaching and clinical investigation for over 25 years has been more than sufficient in reinforcing the adage that more mistakes are made by not looking than not knowing.

This text has been written with the objective of providing, in one book, instructions for carrying out the procedures involved in a general clinical examination and the special examinations of body systems of the horse. The lack of such a book has been apparent during the time this author has been teaching clinical examination techniques to veterinary undergraduates. Although the main objective has been to describe what examinations are necessary and how they can be carried out, an effort has been made to ensure that the reader understands the reason for each test and the significance of the result. A clinician should be aware of the vast array of ancillary diagnostic aids that are available, and they should have a working knowledge of how they function and of the indications for the use of each. More importantly, because the clinician is usually the main or only point of contact for the owner of a patient, a thorough understanding of the significance of the results of extra diagnostic tests is required. For this reason the theoretical basis of the ancillary diagnostic aids, some of which are extremely sophisticated, has been briefly described.

This book is directed primarily towards students, although it is hoped that graduates at all levels will find it a useful reference for occasions when a test or procedure with which they are not familiar must be carried out. The text is not intended to be a text of medicine, although whenever possible the normal findings and results of the various tests are presented in order to facilitate identification of the abnormal.

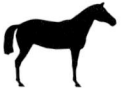

Contents

Handling Horses

INTRODUCTION

A clinical examination is almost always carried out with the horse or foal under some form of restraint. Exceptions to this do occur, for example when the horse is too dangerous, is thought to be suffering from a disease such as rabies, or is running in a paddock and cannot be caught. Under such circumstances the examination cannot be thorough. The general examination requires relatively little restraint, but some of the more invasive components may involve discomfort necessitating a greater level of restraint. In unhandled or fractious animals examination of the hind limbs is more difficult and often dangerous. Although small, foals are often difficult to restrain before they have been educated to human contact and control.

PHYSICAL RESTRAINT OF THE ADULT HORSE

Before an adult horse can be restrained and controlled, it must be caught, which is usually done by the person presenting the horse. Occasionally this is not possible and the veterinarian must catch the animal. At pasture this is often difficult, and relatively few horses will let a stranger approach and place a halter or rope on them. Nevertheless this is the simplest and quickest method when the horse is cooperative. It is usually better to conceal the rope or halter and when possible to carry a tidbit in the form of grass or hay. If required, the horse can be chased into a small yard or corner, which makes capture easier. If there are several horses together, it is better to chase them all into the yard and then to isolate the patient. Horses should always be approached from the left, or "near," side because most are trained to accept an approach and application of equipment from this side. Of course, most horses also tolerate an approach from the other side (the "off" side), but usually not as readily, especially when it is a person they are not familiar with. The approach is best made toward the shoulder. From there it is easy to pass the left arm under and then around the neck, prior to putting a rope around the neck or applying a halter, bridle, or headstall (Fig. 1-1). Once contact is made by passing the arm around the neck, most horses succumb to their training and will not attempt to escape. Many horses will allow an approach directly to the head, but if this is resented, the horse quickly withdraws and the opportunity to catch it is often gone.

If the horse is in a stall or small yard, capture is theoretically easier because it cannot run away. However, confinement also makes it more difficult and dangerous for the veterinarian to move back if the horse panics or becomes aggressive. Aggression is more likely to come from a stallion or from a mare with a foal. It is important that the door or gate is not completely closed so that the veterinarian, but not the horse, can quickly escape if necessary. The method of approach is again to the left shoulder, as described. In most cases this will be successful. Occasionally a horse

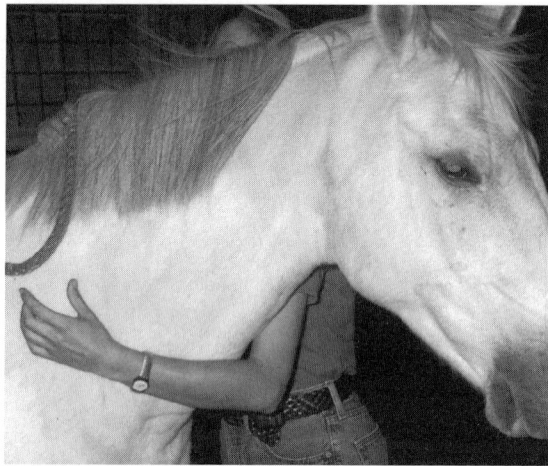

▶ **FIGURE 1-1**

Placing a horse under control. First, an arm is placed around the neck to secure control and prevent the horse from pulling away, and then a lead rope is passed around neck.

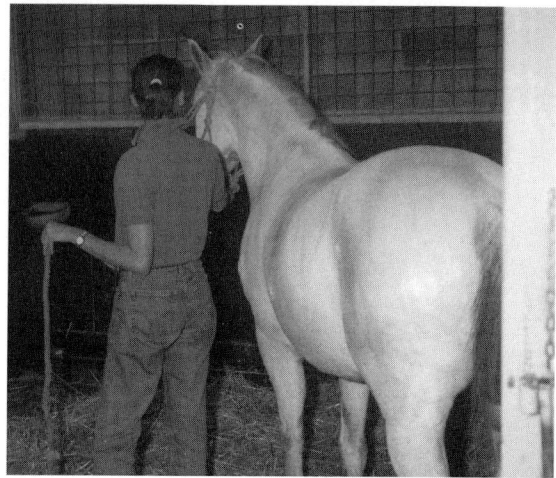

▶ **FIGURE 1-3**

Leading a horse through a doorway. It is important to maintain control by holding the lead as demonstrated and to ensure that the horse is brought completely through the door before being allowed to turn.

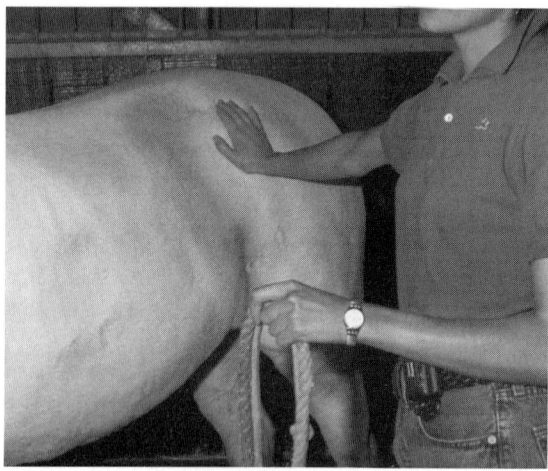

▶ **FIGURE 1-2**

Placing right hand on the left rump to prevent horse from swinging its rear end toward the clinician, sometimes done preparatory to kicking.

will resist by turning away and presenting its rear end. This habit, which can be disconcerting, especially to the inexperienced handler, is usually controlled by placing a hand on the side of the horse to prevent it from swinging its hind quarters toward the handler (Fig. 1-2). Sometimes it is done with the malicious intent of kicking and in such cases great care and some assistance is required. As with all aspects of horse handling, experience slowly provides the extra awareness of which horses are going to cause trouble and how best to avoid or control the situation. *In all cases a sensible, nonheroic attitude is recommended,*

which will ensure a working career relatively free from injury. Stupid or heroic efforts to control horses will sooner or later result in injury that at best may cause a few days away from work but at worst can be fatal.

When returning a horse to a stall or yard, the gate or door should be fully opened, the horse led completely through, then turned around so that the handler is closest to the door or gate. It is unwise to release the horse before the handler can ensure that it cannot run back through the opening before the handler can close it. The horse should be taken straight through the opening and not allowed to "cut the corner," which sometimes results in the horse hitting its tuber coxae on the edge of the doorway. Some horses tend to rush quickly through any opening, and it is wise to ensure that the person leading has good control of the lead rope (Fig. 1-3).

CHEMICAL RESTRAINT OF THE ADULT HORSE

For the normal clinical examination it is better if the horse is not under the influence of any medication that can depress the central nervous system (CNS) because the patient's mental state and response to various stimuli form an important part of the clinical assessment. For some of the more invasive examinations and in certain unruly horses some chemical restraint is sometimes necessary. When chemical restraint is necessary, thought should be given to the pharmacological actions of the drugs used and whether or not they might interfere with the function of the organs being examined (e.g., xylazine administration before abdominal auscultation to evaluate intestinal function or cardiac auscultation to evaluate cardiac sounds). There are other examples, and the use of chemical restraint will be discussed where necessary as each body system is described.

Drugs used for chemical restraint produce varying degrees of CNS depression and analgesia. These drugs are classed as tranquilizers, sedative-hypnotics, and opiates. The basic difference between tranquilizers and the others is that tranquilizers produce CNS depression without analgesia or anesthesia, whereas the others in addition to CNS depression cause varying degrees of anesthesia and analgesia.

Until recently acetylpromazine, a phenothiazine derivative, was the most frequently used tranquilizer in equine practice. It produces alpha-1 blockade and has a mild tranquilizing effect that is maximized if the horse is kept quiet after injection. Horses are easily aroused from its effect, and it is not effective in horses that are already excited. It produces hypotension as a result of the loss of vasomotor tone, which, although usually well tolerated, can be dangerous if the horse is excited or hypovolemic. It lowers the seizure threshold and, therefore, should not be given to horses exhibiting CNS hypersensitivity. There is no specific antagonist. Care should always be exercised when it is used in male horses, particularly stallions, because of the possibility of penile paralysis. Tranquilization in male horses is accompanied by penile prolapse lasting 1 to 2 hours, and each horse should be checked to ensure that penile function has returned and that the penis had retracted into the prepuce. If retraction does not occur, the penis can become edematous, develop permanent paralysis, and incur physical injury necessitating amputation. This problem is more likely to occur if the horse is allowed to run at pasture before the penis has retracted. Therefore, confinement should be maintained until the penis has retracted. If retraction has not occurred after about 2 hours, the penis should be manually placed in the prepuce and prolapse prevented with towel clamps placed in the skin around the prepucial orifice.

The alpha-2 agonist group of drugs, xylazine, detomidine, and romifidine, are the sedative-hypnotic drugs most frequently used in the standing horse, with the latter being more potent and having a longer effect. They are used to produce rapid and reliable sedation, analgesia, and muscle relaxation. They all have a rapid onset of action, within 1 and 5 minutes after intravenous and intramuscular injection, respectively. Duration of effect ranges from 30 to 60 minutes for xylazine to a few hours for romifidine. The duration of analgesia is about half that of sedation. Romifidine has less tendency to cause ataxia than the others. Alpha-2 antagonists such as yohimbine (0.04–0.08 mg/kg IV) can be used to reverse their effects. The major side effects of alpha-2 agonists that are relevant here are bradycardia, first- or second-degree heart block, transient hypertension followed by hypotension, and decreased gastrointestinal propulsive activity.

Opiates are used primarily to provide analgesia when the pain stimulus is expected to be significant, for example during a bone marrow biopsy. They also produce calmness and euphoria. Opioid agonists (morphine, oxymorphone, meperidine) stimulate mu-opioid receptors, opioid agonist-antagonists (pentazocine, butorphanol) and have an affinity for mu- and kappa-opioid receptors with a tendency to block the former, whereas opioid antagonists (naloxone, naltrexone) block

▶ **TABLE 1–1**

SOME DRUGS AND DRUG COMBINATIONS USEFUL FOR ROUTINE STANDING RESTRAINT IN HORSES

Drugs	Intravenous Dose (mg/kg)
Phenothiazine derivatives	
Acetylpromazine maleate	0.04–0.06
Alpha$_2$ agonists	
Xylazine hydrochloride	0.50–1.10
Detomidine hydrochloride	0.01–0.04
Romifidine HCl	0.04–0.08
Opiates	
Meperdine hydrochloride	Not used alone
Butorphanol tartrate	Not used alone
Combinations	
Xylazine HCl-butorphanol tartrate	1.10, 0.02
Xylazine HCl-methadone HCl	0.55, 0.01
Xylazine HCl-meperidine HCl	0.55, 1.10
Xylazine HCl-acetylpromazine maleate	0.55, 0.02
Detomidine HCl-butorphanol tartrate	0.02, 0.02
Romifidine HCl-butorphanol tartrate	0.05, 0.02

Note: Adding opiates provides increased analgesia and sedation.

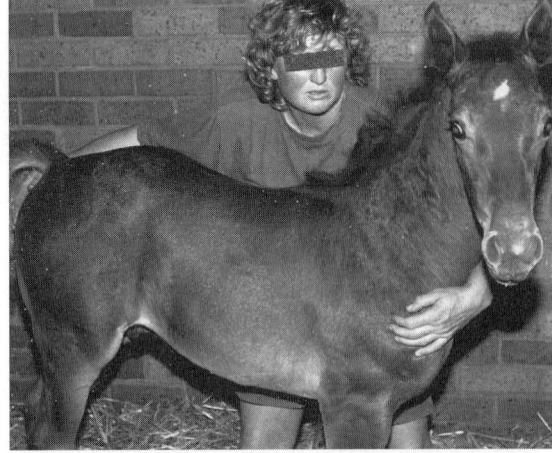

A

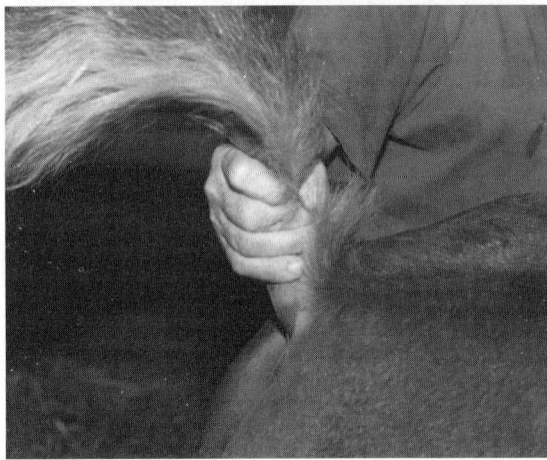

B

▶ **FIGURE 1-4**

Foal restraint. **A.** Standard method with arms around the chest and the thigh. **B.** Holding the base of the tail provides greater security and tends to stop the foal from "sitting down."

the activity of both. Their use is limited by the unpredictable CNS stimulation they often provoke. Therefore they are used most often with or after other drugs that prevent excitement. The opioids have minimal effect on the cardiovascular system but do diminish gastrointestinal propulsive activity. Naloxone is an effective antagonist that, because of its short duration of effect, may require redosing. Of this group of drugs butorphanol tartrate is used most commonly.

No single drug will provide ideal standing restraint under all circumstances, giving rise to a large choice of drugs and drug combinations. Some of these, presented in Table 1-1, having been found useful by the author.

PHYSICAL RESTRAINT OF FOALS

Foals can be very difficult, and even dangerous, to control before they have become used to being handled and controlled because they are so small, are unaccustomed to restraint, and can move very quickly. Although not as dangerous as a large horse, they can still bite and deliver a nasty kick, especially if the veterinarian is squatting down to administer treatment or carry out an examination. When the foal is standing, the best method of restraint is to stand beside it with one hand placed around the chest and the other behind the thigh muscles. In some unruly cases it may be necessary to grasp the base of the tail and elevate it to obtain a little extra control (Fig. 1-4). This way the foal can move neither forward nor backward, and a good, safe level of restraint is ensured.

Foals that have not been trained to lead with a rein or rope attached to the halter can be coaxed along by a noose, made from rope, placed over their rump. The free end of the rope is held by the handler who pulls gently on it while standing beside the foal. In this way the foal feels the pressure from the rear and tends to walk forward away from it, whereas if a lead rope is pulled, the foal resists by pulling backward. *With foals—and adult horses—it is important that whenever the animal pulls backward, the handler does not engage in a "tug-of-war," as this often causes the horse to rear, which can result in its falling over backward and incurring a skull fracture.*

Recumbent foals also need to be restrained. The best method is to have someone sit down and cradle the foal's head in their lap. This allows good control and prevents the foal from throwing its head around and causing self-inflicted injuries.

CHEMICAL RESTRAINT OF FOALS

The essential differences between adults and foals are that foals have a larger volume of distribution for drugs, a lower proportion of body fat, less albumin for drug binding, and less well-developed hepatic and renal clearance mechanisms. Provided these aspects are kept in mind, most of drugs used for adults can be used in foals (Table 1-2). Xylazine is particularly useful as it acts quickly and reliably, has a short period of action, and can be combined with butorphanol to provide a reliable combination for painful diagnostic procedures such as synovial or cerebrospinal fluid collection.

A doseage for Xylazine of 1.1 mg/kg produces recumbency that will last 60 to 90 minutes. Depending on the procedure, a lower dose can be used, or reversal can be achieved with yohimbine (0.1 mg/kg slowly IV). Diazepam (0.05–0.1 mg/kg IV) may be used but may result in recumbency.

▶ **TABLE 1–2**
SOME DRUGS AND DRUG COMBINATIONS USEFUL FOR ROUTINE RESTRAINT IN FOALS

Drugs	Intravenous Dose (mg/kg)
Phenothiazine derivatives	
Acetylpromazine maleate	0.03
Alpha$_2$ agonists	
Xylazine hydrochloride	0.25–1.1
Detomidine hydrochloride	0.01–0.04
Benzodiazepines	
Diazepam	0.05–0.1
Combinations	
Xylazine HCl-butorphanol tartrate	0.55, 0.02

Note: Recumbency will often occur.

AIDS TO RESTRAINT

Twitch

The twitch is an essential piece of equipment for anyone handling horses. There are many different designs, mainly reflecting personal preference. However, the basic structures are a loop of rope or chain attached to a handle (Fig. 1-5). The principle is that the loop is placed over the horse's muzzle and tightened by twisting the handle, thereby distracting the horse and so allowing the examination or treatment to proceed (Fig. 1-6). There are different methods of applying and holding a twitch, but, as it is potentially dangerous to both horse and handler, it is a procedure that must be done safely. If there is a competent handler holding the head of the horse, the veterinarian can use both hands to apply the twitch. The twitch handle is held in the right hand; the fingers of the left hand are inserted partly through the loop and then used to grasp the upper lip and elevate it slightly; the loop is slid down the fingers and onto the lip; and the right hand then tightens the loop by twisting the handle (Fig. 1-6A). For routine restraint the direction in which the handle is twisted is unimportant, but

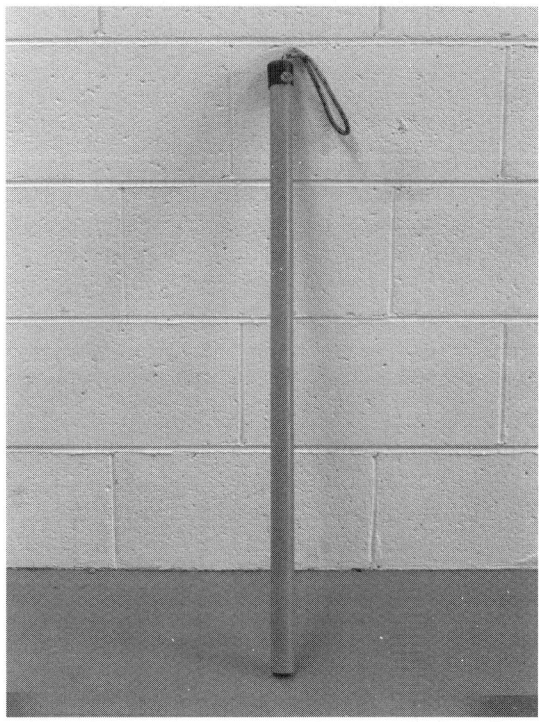

▶ **FIGURE 1–5**
Nose twitch. There are many twitch designs. This is an example of a long-handled twitch with a rope noose.

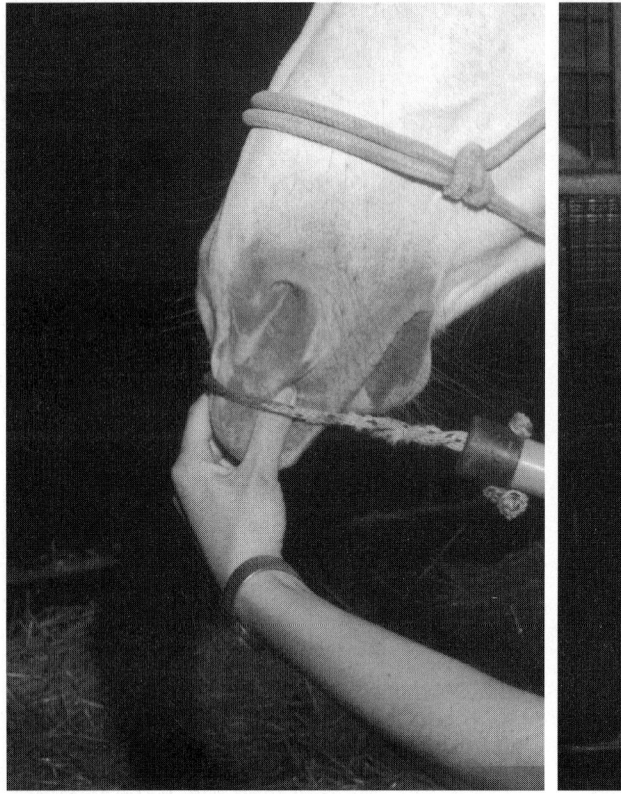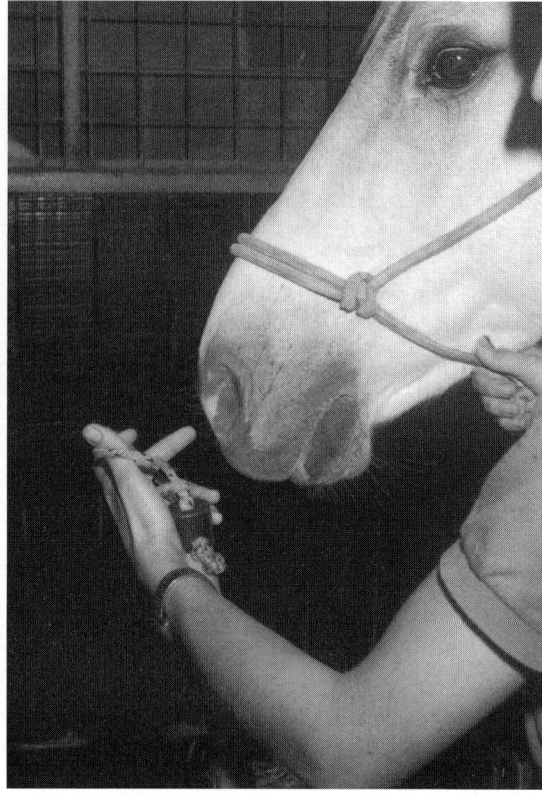

A   B

▶ **FIGURE 1–6**
Application of nose twitch. **A.** Two-handed method, with horse's head controlled by the holder. **B.** One-handed method, in which the clinician must assist with holding the head as well as applying the twitch. Note how the handle of the twitch is held in the palm of the hand.

when an endoscope or stomach tube are to be inserted, it is preferable to rotate it anticlockwise, which tends to open the nostril and make the insertion easier. When competent assistance is unavailable, the clinician must assist with holding the horse and also apply the twitch: In preparation, the loop of the twitch is placed partly over the fingers of the left hand; the handle is twisted so that the loop is just big enough to accommodate the lip; the handle is transferred to the left hand where it is held between the palm and the third and fourth fingers; the right hand holds the headstall, while the fingers of the left hand with the twitch attached are used to grasp the lip, at which time the clinician can use the right hand to twist the handle or, alternatively, this can be done by the helper if the clinician is unable to release the hold on the headstall (Fig. 1–6B).

Whether the loop is made from soft material, such as rope, or of chain, or whether the handle is long or short or made of wood or rubber is a matter of individual preference. There are advantages and disadvantages to all designs, but the

principles of use apply equally. The twitch should not be applied too tightly because it can damage the muzzle and because the horse may resent it and become extremely violent as the pain aspect becomes predominant. The objective is to apply it firmly, then increase pressure just before the invasive or painful procedure is performed, and then reduce the pressure. In this way the maximum effect is obtained without unduly disturbing the horse. As a general rule the person holding the twitch should stand on the same side of the horse as the examiner so that if the horse pulls away or escapes, there is an open escape route for it. The twitch should always be under manual control so that it can be released or tightened as necessary. It is not an uncommon practice to attach the twitch to the head collar, which means that it is not under control and also that if the horse escapes the twitch cannot release. It cannot be stressed enough that the tension in the loop should be under constant control and adjusted as necessary and that the holder should not "go to sleep." In some horses the same effect can be obtained simply by manually squeezing the muzzle.

Neck Squeeze

Horses can often be distracted by grasping with one or both hands a fold of skin at the base of the neck and then firmly rotating the hand so as to put tension in the skin (Fig. 1–7). This may be difficult to do in thick-skinned or strong horses or if the examiner is not strong enough. However it requires no equipment and can be applied quickly and safely.

Ear Hold and Twitch

The horse's head can be restrained by firmly holding the ear and twisting it. To perform this safely, the examiner should stand beside the horse and slide the right hand up the neck until the ear can be grasped. This should be done smoothly and in one coordinated movement. When a horse is familiar with the procedure, it must be done very quickly; otherwise it will lift its head quickly out of reach. The examiner must then keep control of the horse's head by bracing the forearm against the horse's neck. This is very important because, if the horse pulls its head away or attempts to rear, the examiner can be pulled under the front legs and be injured. By bracing the forearm against the neck, the examiner is in a better position to resist. The mechanical advantage is also improved by also holding the headstall with the left hand and ensuring that the horse's head is pulled to the left side (Fig. 1–8). The ear hold is

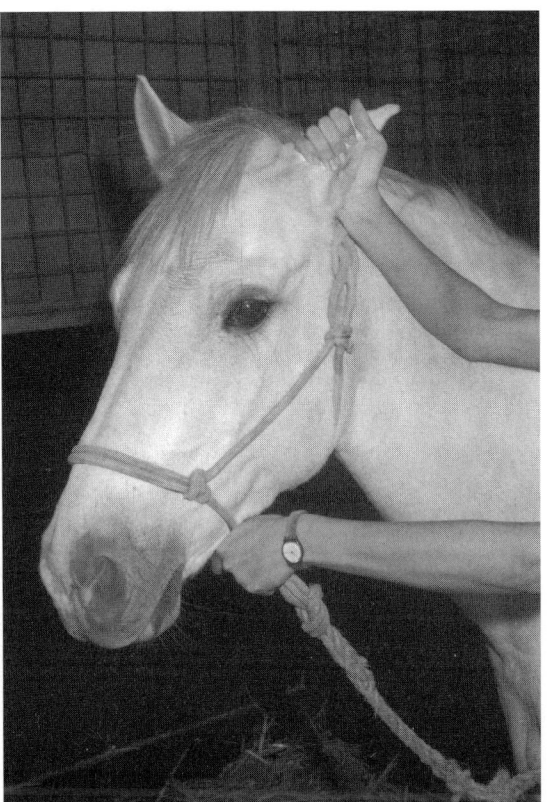

▶ **FIGURE 1–8**

Ear hold. Note that the clinician's arm is braced against the neck and that the head is controlled by the other hand holding the headstall.

not recommended for routine use in all horses because they have a tendency to become "head shy" and will then resent all manipulation around the head. It has particular value for quick restraint and to stabilize the head while a nose twitch is applied or a stomach tube or endoscope are passed into the nasal passage. A twitch can also be applied to the ear, but this is not recommended because of the possibility of injury to the aural cartilage.

Stocks

Stocks are useful for restraining horses that have a tendency to move away from the examiner or to be violent. Placing the horse in stocks restricts activity and makes the examination safer. Some examples of a set of stocks is shown in Figure 1–9. It is important that the examiner get access to the desired region and that the horse be placed in, and removed from, the stocks safely. Ability to release the horse quickly is important if the horse becomes recumbent or violent. A back strap is

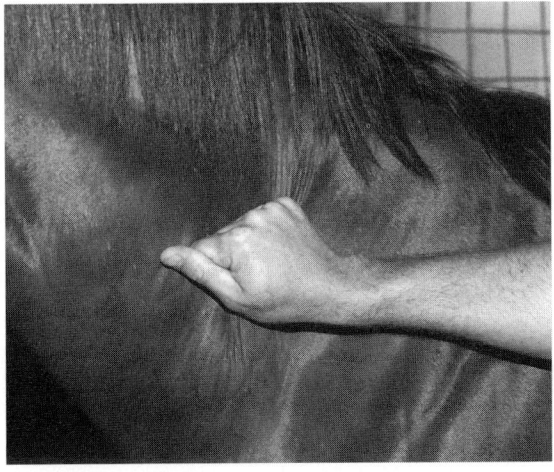

▶ **FIGURE 1–7**

Neck squeeze. This can be a one-or two-handed maneuver. A one-handed method is demonstrated.

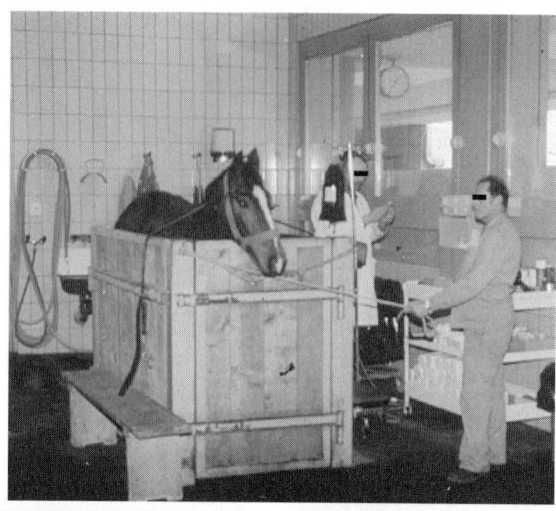

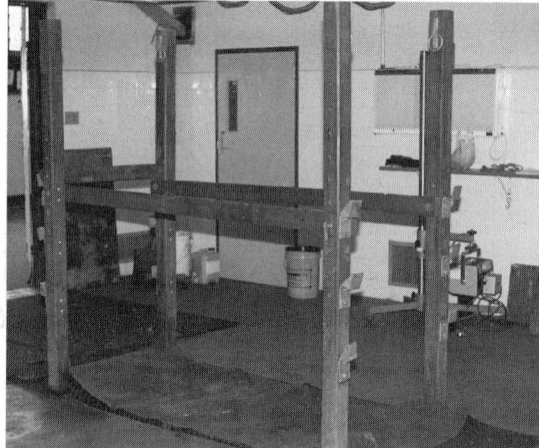
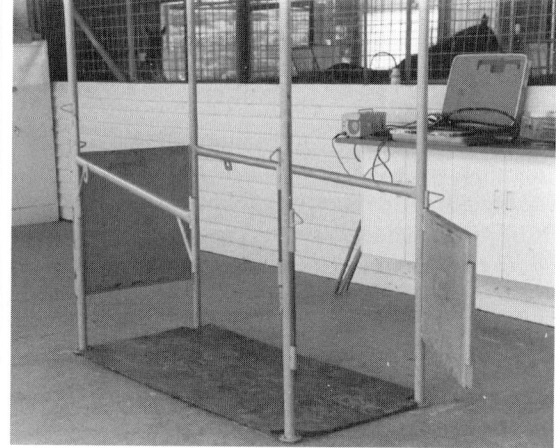

▶ FIGURE 1-9

Stocks. Three different designs are shown, demonstrating varying levels of confinement and restraint. Note that all three pieces of equipment can be opened at either end, and also on at least one side, to allow access for different procedures and also for safety purposes.

useful for preventing a horse from jumping out, but it should be capable of rapid release. Stocks come in many forms, the main variations being the degree to which they are enclosed and whether or not the side doors can be opened. When sides are fixed and cannot be opened, it is important that they are not fully enclosed as it is often desirable to gain access to the lower limbs for radiology or the ventral abdomen for an abdominal paracentesis. Appropriate padding is required to protect the horse from injury if it rears or kicks.

Clinical Examination

2

INTRODUCTION

The clinical examination can include all or some of the following components:

- Identification of the patient
- History taking
- Preliminary visual appraisal
- General physical examination
- Special examination of specific regions or organs
- Use of diagnostic aids (clinical pathology, electrocardiology, etc.)
- Examination of the environment

Although a full clinical examination is not always necessary, a general examination should always be carried out.

IDENTIFICATION

The patient is identified by its signalment, or outward appearance, using features such as breed, age, sex, color, body markings, brands, and tattoos. The requirements for identification vary between countries and breeds, but, as horses move more frequently across borders, uniformity is emerging.

Natural Markings

The natural markings consist of the basic coat color and any extra markings superimposed over the coat color. The whole body, including the mane, tail, and hooves, are included.

Coat Color

Horses come in a range of colors with a very confusing nomenclature that is more complicated in some breeds than in others. Fortunately, because of such difficulty and the increasing worldwide mobility of horses, the terms used to describe horse colors and markings have become simpler and, to a certain extent, more uniform between breeds and countries. Nevertheless, familiarity with the terminology associated with the colors and patterns requires special experience and interest. There are numerous genes and alleles involved in the production of coat color and pattern, some of which play a major role whereas others have a modifying effect. For a more detailed description of the coat color and its modes of inheritance, the reader is referred to the published literature.[1] The different breed registries should also be consulted for specific details.

Assessing color takes into account the general body color, the presence of points and their color, and the patterns of white marking. The *points* consist of the distal part of the limbs, mane, tail, and sometimes the ears. A list of the common colors and patterns follows. The reader is advised that definitions and acceptance of various terms vary greatly among countries, breeds, and horse registries:

- *Black.* A black horse has black pigment throughout its hair, mane, and tail. White markings are permitted.
- *Brown.* Coat hairs are a mixture of brown and black hairs. The limbs, mane, and tail are black.

9

- *Grey.* Grey horses have a mixture of white hairs distributed throughout the colored hairs of the body, mane, tail, and limbs. The colored hairs can be any color. The foal is born colored, and the proportion of white hairs increases progressively with each new coat.
- *Chestnut.* The term *chestnut* is taken to identify the specific dark red horse ("liver chestnut") or as a general term for all red-colored horses so as to include those otherwise known as sorrels. In its specific form it describes a dark red horse with legs and body colored similarly. Mane and tail are usually slightly darker than the body, but are not black.
- *Sorrel.* A sorrel is copper colored and lighter in color than a chestnut. The limbs are usually the same color as the body, but the mane and tail may be the same or often a lighter color, or flaxen. It can be difficult to separate a light chestnut from a darker sorrel, hence the tendency to group them, as mentioned.
- *Bay.* Bay horses have black mane, tail, ear tips, and limbs, with a body color ranging from yellow to red. All bays have red in their coat. According to body color, they are variably described as blood bay, yellow bay, or dark bay.
- *Dun.* Dun is often used to describe all light-colored horses, with or without black points. The terminology of the group is very confusing. A convenient way to consider them is to divide them according to whether they have black or nonblack points, with grullo and buckskin falling into the former group and red and yellow duns in the latter. Red duns have light red to yellow bodies with red, brown, or flaxen points, usually with primitive marks (see later). Yellow duns have a yellow body color with brown points. There are numerous subsidiary terms used for red and yellow duns.
- *Grullo.* A grullo is a blue- to slate grey–colored horse with black points, usually with primitive marks.
- *Buckskin.* A buckskin is a yellow horse with black points. To complicate matters, the presence of primitive marks changes a buckskin to a zebra dun.
- *Palamino.* Palaminos have a coat color that ranges from cream to copper, with light-colored mane and tail. There are also numerous subsidiary terms.
- *Roan.* Roan is used when the body hair is a mixture of white and colored hairs. The white hairs can vary in number from a few to extensive coverage of much of the body, and the base color can be any color, hence red roan, and so on. Unlike grey horses, which also fit this pattern, the white hairs are usually present at birth, although they are most apparent after the first coat has been shed. The white hairs tend to be confined to the body.
- *Asymmetric white spotting patterns.* In the United States asymmetric patterns of white spotting are called *paint* or *pinto*. The white hairs are grouped to produce patches of solid white on any base color, rather than the mixed distribution of the grey and roan. Patterns include *tobiano* and *overo*. The terms *piebald* and *skewbald* also fall into this category. Piebald and skewbald describe black and nonblack horses, respectively, ignoring which of the specific patterns is present. The *tobiano* pattern occurs with any coat color and produces areas of sharply delineated white hair with underlying pink unpigmented skin. The dorsal midline is usually crossed at some point by a patch of white. There are numerous variations but, in general, the white extends from the dorsum, in the region of the crest or withers, ventrally. Usually, the head is colored with white markings, and the limbs are also usually white. At one end of the spectrum exist horses that are almost white with some white spotting, and, at the other, horses that are colored with a little white limited to dorsum and legs. The *overo* pattern, similar to the tobiano, is characterized by a pattern in which the white hair tends to be located ventrally, and extends toward, but not over, the dorsal midline. Legs are usually white and eyes are often blue. Combinations of the overo and tobiano can exist, and these may be complicated by appaloosa spotting.
- *Symmetric white spotting.* The main example of this pattern is the *appaloosa.* The patterns may vary with age and are therefore not reliable as markers for permanent identification. The minimum phenotypic expression of an appaloosa is a mottling of the skin, white sclera, and striped

hooves. The mottling, which consists of regions of unpigmented skin, tends to be concentrated around the genitalia and the muzzle. Several varieties of the Appaloosa pattern are recognized, depending on the extent and location of the spotting pattern and the background. These include leopard, frost, varnished roan, white blanket, spotted blanket, and snowflake. The appaloosa often is characterized by the primary color, hence, for example, a "black appaloosa."

- *White.* There are several forms of white coloration. True albinism, with white hair and complete lack of skin and eye pigment, is a lethal recessive trait, and the fetus dies in utero. Another form of lethal white is found in the white overo foal, which is born with segmental aplasia of a section of the large intestine. White horses also are associated with genes that produce dilution of color, as well as with the extreme forms of the spotting. White or cream horses with pigmented blue eyes and lacking skin pigment are known as *creamellos*. These other forms of white are sometimes, incorrectly, called albino.
- *Dappling.* Dappling is the presence of darker areas superimposed over lighter areas, in horses of any color. They are seen most commonly in greys.
- *Primitive marks.* These include a stripe along the dorsal midline (eel stripe), a transverse stripe over the withers, and horizontal stripes over the carpi and the tarsi (zebra stripes). Although they occur most commonly in dun horses, they can occur in any combination in any colored horse. Their presence is obscured by dark base colors.
- *Foal colors.* Identifying foal colors is often difficult because of the color changes that occur with aging and, especially, those associated with the shedding of the foal coat.
- *Eye color.* Most horses have darkly pigmented eyes. Other colors such as amber (especially in duns) and blue (especially in association with lack of periorbital pigment) exist. Blue eyes are also known as *wall eyes.*

Head Markings

White markings on the head are common and carry specific nomenclature. If they contain a mixture of white and colored hairs, they are classed as *mixed,* and if they are circumscribed by hairs of another color they are classed as *bordered.* Although markings are usually drawn onto a diagram, the clinician must also know how to describe them for occasions when a written report is required. The white markings are described as follows and are shown in Figure 2–1:

- *Star.* Any solid white marking on the forehead. A few white hairs or a patch of mixed hairs should be described as such, and not as a star. The star may be described further as to its specific location, and also according to its shape as oval, diamond-shaped, triangular, and so on.
- *Stripe.* A white marking extending down the face that does not extend laterally beyond the flat surface of the nasal bones. When not associated with a star or a snip, the sites of origin and termination must be described.
- *Snip.* A white marking located between, or in, the nostrils.
- *Combinations of the above.* When any of the above are continuous, they are said to be conjoined (i.e., star and stripe conjoined, or star, stripe, and snip conjoined).
- *Blaze.* A solid white marking, similar to a stripe, but extending laterally beyond the nasal bones.
- *Bald face.* Larger than a blaze, extending to or around the eyes or nostrils.
- *Apron face.* Like a bald face but extends to include the lower jaw.
- *Bonnet.* A white head, often with colored hair around the eyes and ears.
- *Flesh mark.* When there is no skin pigment and the skin is pink or flesh colored.

Leg Markings

Leg markings are also very common and an integral part of identification. As with head markings, they can be both described in written form using standard nomenclature and drawn on to a diagram. Limb markings are described in the following and are shown in Figure 2–2. Descriptions are complicated by the fact that a marking can involve all or part of the circumference of a specific part of the limb.

- *Coronet.* A solid white marking immediately above the hoof. The hoof color usually corresponds to the hair color of the coronet.

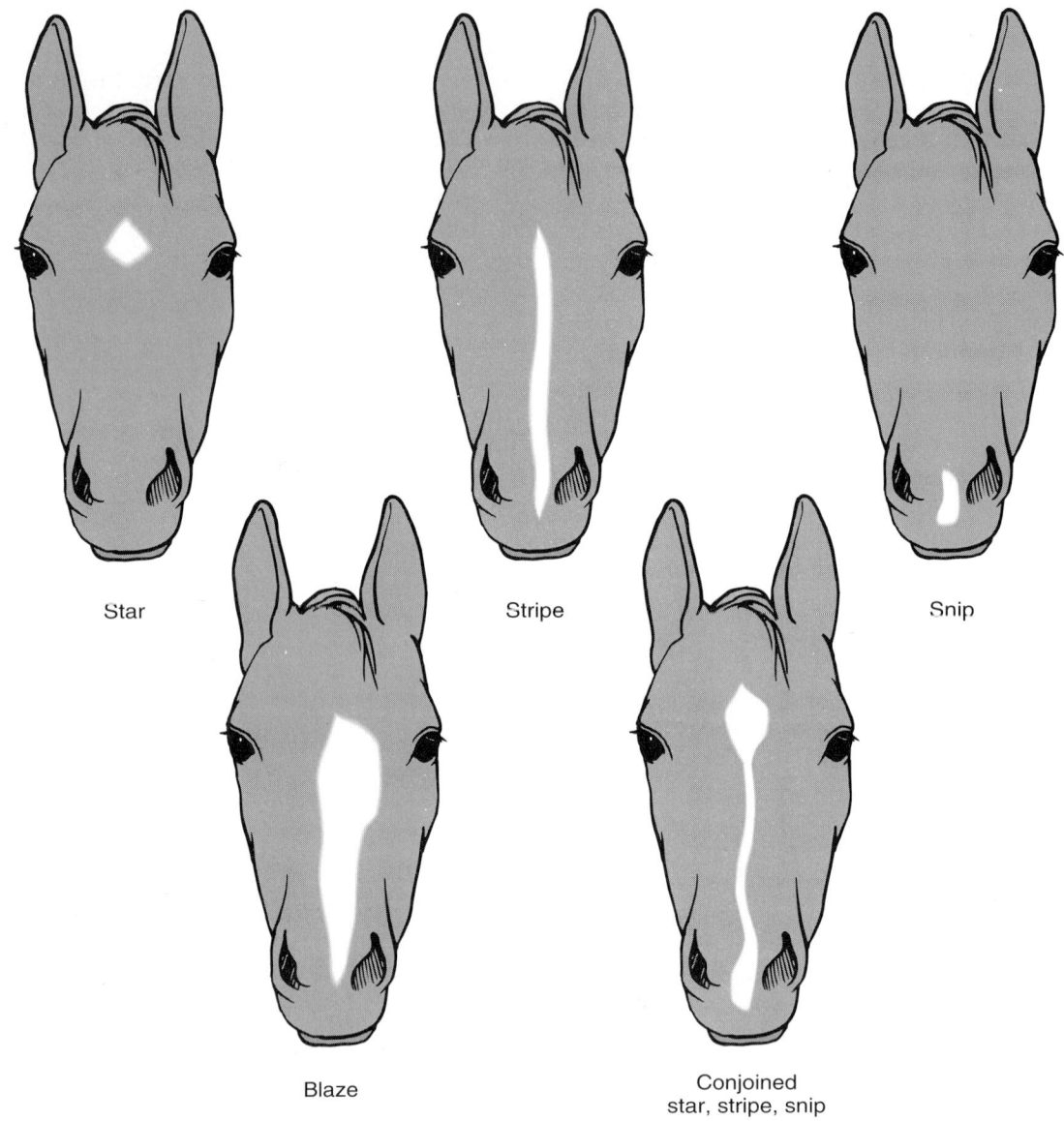

Star

Stripe

Snip

Blaze

Conjoined
star, stripe, snip

A

▶ **FIGURE 2–1**

Nomenclature for describing white markings on the head. **A.** Face. **B.** Head

- *Heel and white spot.* The term *heel* is used to denote a white heel and white spot when the white is located elsewhere on the coronet.
- *Pastern.* White extending proximally to the beginning of the bulge of the fetlock joint. Further described as half, three-quarter, or full pastern.
- *Fetlock.* White marking extending to the proximal bulge of the fetlock joint. Further classed as full or half fetlock.
- *Cannon.* White to proximal metacarpal or metatarsal region. Further classed as half,

three-quarter, or full cannon. A *sock* corresponds to a half cannon.
- *Carpus or tarsus.* White involving the carpus or tarsus. White involving the carpus or tarsus and above is also termed a *stocking.*
- *Black marks.* Spots consisting of black hairs are often found in regions consisting of another color. When the background is white, these are classed as *ermine marks,* otherwise they are called *black marks.* They are usually associated with a dark vertical hoof stripe.

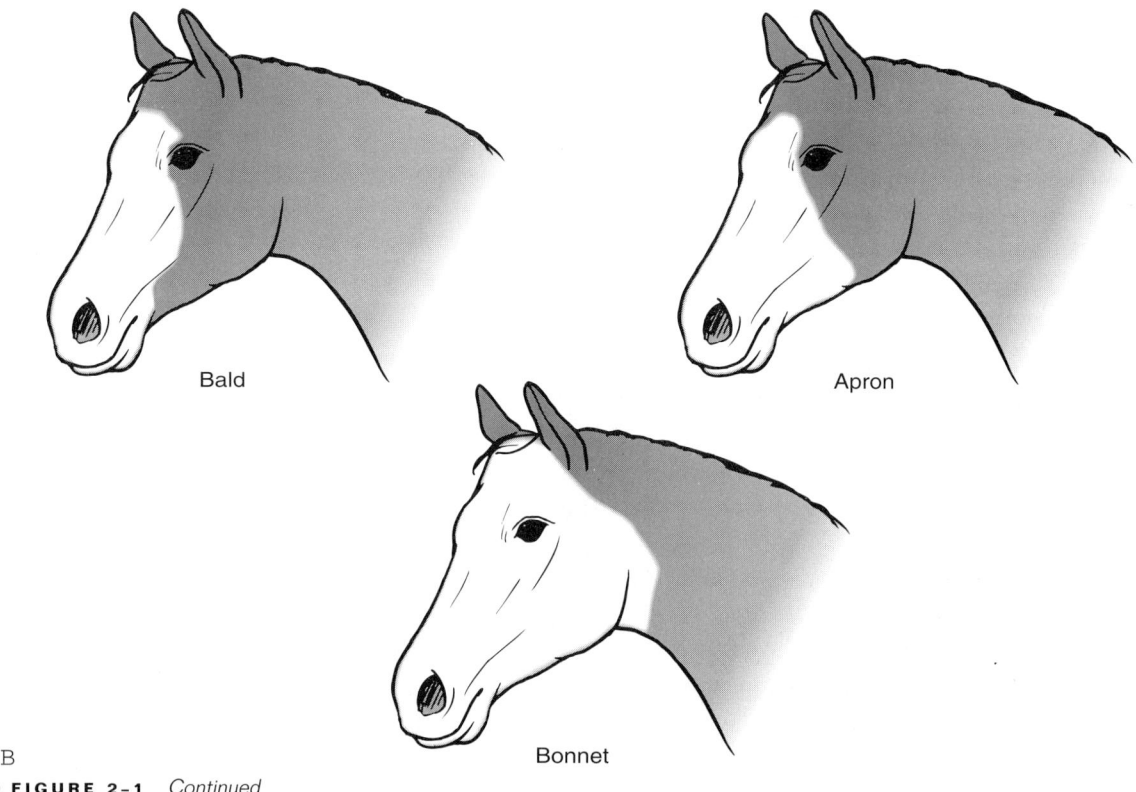

B

▶ **FIGURE 2–1** *Continued*

Hair Whorls

Patterns of hair flow are unique for an individual and are important for identification. Close examination will reveal that, although the hair lies flat over most of the body, not all of it is oriented in the same direction. Furthermore, there are a number of sites where regions of hair oriented in different directions come together, known as *whorls,* where the hair has a tendency to stand erect. At these sites, and depending on the extent of the interface between the hair patterns, the opposing erect hairs are confined to a small region (simple) or extend along the line of demarcation (feathered) (Fig. 2-3). When drawing these on a diagram, as part of an identification process, a simple whorl is drawn as an "x" and the feathering is shown as a line joined to the "x." The number and location of these sites vary greatly. Simple whorls are described as being clockwise or anticlockwise, and feathered whorls are specified according to their direction. For identification purposes it is usual to select the major whorls, such as those from the head, neck, and flank.

Chestnuts

The cornified tissues located on the medial side of each limb at the level of the tarsus and just proximal to the carpus are known as chestnuts. As each is peculiar to each horse, they are useful for identification purposes. However, for a number of reasons, mainly because they can be surgically altered and because they can vary in size and shape up until about 18 months of age, they have no practical use.

Acquired Markings

Scars

Scars are a common finding when identifying horses. Their location and shape should be recorded, although they serve only as supplementary identifiers.

Freeze Branding

Freeze branding is the most frequently used method of producing a mark of identification. It produces a brand consisting of white hairs. The white hairs grow after the melanocytes in the hair follicle have been destroyed by cold. Sometimes the complete follicle is destroyed, resulting in a hairless mark. On white or light-colored horses the brand should be made so that it is hairless, as white hairs will not be visible. The brand is made by applying a cold iron to the skin. It is a relatively painless procedure and produces a well-defined mark. Brands vary from country- or breed-specific systems to the increasingly popular angle system (Fig. 2–4). The numbers 2 to 9 are represented by a right angle, number one by two vertical lines, and zero by two horizontal lines.[2] A straight line

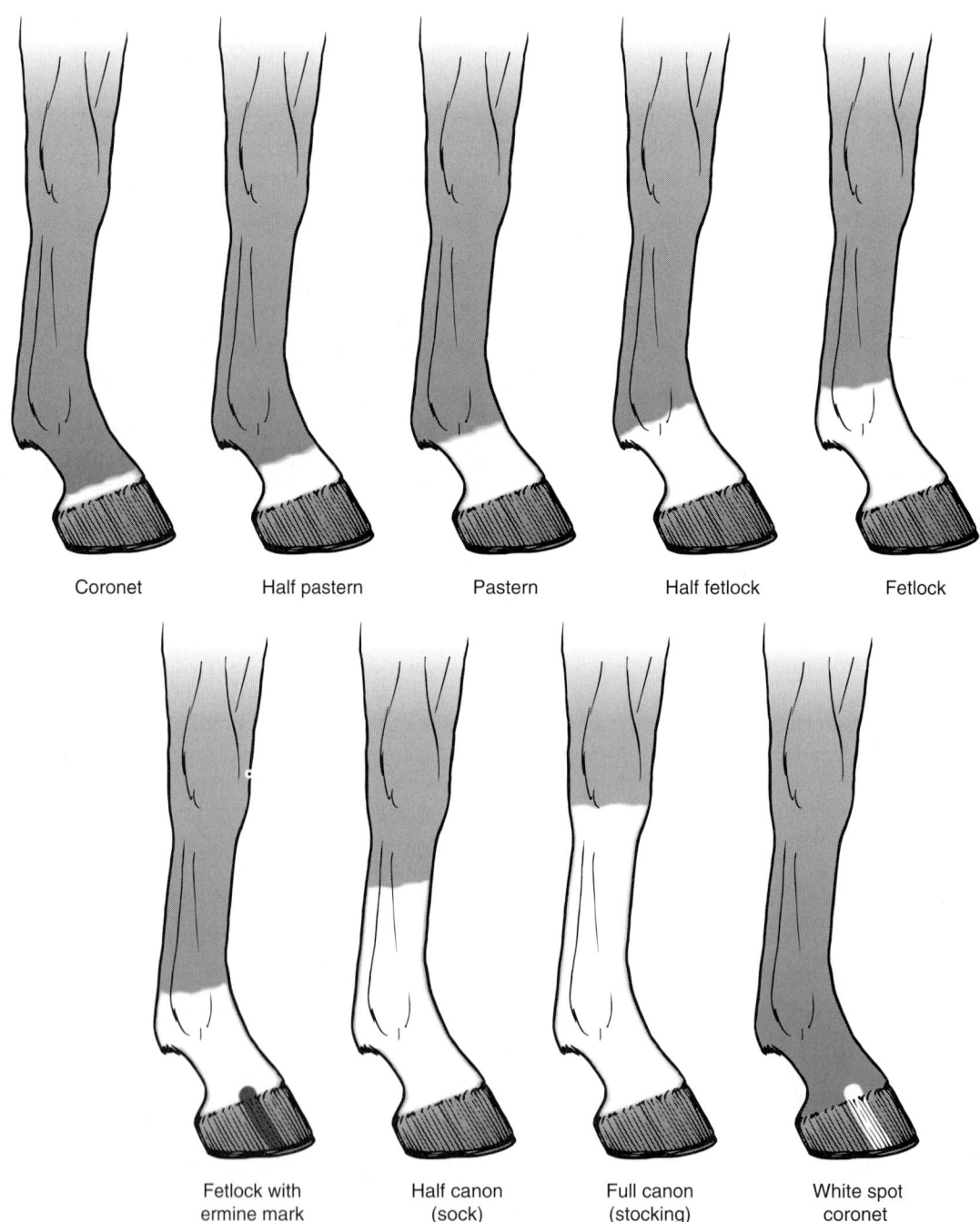

| Coronet | Half pastern | Pastern | Half fetlock | Fetlock |

| Fetlock with ermine mark | Half canon (sock) | Full canon (stocking) | White spot coronet |

▶ **FIGURE 2–2**

Nomenclature for describing white markings on the limbs.

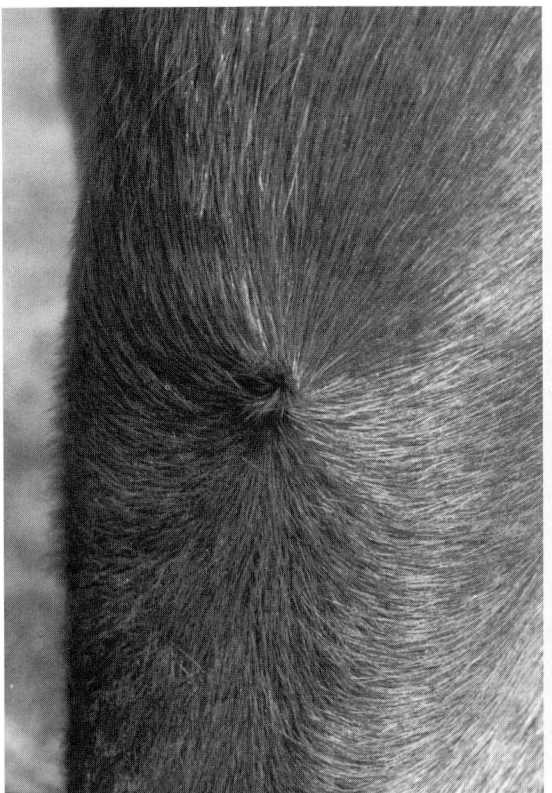 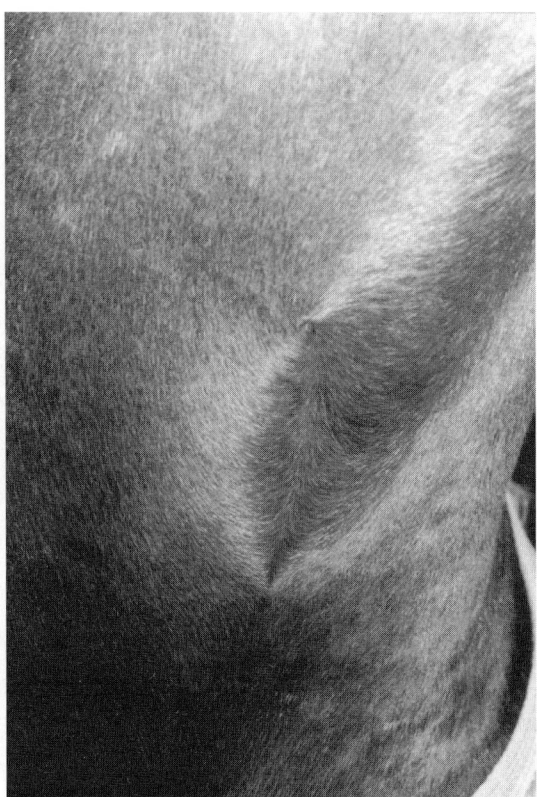

A   B

▶ FIGURE 2-3

Hair whorls. **A.** Simple whorl. **B.** Feathered whorl.

is always placed beneath the angle numbers to indicate whether there has been any distortion as a result of growth. The site of the brand varies with the breed and country, common locations being the shoulders or under the mane.

Fire Branding

Fire branding, usually on the shoulders, has been a common method of identification. Ideally, the process eliminates hair growth, although application of excessive heat produces an ugly scar, whereas insufficient heat results in a poorly defined mark characterized by regrowth of a mixture of normal and white hairs. On aesthetic and humane grounds fire branding is rarely carried out.

Tattoos

Tattooing the inner side of the upper lip has been a popular method of identification in the United States. However, the mark tends to fade, become less distinct, and be smudged by massage. It cannot be used in foals because it tends to be absorbed.

Blood Typing

Blood typing is very important for identification purposes. Although not part of a routine clinical examination, it is frequently required for registration purposes and for parentage verification. Testing involves serological identification of red cell antigens and electrophoretic identification of several protein markers.[3] The tests require clotted and unclotted samples. Although the number of identifiable and useful factors is expanding, recent stimulus has been given to the development of DNA testing.

Electronic Identification

The stimulus for a simple, unalterable method of identification that can interface with computerized data retrieval systems has produced electronic identification.[4] The system involves the implantation of a transponder (microchip) coded specifically for the individual that can then be identified by applying an electronic sensor. Each microchip is encoded with an alphanumeric

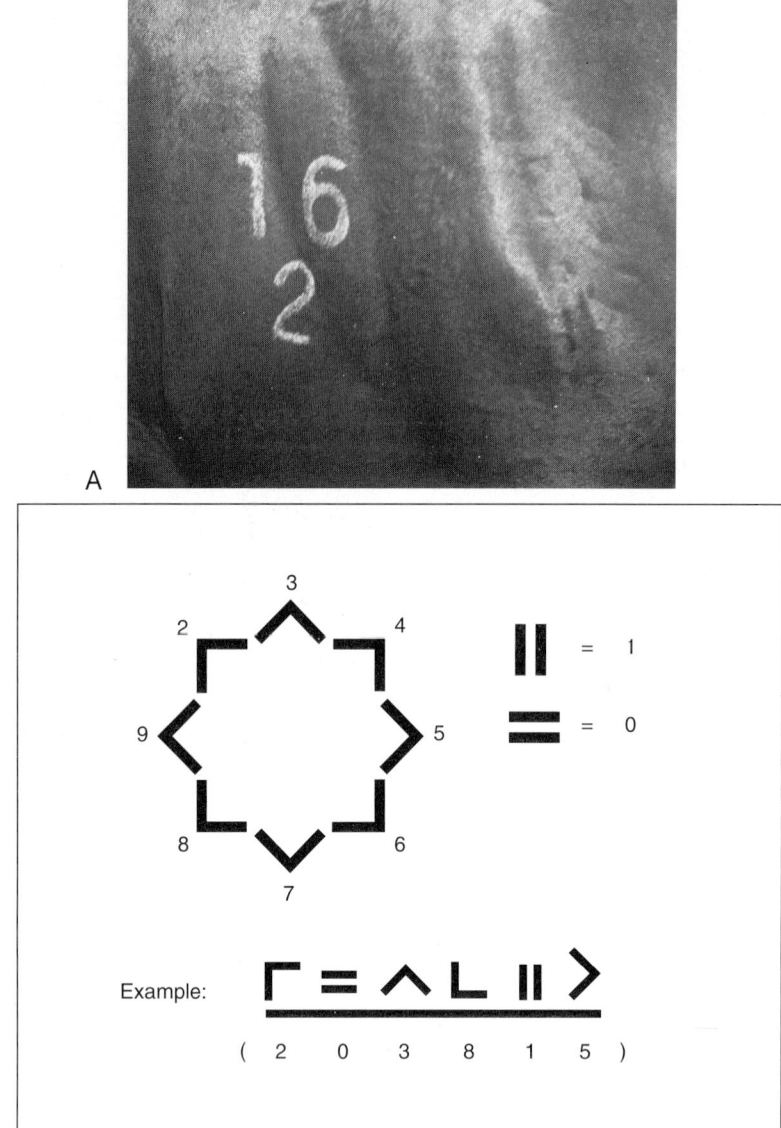

▶ FIGURE 2-4

Freeze brand. **A.** Brand produced by the freeze technique showing the loss of pigment from the hair. **B.** Freeze brand alphabet and how a number is compiled.

combination of characters. Although in use in certain parts of the world, the system is not yet in common use but shows considerable promise.

Aging by Dental Examination

The techniques for examining the teeth and opening the mouth are described in the section Examination of the Teeth and Oral Cavity. Aging by dental examination is not an exact science. However, good approximation is possible if the examination is done carefully by someone who can identify the factors involved in aging. As will

be described, aging is based to a significant extent on recognizing specific features associated with the normal eruption and growth of teeth. Some factors that can alter the normal sequence of events and therefore interfere with accurate aging include trauma or infection, which can result in loss, distortion, or malformation of teeth, and excessive wear, which accelerates the appearance of the various aging landmarks and artificially increases dental age. The pertinent features of dental aging are described briefly here and can be found in greater detail elsewhere.[5]

Dental Formula

The dental formula for horses is shown in the box.

Canine teeth (Fig. 2-5) are almost always present in males and are either small or do not erupt at all in females. The first premolar (PM1), known as the wolf tooth, is usually present, and is usually located in the upper arcades, varying in size from tiny to relatively large (Fig. 2-6).

Sequence of Tooth Eruption

The eruption times of teeth, especially the incisors, are very useful indicators of age.

Coming Into Wear and Incisor Cross-Sectional Anatomy

After the incisor teeth erupt, they continue to grow and lengthen until each lower-jaw incisor

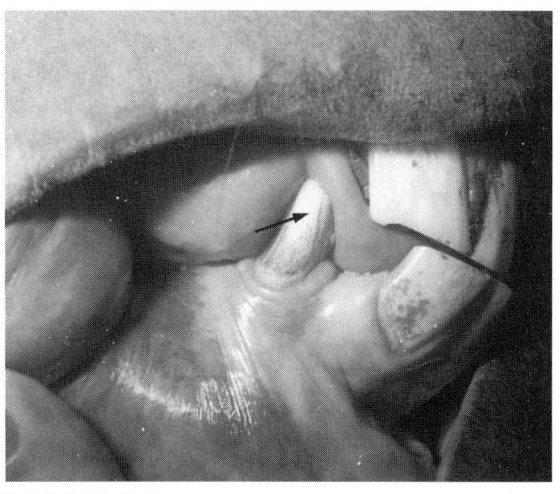

▶ **FIGURE 2-5**
Canine tooth.

meets its opposite number in the upper jaw, approximately 6 months after eruption, a phenomenon known as coming into wear. The incisors therefore come into wear at 3, 4, and 5 years of age. Subsequently, they continue to grow, each undergoing erosion of its occlusal surface with the exposure of increasingly deeper parts of each. The anatomy of an incisor tooth and its appearance in cross section are shown in Figure 2-7. As demonstrated, the shape and appearance of the cross section gradually change. The occlusal surfaces of the first, second, and third incisors are round at approximately 10, 11, and 12

DENTAL FORMULA

- Deciduous teeth
  2(Incisors 3/3, Canines 0/0, Premolars 3/3) = 24
- Permanent teeth
  2(Incisors 3/3, Canines 1/1, Premolars 3 or 4/3, Molars 3/3) = 40 or 42

SEQUENCE OF TOOTH ERUPTION

	Deciduous	Permanent
• Incisors		
First	Birth–first week	2½ years
Second	4–6 weeks	3½ years
Third	6–9 months	4½ years
• Canines	Absent	4–5 years
• Premolars		
First (wolf)	Absent	5–6 months
Second	Birth–2 weeks	2½ years
Third	Birth–2 weeks	3 years
Fourth	Birth–2 weeks	4 years
• Molars		
First	Absent	9–12 months
Second	Absent	2 years
Third	Absent	3½–4 years

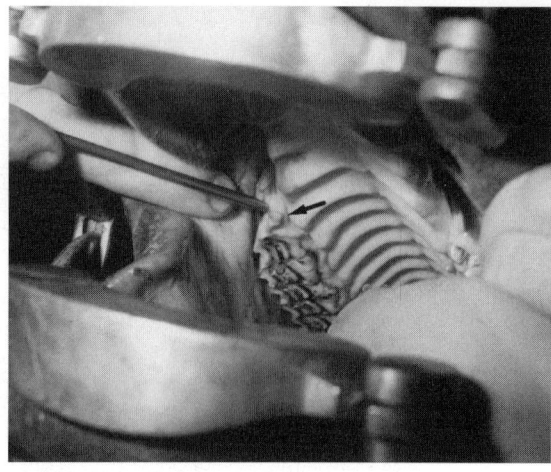

▶ FIGURE 2–6
First upper premolar tooth (''wolf tooth'').

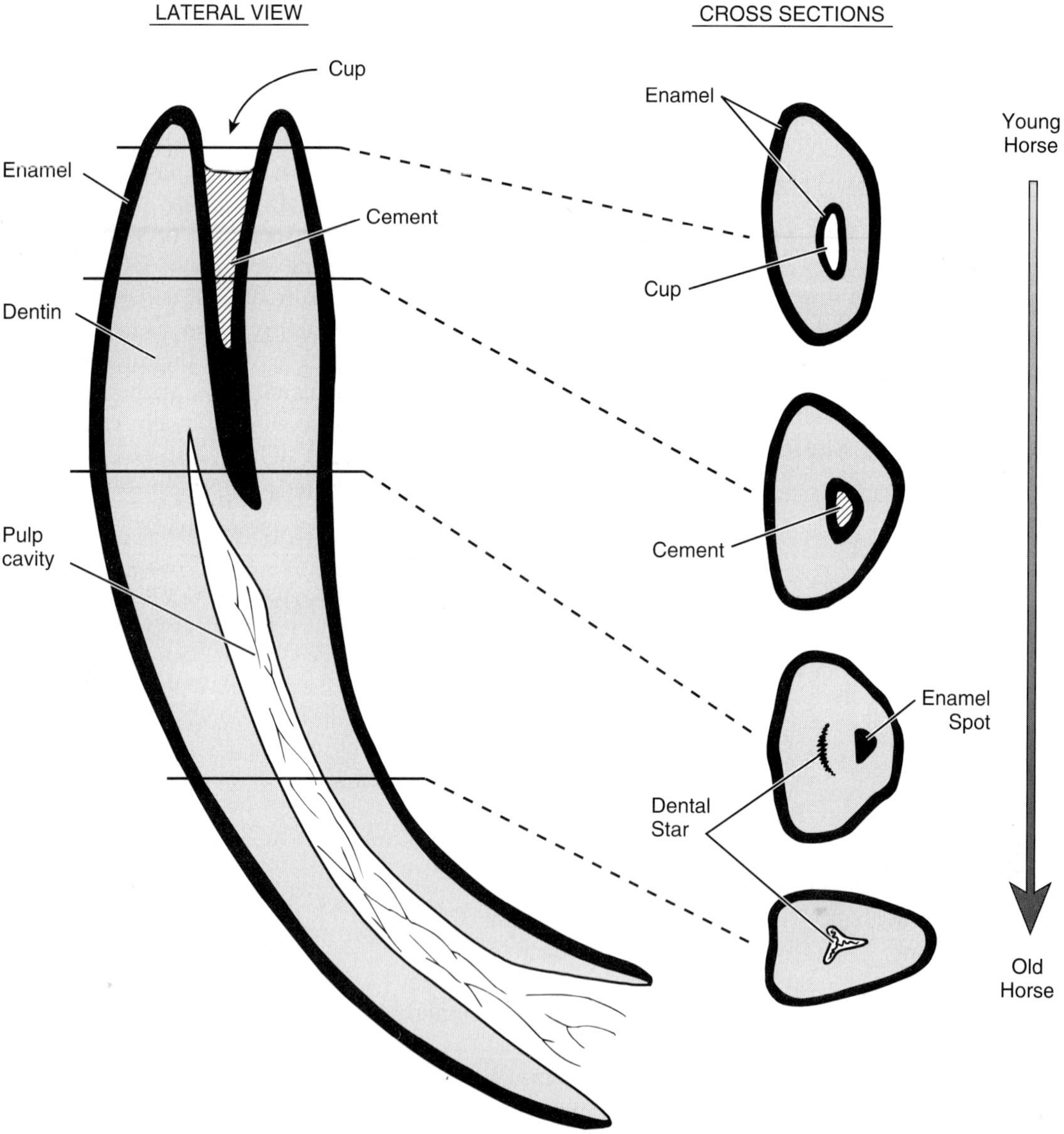

LATERAL VIEW | CROSS SECTIONS

Cup

Enamel

Enamel

Cup

Cement

Dentin

Young
Horse

Cement

Pulp
cavity

Enamel
Spot

Dental
Star

Old
Horse

▶ FIGURE 2–7
Cross-section of an incisor tooth, demonstrating appearance of the occlusal surface as the tooth is worn down during use.

years. The *infundibulum,* or cup, is the cavity in the occlusal surface produced by the invagination of enamel. Later, as the deeper sections of the tooth are exposed by wear, the infundibulum gradually ceases to exist as a cavity and is represented by a circle of enamel filled with cement, known as the *enamel spot* or *mark,* which gradually approaches the lingual surface of the teeth. The occlusal surfaces of lower incisors 1, 2, and 3 lose their cavities and become smooth at 6, 7, and 8 years of age, respectively. Later, the mark is lost in all lower incisors at about 12 to 13 years. As the infundibulum disappears, the pulp cavity is exposed as a yellow-brown transverse mark in the dentin, known as the *dental star,* located toward the labial aspect of each incisor. It appears in the first, second, and third incisors at about 8, 9, and 10 years, respectively.

Incisive Arcades

In young horses, the upper and lower rows of incisors grow directly toward one another and occlude with their long axes forming an angle of about 140°. With age, the teeth tend to protrude further forward from the mouth and occlude with a progressively smaller angle between them, approaching 90° at 20 years. This angle is useful only for quickly differentiating between an old and a young horse.

Galvayne's Groove

Galvayne's groove is a longitudinal depression running down the labial surface of the upper third incisors (Fig. 2-8). It is often stained a dark color by the cement that it contains. This groove appears just below the gum margin at about 10 years of age, extends about half way down by 15 years, and the full distance by 20 years.

Loss of Deciduous Premolars

The second, third, and fourth deciduous premolars are pushed up by the corresponding emerging permanent premolars (remember that the wolf tooth is the first premolar). The deciduous teeth sit on top of the permanent teeth and, accordingly, are known as *caps* (Fig. 2-9).

Seven Year Hook

When the upper and lower third incisors come into wear, at 5 years, it is apparent that the dental tables of the upper teeth are longer than those of the lower teeth. As a result of this, the caudal parts of the upper teeth do not occlude with the lower teeth and are therefore not worn away, as are the rostral portions. As the uneven wear continues, the unworn caudal part forms a projection, or hook, over the caudal part of the lower tooth (Fig. 2-10). This projection is most obvious at seven years, hence the name *seven year hook.* As wear changes, the hook gradually disappears only to reappear later on, in a second cycle, when it is most obvious at about 13 years.

HISTORY

The volume of data actually recorded varies greatly. However, in order to have accurate accounting, exact identification of the patient(s), correct identification, address, and telephone number of the owner, diagnosis, and details of treatments and medications are required as a minimum.

The first phase of the examination involves collecting and assessing all relevant history. This is a most important part of data collection, and it requires a careful selection of questions as well as a thoughtful consideration of the results. Unfortunately, owners are not always aware of the significance of particular pieces of data and may unintentionally, or occasionally intentionally, supply false or misleading information. Although the exact technique for gathering information is a matter of the personal preference of the clinician, the speed with which the process is carried out and the ability to extract the maximum amount of useful information usually improve as experience is gained. The question phase should ultimately produce a database that includes information about the following aspects of the case:

- The owner's description of the problem
- Number of animals affected
- The time of onset
- Details of previous treatment
- Response to previous treatment

History taking is very important and should be diligently carried out. Failure to do so will often mean that, at worst, a problem is not detected or,

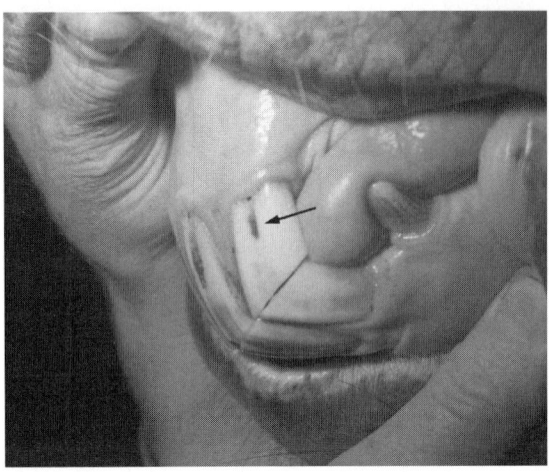

▶ **FIGURE 2-8**
Galvayne's groove.

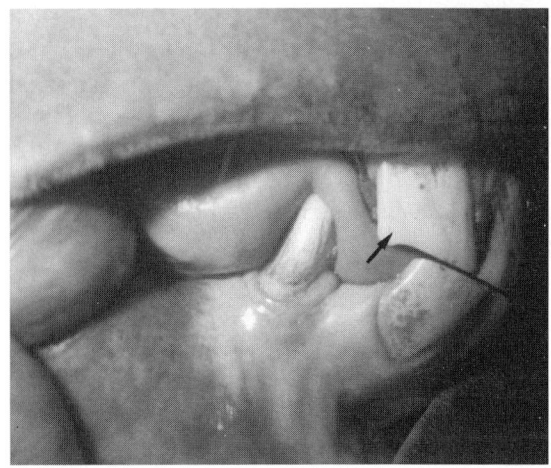

▶ **FIGURE 2-10**
Seven-year hook on caudal aspect of corner or lateral incisor.

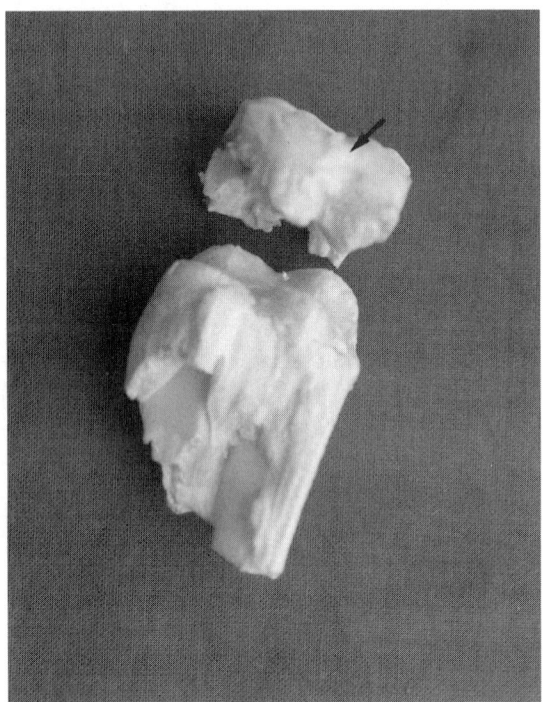

▶ **FIGURE 2-9**
Temporary premolar, or "cap."

at best, is not detected until after considerable time has been devoted to an unrewarding examination of healthy organ systems.

A clinician's job is greatly simplified when the problem is described by an intelligent person with equine experience. This is not always the case, and it is sometimes only with considerable diffi-

culty that the precise circumstances are discovered.

PRELIMINARY VISUAL APPRAISAL

The preliminary visual appraisal is a relatively superficial, but wide-ranging, appraisal of the horse and should be completed before the manual part of the examination is carried out, mainly to ensure that the exam is complete and that the horse is examined in as relaxed a state as possible. Because it is carried out mainly from a distance, the general visual appraisal can be completed almost while talking with the owner and obtaining the history of the case. The visual examination should be systematically performed in any way that suits the clinician and guarantees thoroughness; a logical progression from head through neck, trunk, and limbs should suffice. The following aspects should be noted:

- General body condition and nutritional status
- Demeanor and facial expression
- Posture (including during feeding, urination, and defecation if demonstrated)
- Hair coat and skin
- Voice (if demonstrated)
- Character of respiration
- Presence of wounds and swellings
- Discharges from mouth, nostrils, eyes, ears, vulva, anus, penis, or prepuce

- Muscle development (atrophy, hypertrophy)
- Gait (lameness or ataxia)
- Weakness
- Temperament

GENERAL PHYSICAL EXAMINATION

The general examination is made to identify quickly problems and to localize them to a particular organ system. It is an extremely important component of the clinical assessment because, when correctly performed, it can quickly direct attention to a specific region or body system and, simultaneously, ensure that less obvious or totally unexpected problems are not overlooked. This is an important point because many owners have little or no idea of the specific problem affecting their horse, and, furthermore, the person presenting the animal is frequently a person with no knowledge of the case whatsoever. The physical examination begins with recording of temperature, pulse, and respiration and then concentrates on particular regions of the body.

Temperature

The recording of temperature is simple and is usually taken rectally and occasionally vaginally. The thermometer should be lubricated with a little lubricant, although it is a common, but unesthetic, practice to spit a little saliva on it. To insert a thermometer, the clinician should stand beside the horse and then run the left hand along the horse's back and over its rump to the base of the tail, which is grasped and then elevated slightly and moved away sufficiently to expose the anus. The lubricated thermometer is then inserted gently (Figure 2-11). To avoid being kicked, the clinician should stand beside the hind leg and never behind the horse. If the horse has a tendency to kick, it can be placed beside a doorway and the clinician can work from the other side. The bulb of the instrument should be against the mucosa. Therefore, if fecal balls are present or if the rectum is flaccid, it may be necessary to hold the bulb against the mucosa. Some thermometers can be clipped onto the tail hair while the instrument comes to equilibrium, however there is a tendency to forget them. I prefer to wait

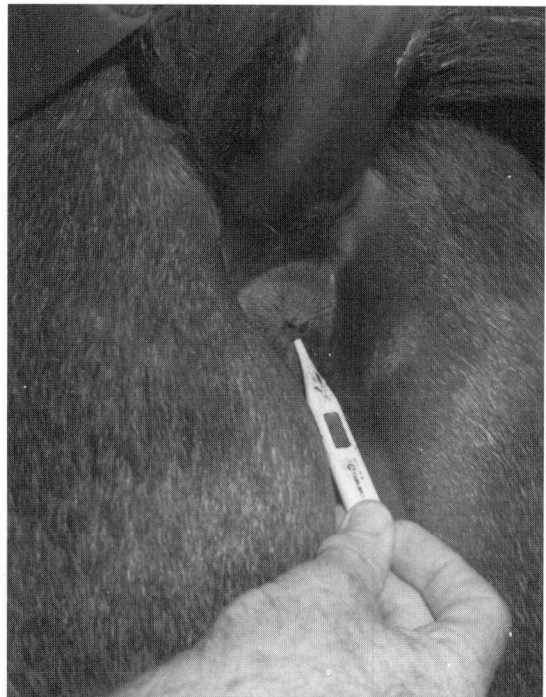

▶ **FIGURE 2-11**
Insertion of a rectal thermometer.

NORMAL TEMPERATURE

- Adult horses: 100.5 ± 1.5°F (38.0 ± 1.0°C)
- Foals, First 4 days of age: 99–102°F (37.2–38.9°C)[6]

---

and read the instrument when it is ready, using the time to continue questioning the owner and discussing the case.

Thermometers are of the mercury or electronic types (Fig. 2-12). Mercury thermometers should be shaken before use to bring down the mercury column. Both types should be left in the rectum for the recommended time. Normal temperature has a diurnal variation (1.0-2.0°F) with the low point occurring in the morning. In addition, it is elevated up to 4.5°F (2.5°C) by severe physical activity, and by up to 3.0°F (1.5°C) when it is hot and humid. Foals have slightly lower temperatures for the first few days of life.[6]

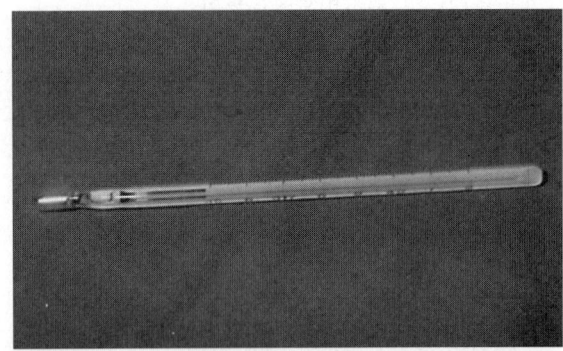

A

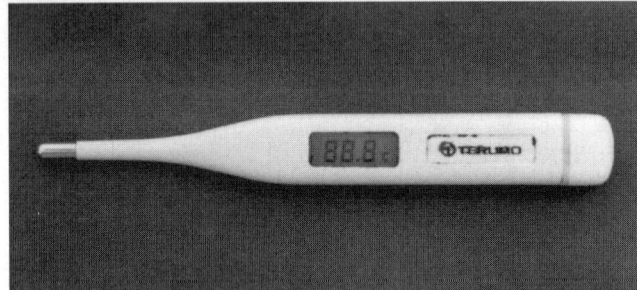

B

▶ FIGURE 2-12
Two rectal thermometers. **A.** Mercury. **B.** Electronic.

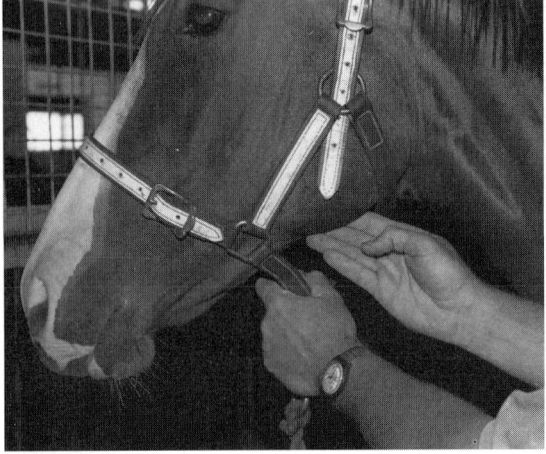

▶ FIGURE 2-13
Counting the pulse from the facial artery along the ventral border of the mandible.

NORMAL PULSE RATE

• Adult horses: 30–40 beats per minute (bpm)
• Foals[6]
   At birth: 40–80 bpm
   First hour (during attempts to rise): 130–150 bpm
   First few days: 70–100 bpm

Pulse Rate

The pulse rate is most easily taken at the facial artery as it curves around the mandible (Fig. 2-13). The pulse also is defined by rhythm and amplitude and can be regular or irregular. Identification of other sites where it can be taken from, as well as discussion on its characterization by rate, rhythm, and amplitude can be found in Chapter 6. The normal pulse rate is shown in the box.

Respiration

Respiration should be recorded when the horse is at rest with background noise kept to a minimum. Movement of the thorax during normal breathing is minimal, and it can be difficult to record a normal rate when a horse is at rest. The rate of breathing is usually recorded by observing the movements of the thorax, abdomen, or nostrils or by listening to air movement through the airways by auscultation and, occasionally, by feeling air movement against a hand positioned adjacent to the nostril or by observing fogging off a mirror held outside a nostril. For auscultation, the phonendoscope is placed just caudal to the point of the elbow, to monitor sounds in the major bronchi or over the base of the trachea. A more detailed description of breathing can be found in Chapter 3.

GENERAL PHYSICAL EXAMINATION OF BODY REGIONS

The head, neck, thorax, abdomen, external genitalia, mammary glands, and limbs are examined using a combination of visual appraisal, palpation, percussion, manipulation, and auscultation. If a specific problem is identified, a detailed examination of the appropriate region or system follows (see individual chapter for specific body systems).

Head Region

- Symmetry, position (height from ground, orientation), mobility
- Eyes and eyelids: inflammation, ocular reflexes, eyeball position, discharge, function of membrana nictitans, color of conjunctivae, corneal lesions and opacities, pain
- Nostrils: odor, discharge, patency, symmetry
- Mouth: excessive salivation, ability to prehend and chew, odor, position, and function of tongue, color and lesions of conjunctiva

Neck Region

- Swelling in throat region (tympany of guttural pouch, lymph node abscessation), lesions of jugular veins (phlebitis, obstruction, engorgement), neck mobility (fracture or arthrosis of vertebrae), deformity of trachea, distension of esophagus

Thoracic Region

- Heart: palpation of apex beat and detection of thrills, auscultation, percussion
- Lung: palpation of intercostal spaces (pleuri-

tis), auscultation and percussion (pneumonia, pleuritis, abscessation, presence of intestinal sounds [diaphragmatic hernia])

Abdominal Region

- Palpation, percussion, and ballottement of abdominal wall (tympany, pain from peritonitis, fetal movement, ascites), auscultation (intestinal movement, tympany)
- Rectal examination. This is not usually a part of the general examination but may be used to localize problems to the intestinal tract (obstruction), urogenital tract (cryptorchidism, neoplasia, calculus, nephritis), or abdomen (neoplasia).

SPECIAL EXAMINATION OF SPECIFIC REGIONS OR ORGAN SYSTEMS

A more detailed examination of a specific system(s) is indicated if the preliminary examination has uncovered information indicating disease or malfunction of a specific system. Examination of specific systems is described in the subsequent chapters.

USE OF DIAGNOSTIC AIDS

Although a diagnosis can often be made without recourse to diagnostic aids, extra assistance is frequently necessary. There are many ways in which the normal and abnormal can be categorized. Relatively commonly used diagnostic aids include clinical pathology, radiology, ultrasonography, electrocardiography, and histology. Details on these aids are presented under each organ system.

EXAMINATION OF THE ENVIRONMENT

Examination of the environment is not so often necessary for horses as it is for the other domestic animals. To complete a competent examination of the indoor and outdoor environment, the clinician must have a sound understanding of animal husbandry as it relates to horses (accommodation, nutrition, general management, stable ventilation, hygiene) and a basic understanding of the interaction between the horse and the environment (botany, environmental and plant toxicology, soil type, topography).

Examination of the environment can include all or some of the following topics:

- *Accommodation.* Horses housed indoors require adequate room in which to move around. Horses kept outdoors should have fencing that minimizes the chance of injury. Fences should be high enough to discourage attempts to escape by jumping out and be constructed so that it is difficult for horses to become entangled in them. Unacceptable fencing materials include barbed wire (injuries) and rubberized compounds that can be chewed and ingested (colic). Gates and doorways should be constructed so that horses cannot open them and escape. Ideally, there should not be any projections, especially sharp ones, that could cause lacerations especially to the eyes, nostrils, and mouth. Feed and water containers should be constructed so that it is impossible for horses to get their teeth or jaws caught in such a way that a fracture or avulsion can occur if the animal pulls back quickly.
- *Ventilation.* Stables should be well ventilated to minimize problems such as chronic obstructive pulmonary disease. Hay and other feed stuffs should not be stored above the stables, unless it is impossible for dust and fungal spores to gravitate down onto the horses.
- *Bedding materials.* Materials used as bedding include straw, peat, wood shavings, and paper. There must always be an adequate supply of bedding to prevent injury to soft tissues overlying bony protruberances, such as bursitis over the olecranon ("capped elbow") or calcaneus ("capped hock"). Bedding should be changed regularly and feces removed to prevent bedding from becoming wet and producing conditions that cause hoof disease (pododermatitis). Bedding materials are occasionally eaten and can lead to colon obstipation, or toxicity (e.g., laminitis from Black Walnut).
- *Water.* Fresh water should always be available. In regions where freezing is likely, precautions should be taken to ensure the continuity of supply by using for example insulated or heated containers.
- *Nutrition.* Nutritional requirements for horses are well documented. However, despite this, over and under feeding as well as feeding an unbalanced ration are common. The frequency of feeding is important. Horses by nature graze frequently during waking hours, a habit that is severely disrupted by enclosure and dependence on being fed by hand. Another potential problem is that the frequent use of highly concentrated pelleted rations means that a horse can eat its daily allowance in a few minutes. This can contribute to digestive problems (gastric distension) but, more important, it eliminates an activity that appears to be vital to a horse's psychological health. A variety of stereotypic behavioral patterns are recognized, such as "weaving" (moving the head, neck, and thorax from side to side while shifting the body weight from one front foot to the other), "cribbing," and "wind sucking" (chewing on materials in the stall and swallowing air). The exact cause of these is not known, but boredom appears to be significant.
- *Examination related to intoxication.* There are numerous aspects in addition to the clinical syndrome that need to be evaluated when intoxication is suspected. These include animal movement, addition of new animals, what other animals are affected, sources and delivery dates of food, water, bedding, food for other species that might contain substances such as monenesin or antibiotics, geographical proximity to sources of industrial toxins (lead, insecticides) or plant or hedge clippings such as oleander (*Nerium oleander*). Food and water samples need to be collected. Stable and pasture surrounds should be carefully examined for the presence of toxic plants or industrial waste.

The samples that should be collected for analysis vary with the problem at hand but will be selected after the appropriate environmental, clinical, and postmortem examinations have been completed. Some details of which antemortem and/or postmortem samples may be required for toxicological analysis, as well as methods of storage, can be found in Table 2-1.

▶ TABLE 2–1

SAMPLES NEEDED FOR TOXICOLOGIC ANALYSIS

Sample	Amount	Condition	Examples
Antemortem Samples			
Whole blood	5–10 ml	EDTA anticoagulant	Lead, arsenic, selenium, acetylcholinesterase
Urine	100 ml	Plastic screw-capped vial	Drugs, some metals
Serum	10 ml	Remove from clot; use special trace element tubes	Trace elements, drugs, nitrates
Cerebrospinal fluid	1 ml	Clot tube	Sodium
GI contents	500 gm	Obtain representative sample	Pesticides, plants, metals; feed-associated toxicants
Hair	—	Rarely useful, call laboratory; wash prior to sampling	Occasionally chronic selenosis
Postmortem Samples			
Urine	100 ml	Plastic screw-capped vial	Drugs, some metals
Serum	20 ml	Remove from heart clot	Drugs, nitrates, electrolytes
Liver	250 gm	Plastic (foil if organics)	Pesticides, metals, botulinum
Kidney	250 gm	Plastic (foil if organics)	Metals
Brain	50%	Split sagitally, send half in formalin to pathologist, half frozen in plastic to analyst	Organochlorides, sodium, acetylcholinesterase
Fat	250 gm	Foil inside plastic	Accumulated organochlorines
GI contents	500 gm	Obtain representative sample	Pesticides, plants, metals, feed-associated toxicants
Ocular fluid	0.5 ml	Entire eye	Nitrates, magnesium
Bone	100 gm	One long bone	Fluoride
Miscellaneous	—	Injection sites, spleen	Some drugs
Environmental Samples			
Baits, etc.	200 ml or 200 gm	Clean mason jar (liquid, plastic)	Unidentified chemicals, feed additives
Concentrates	1 kg or more	Plastic sack, box; representative sample is imperative	Mycotoxins, feed additives, plants, pesticides, botulinum
Forage	1 kg or more	Plastic sack, box; representative sample is imperative	Plants, pesticides, botulinum
Plants	Plant	Fresh, or pressed and dried; send all plant parts	
Water	1L	Clean mason jar, foil under lid for metals, plastic if organics	Metals, nitrates, pesticides, algae, sulfate

Note: With the exception of whole blood and very dry samples (e.g., some feeds), all samples should be submitted frozen. When available, appropriate tissue samples, fixed in formalin, should also be submitted for histological analysis. Do not submit material in syringes. (Source: Galey FD: Diagnostic Toxicology In Robinson NE (ed) Current Therapy in Equine Medicine Philadelphia, Saunders, 1992, Section 8, p 339. Reprinted with permission.)

R E F E R E N C E S

1. Jones WE: Coat color inheritance. *In* Jones WE (ed), Genetics and Horse Breeding. Philadelphia, Lea & Febiger, 1982, ch 9, p 220.
2. Farrell RK, Norman WH: 1972 Permanent International Horse Identification. Proceedings, Horse Identification Seminar, Washington State University, Pullman, 1972, p 57-72.
3. Stormont CJ: Identification and parentage verification of individual horses by blood typing tests. Equine Vet Sci 1988; 8:176.
4. Gabel AA, Knowles RC, Weisbrode SE: Horse identification: A field trial using an electronic identification system. Equine Vet Sci 1988; 8:172.
5. Fort Dodge Laboratories: Official Guide for Determining the Age of the Horse. Fort Dodge Iowa, 1966.
6. Koterba AM: Physical examination. *In* Koterba AM, Drummond WH, Kosch PC (eds), Equine Clinical Neonatology. Philadelphia, Lea & Febiger, 1990, ch 6, p 71.

The Respiratory Tract

3

COMPONENTS

The respiratory tract is made up of the nostrils, nasal passages, nasal septum, paranasal sinuses, nasopharynx, larynx, guttural pouches, soft palate, trachea, bronchi, small airways, lungs, and pleural cavities.

MANIFESTATIONS OF DISEASE

The main manifestations of disease in the respiratory system are the result of obstruction, reduced exchange of oxygen and carbon dioxide, inflammation, septicemia, toxemia, and neoplasia and include:

- Abnormal respiratory sounds (obstruction)
- Reduced exercise tolerance (reduced delivery of oxygen to tissues)
- Fever (infection)
- Nasal discharge (infection, neoplasia)
- Epistaxis (neoplasia, ethmoidal hematomata, pulmonary hemorrhage)

GENERAL CLINICAL EXAMINATION

The general examination of the respiratory tract should be conducted when the horse is at rest.

Patterns of Breathing

When a horse is at rest, the movements associated with the transfer of air into and out of the lungs are barely visible. Normal breathing at rest is composed of a regular sequence of inspiratory and expiratory movements with a pause in between. The ratio between times of expiration and inspiration is 2 to 1. Inspiration is an active process, and during normal resting breathing expiration is a passive act, based on the tendency of the thorax, diaphragm, and lungs to recoil. As demand increases, the expiratory pause becomes shorter and eventually disappears as inspiration and expiration become continuous. In normal adults thoracic movements are difficult to see, and, accordingly, the rate of breathing is more difficult to count. In response to increased stimulus, the rate of thoracic and abdominal movements increase and the external nares begin to participate by opening and closing. If movement of the thorax is painful (pleuritis), air transport is accomplished by reducing movement of the thorax and increasing the abdominal component, so-called "abdominal respiration." When there are extensive abdominal and diaphragmatic movements, the anus can be seen moving in and out. The presence of airway obstruction causes turbulent flow and increased noise production, with the noise being audible during inspiration, expiration, or both, depending on which phase of breathing is affected. When there is a desperate need for oxygen, the horse will extend its head and neck to reduce airway resistance as much as possible. Normal breathing rates are presented in the box.

In its broadest sense respiration refers to the exchange of gases between the atmosphere and body cells, and breathing refers to air movement in and out of the respiratory tract. Therefore, any change in the efficiency of respiration will alter the pattern of breathing. Rate is easily evaluated, but respiration requires measuring oxygen consumption and carbon dioxide production. To facilitate the clinical description, the rate and apparent tidal volume can be described as decreased, normal, or increased and the difficulty of breathing as labored or difficult. Terms such as *dyspnea, hyperpnea, polypnea, hyperventilation,* and *hypoventilation* are used to describe respiration and breathing, but they are subjective parameters and, when used as part of the early clinical exam, they imply changes in ventilation that may not exist. Ventilation refers to air movement into and out of the alveoli and is best measured by arterial blood gas analysis as it cannot be categorized simply by extrapolating from the supposed ease, rate, and depth of breathing.

Although breathing is involved primarily in gas exchange, changes may be seen in response to local (e.g., obstruction) or systemic factors (e.g., paralysis of muscles of respiration by botulinum toxin) and may be a primary (influenced by problems located in the respiratory system) or a secondary response to disease in another part of the body (e.g., compensation for metabolic acidosis).

Nasal Discharge

The nasal passages are usually covered by a thin, transparent, glistening film of moisture. The external nares may be dry or moist depending on prevailing conditions; they are often moist in cold weather, after transport, and when housed in dusty environments with associated mucosal irritation. Nasal secretions can be categorized depending on their appearance. A *serous* secretion is thin and transparent and is characteristic of a response to a mild stimulus as well as the early stages of viral infections and, as such, is usually bilateral. *Purulent* discharges are viscid, opaque, and yellowish on account of the increased white cell content. Purulent discharges are present whenever there is an adequate stimulus to white cells such as bacterial infection and presence of foreign bodies. When blood is present, the term *sanguineous* is used. Blood may be in small volumes in the presence of neoplasia, ulceration, foreign bodies, or ethmoidal hematomata or in larger volumes in association with lesions in the guttural pouch or the lungs. It is common to have a combinations of the above (e.g., serosanguineous, mucopurulent).

Contamination with Food, Water, and Saliva

Functional abnormality of the swallowing mechanism, obstruction of the pharynx or esophagus, or anatomical malformation can result in food, water, milk or saliva being passed back out through the nasal passages after attempts to swallow.

Odor

A foul odor usually indicates the presence of necrosis and anerobic bacteria such as commonly occurs with pneumonia, foreign body, and sinus infections associated with fistulae into the mouth.

Side of Discharge

Lesions localized to one nasal passage usually have a predominantly unilateral discharge. However, exercise and coughing can result in aspiration of material into the nasopharynx with expulsion through both nostrils. Discharges related to inflammation, infection, and bleeding of tissues caudal to the nasal septum can pass down both nasal passages and are therefore usually bilateral. Chronic nasal discharge causes a localized dermatitis that often produces a depigmentation of the skin affected by the discharge.

Quantity

The quantity of discharge depends largely on the extent of the stimulus. However, significant volumes are usually associated with diseases of the paranasal sinuses and the guttural pouches. Whenever there is fluid accumulation in these cavities, and they have patent openings, there will be an increased flow of fluid whenever the animal lowers its head and also when breathing rate increases during exercise.

Evaluation of Nasal Discharge

Collection and analysis of nasal discharges can be of diagnostic value. Because discharge can originate from anywhere in the respiratory tract, and because the airways are not sterile, results must be interpreted with caution. Nevertheless, evaluation of cells, identification, culture and sensitivity testing of bacteria, and identification of viruses may be useful. Although shedding of virus usually coincides with pyrexia, it may precede the onset of clinical signs by a few days, indicating that virus identification is best carried out in samples collected around the time of onset of clinical signs. Samples may be collected by nasal swabbing, nasal scraping, or nasopharyngeal swabbing.

Identification of viruses causing respiratory disease is done by culturing secretions, serologically, or by direct identification of viral antigen using procedures such as enzyme-linked immunoabsorbent assays (ELISA) or immunofluorescent staining (IFA) techniques. The disadvantages of virus isolation is that live virus is required, necessitating careful sample collection, preservation, and transport—and also considerable time. The immunostaining methods do not require live virus and are therefore useful when the presence of live virus cannot be guaranteed.

NASOPHARYNGEAL SWABBING. The purpose of this method is to collect samples from the nasopharynx for viral identification.[1]

Procedure. The sample is collected by passing the guarded swab into the nasopharynx through the ventral meatus. The sample is collected by extending the swab from its protective cover and then rubbing it against the pharyngeal

---

Materials for Nasopharyngeal Swabbing

▶ Sterile swabbing device
    Guarded culturette
    Gauge swab (2 × 2-inch) tied to stiff wire inserted through rubber or plastic cannula

▶ Virus transport media (commercial preparation or medium prepared by adding gentamicin [50 μg/mL] to normal saline containing 5% bovine serum albumin)

Materials for Nasal Lavage

▶ Syringe (50 ml)
▶ 0.01 M phosphate buffered saline (pH = 7.4, 30 mL)
▶ Plastic beaker
▶ Catheter (30 cm)

---

mucosa. Samples are placed immediately in the transport medium that contains antibiotics to inhibit bacterial growth and proteins to stabilize virus. Samples should be maintained between 0°C and 4°C and arrive at the laboratory within 24 hours.

NASAL LAVAGE. This collection method requires that lavage fluid be deposited in the caudal nasal passage and then collected as it flows back from the nostrils by gravity.[2]

Procedure. With the horse under appropriate restraint, the catheter, with the syringe containing the buffered saline attached, is passed up one nasal passage so that its tip is located in the caudal nasal cavity. The correct location for deposition of the fluid is at a point approximately halfway between the medial canthus of the eye and the nasomaxillary notch. The beaker is placed against the nostril, and after ensuring that the head is not elevated, the fluid is injected and then collected in the beaker as it flows from the nose. Approximately half of the fluid is usually recovered. Evaluation consists of a total cell count, and, after centrifugation, a cytological examination is conducted on a stained smear. Some values derived from normal horses are listed in Table 3–1.

NASAL SCRAPING. A simple, but useful, method of obtaining some information about the possible etiology of respiratory disease is to analyze the material collected by nasal scraping.[3] A nasal scraping is most easily collected with a wooden tongue depressor, but any other flat instrument is adequate. The procedure is relatively innocuous, and only minimal restraint is necessary. The sample is collected by firmly scraping the depressor along the floor of the nasal passage and then preparing a smear. An evaluation of the numbers and relative proportions of eosinophils and neutrophils may be of assistance in separating diseases into allergic or infectious categories.

Nasal Patency

One or both nasal passages may become obstructed by space-occupying lesions that originate either in the nasal passages (ethmoidal hematomas, neoplasia) or in the paranasal sinuses (cysts, chronic sinusitis). A lesion in a sinus does not have to invade the nasal passage to cause obstruction, because the ventral conchal sinus, which constitutes part of the medial wall of the maxillary sinuses, is easily pushed medially by an enlarging intrasinus lesion. Similarly, by causing displacement of the nasal septum, an expanding lesion in one nasal passage can obstruct the contralateral nasal passage.

Patency can be tested by obstructing each nostril in turn and estimating the volume of air passing through the other nasal passage. Normally, this causes no discomfort and no increase in respiratory sounds, but, when obstruction is present, resentment and increased sounds are present in proportion to the level of obstruction. Passage of a nasogastric tube can also be useful in demonstrating obstruction of the ventral meatus, although care should be taken not to traumatize the tissues and cause epistaxis.

Symmetry and Contour of Facial Bones

The bones overlying the paranasal sinuses and nasal passages should be examined visually and by palpation and percussion. Swelling, fistulae, and asymmetry can be detected visually. Palpation allows the identification of pain and of the extent of edema. Percussion identifies pain and theoretically allows the detection of space-occupying lesions that reduce the normal resonance. However, it often is unreliable.

Examples of lesions producing asymmetrical swelling are unilateral obstruction of sinus drainage to the nose, neoplasia, and periapical dental abscessation. Examples of lesions producing symmetrical swellings include osteodystrophy and alveolar periostitis.

Lesions of the maxilla may obstruct the nasolacrimal duct with the subsequent overflow of lacrimal fluid down the horse's face (epiphora). Patency of the nasolacrimal duct should be checked if this complication is suspected (see Evaluation of Nasolacrimal Duct Patency).

Evaluation of the Nasal Septum

A number of different conditions can affect the nasal septum, resulting in inflammation, distortion, thickening, or deviation. Chronic mycotic chondritis is one cause of thickening and distortion. As described, space occupying lesions in the nasal passages can, if large enough, produce deviation of the septum to one side even though the septum itself is free of disease. The cranial portion of the septum can be examined by holding the nostril open, and it can also be palpated. More extensive examination requires the passage of an endoscope that allows the complete septum to be evaluated. A ventrodorsal radiograph, which may sometimes require a general anesthetic, is also useful for evaluating the thickness and extent of deviation of the septum.

Percussion of Paranasal Sinuses

Percussion of a sinus cavity that is filled with fluid, tissue mass, or inspissated purulent material elicits a dull sound, rather than the more resonant normal note. Bilateral abnormality is more difficult to detect because the abnormal note cannot be compared with that from the normal, contralateral side. Occasionally, when acute sinusitis is present, percussion will cause pain and is resented by the horse. Percussion is done by tapping the sinus region with the fingers (Fig. 3–1). Left and right sides are percussed alternately in order to detect any difference between the sides.

▶ **TABLE 3–1**

REFERENCE VALUES FOR CELLULAR CONTENT OF NASAL FLUID OBTAINED FROM HORSES BY LAVAGE: TOTAL ($\times 10^5$/CELLS/ML) AND DIFFERENTIAL (% ± 1 SD) CELL COUNTS ($n = 42$)

Total cells	1.9 ± 0.8
Epithelial cells	80.9 ± 12.2
Squamous cells	14.4 ± 11.9
Macrophages	2.3 ± 2.0
Lymphocytes	1.5 ± 1.4
Neutrophils	0.9 ± 0.8
Eosinophils	0
Mast cells	0

Source: Extracted from Mair TS, Stokes CR, Bourne FJ: Cellular contents of secretions obtained by lavage from different levels of the equine respiratory tract. Equine Vet J 1987;19:458.

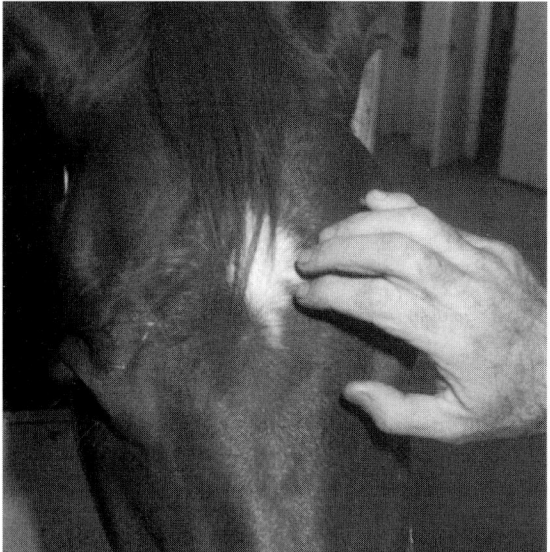

▶ FIGURE 3–1
Percussion of paranasal sinuses.

Palpation of the Trachea and Larynx

The trachea should be carefully palpated from proximal to distal to identify any distortion indicative of previous trauma, previous surgery, or congenital malformation. It should be firmly squeezed to evaluate sensitivity associated with infection (laryngitis, tracheitis). Increased sensitivity will often cause the horse to cough. Palpation to test for sensitivity is done by squeezing the larynx or trachea between the thumb and fingers of one hand. Palpation done to check the laryngeal musculature is best done by palpating both sides simultaneously with the index fingers

of both hands, partly to allow one hand to provide support while the other is used to palpate, and partly so that one side can be used as a comparison for the other, which is particularly useful for assessing muscle atrophy. Access to the larynx is easier if the horse's head is extended by resting the horse's lower jaw on the shoulder of the examiner who stands facing the horse.

Palpation of the Thorax

The thorax is examined by carefully palpating each rib and the costochondral junctions to detect deformity indicative of fracture and metabolic bone disease. Deep firm palpation in the intercostal spaces can elicit a pain response when pleuritis is present. In emaciated horses excessive accumulation of pleural fluid sometimes causes the intercostal spaces to bulge outward.

SPECIAL EXAMINATION PROCEDURES

Auscultation of the Thorax and Upper Airways

The upper airways and thorax should be auscultated in a quiet environment. Auscultation is the science of listening to and interpreting sounds, in this case, sounds originating in the respiratory tract. The stethoscope is the instrument of most use in allowing the thoracic sounds to be heard and evaluated. An example of a simple stethoscope demonstrating the basic components is presented in Figure 3-2. For large animal work a

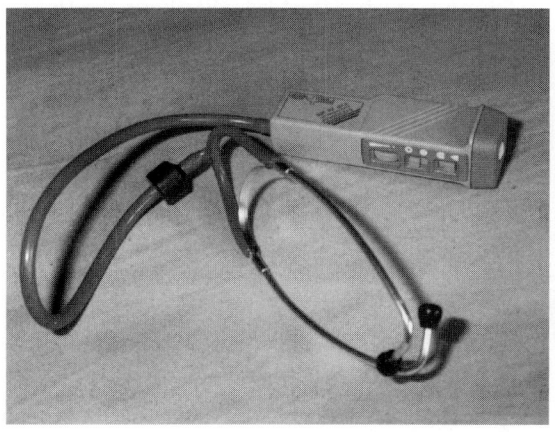

A

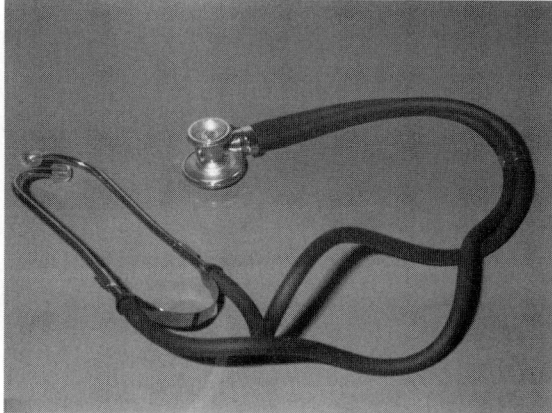

B

▶ FIGURE 3–2
Stethoscopes. **A.** Electronic. **B.** Sprague.

stethoscope with an interchangeable 2"- (5-cm) diameter phonendoscope and a smaller bell chestpiece are generally used. Correct interpretation of lung sounds requires knowledge of how such sounds are generated as well as how they are modified by different tissues and disease processes.[4-6] Normal breath sounds are produced by turbulent flow in airways that have diameters greater than 2 mm. They are loudest over the trachea and quietest over the diaphragmatic lobes of the lungs. Their loudness is a function of production and transmission, with sound being attenuated during transmission through the lung and thoracic wall. The greatest reflection, and hence attenuation, of sound occurs at the interface between tissues of markedly different densities or acoustic properties. Fluid or air decrease sound transmission to a greater degree than consolidated tissue (e.g., abscess) because of the greater similarity of consolidated tissue to the tissues of the thoracic wall. Respiratory sounds are less audible in obese or large horses. The intensity of normal sounds increase as turbulence rises with increased velocity of air flow or decrease in airway diameter. It is not easy to describe respiratory sounds, however, a useful working system is as follows.

Normal Lung Sounds

These are the soft, rustling sounds, often termed *vesicular,* or *bronchovesicular,* sounds heard over the lung fields in foals and thin horses and over the hilar regions in most horses. These sounds become louder when breathing increases and when transmission is increased in the presence of lung consolidation. Sound is diminished by reduction in breathing and by space-occupying lesions (fluid and air) in the pleural cavities.

Abnormal Lung Sounds

Included in this group are increased breath sounds, crackles, wheezes, and friction rubs. *Crackles* are sharp clicking sounds produced when there is sudden equalization of pressures between different parts of the lung. *Wheezes* are sounds of longer duration and more musical character that are produced by the vibration of thick material within the airways or by the vibration of the airways themselves. Wheezes from different sites are likely to have different tones—therefore any variation in tone should be noted. Because of the tendency for intrathoracic airways to collapse on expiration and open on inspiration, expiratory wheezes are likely to originate in intrathoracic airways. The reverse situation applies to extrathoracic airways. *Friction rubs* are sounds produced when the normal lubrication between pleural and also pericardial surfaces is reduced in association with pleuritis or pericarditis, respectively. Usually pleural friction rubs are coordinated with breathing and pericardial friction rubs with the heart beat. When fluid accumulates in the cavity, or adhesions restrict movement between adjacent layers, the sound disappears.

Absence of Breath Sounds

This occurs when there is no air passing through the airways, when space-occupying lesions, such as a diaphragmatic hernia, interfere with the transmission of sound, and when airflow is very slow, such as during shallow breathing associated with the pain of pleuritis or a rib fracture.

Miscellaneous Sounds

Because of the domed shape of the diaphragm, much of the abdominal viscera is located under the ribs, and auscultation will often detect intestinal sounds, especially after feeding. It is important to differentiate such sounds from those occurring with a diaphragmatic hernia. It often is possible to hear sounds that have been transmitted from the upper respiratory tract if they are particularly loud. The sounds generated by movement of the phonendoscope on skin and hair often interfere with breath sounds.

Methods of Stimulating Breathing

Despite every effort to eliminate extraneous noises and to use good equipment, evaluation of

---

METHODS OF STIMULATING BREATHING

- Rebreathing from a plastic bag
- Addition of carbon dioxide to inspired air
- Respiratory stimulants Doxapram hydrochloride ("Dopram"), Lobeline hydrochloride ("Lobelin")
- Manual obstruction of nostrils

intrathoracic disease through interpretation of breath sounds is impossible if the sounds generated are not of sufficient loudness to be detected. There are several ways to stimulate breathing so that a more thorough auscultation can be carried out:

- *Rebreathing of expired air.* This is most easily done by covering the nostrils with a plastic bag, such as a rectal examination glove.
- *Addition of carbon dioxide to inspired air.* This is also done most easily by using a plastic bag placed over the nostrils and then adding carbon dioxide by tube.
- *Respiratory stimulants.* Intravenous administration of a respiratory stimulant will cause a rapid increase in rate and depth of breathing. Doxapram hydrochloride (0.5–1.0 mg/kg IV) and Lobeline hydrochloride (0.2 mg/kg IV) are used for this purpose and produce hyperventilation of 1 to 2 minutes' duration.
- *Obstruction of the nostrils.* Manual obstruction of the nostrils is a simple way of increasing breathing. Simply covering the nostrils is not sufficient and both nostrils must be squeezed closed. The clinician stands in front of the horse and uses the left hand for the right nostril and the right hand for the left nostril. Care should be taken because some horses resent the procedure, and all horses become agitated as they strive to inhale.

Percussion of Thorax

Thoracic percussion is an examination technique based on the interpretation of sounds and the vibrations elicited by striking the thoracic wall sharply. Practice is necessary to develop the skill necessary to perform and interpret the procedure simultaneously.[7] *Direct percussion* consists of striking a rib directly with the finger, usually the second, or a hammer (plexor). *Indirect percussion* relies on a flat object, the pleximeter, which is placed against the thoracic wall and then struck with a second instrument, the plexor. The plexor–pleximeter combination is often a finger and hand, although a special set of instruments is available (Fig. 3-3). The pleximeter is placed in the intercostal space.

With both techniques the plexor is struck firmly against the pleximeter in a series of sharp blows. The thoracic wall is covered systematically, usu-

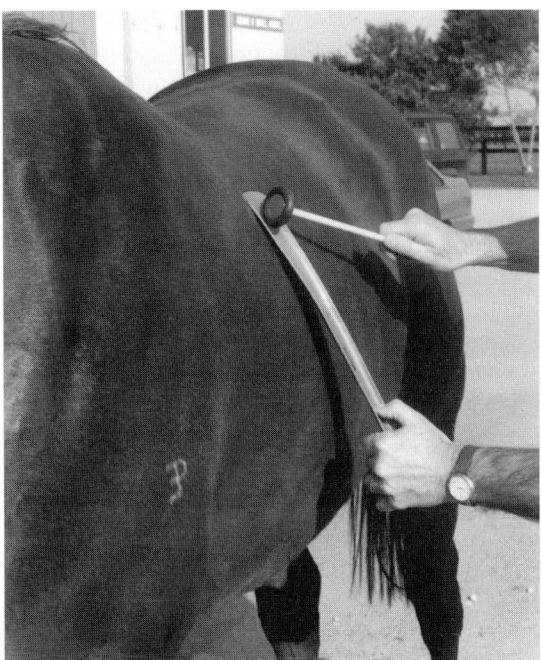

▶ **FIGURE 3-3**
Plexor and pleximeter for carrying out thoracic percussion.

ally in a dorsal to ventral direction, and two to four blows should be delivered before moving the pleximeter. Percussion elicits an audible and tactile frequency response, the propagation and transmission of which depends on the force of the blow, the density of the medium, and the number of tissue interfaces. The degree of propagation is known as *resonance,* and air and gases being more resonant than solid tissues. The objective of percussion is to identify any abnormal sound(s) and then to interpret the information in order to assist in establishing a diagnosis. Useful percussion requires practice, and skill is developed best by taking every opportunity to compare the results of percussion with the findings of radiography, ultrasonography, and necropsy. Percussion findings can be described as follows:

- *Resonant.* Percussion over normal expanded lung tissue produces a resonant sound that is of moderate pitch and easily heard.
- *Hyperresonant.* In young animals with little fat or muscle and during deep inspiration a hyperresonant response, which is normal, can be elicited. Occasionally, a similar response is found when a greater than normal volume of air is present (e.g., pulmonary emphysema).

- *Tympanitic.* When there is air under increased pressure in the thorax (tension pneumonthorax), a tympanitic sound is elicited. It is clear and high-pitched, rather drumlike in character.
- *Dull.* As the content of air decreases and the content of tissue and fluid increases (lung consolidation, abscess), percussion elicits a sound that is of lower pitch without a well-defined vibrant quality. A dull note is normal over the heart.
- *Flat.* When there is no air present, such as with a pleural effusion, the sound is very dull and flat.

The technique is limited by the skill of the clinician, its subjective nature, the thickness of tissues in the thoracic wall, environmental background noise, and because useful sounds penetrate only a few centimeters and lesions less than a few centimeters in size cannot be detected at all. Comparison of one side of the thorax with the other is useful. Despite these limitations, large lesions such as abscesses, neoplasms, pulmonary consolidation, emphysema and pneumothorax, and horizontal interfaces between fluid and air are relatively easily detected. The limits of percussible lung fields are shown in Figure 3–4.

Endoscopic Examination of the Airways

Endoscopy is a technique regularly used to evaluate the status of the airways. The major development in the last twenty years has been the change from a rigid instrument with a light source in the distal end and with image transmission

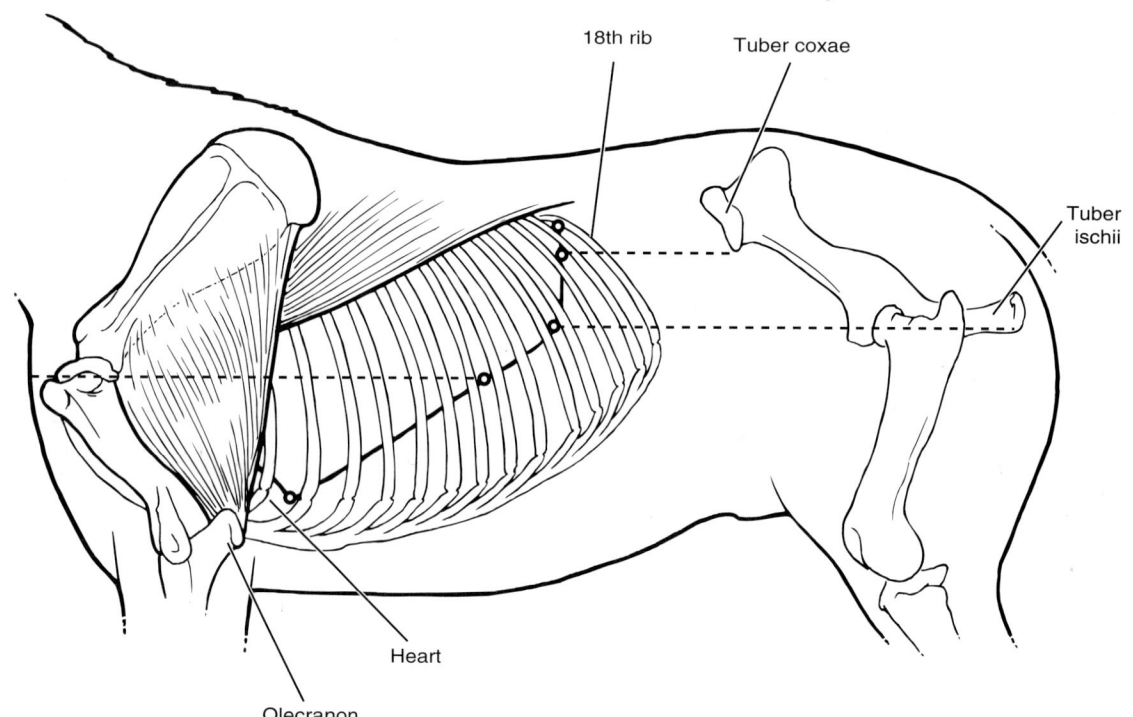

Borders of Percussable Lung
- Cranial border – shoulder musculature
- Dorsal border – back musculature
- Caudoventral border
  - 17th intercostal space adjacent to back musculature
  - 16th intercostal space at level of ventral border of tuber coxae
  - 14th intercostal space at level of tuber ischii
  - 11th intercostal space at level of point of shoulder

▶ **FIGURE 3–4**

Approximate limits of percussable lung.

Materials for Endoscopy

▶ Restraining stocks
▶ Nasal twitch
▶ Chemical restraint
▶ Endoscope

based on reflection via prisms to the flexible fiber-optic and video systems (Appendix 1).

Procedure

Although not all horses require extensive restraint the value of the instrumentation, particularly the videoendoscope, dictates that reasonable care be taken. Alternatively, in a busy environment where the clinician moves quickly between well-managed horses, such as in a training establishment, only minimal restraint is feasible or generally necessary. For the optimum safety of patient, personnel, and equipment the horse is placed in stocks and sedated as necessary. Most horses can be examined without a twitch. However, an examination can be performed faster and with less movement by the horse when a twitch is used. The effect that chemical and twitch restraint might have on the interpretation of subtle laryngeal function is mentioned in the section on the larynx. General anesthesia is occasionally necessary because of temperament or the circumstances under which the examination is initiated. However, recumbency produces nasopharyngeal vascular engorgement, that can interfere with interpretation. At least two people are required to conduct an examination, one to hold the horse, the twitch, and the endoscope, once it has been inserted, and a second to insert the endoscope and conduct the examination. Preferably, there will be a third person who is responsible for inserting and holding the endoscope. Figure 3-5 shows an endoscopic examination of the respiratory tract in progress.

Nasal Chambers

An endoscope with an external diameter of 11 mm is adequate for adult, full-size horses but, for ponies and foals a smaller diameter of about 8 mm often is necessary. The endoscope should

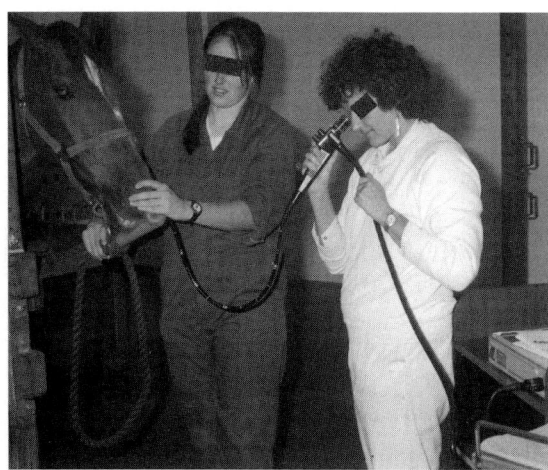

▶ **FIGURE 3-5**
Upper respiratory tract endoscopy with a flexible endoscope, twitch, and stocks restraint.

be inserted quickly and smoothly into the ventral meatus while the nostril is held open. This is necessary because the horse will usually resent passage of the endoscope through the most rostral section. Because of this rapid insertion, thorough examination of this region is impossible at this time and should be conducted when removing the endoscope, which can be done slowly. Although complete examination may require that the endoscope be retracted and inserted a number of times, it is recommended that, after the initial rapid insertion, the ventral meatus, ventral conchus, and ventral aspect of the nasal septum are examined during insertion, and the dorsal structures during withdrawal. The clinician needs to be aware of the normal anatomy of the region and be able to identify the ventral and dorsal conchae, nasal septum, dorsal, middle, ventral, and common meati, the endoturbinates of the ethmoidal labrynth, and the site where exudate coming from the nasomaxillary opening can be seen.[8] Some of these structures are shown in Figure 3-6. Whenever lesions of the nasal passages are suspected, examination of both nasal passages should be conducted. When the more distal regions of the respiratory tract are to be examined, it is usual to examine only that nasal passage through which the endoscope is passed. This procedure carries the risk that an unsuspected lesion in the unexamined nasal passage will go undetected, and, for this reason, the clinician should be aware that a calculated risk is being taken. The objective of examining the nasal passage is to detect diseases

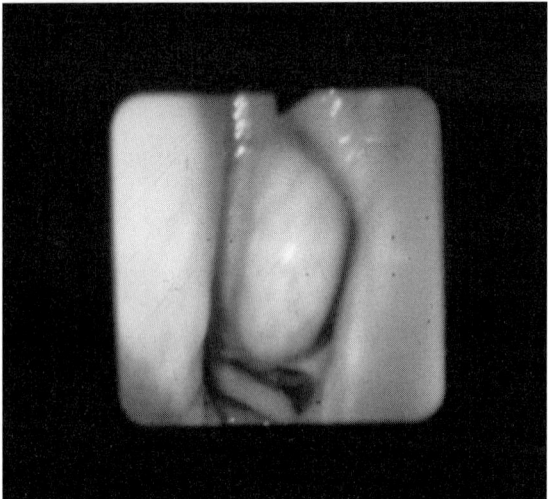

FIGURE 3-6

Endoscopy of the nasal passage. Note the large bulbous endoturbinatell, located in the dorsocaudal nasal cavity. It is bounded by the dorsal conchus and the nasal septum.

such as infection, neoplasia, foreign body, developmental problems, and trauma (Figure 3-7).

Paranasal Sinuses

Endoscopic examination of the paranasal sinuses can be carried out for diagnostic and therapeutic purposes. The procedure is usually possible in the standing position with the horse sedated, but general anesthesia may be necessary for horses that are not sufficiently tractable.

Procedure. The procedure is carried out with the horse under appropriate chemical and

Materials for Paranasal Sinus Endoscopy

- Endoscope
    Arthroscope (e.g., 4.0 mm) with flexible light cable and light source or
    Flexible fiber-optic or videoendoscope with light source
- Instrument for opening the sinus
    Bone drill, Steinmann pin, or trephine
- Polyionic lavage fluid and administration set
- Local anesthetic—2% lidocaine hydrochloride, 2% mepivacaine hydrochloride
- Chemical restraint (See Chapter 1, Chemical Restraint of the Adult Horse

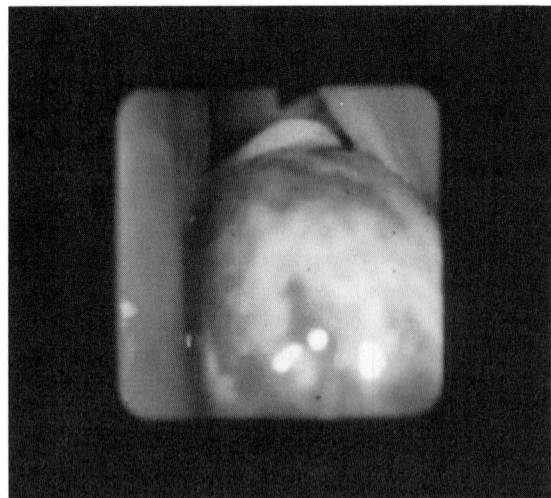

FIGURE 3-7

Ethmoidal hematoma in the dorsal aspect of the caudal nasal passage.

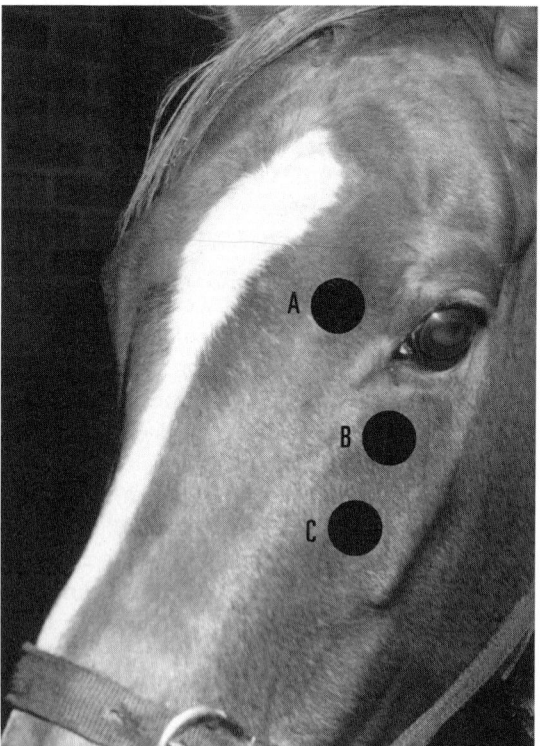

FIGURE 3-8

Location of sites for trephination of the paranasal sinuses. **A.** Frontoconchal sinus. **B.** Caudal maxillary sinus. **C.** Rostral maxillary sinus.

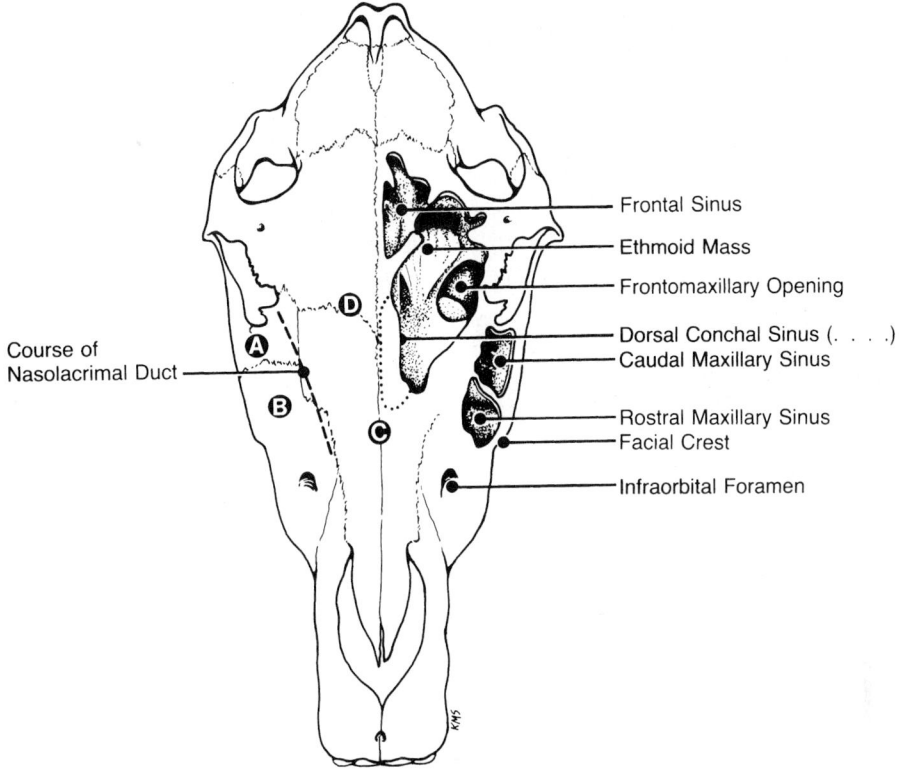

Course of Nasolacrimal Duct

Frontal Sinus

Ethmoid Mass

Frontomaxillary Opening

Dorsal Conchal Sinus (. . . .)

Caudal Maxillary Sinus

Rostral Maxillary Sinus

Facial Crest

Infraorbital Foramen

▶ **FIGURE 3-9**

Anatomy of the paranasal sinuses. (From Haynes PF: Surgery of the equine respiratory tract. *In* Jennings PB (ed), The Practice of Large Animal Surgery, vol 1. Philadelphia, Saunders, 1984, p 40. Reprinted with permission.)

physical restraint. A rigid arthroscope is preferred, in which case a Steinmann pin or bone drill of appropriate diameter is used to make an opening into the sinuses. If a flexible endoscope is used, the openings into the sinuses need to be larger and these are usually made with a trephine. The locations of the openings are similar to those for routine trephination of the sinuses (Fig. 3-8).[9] The techniques for both small and larger openings are similar and consist of infiltration of local anesthetic, skin incision, and creation of a hole in the bone with pin, drill, or trephine. When using the trephine it is usual to incise and reflect or resect the periosteum. The examination is carried out while lavaging the sinuses with the polyionic fluid.

Results. In some clinical cases the sinuses are full of exudate that must be flushed out before an examination is possible. Furthermore, the presence of space-occupying lesions, such as neoplasia or grossly thickened mucosae, can limit a complete examination. The normal anatomy is demonstrated in Figure 3-9. Causes of sinus disease include infection (primary sinusitis, dental

sinusitis), neoplasia, and developmental abnormalities (paranasal cysts).

Pharynx

Examination of the pharynx requires a thorough understanding of the anatomy of the region as well as its function.[10] The pharynx is divided into dorsal and ventral parts by the soft palate. Rostrally the dorsal and ventral parts are known respectively as the naso- and oropharynx, and caudally as the dorsal laryngopharynx and ventral laryngopharynx. The endoscope first enters the nasopharynx from where the soft palate is visible ventrally. It then progresses to the dorsal pharyngeal recess and openings to the auditory tubes dorsally and dorsolaterally, respectively (Fig. 3-10). The larynx is usually visible in the background and is examined by moving the endoscope deeper into the pharynx (Fig. 3-11). The observer should be familiar with the structure of the soft palate and the manner in which the rostral larynx (epiglottis and corniculate processes of the arytenoid cartilages) is inserted through the intrapharyngeal opening in the soft palate (Fig. 3-12).[11]

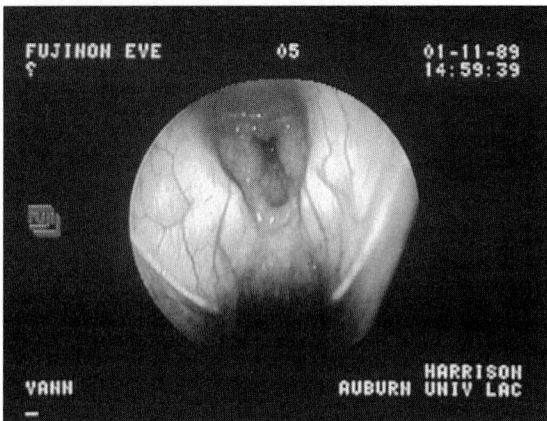

▶ **FIGURE 3-10**

Endoscopic view of the nasopharynx showing the pharyngeal openings to the left and right auditory tubes and in the dorsal midline the dorsal pharyngeal recess.

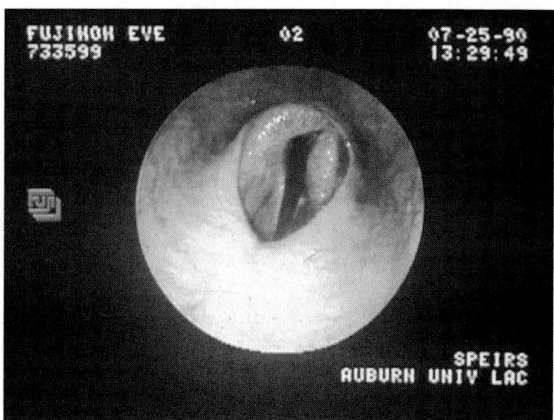

▶ **FIGURE 3-12**

Elliptical fenestration in the soft palate, the intrapharyngeal ostium, through which the larynx (epiglottis and corniculate processes of the arytenoid cartilages) are normally inserted. (Note that left laryngeal hemiplegia is also present.)

Examination of the oropharynx and ventral laryngopharynx is more difficult but may be achieved by advancing the endoscope further into the nasopharynx and then bending it ventrally so that the distal end passes through the intrapharyngeal ostium. This procedure can be performed in a conscious horse but is most safely done under general anesthesia. They can also be examined by passing the endoscope through the mouth, which, although best done under general anesthesia, can also be carried out in a well-restrained, conscious horse with a mouth gag in place. Of course, this places the instrument at risk of damage. Some protection can be afforded the endoscope if it is inserted inside a tube such as an endotracheal tube or a metal cannula. The endoscope can also be inserted through a laryngotomy or tracheotomy incision, with viewing made in a

caudal to rostral direction. Such incisions are not usually made for this purpose but can be used if they are present.

The objectives of examining this part of the respiratory tract are to evaluate visible lesions and the functional competence of structures such as the soft palate and larynx. Horses often swallow during examination, and the examiner should be familiar with the endoscopic appearance of the pharyngeal region during this maneuver. When the tip of the endoscope is in the rostral portion of the nasopharynx during swallowing the following changes will be seen:

- Rostrodorsal movement of the soft palate and constriction of the nasopharynx with immediate loss of view of the larynx, caudal nasopharynx, and dorsal laryngopharynx. These movements are followed immediately by medial displacement of the cartilaginous flaps of the entrances to the auditory tubes, which meet in the midline.
- Reappearance of the obscured structures in their normal positions and full abduction of both arytenoid cartilages. The position of the soft palate relative to the epiglottis and corniculate processes of the arytenoid cartilages are of particular importance in the diagnosis of soft-palate displacement and malfunction of the swallowing mechanisms. The ability of the larynx to abduct fully after swallowing is important when evaluating laryngeal function.

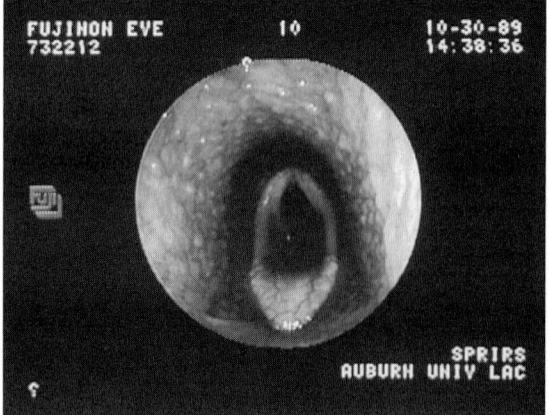

▶ **FIGURE 3-11**

Endoscopy of the dorsal laryngopharynx, viewed from the rostral nasopharynx. The larynx is visible in the background.

Conditions that affect the pharynx include pharyngeal lymphoid hyperplasia, dorsal displacement of the soft palate, bacterial, fungal, and viral infections, paresis or paralysis, and developmental conditions such as cysts and cleft palate. Some of these are shown in Figure 3-13.

Auditory Tube Diverticulae

To examine auditory tube diverticulae (ATD), also called guttural pouches, the endoscope must first be inserted through the nasopharyngeal openings of the auditory tubes that are located on the dorsolateral walls of the pharynx, rostral and ventral to the dorsal pharyngeal recess.[12] Each opening is slitlike and covered medially by a triangular flap of cartilage. These flaps are normally closely apposed to the lateral pharyngeal walls (except during swallowing), and a blunt straight instrument cannot usually be inserted beneath them. There are various ways to gain entry to the ATD, but each requires practice.

FLEXIBLE ENDOSCOPE. Inserting a flexible endoscope into the ATD is most easily done with the assistance of a flexible biopsy forceps passed through the biopsy channel. The endoscope, with biopsy forceps in place but not protruding from the distal end, is inserted into the ipsilateral nasal passage and advanced into the nasopharynx to a level just rostral to the opening of the auditory tube. The forceps are then extended from the endoscope for about 2 cm and directed under the

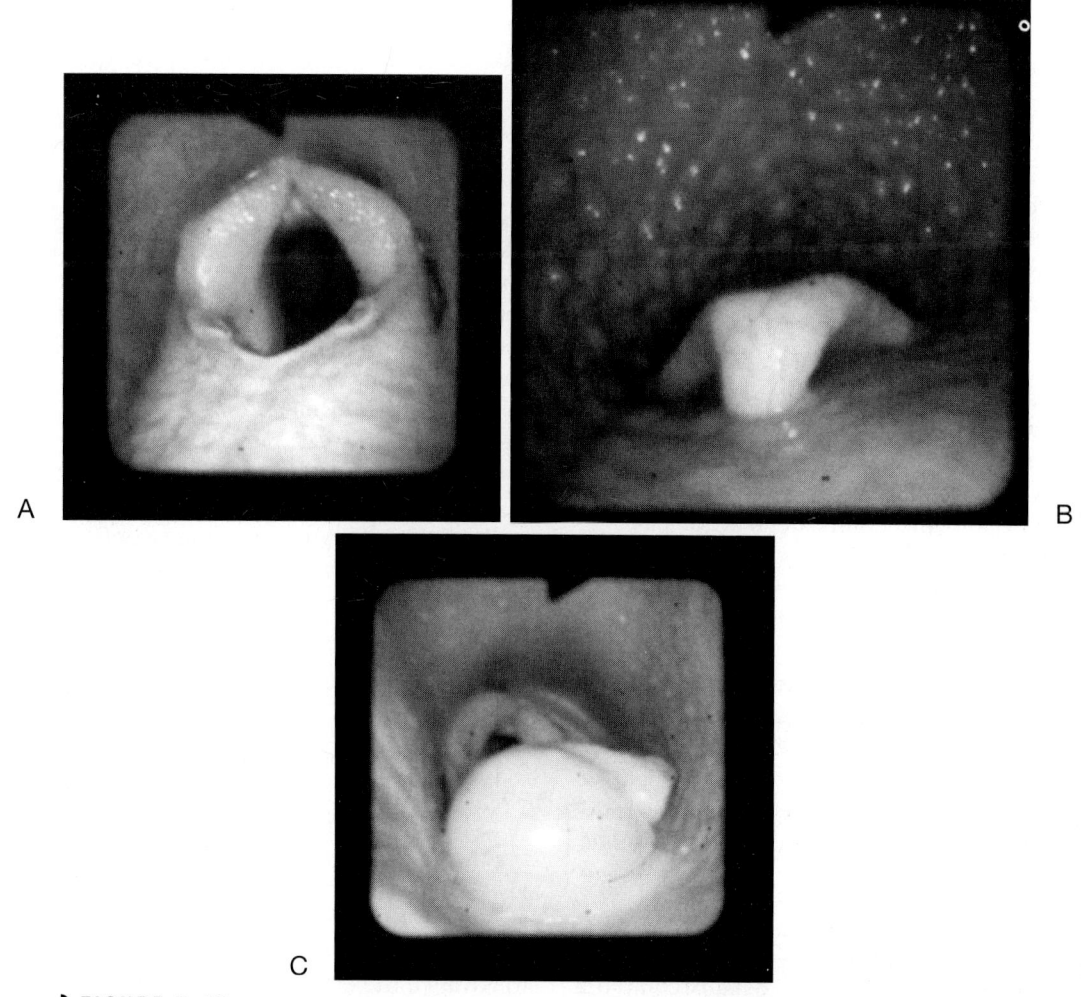

A

B

C

▶ **FIGURE 3-13**

Endoscopic photographs of some pharyngeal abnormalities. **A.** Dorsal displacement of the soft palate. Note that the epiglottis cannot be seen and also the ulcers present on the rostral border of the ostium. **B.** Pharyngeal lymphoid hyperplasia. Note the extensive proliferation of nodules on the dorsum and walls of the pharynx. Normally the larynx would be visible, but in this case the inflammatory response and associated swelling is so marked that only the epiglottis can be seen. **C.** Subepiglottic cyst. A cyst is located beneath the epiglottis, the apex of which can be seen lying on the left dorsolateral surface of the cyst. A coexisting left laryngeal hemiplegia can also be seen.

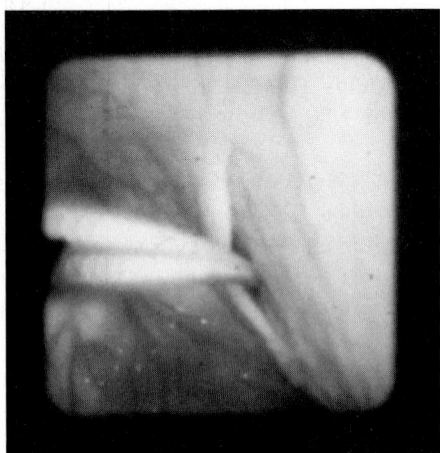

▶ **FIGURE 3–14**

Insertion of a flexible endoscope into the auditory tube. The flexible biopsy forceps has been passed beneath the cartilaginous flap covering the opening of the auditory tube, thus elevating it and allowing the insertion of the endoscope.

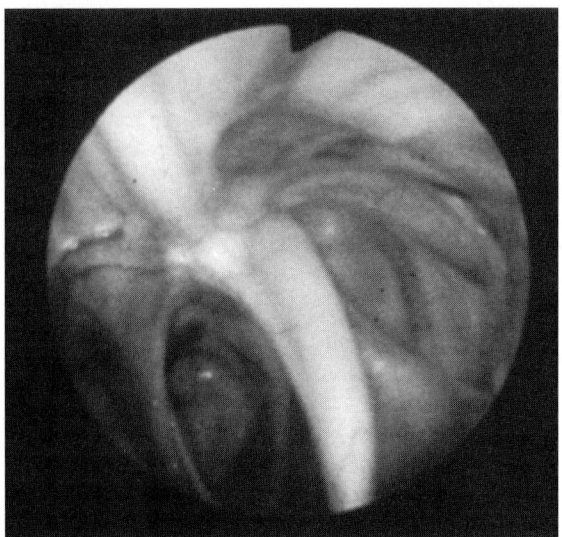

▶ **FIGURE 3–15**

Endoscopic photograph of the interior of the normal auditory tube diverticulum.

cartilage flap as the endoscope is slowly advanced (Fig. 3–14). After successful entry, the endoscope is guided beneath the flap and into the ATD. This maneuver requires some manipulation and finesse, which is acquired only with practice. The cartilage flap is elevated most easily if, during insertion, the endoscope is rotated so that the biopsy probe, which is located in the eccentrically positioned instrument channel, is positioned medially (i.e., closer to the flap than to the wall of the pharynx). Although the left and right diverticulae can be examined without reinserting the endoscope into the contralateral nasal passage, this is not always possible, and it is usually a little more difficult. For this reason, it is recommended that each ATD be examined with the endoscope in the ipsilateral nasal passage.

The cartilage flap can also be elevated with a stiff, bent-tipped catheter passed up the same nasal passage as the endoscope. Insertion of the catheter is done under direct vision through the endoscope. Once the flap is elevated, the endoscope can be advanced into the ATD, also under direct vision.

RIGID ENDOSCOPE. Prior to the advent of the flexible endoscope, examination of the ATD was done with a rigid endoscope, which required a totally different insertion technique. With a rigid endoscope it is more important to have excellent restraint because any sudden movement by the horse can result in damage to the instrument or the most profuse epistaxis. For restraint, a nose

twitch is necessary, and, occasionally, chemical restraint is required as well. To facilitate insertion beneath the cartilage flap, the endoscope should possess an angled tip. The instrument, with its tip angled downward, is passed carefully up the ventral meatus while maintaining firm and gentle contact with the floor of the nasal passage. When it reaches the level of the caudal hard palate perceived as a small bump on the floor of the caudal nasal passage, it is rotated 90° to direct the tip laterally. With the tip held against the lateral wall of the pharynx, the endoscope is slowly advanced, allowing the tip to slide beneath the cartilaginous flap and then into the ATD. With experience the clinician can detect when the instrument contacts the flap. If the instrument fails to enter the ATD, it passes caudally and contacts the caudal pharynx, which provides a spongelike sensation. The technique is not easy and also requires practice. If one is lucky enough to have two endoscopes, then the second, passed up the opposite nasal passage, can be used to visualize the insertion of the first. These methods also apply to the anesthetized horse.

With any of these techniques, it is important to advance the endoscope very carefully to avoid damage to any of the structures within the ATD, especially whenever there is a possibility of mycosis.

The endoscopic appearance of the ATD is demonstrated in Figure 3–15. Some conditions frequently diagnosed are empyema, sometimes with accumulation of inspissated exudate known as chondroids; mycosis, with or without bleeding from an associated vessel; and tympany. Some abnormalities are shown in Figure 3–16. If the ATD is full of blood or exudate, the endoscope will be submerged and it will be impossible to view anything.

Larynx

The larynx is examined by advancing the endoscope further into the nasopharynx. The examiner must understand the normal anatomy of the larynx and its constituent cartilages and be able to detect static as well as functional abnormalities.[13] Evaluation of the ability of the aryte-

noid cartilages to abduct is particularly important because of the high incidence of laryngeal hemiplegia and the condition known as laryngeal paresis, or the asynchronous larynx. Horses undergoing endoscopy are usually at rest and therefore are breathing very quietly, which often makes it impossible to assess abductor and adductor function. Some simple and reliable techniques for inducing increased laryngeal activity in the stationary horse follow.

INDUCTION OF SWALLOWING. In normal animals swallowing is followed immediately by full, bilateral abduction. If there is an abductor defect present, it can usually be detected at this time. Swallowing is most easily induced by introducing

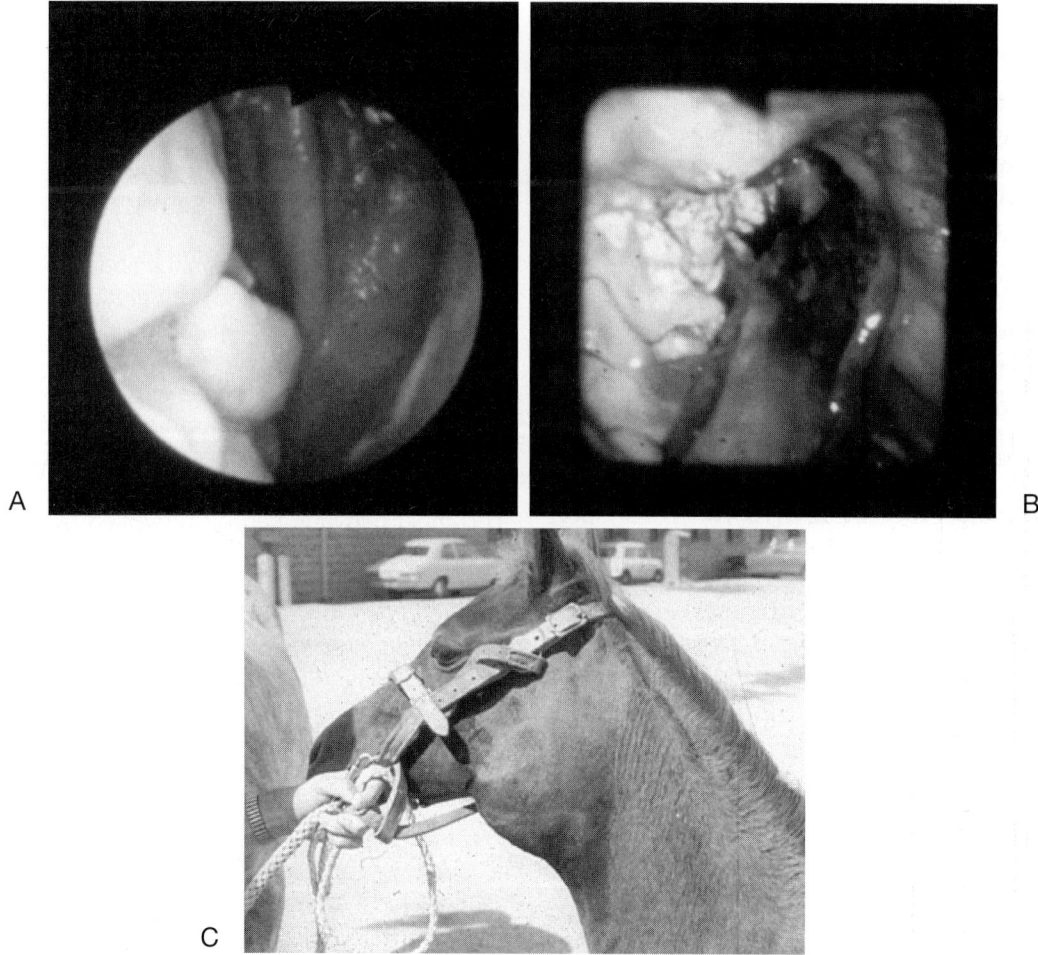

A

B

C

▶ **FIGURE 3–16**

Endoscopic photographs of some examples of abnormalities of the auditory tube diverticulum. **A.** Chondroids. Note the presence of the rounded chondroids, composed of inspissated exudate. **B.** Mycosis. Note the hemorrhagic mucosa and the fungal hyphae. **C.** Tympany. The auditory tube diverticulum is distended with air and manifests as a tympanitic swelling in the parotid region.

a few milliliters of water through the flushing channel of the endoscope. Another method is to briefly touch the epiglottis with the tip of the endoscope or a biopsy forceps protruding from the endoscope.

NASAL OCCLUSION. Occlusion of both nostrils during examination induces both adduction and partial abduction. However, the procedure may be resented by the patient, thus causing a violent response.

SLAP TEST. A slap test in a horse with normal spinal reflexes and not suffering from laryngeal hemiplegia, will stimulate arytenoid adduction. The test consists of sharply slapping the horse just behind the withers with the open hand. A normal response consists of a momentary adduction of the contralateral arytenoid. Unfortunately, the test is limited because the response is poor or absent in nervous or tense horses.

REBREATHING. Breathing and laryngeal movement increase if a plastic bag is placed over the nose and mouth (see Methods of Stimulating Breathing). An endoscope inserted through a hole in the bag will allow observation of the increased laryngeal activity as the horse responds to being forced to breath increasingly higher concentrations of carbon dioxide.

CHEMICAL STIMULATION. Chemical stimulation of respiration is a useful method of stimulating laryngeal movement (see Methods of Stimulating Breathing).

POSTEXERCISE EXAMINATION. For a short time after exercise horses continue to breathe deeply and rapidly. However, this activity subsides within a few minutes. If exercise is continued until the horse is breathing at a rate of about 100 bpm, there will be sufficient time afterward to conduct an endoscopy provided the examination is carried out immediately.

VIDEOENDOSCOPY DURING EXERCISE. In appropriately equipped facilities it is now possible to evaluate upper respiratory function in horses while they are moving on a high-speed tread mill. This is particularly valuable to detect dynamic collapse of the arytenoid and to evaluate subtle abnormalities. This is described under Endoscopic Evaluation of the Upper Respiratory Tract during Exercise.

As most horses are at rest, at least for the first examination, a system of grading laryngeal function in resting horses that can be extrapolated to the horse during exercise is necessary. One such system is described in the box.[14] Evaluation of symmetry and arytenoid abduction in the resting larynx is subjective and can vary with sedation, application of a twitch, viewing through the opposite nostril, and between examinations. Therefore, in the interest of consistency, the examination should be carried out without sedation and with the endoscope always inserted into the same nasal passage. On occasions it becomes necessary to compare the image of the larynx from both the left and the right nasal passages. As stated, a twitch often is necessary, and it should be remembered that both twitch and sedation tend to reduce laryngeal movement and the extent of asynchronous movement.

Figure 3–17 demonstrates the normal larynx as well as some abnormalities.

GRADING SYSTEM FOR LARYNGEAL FUNCTION

- *Grade 1.* Synchronous full abduction and adduction of left and right arytenoid cartilages. Full abduction occurs during exercise.
- *Grade 2.* Asynchronous movement (hesitation, flutter, abductor weakness) of the left arytenoid cartilage during any phase of breathing. Full abduction of the left arytenoid cartilage can be provoked by nasal occlusion or swallowing. Full abduction occurs during exercise.
- *Grade 3.* Asynchronous movement (hesitation, flutter, abductor weakness) of the left arytenoid cartilage during any phase of breathing. Full abduction cannot be provoked. Full abduction occurs during exercise in most of these horses, but some undergo dynamic collapse of the arytenoid cartilage. Exceptions cannot be predicted on the basis of resting interpretation.
- *Grade 4.* Marked asymmetry of the larynx at rest without significant movement during any phase of breathing. All horses undergo dynamic collapse of the arytenoid.[14]

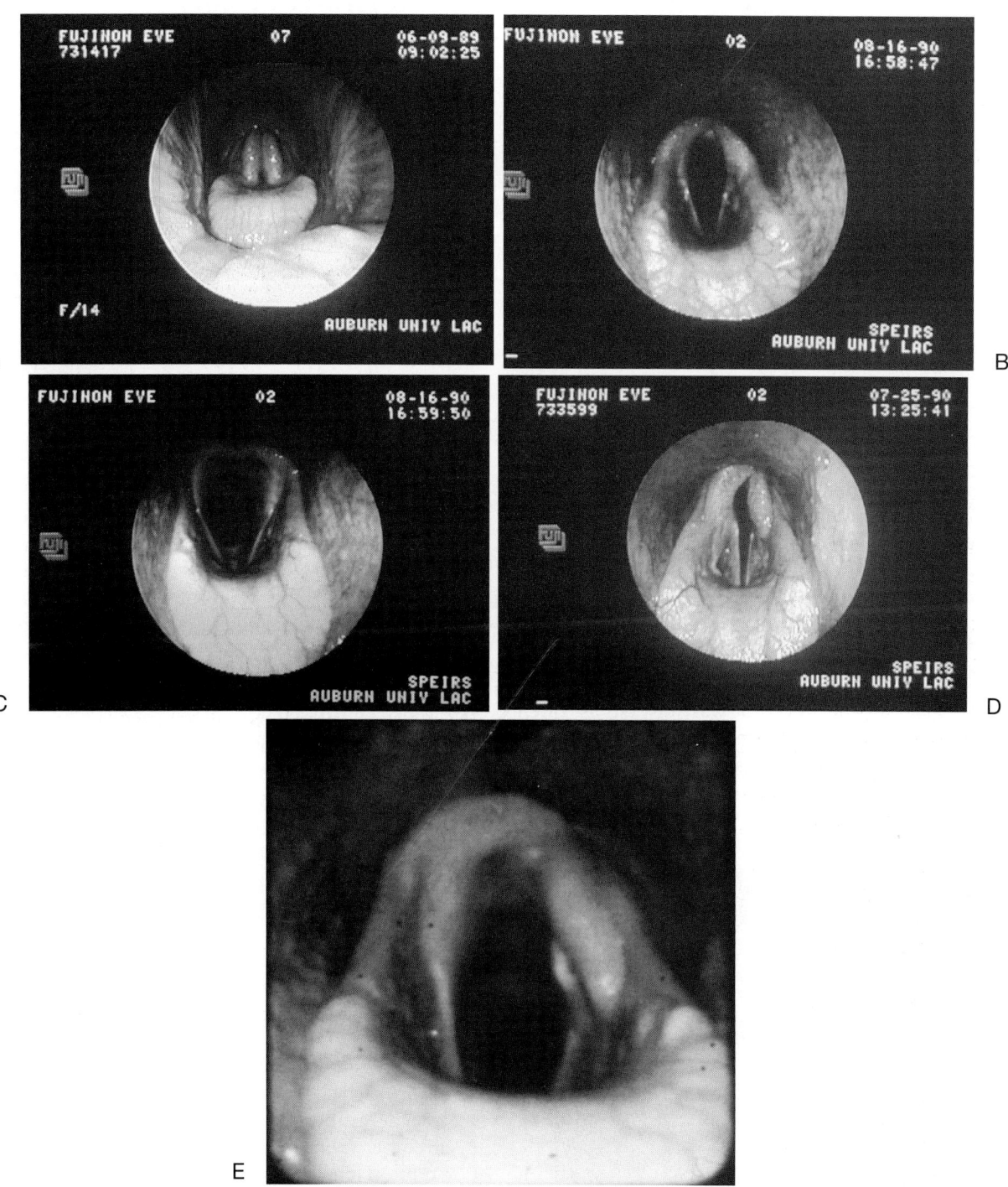

▶ **FIGURE 3-17**

Endoscopic photographs of the larynx. **A.** Adduction. The left and right corniculate processes are fully adducted and are opposed to one another in the midline. **B.** Asynchrony. Note that the left corniculate process is not abducted as far as the right side. **C.** Full abduction. This is the same horse as depicted in part B following stimulation of swallowing. **D.** Laryngeal hemiplegia. The left corniculate process and vocal cord are positioned almost in the midline and demonstrate the absence of abduction. **E.** Chondritis. Note the distortion of the left corniculate process and the swelling on the medial surface of the arytenoid cartilage.

Trachea and Bronchi

The trachea and major bronchi can be examined with the horse restrained in stocks.[15] A nose twitch is useful for restraint, and occasionally chemical restraint also is necessary. The use of a drug such as xylazine hydrochloride is also useful because it reduces coughing. Most horses allow the flexible endoscope to be passed into the proximal trachea without evidence of discomfort. Examination of the bronchi requires an endoscope with a minimum length of 150 cm. In foals and small horses a shorter endoscope may be adequate. As the endoscope is advanced into the distal trachea and the region of its bifurcation into the right and left principal bronchi, a cough reflex is usually induced. Coughing is minimized by spraying a few milliliters of local anesthetic through the biopsy channel of the endoscope as it is advanced down the airway. Examination should be systematic and each major bronchus should be examined. Endoscopes with a diameter of about 12 mm pass easily into the major bronchi and also many of the smaller segmental ones. The normal airway is shown in Figure 3-18.

Collection and Evaluation of Lower Airway Secretions

Diagnosis of lower airway disease is often enhanced by cytological and microbiological evaluation of respiratory secretions. To do this, a sample of the secretion is collected from the trachea and lower airways.

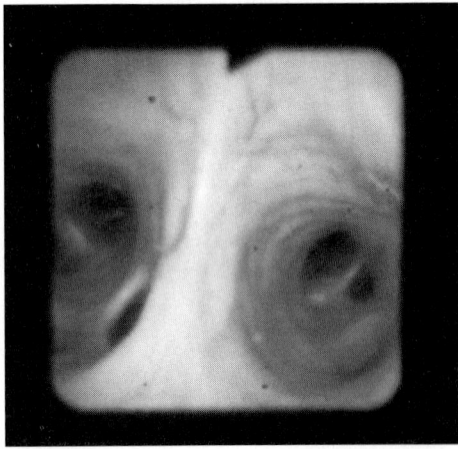

▶ FIGURE 3-18

Endoscopic photograph of the normal tracheal bifurcation. Note the left and right principal bronchi, separated by the carina. The smaller accessory lobe bronchus can also be seen lying ventromedially just inside the right principal bronchus.

```
METHODS OF COLLECTING
LOWER AIRWAY FLUIDS
.............................................................
• Percutaneous transtracheal washing and
  aspiration (PTW)
• Percutaneous transtracheal aspiration
  (PTA)
• Endoscopic transtracheal washing and as-
  piration (ETW)
• Endoscopic transtracheal aspiration (ETA)
• Bronchoalveolar lavage (BAL)
```

Tracheal Fluids

Secretions within the trachea can be collected under direct vision by using an endoscope passed via the nasal passage into the trachea or blindly by inserting a catheter percutaneously. In either case it is possible to collect a sample by simple aspiration or by aspiration after injecting a lavage ("wash") solution. Regardless of which method is preferred by the examiner, it is necessary to obtain a sample of sufficient volume for analysis.

PERCUTANEOUS TRANSTRACHEAL WASHING AND ASPIRATION. Percutaneous transtracheal washing and aspiration (PTW) refers to the collection of fluid from within the tracheobronchial tree using a percutaneous technique to inject lavage fluid and to then collect it by aspiration. Percutaneous transtracheal aspiration (PTA) refers to the same method performed without injecting lavage fluid. The principle is demonstrated in Figure 3-19.

Procedure. An area approximately 5 × 5 cm centered over the middle third of the trachea is clipped and surgically prepared.[16] With appropriate restraint 5 ml of local anesthetic solution is injected subcutaneously and between a pair of adjacent tracheal rings. A small stab incision is then made in the skin and the needle or trochar inserted between the tracheal rings and directed down the trachea. Care should be taken to avoid traumatizing the opposite wall of the trachea, and the bevel of the needle should face down the airway to minimize the chances of the catheter being cut accidentally.

When using the homemade system, the catheter is inserted through the needle or trochar, and when using the commercial system the catheter is simply advanced through the needle. In all cases the catheter is advanced until it reaches just beyond the thoracic inlet. It is important to avoid withdrawing the catheter with the needle in situ, because the cutting edge of the needle can quickly sever the catheter, leaving a piece within the trachea. To perform PTW, the sterile saline is injected quickly and immediately aspirated. When using the Intracath system, the stylet must be removed before injecting the fluid. Sometimes the procedure will require several repetitions before a satisfactory volume of aspirate is obtained. For PTA, secretions are simply aspirated without first injecting a wash fluid, although this is successful only when a copious volume of secretion is present. It is usual to retrieve less than the infused volume of fluid. Frequent repetition is often associated with coughing, which can displace the tubing proximally into the pharynx, although this is not so likely if thick tubing is used. Finally, the catheter is removed, and although

the stab incision can be sutured and a neck bandage applied, neither of these procedures is necessary.

The sample should be submitted for cytological and bacteriological evaluation, as described in Appendix C.

Complications. The procedure is relatively innocuous, but has the potential for complications:

- Leakage of air from the trachea is common, and may be seen, rarely, as obvious subcutaneous emphysema or, more commonly, on radiographs as mediastinal emphysema. It is usually of no clinical significance. Its incidence can be reduced by applying pressure to the puncture site for a few minutes after the procedure.
- Chondritis may occur after damage to the cartilage, however it is rare and easily avoided by careful technique.

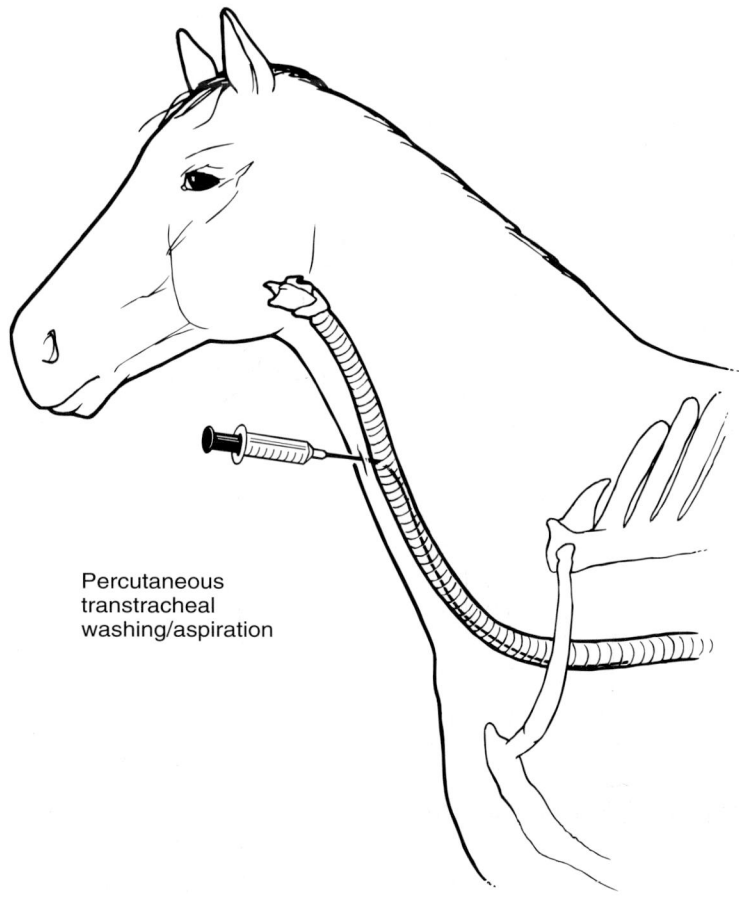

Percutaneous
transtracheal
washing/aspiration

▶ **FIGURE 3–19**

Percutaneous collection of lower airway secretions. Note that a catheter has been inserted percutaneously into the trachea.

Materials for Percutaneous Transtracheal Washing and Aspiration

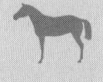

▶ Local anesthetic solution (2% lidocaine hydrochloride, 2% mepivacaine hydrochloride)

▶ Scalpel blade (#22)

▶ Collection devices

    Commercially available prepackaged and sterilized system consisting of a 16-gauge through-the-needle catheter 58 cm long

    "Homemade system" using a 16- or 14-gauge cannula with polyethylene tubing (PE 240) and attached needle

    Trochar (5–6 cm, 8–10 G) and PE 240 tubing or similarly-sized canine urinary catheter

▶ Syringe (50 ml) with sterile saline

▶ Sterile gauze sponges and gloves

▶ Collecting tubes

• Subcutaneous infection is not uncommon, and although it is usually of no significance it can develop into a local abscess or extend down the neck and create a septic mediastinitis, which is potentially very serious.

• Loss of a section of catheter. If the catheter is inadvertently severed and a piece left in the airway, it has been shown that it is expelled by coughing within a few minutes.[17] However reassuring this might be, it is preferable to avoid the complication by ensuring that the catheter is never withdrawn from the needle while the latter is within the airway.

Cytologic Results. Tracheobronchial fluids from normal horses contain mainly ciliated columnar epithelial cells, macrophages, small lymphocytes, and neutrophils.[18] Some data from cytological evaluation of tracheal fluids gained by PTW from clinically normal horses are presented in Table 3–2.[2,19,20]

The data are presented in percentage form because the use of the lavage method introduces an unknown dilution factor. In general little mucus is present and the predominant cells are the pulmonary alveolar macrophage and the epithelial cell. Some variation can be seen, which is probably related to collection and interpretation techniques, and to the difficulty in selecting healthy horses with which to establish reference values. The difficulty in selecting healthy horses to establish reference values has been demonstrated.[20]

The predominant cell type varies with the type of disease present. The following broad categories are recognized:

• Increased proportion of neutrophils associated with inflammation (chronic respiratory disease, pneumonia, pleuropneumonia)
• Increased number of hemosiderophages associated with exercise-induced pulmonary hemorrhage
• Increased eosinophils associated with allergic disease

An earlier study using PTA also noted the dominance of epithelial cells in normal secretions and the trend for increasing numbers of neutrophils and lymphocytes in horses with chronic respiratory disease and eosinophils in allergic disease.[21]

However the cytological findings do not always agree with results from histological examination of the lungs.

Bacteriological Results. The upper airways are not sterile, and their flora may vary with the environment, with increased numbers of bacteria and fungi likely to be isolated from hospital and barn environments, respectively. An example of results of culture from healthy horses follows.[22]

• From housed racehorses ($N = 50$)
    Aerobic bacteria of recognized pathogenicity (8%)
    Transient bacteria (24%)
    Negative (74%)
• From pastured racehorses ($N = 36$)
    Aerobic bacteria of recognized pathogenicity (8%)
    Transient bacteria (64%)
    Negative (28%)

In 12 cases when anaerobic cultures were performed no positive culture resulted. Fungal culture was not done but fungal growth was observed on 16% of the blood agar plates in both groups. Likewise, *Nocardia* spp was observed in 4% of housed and 19% of pastured horses.

▶ **TABLE 3-2**

SOME REFERENCE VALUES FOR CELLULAR CONTENT OF TRACHEOBRONCHIAL FLUID OBTAINED BY PERCUTANEOUS TRANSTRACHEAL ASPIRATION WITH LAVAGE:
TOTAL ($\times 10^5$/CELLS/ML) AND DIFFERENTIAL (% ± 1 SD) CELL COUNTS

Number of Horses	Total Cells	Squamous Cells	Epithelial Cells	Macrophages	Lymphocytes	Neutrophils	Eosinophils	Mast Cells	Plasma Cells	Alveolar Cells	References
15	4.9 ±2.7	0	19.8 ±6.1	65.0 ±13.7	7.4 ±3.8	6.4 ±5.5	1.2 ±1.4	0.2 ±0.4	—	—	2
92	—	2.3 ±2.6	13.0	34.0 ±18.0	4.9 ±3.1	39.0 ±21.0	3.5 ±2.0	1.6 ±1.9	2.2 ±3.4	10.7	19
66	—	—	30.4 ±24.4	44.1 ±23.2	5.4 ±4.1	17.8 ±21.8	0.7 ±2.2	—	—	—	20

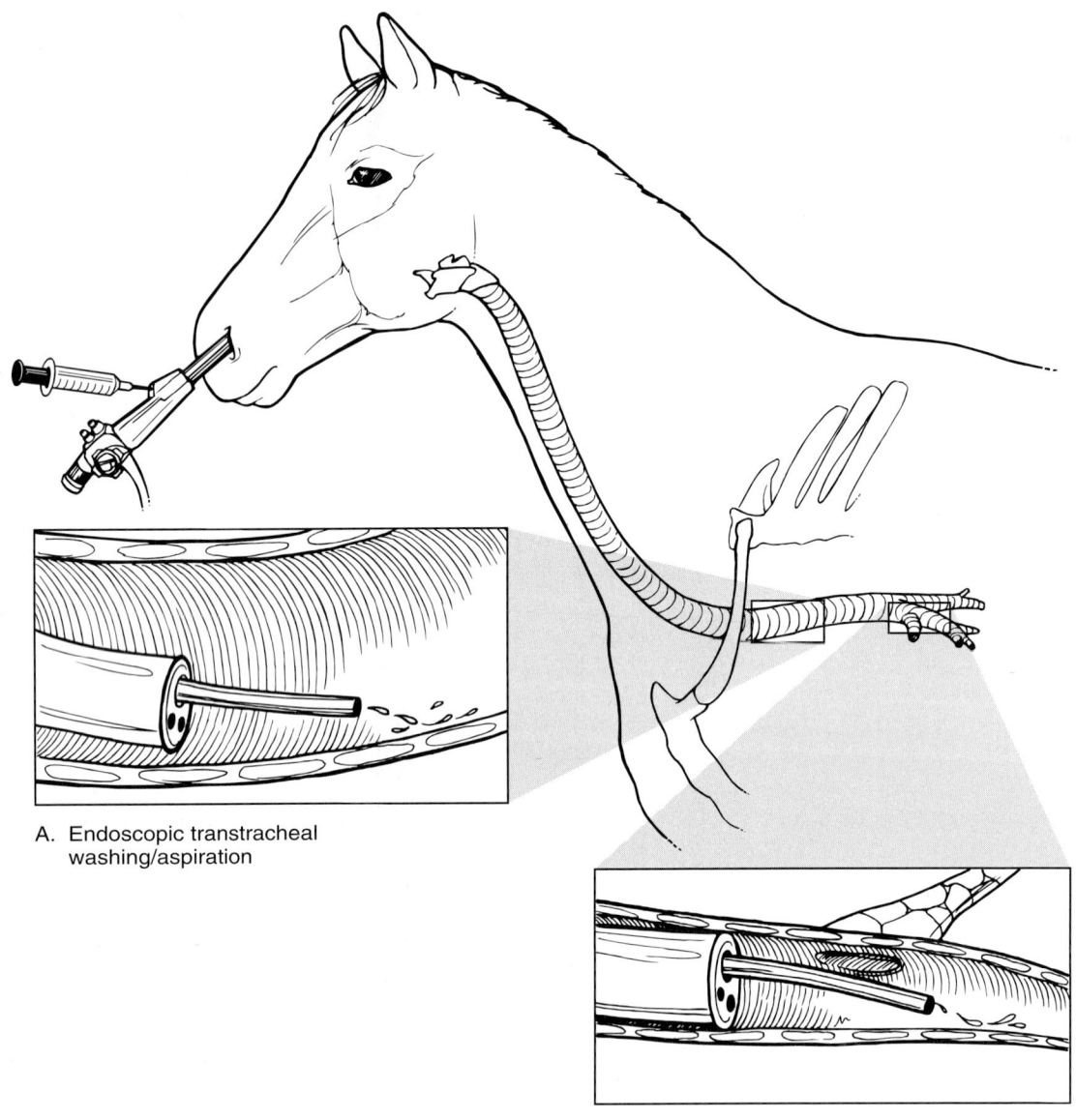

A. Endoscopic transtracheal
   washing/aspiration

B. Bronchoalveolar lavage

▶ **FIGURE 3-20**

Endoscopic transtracheal collection of lower airway secretions. Note that the catheter is inside an endoscope that has been passed through the nasal passage and then into the trachea. **A.** Endoscopic transtracheal aspiration or washing. Note that the tip of the endoscope has not been fully inserted. **B.** Bronchoalveolar lavage. Note that the endoscope has been inserted until it is wedged in a distal airway.

The significance of microorganism isolation is therefore sometimes difficult to judge. However, bacteria causing disease are likely to be present in large numbers, to have recognized pathogenicity, and be found intracellularly in association with cellular evidence of inflammation.

ENDOSCOPIC TRANSTRACHEAL WASHING AND ASPIRATION. With these methods, access to the airway secretions is achieved with a flexible endoscope passed into the trachea through a nasal passage (Fig. 3-20A). The secretions are collected under direct endoscopic vision with lavage, or "wash," fluid (endoscopic transtracheal wash (ETW) or without fluid (ETA).

Technique. After the horse has been appropriately restrained, the endoscope, which contains a catheter in the biopsy channel, is passed transnasally and then down the trachea to a position just proximal to the thoracic inlet. For

ETW, 30 ml of the sterile buffered saline are injected through the catheter. The saline tends to pool in the region of the thoracic inlet. The endoscope is then advanced, under direct vision, until its tip is close to the fluid that is then aspirated using the catheter and syringe. For ETA the airway secretions are aspirated under direct vision without dilution by saline lavage fluid. The procedure can be extended by passing the catheter into a bronchus. As much of the fluid as possible is collected to evaluate total and differential cell count and for bacteriological assessment.

Cytologic Results. Some reference values for tracheal secretions are presented in Table 3-3.[2,23,24] Not surprisingly, the cytological responses to disease in secretions obtained endoscopically are similar to those just described for the percutaneous technique. Again, there is an increase in the proportion of neutrophils in association with pneumonia and chronic respiratory disease, an increase in eosinophils in association with lung worm, and an increase in degenerate neutrophils when infection is present.

Bacteriological Results. The main advantages of this method are that secretions, even when scant, can be collected under direct vision. It also is easy to perform, is quickly carried out, and avoids trauma to the trachea. The main disadvantage is that without special precautions contamination of the sample with upper airway microorganisms usually occurs.

The significance of the presence of microorganisms is not always easy to establish, and in one study of normal horses 30% of samples yielded organisms regarded as potential pathogens.[25] In another there was good agreement between PTA and a simple guarded swab (single-catheter brush)

Materials for Endoscopic Transtracheal Washing and Aspiration

▸ Flexible fiber-optic endoscope that has been cleaned or sterilized (see Appendix A).

▸ Polyethylene or Teflon catheter with adaptor

▸ Phosphate buffered saline

▸ Sample collecting tubes

---

technique in their ability to isolate aerobic and anaerobic bacteria as well as transient bacteria and fungi from both horses that did and did not have pneumonia.[26]

To circumvent the problem of contamination with organisms from the upper airway, a number of methods have been described with the objective of isolating the swab from the upper airway. In man, comparing the single-catheter brush method with other catheter brush techniques, such as the distal occluded and unoccluded and double sheathed methods, revealed that 92% were contaminated.[27] A more reliable method of protection is the double-sheathed protected catheter,[28] which produces results that correlate with isolates from lung,[29] blood,[30] percutaneous aspirates,[31] and bronchoalveolar lavage. Although the relevance of these methods in horses remains to be decided, it has been shown that using a double-sheathed, protected aspiration catheter more closely approximated the results obtained percutaneously than by a protected catheter brush.[32]

To differentiate between bacterial colonization and infection, quantitative analysis of gram stains and culture as well as assessment of the cytological responses are probably necessary. Microorganisms commonly regarded as pathogenic include:[17] Hemolytic *Streptococcus* spp, *Pseudomonas aeruginosa*, *Pasteurella* spp, *Escherichia coli*, *Bacillus bronchisepticus*, *Streptococcus equi*, *Klebsiella pneumoniae*, *Staphylococcus aureus*.

BRONCHOALVEOLAR LAVAGE. Bronchoalveolar lavage (BAL) involves lavaging the lower airways by means of an endoscope or catheter that has been passed down the trachea and wedged in a bronchus (Fig. 3-20B). Depending on where the tip of the endoscope is lodged, how vigorously the lavage is carried out, the volume of the lavage, and whether or not a catheter is advanced into the smaller airways, the method may yield bronchial or bronchoalveolar samples.

Procedure. After the horse has been appropriately restrained, the endoscope is passed down the trachea until it lodges in a bronchus.[33] The topical anesthetic is infused if the horse coughs. The PBS is then infused in two to three 100-ml aliquots, and aspiration is carried out after each infusion. If no endoscope is used, the catheter is passed into the nares and then down the trachea as far as it will go. To facilitate the passage of the

▶ TABLE 3-3

Some Reference Values for Cellular Content of Tracheobronchial Fluid Obtained by Endoscopic Transtracheal Aspiration with Lavage: Total (×10⁵/cells/L) and Differential (% ± 1 SD) Cell Counts

Number of Horses	Total Cells	Squamous Cells	Epithelial Cells	Macrophages	Lymphocytes	Neutrophils	Eosinophils	Mast Cells	Plasma Cells	Alveolar Cells	References
4	5.8 ±5.6	0.3 ±0.6	49.1 ±11.5	43.0 ±10.7	2.2 ±2.8	4.6 ±4.9	0.7 ±0.4	0.1 ±0.2	—	—	2
10	—	—	34.0 ±6.6	24.0 ±4.0	8.2 ±1.9	32.0 ±8.9	<1.0	—	2.2 ±3.4	10.7	23
20	—	—	26.0 ±25.0	53.0 ±20.0	8.0 ±6.0	9.0 ±12.0	2.0 ±4.0	3.0 (Monocytes)	—	—	24

Materials for Bronchoalveolar Lavage

- ▶ Collection device (choice of the following)

  Flexible endoscope (2 m)

  Equine BAL catheter (Bivona Inc., Gary, IN)

  "Homemade" system using plastic tubing

- ▶ Topical anesthetic (2% lidocaine hydrochloride, 2% mepivacaine hydrochloride)

- ▶ Sterile phosphate buffered saline (PBS) 500 ml

- ▶ Suction device (syringe or pump)

- ▶ Chemical and physical methods of restraint

catheter into the trachea, the horse's head should be extended. With the BAL catheter a small cuff is inflated to create a seal. This is an easier but less selective technique as the location of the catheter tip is not known.

Sample Preparation. Straining the sample through gauze swabs has been recommended, but this is unnecessary and may compromise the sample. Samples for cytological evaluation can be placed in EDTA or an equal volume of 50% ethyl alcohol, prepared by cytocentrifugation and then smears made from the sediment.

Results, Cytology. Comparison of data is made difficult by the variations in collection technique. Some reference values for cytology are shown in Table 3-4.[2,34-36] Macrophages and lymphocytes are the dominant cell types (about 60% and 30%, respectively). In young foals the situation is different,[33] as approximately 80% to 90% of cells recovered at first are alveolar macrophages. Over the first 2 months of life the proportion of macrophages decreases and lymphocyctes increase from approximately 5% to 10% to 30%.

The introduction of racehorses into training and racing increases the proportions of erythrocytes, neutrophils, and hemosiderophages.[34] The presence of coughing is associated with an increased proportion of lymphocytes.[34,35]

The significance of the cytological results relative to pulmonary disease has been assessed by comparing pulmonary histological findings with cytological evaluations of secretions obtained directly from the airways and by BAL in normal horses and in those with pulmonary disease:[37] In normal horses BAL values are an accurate indicator of normal pulmonary histology. Increased neutrophils are observed in horses with diffuse lung disease, such as interstitial pneumonia and chronic respiratory disease. Eosinophils may be present with pulmonary eosinophilic infiltration, *Dictyocoulus arnfieldi,* or pulmonary larval migrans. Despite these findings, the type and severity of disease are not always apparent.

A potential problem with BAL is that because only a section of lung is sampled the results may not be representative of the remainder, especially with disease processes that are localized in another section of the lung.[23] This is the probable explanation for the report that PTW or PTA are more reliable than BAL for detecting the presence of pneumonia or pleuropneumonia, where localized abscessation is common.[38]

The volume of the lavage fluid, and the region of lung lavaged probably influence the cytological evaluation. To avoid this methodological error, it is recommended that a volume of 300 ml be used, either as a single procedure or as three separate procedures in which three 100-ml volumes are successively infused and aspirated.[39]

Thoracic Radiology

Although the size of adult members of the larger breeds does impose technical limitations, radiology provides a useful, noninvasive means of evaluating the thorax and its contents. Most thoracic radiography is carried out in institutions with high-powered equipment, but the air-gap technique, rare earth screens, and high-speed film allow diagnostic radiology to be carried out with intermediate-output (100–800 mA) and, for foals, even low-output generators (<30 mA). When high-powered equipment is available and output is not a limiting factor, grids can be exchanged for the air-gap technique.

With foals the complete thorax can usually be examined with one lateral exposure. A ventrodorsal exposure is often also possible. This is not the case with larger horses where more exposures are necessary and where ventrodorsal views are not possible in the conscious animal and seldom done

▶ **TABLE 3-4**
Some Reference Values for Cellular Content of Bronchoalveolar Fluid: Total and Differential (mean % ± 1 SD) Cell Counts

Number of Horses	Squamous Cells	Hemosiderophages	Epithelial Cells	Macrophages	Lymphocytes	Neutrophils	Eosinophils	Mast Cells	Erythrocytes	References
15	—	2.0 ±7.0	—	72.0 ±10.0	18.0 ±3.0	5.0 ±4.0	2.0 ±4.0	1.0 ±1.0	—	36
10	0	—	14.3 ±13.4	70.3 ±15.2	7.6 ±3.9	6.2 ±5.0	1.0 ±1.4	0.6 ±1.4	—	2
42	0.1 ±0.4	—	32.5 ±10.9	55.5 ±12.9	3.4 ±2.6	8.4 ±5.9	0	0.1 ±0.3	—	2
62	831.5* ±577.6	19.7† ±23.8	0.4 ±0.8	59.0 ±9.7	31.3 ±9.3	8.8 ±6.4	0.5 ±3.1	—	10.3‡ ±17.7	34
8	—	—	0.8 ±1.3	65.1 ±12.1	28.9 ±11.5	3.6 ±2.2	0.1 ±0.2	1.4 ±1.6	—	35

*Total (×10⁶/L) nucleated cells.
†Percentage of macrophages.
‡Percentage of all cell types.

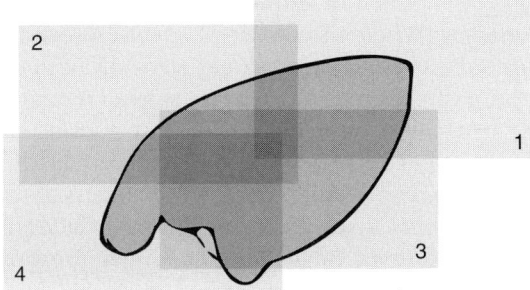

▶ **FIGURE 3-21**

Thoracic radiography. Method of overlapping exposures to ensure a complete thoracic examination.

under anesthesia. With bigger horses multiple exposures are usually necessary, the film being positioned so as to have four overlapping radiographs: caudodorsal, craniodorsal, caudoventral, and cranioventral (Fig. 3-21), termed fields 1, 2, 3, and 4.[40] To improve visualization, the exposure should be made during inspiration and with the radiographic film placed against the hemithorax closest to the lesion or region of interest. Magnification and parallax interfere with interpretation of fields 1 and 3. This can to a certain extent be remedied by taking exposures from the left and right sides, as structures closer to the film will be sharper whereas those closer to the tube will be magnified and not as clear. This approach often is useful in localizing a lesion. Occasionally exposure is made during expiration to evaluate the change in airway diameter or lung dimension related to breathing. The techniques have been well described elsewhere.[40-44]

Structures that can be expected to be seen in the different fields of view are as follows, bearing in mind that the extent of overlap between plates means that certain structures will be present in more than one radiograph:

- *Field 1.* A large portion of the caudal lung lobes, middle and distal airways, pulmonary arteries and veins, descending aorta (depending on positioning and exposure), caudal vena cava, diaphragm (including left and right crura), caudal thoracic vertebrae, and ribs.
- *Field 2.* Dorsal aspect of heart, aorta, main pulmonary arteries and veins, dorsal border of caudal vena cava, trachea, tracheal bifurcation, main bronchi, ribs, and some thoracic vertebrae.
- *Field 3.* Caudal part of the heart (left atrium and ventricle), pulmonary vessels, caudal

vena cava, ribs, ventral diaphragm, trachea, and tracheal bifurcation
- *Field 4.* Major part of heart, aorta, cranial vena cava in cranial mediastinum, trachea, ribs, scapula, humerus. This is the most difficult view to obtain because of the mass of overlying muscle and the scapula and humerus.

Structures that should be examined are lung tissue, blood vessels, airways, ribs, diaphragm, mediastinum, and heart. Structures within the mediastinum such as esophagus, lymph nodes, thymus, and cranial vena cava are not normally visible, although, if sufficient contrast is present, such as when the mediastinal space contains air (pneumomediastinum), these structures can be seen. The objectives of radiology are to identify changes in tissue density, presence of tissue masses, pleural fluid lines, displacement of trachea, patency of the diaphragm, cardiac abnormalities, vertebral or rib problems, and whether lesions are diffuse or localized. Examination should be systematic.

Disease of the pulmonary parenchyma is generally characterized by increased density that occurs in different patterns described as alveolar, bronchial, and interstitial.[43,45] The interstitial pattern is frequently seen in the early stages of most pulmonary disease processes. The interstitial pattern can be divided into the subtypes of unstructured, hazy, infiltrate (UHI), irregular linear interstitial infiltrate (ILI), and nodular interstitial infiltrate (NII). The bronchial pattern is characterized by increased definition of the walls of the bronchi whose outlines can be rather clear (bronchial pattern) or less well defined (peribronchial pattern). A bronchial pattern is often associated with bronchopneumonia and chronic airway disease. The increased thickness of bronchial walls may be due to peribronchial infiltrates, not to be confused with the intraluminal exudate that lines the walls and produces a loss of luminal definition. Bronchiectasis alters the shape and increases the size of bronchi. Bronchography is the term used to describe specific imaging of the bronchi. Use of barium sulphate powder[46] and tantalum dust[47] has been described, and, although the technique allows evaluation of the airway walls down to the seventh or eighth generation, its clinical usefulness is unclear. An alveolar pattern is used to describe the change in density seen when alveoli are filled with fluid,

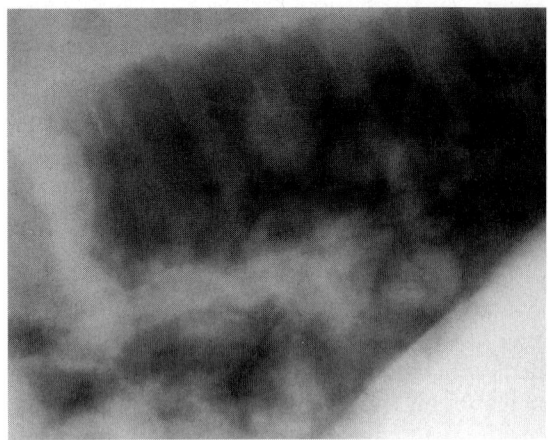

▶ FIGURE 3-22

Pulmonary abscessation. Note the numerous circumscribed regions of increased density.

such as exudate or edema fluid, that eventually causes the bronchi to become visible (air bronchograms) as dark tubular structures seen against an increased background density. Some abnormal findings are shown in Figure 3-22.

Thoracic Ultrasonography

Ultrasonographic examination of the thorax often provides useful information that either cannot be obtained by other means or requires confirmation. Ultrasonography is indicated for the detection, localization, and characterization of fluid, the detection of masses such as abscesses, and the localization of fluid and masses as a preliminary to biopsy. Competent ultrasonography requires a thorough knowledge of the normal appearance of the intrathoracic structures and ultrasound physics.[48-51] A sector scanner is preferred for thoracic scanning because the small, generally hemispherical, head of the instrument fits easily between the ribs. Linear array transducers are usually flat and elongated and are not suited to the curved and narrow intercostal space. Convex linear array scanners do not suffer this disadvantage. Basic information regarding ultrasonography is located in Appendix B.

Procedure

The skin is prepared as described in Appendix B. When a general examination of the thorax is necessary, a suitable procedure is to examine fully each intercostal space before moving on to the next one. For consistency, it is suggested that the examination begin in the cranial thorax and then move caudally, examining each space in a dorsal

to ventral direction with the scan plane oriented vertically. When a structure of special interest is located, its three-dimensional structure can be more easily appreciated if the transducer is rotated 90° to change the orientation of the scan plane. To evaluate specific regions, a complete examination of the thorax may not be necessary. Access to the cranial thorax is best made from the right side and can be improved by moving the foreleg forward.

Results

Normal pleural surfaces are smooth and highly echogenic. Therefore, lung tissue is penetrated poorly by the sound wave, most of which is reflected (Fig. 3-23). The reflected sound is seen as concentric reverberation artefacts deep to the pleural surface. If the surface is irregular, as a result of pneumonia or pleuritis, for example, the reverberation artefact is linear rather than concentric and radiates out from the pleural surface. Because of the high echogenicity of the pleural surfaces, pulmonary abscessation, pulmonary consolidation, and adhesions are visible only when they are in direct continuity with the thoracic wall.

If a pleural effusion is present, it is represented as a nonechogenic region in the pleural space and structures deep to the pleurae become easier to visualize. A small volume of fluid in the ventral aspect of the pleural cavity is often a normal finding. Debris, cells (leucocytes and erythrocytes), adhesions, and fibrin increase the echogenicity within the effusion. Free gas, seen as small, highly echogenic particles, may indicate an anaerobic infection or a bronchopleural fistula.

Adhesions between the visceral and parietal pleura, as well as fibrin strands, are often present. However, these should not be confused with the pericardial diaphragmatic ligament that lies caudal to the heart, is usually thicker, and moves freely in the pleural fluid.

Materials for Thoracic Ultrasonography

▶ Ultrasound machine (sector scanner with a frequency of 3.0–5.0 MHz is preferable)

▶ Ultrasound coupling gel

▶ Hair clipper with #40 blade

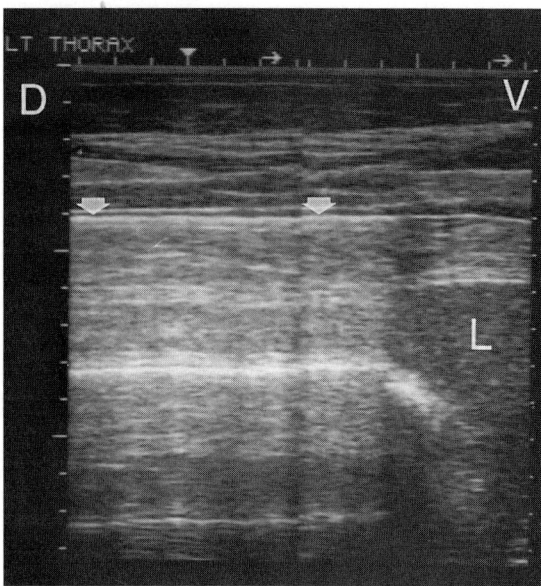

▶ **FIGURE 3-23**

Normal lungs and adjacent right liver. Transverse intercostal ultrasonogram made with a 5-MHz linear array transducer midway along the right 12th intercostal space of a normal quarter horse (*D* = dorsal, *V* = ventral). The echogenic surface of the aerated lung *(arrows)* generates a repeating reverberation artifact deeper in the image. The dorsal edge of the adjacent normal liver *(L)* can also be seen ventral to the lungs. (Courtesy R. H. Wrigley.)

When a region of lung tissue that is not separated from the thoracic wall by air becomes consolidated, most commonly as a result of pneumonia, it also becomes more echogenic and can, therefore, be seen in the scan. As lung tissue is likely to contain some patent airways, there often is an enhanced reflection at the interface between the consolidated parenchyma and the airways. The appearance of such lung tissue varies with the degree of consolidation and the variable presence of blood vessels and patent airways.

Abscesses are a frequent finding, and because of great variation in size, location, and consistency, their ultrasonographic appearance also varies considerably. Usually, no internal airways or vessels are seen, and images are hypoechoic to anechoic, frequently with cavitation and a well-developed capsule. Abscesses also often contain gas, which is seen dorsally. Some examples of abnormal thoracic sonograms are presented in Figure 3-24.

Thoracentesis

It is frequently necessary to collect a sample of pleural fluid to improve the chances of recognizing a disease process in the thoracic cavity.

Procedure

Thoracentesis[52] is carried out in the standing animal on one or, usually, both sides of the thorax. The site for insertion of the needle or cannula on the left side is the eighth or ninth intercostal space approximately 1 to 2 in. above the olecranon. On the right side the needle is inserted in the sixth or seventh intercostal space at about the level of the elbow joint. These sites can be varied if it is necessary to examine a specific region of the thorax, for example, an abscess cavity that has been localized by other means such as radiography or ultrasonography. Utilizing appropriate restraint, the hair is clipped from a 4×4-in. area centered on the chosen site, which is then prepared for sterile puncture. To render the procedure painless, local anesthetic solution is injected subcutaneously and then infiltrated in the deeper tissues, including the parietal pleura. Regardless of the site chosen, it is important to avoid the lateral thoracic vein that traverses the thorax ventrolaterally. If a larger catheter or trochar is used, the possibility of pneumothorax can be minimized by ensuring that the openings in the skin and the underlying muscle layers are not contiguous. This is done by making the skin incision with the scalpel over the rib cranial or caudal to the desired intercostal space and then sliding the skin so that the incision overlies the site for entry into the pleural cavity.

The cannula, with stopcock and syringe attached, is then inserted carefully and slowly immediately cranial to the rib to avoid the intercostal nerves and vessels that lie caudal to each rib. It is not vital to have the syringe attached. When a syringe is attached, entry can be ascertained by intermittently applying negative pressure and checking whether air or fluid is aspirated and, without a syringe, by observing outflow of fluid or hearing passage of air in or out of the cannula. A "popping" sensation is usually felt as the cannula, and sometimes the needle, enters the pleural cavity. The sample is collected into the syringe and transferred to the appropriate containers for evaluation. The procedure is demonstrated in Figure 3-25. If neoplasia is suspected, and no fluid has been obtained, the pleural cavity can be lavaged with warm saline and a sample retrieved for cytological examination.

PROCESSING OF SAMPLES. The sample is transferred into different containers for cytology (purple-top Vacutainer), biochemistry (red-top Vacutainer), glucose (grey-top Vacutainer), and into transport media or in the original syringe, sealed, for microbiological examination. The minimum protocol is to evaluate the sample for smell, color, volume, clot formation, and turbidity, which may be all that is necessary when the diagnosis is obvious, such as advanced pleuritis. As bacteria often are difficult to isolate, it is useful to add some of the fluid to a bacterial enrichment media, for later plating and more successful identification. If chylothorax is suspected, triglyceride and cholesterol analysis can be requested. The appropriate procedures for handling samples are described in Appendix C.

Materials for Thoracentesis

- Scalpel blade (#22)
- Blunt teat cannula (6 cm) or needle (14 gauge, 10 cm)
- Three-way stopcock
- Syringe (20 ml)
- Local anesthetic (2% lidocaine hydrochloride), 20-ml syringe, and 20-gauge needle
- Surgical gloves
- Collection containers
- Transport media

A

B

C

D

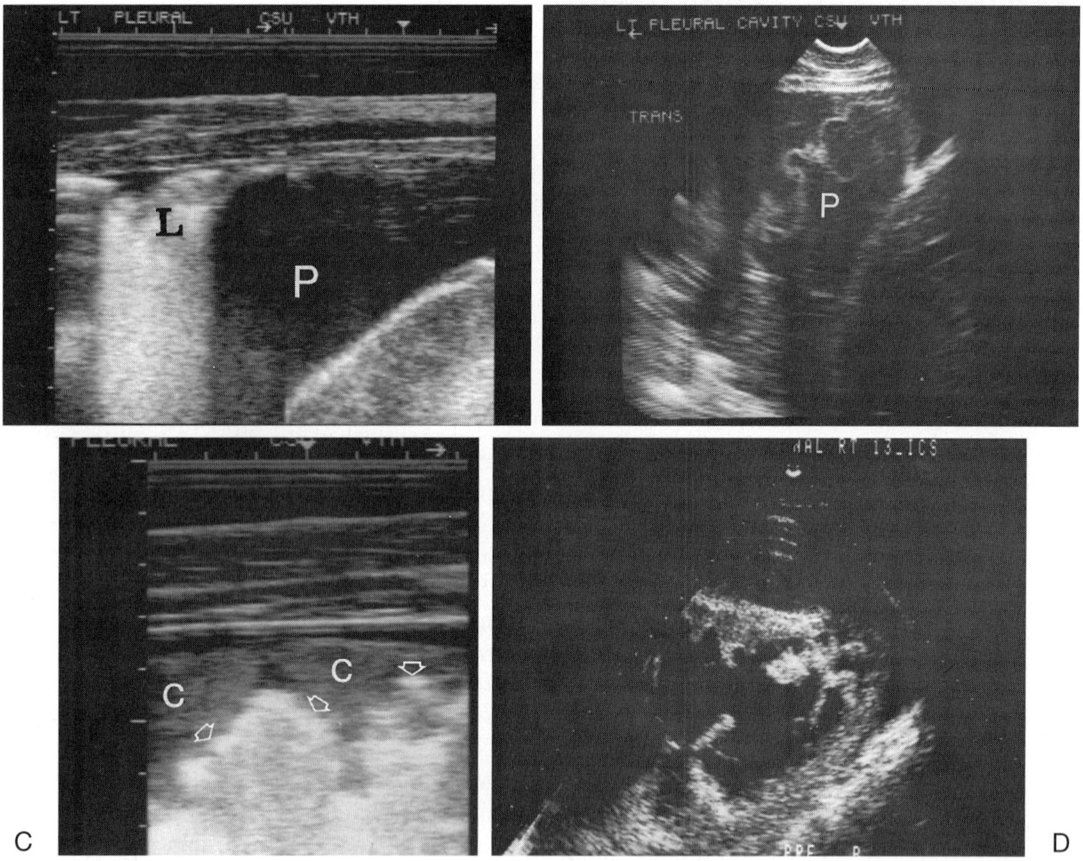

▶ **FIGURE 3-24**

Abnormal thoracic ultrasonograms. **A.** Pleuropneumonia. A ventral transverse intercostal ultrasonogram of the left chest shows dorsal displacement of the lungs (L) by a pleural effusion (P). (Courtesy, R. H. Wrigley.) **B.** Fibrinous pleuritis. A ventral transverse intercostal ultrasonogram made with a 3.5-MHz sector transducer of the ventral left chest of a 4-year-old thoroughbred gelding. A echogenic pleural effusion (P) was present. Many fibrin stands traverse the pleural effusion. (Courtesy, R. H. Wrigley.) **C.** Pneumonia. Transverse right intercostal ultrasonogram made with a 5-MHz linear array transducer of a 1-year-old thoroughbred colt. Dyspnea had been present for 5 days. Lung sounds were dull. The aeration of the lungs was irregular, with echogenic aerated lungs (arrows) interspersed between hypoechoic regions of consolidated (C) lungs. (Courtesy R. H. Wrigley.) **D.** Lung abscess. A dorsal ultrasonogram made with a 3.5-MHz sector transducer of the 13th intercostal space on an 11-month-old American Paint filly. Eight centimeters deep to the skin a large accumulation of hypoechoic fluid was contained by an irregular wall. Partial echogenic separation was present to the fluid. The deeper location suggested that the fluid was not pleural in nature. (Courtesy R. H. Wrigley.)

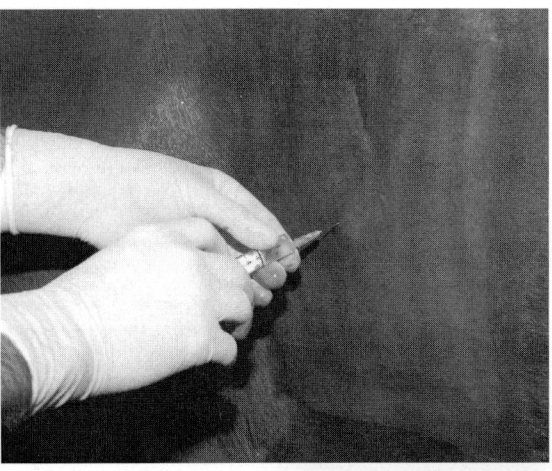

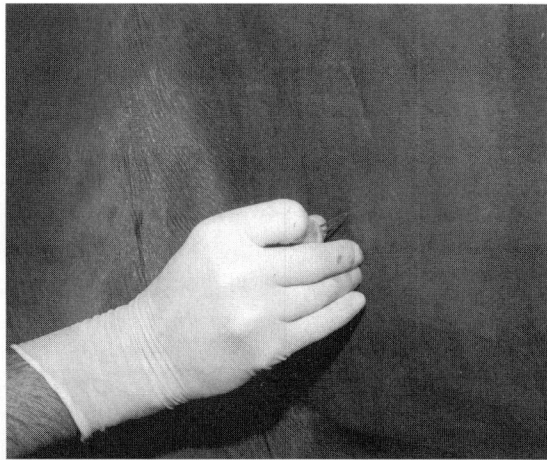

A

B

C

▶ **FIGURE 3-25**

Technique of thoracentesis. **A.** Injection of local anesthetic. **B.** Making a stab incision with a small scalpel blade. **C.** Insertion of needle/cannula attached to a syringe and three-way stop cock.

Results

NORMAL FINDINGS. Some values and characteristics for normal pleural fluid[53] are shown in Table 3-5. In healthy horses only a few milliliters of transparent, clear to yellowish fluid with no odor and no tendency to clot are obtained. If the rates of production or removal of pleural fluid are altered, than an abnormal volume of fluid may exist: Some factors that will increase volume are elevated hydrostatic and decreased osmotic intravascular pressures, increased permeability of capillaries, pleurae, and lymphatics, and obstruction to lymphatic drainage; decreased volume may accompany decreased intravascular hydrostatic pressure. Apparent normal volume does not preclude the possibility of pleural disease.

Classification of pleural fluid on the basis of total protein and total nucleated cell counts[54] as

▶ **TABLE 3-5**

NORMAL VALUES AND CHARACTERISTICS
OF PLEURAL FLUID

Parameter	Value
Total nucleated cell count ($\times 10^9$/L)	3.990 (0.800–12.100)
Neutrophils ($\times 10^9$/L)	2.967 (0.448–10.285)
Monocytes ($\times 10^9$/L)	0.804 (0.048–2.624)
Lymphocytes ($\times 10^9$/L)	0.211 (0–0.675)
Eosinophils ($\times 10^9$/L)	0.013
Total protein (g/L)	1.8 (0.2–4.7)
Erythrocytes	Rare
Turbidity	Transparent
Tendency to clot	None
Volume	Few milliliters
Odor	Odorless
Color	Colorless to yellowish

Source: Modified from Wagner AE, Bennet DG: Analysis of equine thoracic fluid. Vet Clin Pathol 1983; 11: 13.

transudates, modified transudates, and exudates is described in Appendix D. Although of diagnostic significance, these parameters are not reliable prognosticators because of cell sedimentation and variable dilution.

ABNORMAL FINDINGS

- *Sepsis.* Sepsis is characterized by an exudate (total nucleated cell count > 10×10^9/L and total protein > 25 gm/L) and a large volume of cloudy, yellowish fluid that often contains fibrin clots. Presence of erythrocytes as a result of vascular damage will render the fluid reddish. A fetid odor frequently accompanies anaerobic infections. Sepsis implies the presence of bacteria. However, for a number of reasons, including concurrent antimicrobial therapy, isolation often is difficult. Bacteria may be intra- or extracellular and neutrophils are usually degenerate.
- *Neoplasia.* If a neoplasm causes lymphatic obstruction, it will be characterized by an increase in fluid volume with normal to slightly elevated values for total nucleated cell count and total protein (transudate-modified transudate). If there is necrosis and ulceration, these parameters will probably be elevated (nonseptic exudate), and the fluid will be reddish because of the presence of erythrocytes. Bacteria and degenerate neutrophils are not present. Exfoliation of tumor cells often occurs, and the presence of these cells in the fluid can be used as a means of diagnosis.
- *Blood-stained fluid.* Blood can be present because of the primary problem (abscess, neoplasia, trauma) or because of contamination of the sample at the time of collection (see Appendix E for the difference between contamination and true hemorrhage).
- *Milky fluid.* An opalescent, sometimes reddish milky fluid is characteristic of a chylous or pseudochylous effusion.

Pleuroscopy

Pleuroscopy is the technique of examining the pleural space with either a rigid or a flexible endoscope.[55,56] The examination can be carried out in the standing, sedated horse to evaluate suspected intrathoracic lesions, such as pleuritis, abscessation, adhesions, and neoplasia.

Materials for Pleuroscopy

- Endoscope. Rigid (arthroscope or laparoscope) or flexible endoscope (e.g., bronchoscope, gastroscope) with light source
- Restraining stocks
- Suction unit
- Local anesthetic (2% lidocaine hydrochloride) with needle and syringe
- Chemical restraint and analgesic (see Chapter 1. Chemical Restraint of the Adult Horse)
- Suture material
- Scalpel blade (#15)
- Teat cannula

Procedure

The horse is placed in restraining stocks and tranquilized as necessary. When pleuritis is present, the procedure may be unduly painful, in which case an analgesic is required. For routine examination a 12- × 12-inch site, centered over the tenth intercostal space about midway between the points of the hip and the shoulder, is clipped and aseptically prepared. The skin and all underlying tissues, including the parietal pleura, are infiltrated with local anesthetic solution using a 1.5-inch, 22-gauge needle. A stab incision is made through the skin and subcutaneous fascia with a #15 scalpel blade, and a teat cannula is carefully inserted in the pleural space. The cannula is used to remove any fluid that is present in cases of pleuritis and to allow air to enter and collapse the ipsilateral lung so that the endoscope can be safely inserted. When using a rigid endoscope, the cannula with a blunt obturator is then introduced into the pleural cavity, the obturator is removed, and the endoscope inserted. If a flexible endoscope is to be used, it must first be sterilized, which is best done by soaking the section to be inserted (or by full immersion for immersible endoscopes) and flushing the biopsy, flushing, and suction channels with a sterilizing solution recommended by the manufacturer (see Appendix A). Inserting a flexible endoscope is a little more complicated as it is necessary first to make an opening through which to insert it, or, alternately, a larger cannula can be used. An opening through the subcutaneous tissues, muscle layers, and parietal pleura over the cranial border of the rib (to avoid intercostal vessels and nerves) is easily made with a pair of hemostats or forceps. When using a flexible endoscope, the possibility of creating a significant pneumothorax is present, and, to have some control over this, a purse-string suture can be placed in the skin around the endoscope. After the rigid endoscope is removed, a teat cannula is inserted and intrapleural air is removed. If a flexible endoscope is being used, air can be evacuated through the suction channel as well as later with a teat cannula if necessary. The skin incision, as well as the muscle layers if a flexible endoscope was used, are then closed to achieve an airtight seal. If residual air is a problem, it can be aspirated by needle.

Results

When a normal horse is viewed from the right side, it is possible to see the diaphragm, the aorta and azygos vein with their intercostal branches, the esophagus, the lung and its dorsocaudal attachment to the parietal pleura, the ribs and intercostal vessels, the cardiac notch, the heart, the pericardium and cardiac vessels, and the myocardium within the pericardial sac. From the left side, the findings are similar except that the azygos vein is absent. Abnormalities that may be visible are accumulations of effusions, abscesses, neoplasms, and adhesions. Although examination of the opposite side of the thorax can be carried out immediately the first procedure is completed, it is not recommended because it is more stressful and increases the chances of complications related to pneumothorax.

Complications

The technique is relatively free of complications, and under normal circumstances antimicrobial prophylaxis is not necessary. Collapse of the contralateral lung is a potential problem, but this occurs rarely and, provided it is recognized, it is easily managed by removing the air with a suction pump. Although respiratory embarrassment is an uncommon complication, the clinician should always be alert for signs of it and should always have a fully prepared suction apparatus available. Pneumothorax is usually present after the procedure, but it is not a problem and resolves spontaneously over a few days. However, if the clinician is concerned, the air can be removed by suction, as described, or by inserting a temporary indwelling tube connected to a stopcock or one-way valve (Heimlich chest drain, Bard-Parker).

Percutaneous Lung Biopsy

There are at least five different methods for obtaining a lung biopsy: (1) percutaneous trephination with a high-speed drill; (2) transbronchial forceps; (3) thoracotomy; (4) percutaneous needle aspiration; and (4) percutaneous needle biopsy. The technique should allow safe collection of a sample from a selected region of lung, and the sample should retain its normal three-dimensional structure so as to facilitate histological examination. Percutaneous needle biopsy fulfills these requirements and can be useful in diagnosing pulmonary lesions that are generalized or can be localized with the assistance of ultrasonography or radiology. The biopsy is carried out on the standing animal using restraint sufficient to ensure that the horse cannot move around and is breathing quietly.[57]

Procedure

To obtain a sample from either the left or right lung, the usual site for biopsy is the seventh or eighth intercostal space, approximately 3 inch dorsal to a horizontal line drawn through the elbow joint. The site will be different if the lesion has been localized to another region. An area

---

Materials for Percutaneous Lung Biopsy

- Restraining stocks
- Biopsy needle. Tru-Cut Biopsy Needle (Travenol Laboratories, Inc. Deerfield, IL) or Temno biopsy Needle (Products Group International, Inc., Boulder, CO)
- Pins and backing (wooden tongue depressor)
- Scalpel blade (#15)
- Local anesthetic solution (2% lidocaine hydrochloride, 2% mepivacaine hydrochloride), syringe, and needle
- Fixative. 10% neutral buffered formalin

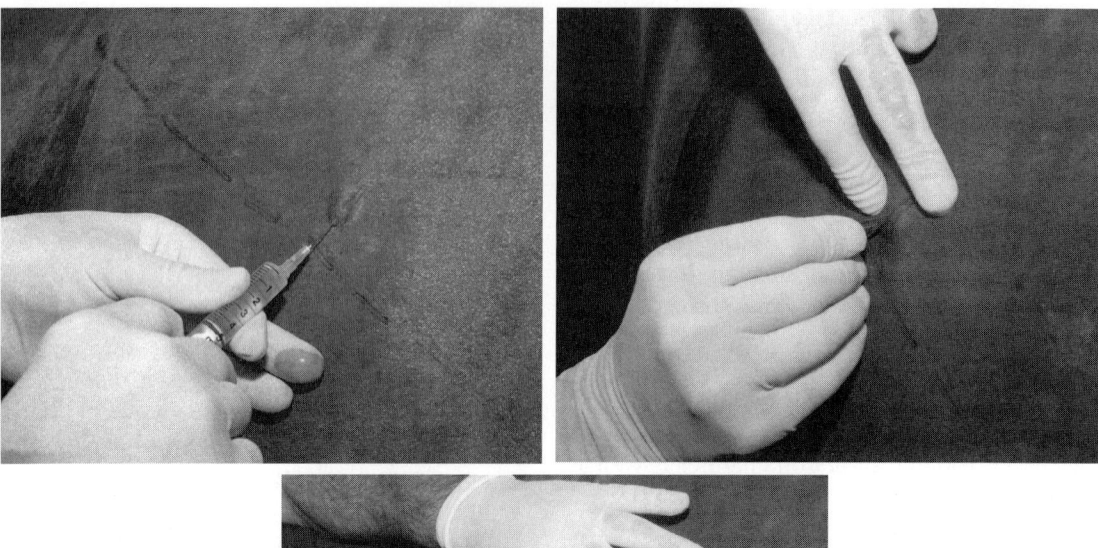

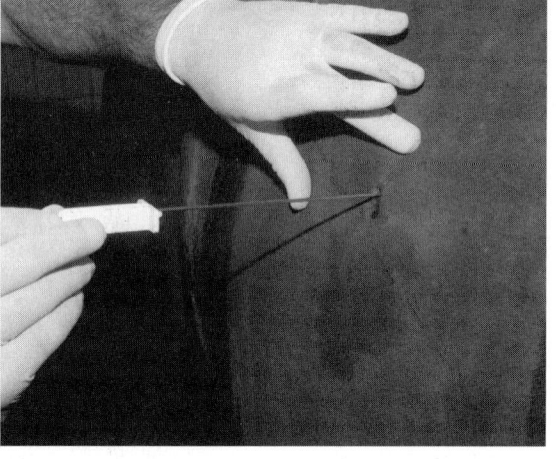

▶ **FIGURE 3-26**

Lung biopsy. **A.** Injection of local anesthetic. **B.** Making a stab incision with a small scalpel blade. **C.** Insertion of biopsy needle (Tru-Cut).

4×4 in. centered over the biopsy site is clipped and aseptically prepared. The subcutaneous tissue, intercostal muscles, and parietal pleura in the selected intercostal space and the subcutaneous tissue over the next most caudal rib are infiltrated with the local anesthetic solution. A small stab incision is made through the skin with the #15 scalpel blade and the biopsy needle is inserted through the incision and then advanced into the lung. The exact procedures for using the Tru-Cut Needle or the Temno Automatic Needle are described in Appendix F. The sample is carefully removed from the needle, transferred to the tongue depressor to which it is attached with a pin at either end, and the sample and depressor are then placed in the fixative. The specimen is placed on the tongue depressor to avoid contraction during fixation. The procedure is demonstrated in Figure 3-26.

Results

The technique allows the collection of samples that regularly contain alveolar tissue, blood vessels, and bronchioles. Occasionally there will be pieces of diaphragm, liver, or gut. However, the tissues are suitable for histology, the histologist should be alert for artefacts such as alveolar collapse and the presence of erythrocytes and tissue fluid.

Complications

The method allows a lung biopsy to be carried out with little risk of serious complication. A small trickle of blood is often seen at the external nares, especially if the horse coughs. Endoscopic examination of the trachea usually reveals some blood. Unless there has been a significant laceration of the lung, the bleeding is without significance. The possibility of lung laceration is higher if the horse is moving around or has a high breathing rate. At a subsequent necropsy examination the site of biopsy is usually characterized as a small wound in the visceral pleura sometimes associated with a zone of hemorrhage. Some other possible complications are pneumothorax, hemothorax, and air embolism. Contraindications for biopsy are elevated breathing rate, an excitable horse, coughing, cystic or bullous lung disease, and clotting abnormalities.

Pulmonary Function Testing

Pulmonary function testing (PFT) is a useful and common procedure in people. However, because many tests require considerable patient cooperation and expensive equipment, the full range of tests cannot be performed in horses. The objectives of the PFT are to measure parameters that indicate the effectiveness of respiration. Although some equipment is simple, accumulation of much of the necessary data requires sophisticated technology.

Some of the available tests and methodology will be described briefly. An overview with more detailed descriptions of pulmonary function testing is available elsewhere.[58]

Measurements of Ventilatory Volumes and Gas Flow Rates

INTEGRATED PNEUMOTACHOGRAPHY. This is the most commonly used method to evaluate volume and flow.[59] Flow is measured by pneumotachography that is then integrated by an electronic circuit or computer program to produce volume data. The pneumotachograph, through which all inspired and expired air must pass, is a tubular device that contains a small resistance (wire mesh or a series of tubes) and is attached to a tight-fitting face mask. As air passes across the resistance, there is a fall in pressure that, provided flow is laminar, is proportional to flow and gas viscosity. The pressure difference is measured by a differential pressure transducer connected to tubes at each end of the resistance. Use of a single Fleisch or Lilly pneumotachograph is limited to horses at rest because their output is not linear for high-flow rates. This problem is overcome by inserting two of the instruments in the mask. Ultrasonic phase-shift flow meters have a number of advantages over the pneumotachograph, particularly their usefulness at higher flow rates.[60]

The face mask should be constructed to avoid leakage of air and have minimal dead space. There are numerous designs, and generally they consist of a circular metal or plastic tube that fits over the horse's nose. A rubber flange with appropriate padding is fitted proximally to ensure an airtight seal with the head. Distally, the mask is made small enough to avoid excess dead space but not so small as to compress the nostrils. The pneumotachograph is attached to a mount at the distal end so that all air flows through it.

SPIROMETRY. Spirometry, which uses a water-sealed bell spirometer, is an accurate and simple method of measuring volume. It involves breathing into a spirometer and recording displacement, which is proportional to tidal volume. All air must pass through the device, which is ensured by using a face mask, nasal endotracheal intubation, or tracheostomy. Unidirectional valves and carbon dioxide absorption are necessary if rebreathing studies are to be conducted. The bell spirometer can be changed to a "bag-in-box" system rather than be water-sealed. The main application of spirometry is to measure functional residual capacity, using helium dilution or nitrogen washout procedures. Otherwise, spirometry is not used often. Although volume data are extremely accurate, the technique is cumbersome and other methods produce much more information.

Helium Dilution Test. The horse breathes through a closed circuit that consists of a spirometer, tight-fitting face mask, tubing containing unidirectional valves, and facility for carbon dioxide absorption.[58,61] Oxygen is added to maintain a constant volume while the horse breathes from the spirometer, to which a known quantity of helium has been added. Rebreathing continues until equilibrium is achieved after about 5 to 7 minutes. The proportion of helium in the gas mixture before and after rebreathing is measured and functional residual capacity (FRC) is calculated from the equation:

$$\text{FRC (L)} = V \times \frac{(C_1 - C_2)}{C_2}$$

where

V = initial volume of gas in the spirometer,
C_1 = initial helium concentration,
C_2 = final helium concentration

Nitrogen Washout Test. Functional residual capacity can also be measured using the multiple breath nitrogen washout test.[58] This test can be done using an open circuit. The spirometer is flushed with oxygen, adjusted to zero, and nitrogen concentration is measured. The system is constructed so that at the end of expiration the horse will inhale pure oxygen, and then all expired gas is collected until a specified endpoint is reached, namely, after 600 L of oxygen has been administered into the system[62] or until end-tidal nitrogen concentration is under 1%.[63] The spirometer's final nitrogen concentration and volume are recorded after the test and used to calculate the volume of exhaled nitrogen. After correction for any nitrogen contamination from nonlung tissue or dead space and correction of gas volumes to body temperature and pressure saturated (BTPS), the FRC is calculated as follows:

$$FRC(L) = \frac{N_2 \text{ exhaled (L)}}{0.81 - \text{end-tidal } N_2\% \text{ at end of washout}}$$

Functional residual capacity is related to body weight (BW) according to the following equation:[58]

$$FRC(L) = 2.63 + 0.03 \text{ BW(kg)}$$

This test is also useful for measuring pulmonary nitrogen clearance during oxygen breathing. In poorly ventilated alveoli nitrogen is less effectively cleared. Normal end-tidal values for nitrogen are under 2%. A washin test is also described, but it is used less often.

RESPIROMETERS. Respirometers, in which the expired air moves a series of blades or wind vanes, have been used in small ponies and foals,[64] but the available equipment is too small for larger horses.

PLETHYSMOGRAPHY. This technique involves placing a horse in an airtight, nonexpansible chamber and then having it breathe through tubing connected to the exterior. A transducer inside the chamber is used to record the pressure changes that result from changes in thoracic volume, and a second transducer records pressure in the conducting airway. Parameters such as resistance, compliance, gas volumes, pulmonary gas flow, and FRC can be derived with this equipment. For FRC, this technique avoids the problems associated with gas distribution in the helium dilution and the nitrogen washout methods. Although it is possible to use this technique

for horses, it is not easily done and the equipment is cumbersome.

The thoracic volume can be measured in other ways such as by using change in abdominal and thoracic movement as an index of tidal volume (inductance plethysmography) or by recording changes in impedance across the thorax, which are proportional to changes in volume.

Measurement of Intrapleural Pressure

Resistance to inspiration or expiration is associated with a change in intrapleural pressure that therefore is a useful index of pulmonary pathology and function. Intrapleural pressure can be measured directly with a transducer attached to a catheter placed in the pleural space or more commonly, indirectly, by attaching it to a thin-walled balloon placed in the intrathoracic esophagus. Although actual pressure (P_{pl}) can be measured, the usual practice is to use a differential pressure transducer to measure pressure relative to the airway opening, such as transpulmonary pressure (P_{tp}), and to record the change in pressure (ΔP_{tp}) during breathing. The P_{tp} can be measured relative to atmospheric air by opening the transducer to the exterior or, relative to air within the face mask, by connecting it to the face mask. The latter method avoids error associated with resistance in the face mask.

Regional differences in pleural and esophageal pressures exist, with pleural pressure increasing as the measurement site is moved ventrally in the thorax and esophageal pressure increasing as the measurement site is moved cranially.[65] Significantly, pressure changes in the middle and caudal portions of the thoracic esophagus are similar to those measured in the dorsal thoracic position. Therefore, in order to facilitate comparisons among data from these different sites, esophageal pressure should be measured just caudal to the heart, and pleural pressure in the dorsal pleural space.

INDIRECT MEASUREMENT OF INTRAPLEURAL PRESSURE WITH AN ESOPHAGEAL BALLOON. The balloon commonly used is a condom, which is attached to the end of a 220-cm polyethylene tube (internal diameter, 4.0 mm; outside diameter, 6.0 mm) containing a few side holes in the distal end. First, a short piece of a normal stomach tube is inserted through the nasal passage into the proximal esophagus, and the smaller tube with the attached condom is inserted through it. If the tubing is stiff enough, the stomach tube can be dispensed with. The stomach tube is then removed and swallowing movements carry the balloon catheter further into the esophagus so that the balloon is positioned just caudal to the heart, as measured before the procedure by holding the catheter alongside the horse. The catheter is then inserted through the face mask, inflated with a predetermined volume of air and attached to the transducer.

DIRECT MEASUREMENT OF INTRAPLEURAL PRESSURE. Direct measurement is made by inserting a catheter through an intercostal space and into the pleural cavity. The insertion site is on the left or right side in about the 10th to 14th intercostal space on a line joining the tuber coxae and the point of the shoulder. The hair is clipped from the chosen site, which is prepared for sterile puncture. A small incision is made in the skin to facilitate relatively friction-free insertion, and the catheter with stilette in place is inserted. The stilette is removed, and, if the catheter is correctly placed, the inrush of air will be heard. The catheter is connected to the transducer and recording can begin. Sometimes the recording is affected by the catheter rubbing on the pleurae, which may be controlled by rotating the catheter or by injecting a few milliliters of air or by recording while saline is being slowly injected.

Pressure-Volume and Flow-Volume Loops

Pressure-volume loops are created by relating P_{pl} to tidal volume, with the area inside the loop being equal to the nonelastic work of breathing. This technique has been used to investigate chronic obstructive pulmonary disease in horses, but, because its main benefits are related to forced voluntary breathing maneuvers, it is not as useful as it is in man. Similar loops can be constructed to express the relationship between flow and volume. However, these also require forced voluntary breathing for maximum value. Recent studies have used these techniques to investigate flow and resistance in the upper respiratory tract during exercise, so that maximal respiration can be used.

Compliance

Compliance, both static and dynamic, is a measure of the distensibility, or stiffness, of the lung. In horses, only dynamic compliance can be measured as it does not depend on the active cooperation of the patient. Compliance is obtained by dividing the change in lung volume by the change in pleural pressure between the end of inspiration and the end of expiration (i.e., when there is zero flow).

Airway Resistance

Resistance is obtained by dividing the pressure difference across a segment of airway by airflow. For total respiratory resistance P_{tp} is used, whereas specific sections of the airways can be evaluated by varying the sites of pressure measurement. The ability to partition airway resistance is useful to evaluate upper and lower airway diseases separately.

Tracheal Pressure

Tracheal pressure can be measured by inserting a catheter percutaneously or transnasally into the trachea. The ability to measure tracheal pressure allows airway resistance to be partitioned into its various anatomical components. Traditionally, this has been directed toward identifying upper and lower airway resistances, but in recent times, it has been applied to the investigation of specific upper airway problems such as laryngeal hemiplegia and soft palate displacement. This is particularly useful for studies involving laryngeal hemiplegia. The most useful application of tracheal pressure is in horses during exercise. There has been a movement from studies conducted at rest during chemical stimulation of respiration,[66] to exercise studies using a treadmill,[67-70] to studies with free-running horses.[71-73] (see Exercise Testing to Evaluate Respiratory Function).

Impedance

Respiratory impedance is the term used to describe the total opposition to movement of air in the respiratory tract. Under certain specific conditions, it includes resistance, compliance, and inertance. It is based on the superimposition of a low-level oscillating airflow on normal respiration and on the calculation of airway pressure and flow after removing the effects of the animal. The impedance is finally obtained by dividing the remaining pressure by the flow. The advantage of this form of measurement is that it does not require patient cooperation to carry out special voluntary breathing maneuvers. A further advantage is the ability to investigate changes in resistance associated with higher frequencies. Measurement of total respiratory impedance in horses using forced random noise has been described.[74]

Measurement of Gas Distribution in the Lung

Optimum gas exchange across the alveolar-capillary membrane requires the coordination, or matching, of alveolar ventilation and capillary blood flow. This relationship is known as the ventilation-to-perfusion ratio (V_A/Q) and is efficient from 0.8 to 1.0. There is uniformity throughout the lung at rest, and there is very little variation during exercise. Disease, especially variation in ventilation, produces mismatching. Considerable abnormality may be present before clinical signs are present, which thus presents an opportunity for early diagnosis.

Techniques to measure the ratio include the single-breath inert gas elimination method, the multiple inert gas elimination method, and lung imaging. Single-breath method, in horses as in people, requires active patient participation and is therefore unsuitable for conscious animals. The multiple inert gas elimination method uses a gas chromatograph to measure the steady-state concentration of infused inert gases in pulmonary and carotid artery blood and in mixed expiratory gases. The data obtained allow a continuous record of the V_A/Q as well as of the pulmonary dead space and shunt.[75]

Lung Imaging

The evaluation of ventilation and pulmonary perfusion by imaging with radioactive isotopes is described elsewhere (see Nuclear Imaging to Evaluate Ventilation and Perfusion). The technique involves the scintigraphic measurement of the topographical distribution of the V_A/Q during intravenous infusion and the inhalation of a radioisotope.[76,77]

Blood Gas Analysis

Measurement of arterial oxygen (P_AO_2) and carbon dioxide (P_ACO_2) is a useful overall index of pulmonary gas exchange. Arterial samples can be collected from various sites, although the carotid or transverse facial arteries are favored in the standing horse. Hypoxemia is defined as $P_AO_2 < 80$ mm Hg, and hypercapnia as $P_ACO_2 > 45$ mm Hg. Because of the increased solubility of carbon dioxide and the shape of the oxyhemoglobin dissociation curve, abnormalities of function tend first to cause a reduction in P_AO_2 and then later an elevation of P_ACO_2, the latter being particularly associated with mismatching of ventilation and perfusion. Hypoventilation causes an increase in P_ACO_2 and a decrease in P_AO_2. The reverse applies to hyperventilation.

A reduction in oxygen transport across the alveolar-capillary membrane, for whatever reason, can be quantified approximately by calculation of the difference in oxygen tension between arterial blood and alveolar air. This is termed the Alveolar-arterial oxygen difference $(A - a)DO_2$.

$$(A - a)DO_2 = P_AO_2 - P_aO_2$$

Alveolar oxygen is calculated by measuring end-tidal oxygen with a mass spectrometer or by the following equation:

$$P_aO_2 = P_iO_2 - (P_ACO_2 \div V_A/Q)$$

where

---

pH AND BLOOD GAS VALUES

Normal

Adults[58]
- pH 7.38 ± 0.01
- P_AO_2 83.6 ± 1.7 mm Hg
- P_ACO_2 42.2 ± 0.8 mm Hg

Abnormal (chronic obstructive pulmonary disease)

Adults[58]
- pH 7.37 ± 0.01
- P_AO2 63.3 ± 2.6 mm Hg
- P_ACO2 47.0 ± 1.7 mm Hg

Foals[78]
- pH 7.354 ± 0.011
- P_AO_2 80.0 ± 3.8 mm Hg
- P_ACO_2 47.5 ± 2.6 mm Hg

SOME RESPIRATORY VALUES IN NORMAL FREE-RUNNING THOROUGHBREDS ($N = 4$)

- Velocity (m/min) 831 ± 59
- Tidal volume (L) 10.1 ± 1.1
- Mean and peak inspiratory flows (L/s) 51.2 ± 4.9 and 61.3 ± 3.4
- Mean and peak expiratory flows (L/s) 48.0 ± 4.5 and 70.5 ± 3.9
- Time for inspiration (msec) 198 ± 23
- Time for expiration (msec) 212 ± 21

- Velocity (m/min) 805 ± 42
- Respiratory rate (min) 131 ± 6
- Tidal volume (L and mL/kg) 11.8 ± 1.1 and 29.5 ± 1.7
- Pulmonary ventilation (L/min and L/kg/min) 1540 ± 129 and 3.84 ± 0.21

Note: Upper and lower data were derived separately).[79]

$$P_iO_2 = (P_b - P_{H2O})F_iO_2$$

P_b = barometric pressure

P_{H2O} = water vapor pressure at animal's body temperature

F_iO_2 = fraction of oxygen in inspired gas

Exercise Testing to Evaluate Respiratory Function

Exercise testing applies particularly to the equine athlete and ranges from simple measurements of heart and respiratory rates after exercise to continuous monitoring of many functions during high-speed treadmill exercise. The introduction of the high-speed treadmill has enabled a level of controlled investigation not previously available. Although optimal performance requires that many physiological systems be functioning at peak capacity, evaluation of the response to exercise especially involves the cardiorespiratory (CR) and musculoskeletal (MS) systems. In addition to obvious factors, such as lameness and respiratory infections, performance is limited by many other subtle factors, including the increased metabolic cost of locomotion or breathing associated with lameness and respiratory obstruction, respectively, and by reduced pulmonary gas exchange associated with pulmonary pathology. Exercise testing is best done when horses are performing at peak levels, as it is only under such conditions that minor abnormalities become apparent.

Simple Exercise Testing

The simplest form of exercise test available to clinicians usually consists of pre- and postexercise recording of heart and respiratory rates, best done after the completion of a standardized piece of exercise. In performance horses this can be termed the *track or field test.* Obvious abnormality of the cardiorespiratory systems will be detected by this method. Relatively simple refinements include continuously recording heart rate with an on-board heart rate meter, measurement of arterial blood gases and venous lactate in blood samples collected after exercise. A more sophisticated technique that uses telemetry to record data generated by a mask-mounted device with a flag located in the airway to sense flow has been developed.[79] This system allows the calculation of tidal and minute volumes, inspiratory and expiratory times, respiratory rate, and inspiratory and expiratory flow rates.

Standardized Incremental Exercise Test

This test measures the response to short periods of exercise repeated at regular intervals at successively higher levels of intensity.[80,81] There are a number of test procedures described and the values derived depend mainly on whether or not equipment to measure flow is available.

Procedure. One form of the routine test consists of 10 tests performed with the treadmill inclined at 6° to the horizontal.[80] The number of steps and the times at each step may vary between laboratories. Some horses require a training period to become accustomed to the treadmill before testing can be performed, this applies especially to thoroughbreds and to younger, less experienced horses. The training or acclimatization period consists of a period of walking followed by a step-wise increase in speed so that the horse begins to trot (at about 4 m/s) and then canter (at about 6 m/s).[81] Each step occupies 3 to 4 minutes, and it is important that the horse be encouraged to work at the front of the machine.

The jugular vein or transverse facial artery are catheterized to collect venous or arterial blood samples. Arterial samples are required to measure arterial blood gases. The horse is placed on the treadmill, and all the apparatus is placed in position. The closed-mask system has the disadvantages that it must be close fitting, is not so well accepted by horses not used to the procedure, and increases resistance in the system, but it makes it possible to measure ventilation and flow rates. Treadmill velocity ranges from 1.8 to 13 m/s (or 15.00 to 2.00 min/mile), with the speed being increased at 1-minute intervals within this range. The test is finished after the sequences are completed or if the horse cannot maintain its position on the front of the treadmill. The treadmill is then returned to the horizontal position, and the test finishes with a cool-down phase of 15 minutes at 1.8 m/s. Oxygen consumption, carbon dioxide production, respiratory exchange ratio, venous blood lactate, heart rate, hematocrit, and total plasma protein are recorded during exercise and again at 1, 5, and 15 minutes. If arterial blood is

collected, arterial blood gases can be measured. Serum samples are taken before and after testing to measure creatine kinase as an index of muscle injury.

Results.   The key biochemical steps in producing the energy necessary for muscle contraction is the hydrolysis of adenosine triphosphate (ATP) to adenosine diphosphate (ADP) and the subsequent restoration of the ATP from phosphocreatine (PC), anaerobic glycolysis, and aerobic metabolism. Evaluation of the energy produced by creatine phosphate requires muscle biopsy (see Muscle Biopsy), which is not a practical clinical procedure. During ATP regeneration by anaerobic glycolysis, lactic acid is produced, and venous blood lactate can be used as an index of the contribution of anaerobic metabolism to energy production and the ability to tolerate high levels after exhaustive exercise in a measure of anaerobic endurance. Aerobic metabolism requires oxygen transported by the cardiopulmonary system, and measurements of oxygen consumption and carbon dioxide production are used to evaluate this pathway.

When compared with fit horses, unfit horses have a higher oxygen consumption for a given speed, achieve a lower maximum oxygen consumption, have early elevation of blood lactate, are inable to complete all levels of the test, and arrive at peak hematocrit and heart rates earlier. Lack of physical effort is characterized by failure to achieve maximum oxygen consumption, no decrease in slope of the oxygen consumption versus velocity curve, low heart rates, no marked elevation of blood lactate, and suboptimal values for carbon dioxide production compared to oxygen consumption. Minor levels of pulmonary pathology are reflected under heavy workload by sudden reduction in the slope of the curve of oxygen consumption versus velocity or by early achievement of maximum oxygen consumption and lactate levels, and cessation of effort. Arterial oxygen and carbon dioxide values are useful in identifying horses with disease localized to the respiratory tract. Some data are presented in Table 3–6.

Intrapleural Pressure

Increased airway resistance is associated with increased respiratory effort and abnormally high and/or low pleural pressures depending on whether the resistance is inspiratory, expiratory, or both. Intrapleural pressure (IP) can be mea-

---

Requirements for Standardized Exercise Test Conducted on a Treadmill

- High-speed treadmill. Capable of speeds of up to 14 m/s and a maximum inclination of 10% (6°) (e.g., Säto or Mustang)
- Closed-face mask or open-flow respirometry systems
- Oxygen and carbon dioxide analyzers
- Sample tubes for hematocrit, total protein, blood lactate
- Intravenous and intraarterial catheters
- Heart rate monitor (e.g., Hippocard or EQB)
- Equipment for telemetric electrocardiography (adhesive electrodes, telemetric transmitter and receiver)

▶ **TABLE 3-6**

BLOOD GASES: EFFECTS OF EXERCISE AND DISEASE
ON ARTERIAL OXYGEN (PaO_2) AND
CARBON DIOXIDE ($PaCO_2$)

GROUP	PARAMETER (MM HG)		
	PaO_2	$PaCO_2$	REFERENCES
Resting values	96.2 ± 6.0	44.5 ± 1.6	86
Postexercise	61.5 ± 2.1	50.8 ± 4.3	86
Laryngeal hemi-plegia	53.2	58.1	86
Chronic obstructive pulmonary disease	73.1 ± 8.8	49.4 ± 8.2	87

sured directly by inserting an intrapleural catheter or needle, but this is invasive and not well suited to measurement during high-speed exercise. The alternative method is to measure the intraesophageal pressure using a pressure-sensitive balloon attached to the end of a small tube passed through the nasal passage and into the thoracic esophagus (see Measurement of Intrapleural Pressure). Normal resting intrapleural pressures range between approximately −3 and +3 cm of H2O.

Tracheal Pressure

Measuring tracheal pressure during exercise is a viable procedure and avoids the necessity of the extra equipment required for measuring flow and tidal volume. Methods for percutaneous and transnasal placement of the catheter have been developed, both of which appear to be clinically acceptable. The usefulness of tracheal pressure to diagnose and to evaluate the response to surgery of conditions such as laryngeal hemiplegia and dorsal displacement of the soft palate has been demonstrated.[69,70-72,82,83] An example of results obtained with a percutaneous catheter is presented in Figure 3–27.

Pulmonary Flow-Volume Loops

Pulmonary flow-volume loops are frequently used when examining human patients with pulmonary disease. However, cooperation in producing full maximal expiration after maximal inspiration is necessary. As this is not possible with horses, compromise, in the form of loops constructed from data obtained during exercise, is necessary.[84] Similar data can be obtained during chemically induced hyperventilation, but flow rates are insufficient to allow the identification of subtle or even relatively obvious lesions.[66] Con-

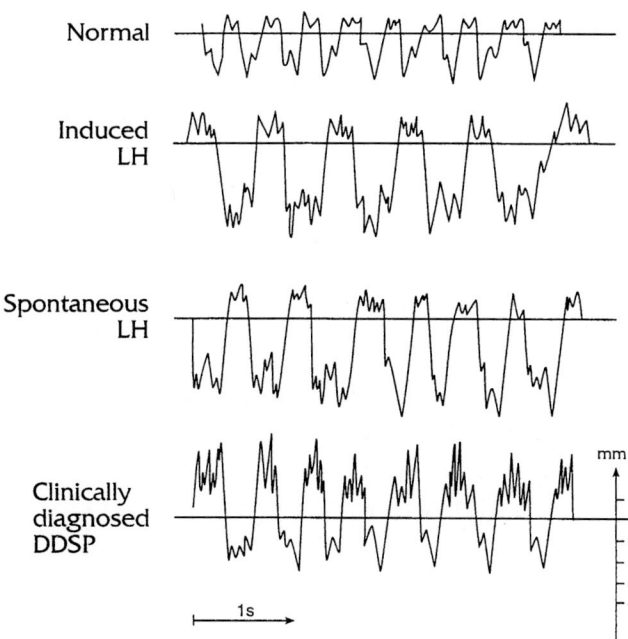

Normal

Induced LH

Spontaneous LH

Clinically diagnosed DDSP

1s

mm Hg
10
0
-10
-20
-30
-40

▶ **FIGURE 3-27**

Tracheal pressure recorded with a percutaneous transtracheal catheter. The difference between a recording from a normal horse and those from horses with laryngeal hemiplegia (induced and spontaneous) and dorsal displacement of the soft palate can be seen. (From Roethlisberger-Holm K: Transtracheal Pressure Recordings in the Exercising Horse. Doctoral Dissertation, Swedish University of Agricultural Sciences, Uppsala, Sweden, 1995. Reprinted with permission.)

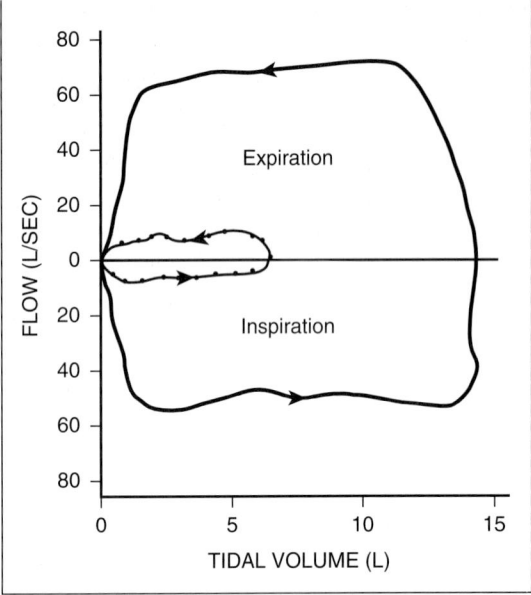

FIGURE 3-28

Flow-volume loops at rest and during exercise.

struction of flow-volume loops requires continuous data for inspiratory and expiratory flow and tidal volume, which can be provided by using the traditional mask and pneumotachograph or by one of the other systems for sensing flow described. There is no need for measuring pleural pressure.

Small airway disease is associated with collapse of the airways during expiration, thus limiting expiratory flow. Horses with laryngeal obstruction also suffer flow limitation, but this occurs during inspiration when there is tendency for the airway to become narrower, a process known as *dynamic collapse*. An example of a flow-volume loop is shown in Figure 3-28.

Arterial Oxygen and Carbon Dioxide Partial Pressures

Measuring blood gases at rest is of little value in the detection of minor lesions. However, this is improved during exercise. During strenuous exercise horses become hypoxemic and marginally hypercarbic,[85] even more so when impairment such as laryngeal hemiplegia[86] or lower airway disease are present.[87] The data vary depending on the exercise protocol and equipment and each laboratory should establish its own reference values. Some reference values are presented in Table 3-6.

Endoscopic Evaluation of the Upper Respiratory Tract During Exercise

As described, endoscopic examination of the upper respiratory tract is a common procedure, although, because it is usually performed with the horse at rest or shortly after exercise, it is most suited to detecting static, rather than dynamic, abnormalities. This is a disadvantage mainly in performance horses where early diagnosis of subtle airway obstruction, evaluation of surgery, and detection of functional lesions manifest only during exercise are required. This situation has been greatly improved by the availability of treadmills and flexible endoscopes with which the upper respiratory tract can be evaluated during exercise.

Procedure. Horses should undergo routine endoscopy before exercise testing and should be exercised with as much of their normal head tack in place as possible.[88] This especially includes bridle, bit, and nosebands for all horses, and head checks for harness horses. This is important, because such equipment and the position and carriage of the head often are associated with functional abnormalities during exercise. Insertion of the endoscope is done after the horse has had a preliminary warm-up exercise and is apparently tolerating the treadmill procedure. The endoscope should be inserted into the nasopharynx through the ventral meatus, positioned with its tip about 6 cm from the epiglottis, and then attached to the noseband. As it is important to be able to remove the instrument quickly, a quick release attachment is required, such as a rubber band or Velcro strap. The objective is to create test conditions that simulate strenuous exercise, done best with the treadmill inclined at 6° for horses that gallop and 3° for horses that trot or pace. The speed of the treadmill is adjusted to

---

Materials for Endoscopy during Exercise

- Endoscope (videoendoscope or standard fiber-optic endoscope with a video camera and monitor)
- High-speed treadmill, with adjustable slope and speed capability of 14 m/s
- Tape recorder
- Microphone

produce a heart rate above 220 beats per minute, and, although the final speed achieved will vary with the horse, its state of fitness, and the extent of the performance-limiting factors, a treadmill speed of the order of 9 to 14 m/s is usually necessary.

Audio recordings are useful for correlating gait and endoscopic appearance, although the noise from the treadmill usually precludes evaluating all but the loudest respiratory sounds. Posttest endoscopy is carried out 1 hour later to identify abnormal airway discharges, such as blood, mucus, or purulent exudate.

Results. Evaluation of the resting airway is described under Endoscopic Examination of the Airways. Conditions such as persistent dorsal displacement of the soft palate, persistent entrapment of the epiglottis, and laryngeal hemiplegia can be seen at rest and are, of course, still visible during exercise. Conditions such as intermittent dorsal displacement of the soft palate, generalized collapse of the nasopharyngeal soft tissues, prolapse of the lining of the lateral saccule, and dynamic collapse of the arytenoid cartilage in cases of laryngeal hemiplegia and some cases of laryngeal hemiparesis can be diagnosed during exercise endoscopy.

Nuclear Imaging to Evaluate Ventilation and Perfusion

Nuclear imaging techniques allow some of the functional aspects of the lungs and blood circulation to be defined. In comparison, radiographic examination provides information more related to the structural changes. Nuclear imaging involves the intravenous or aerosol administration and subsequent monitoring of a radioactive compound that has been converted to a radiopharmaceutical by labeling it with a tracer material, in order to study functional and biochemical changes.[89] The unstable isotope emits gamma rays or particles that are recorded with a special detector.

Although there are a number of isotopes of potential use, ^{99m}Tc-diaminetriaminepentaacetate (^{99m}Tc-DTPA), with an energy of 140KeV and a half-life of 6 hours, is the agent that has been used most extensively in veterinary medicine for ventilation studies.

Perfusion Studies

It is sometimes important to know how effectively the lungs are being perfused by their blood supply. The distribution of the radioactivity in the lung scan is an index of pulmonary arterial blood flow. Pulmonary perfusion in horses has been investigated by monitoring microspheres of serum albumin labeled with ^{99m}Tc-DTPA.[90,91] Perfusion has also been evaluated with ^{81m}Krypton, a radioactive gas whose elimination through the lungs also is a measure of pulmonary blood flow. However it is technically difficult to use.[92] In man, an aerosol of ^{99m}Tc-DTPA is replacing ^{81m}Kr, and its use has also been described in the horse.[91] Perfusion studies have proved to be of value in evaluating horses with exercise-induced pulmonary hemorrhage, where an abnormality of flow in arterial blood flow is thought to occur.[91]

Ventilation Studies

Ventilation studies can be carried out using nongaseous radiopharmaceuticals administered in an aerosol. It is important to use the correct nebulizer to ensure that appropriately sized droplets are delivered. A method of using this technology has been described.[93]

Airway patency and pulmonary deposition and mucociliary clearance of inhaled particles can also be evaluated using inhalation of aerosols of ^{99m}Tc-DTPA-labeled polystyrene particles.[94] Simpler equipment has been described for evaluation of mucociliary clearance.[95]

Ventilation-to-Perfusion Ratio

Ventilation and perfusion data can be combined to produce a ventilation-to-perfusion ratio, and the combined procedure, beginning with a ^{99m}Tc-DTPA ventilation scan followed by a ^{99m}Tc-macro-aggregated-albumin (^{99m}Tc-MAA) perfusion scan, is well described.[91] The combination of scans is particularly recommended for horses that display clinical evidence of lung disease but that exhibit little or no radiological abnormality, and for those with diffuse focal or generalized radiographic changes.[96]

R E F E R E N C E S

1. Crawford TB: Diagnostic virology in equine practice. *In* Proceedings of the 24th Annual Convention of the American Association of Equine Practitioners, 1978, p. 49.
2. Mair TS, Stokes CR, Bourne FJ: Cellular content of secretions obtained by lavage from different levels of the equine respiratory tract. Equine Vet J 1987; 19:458.
3. Mansmann RA, Mansmann JA: Cytology of equine nasal secretions. J Am Vet Med Assoc 1969; 154:1037.

4. Curtis RA, Viel L, McGuirk SM, et al: Lung sounds in cattle, horses, sheep, and goats. Can Vet J 1986; 27:170.

5. Kotlikoff MI, Gillespie JR: Lung sounds in veterinary medicine: Part 1. Terminology and mechanisms of sound production. Compend Contin Educ Pract Vet 1983; 5:634.

6. Kotlikoff RA, Gillespie JR: Lung sounds in veterinary medicine: Part 2. Compend Contin Educ Pract Vet 1984; 6:462.

7. Roudebush P, Sweeney CR: Thoracic percussion. J Am Vet Med Assoc 1990; 197:714.

8. Nickels FA: Nasal Cavity. In Traub-Dargatz JL, Brown CM (eds), Equine Endoscopy. St Louis, Mosby, 1990, ch 3, p 25.

9. Ruggles AJ, Ross MW, Freeman DE: Endoscopic examination of normal paranasal sinuses in horses. Vet Surg 1991; 20:418.

10. Bertone JJ: Pharynx. In Traub-Dargatz JL, Brown CM (eds): Equine Endoscopy. St Louis, Mosby, 1990, ch 4, p 33.

11. Cook WR: Specifications for speed in the racehorse. In The Airflow Factors. Menasha, WI, Russell Meerdink, 1989.

12. Caron JP: Guttural Pouch. In Traub-Dargatz JL, Brown CM (eds), Equine Endoscopy. St Louis, Mosby, 1990, ch 5, p 47.

13. Haynes PF: Larynx.In Traub-Dargatz JL, Brown CM (eds): Equine Endoscopy. St Louis, Mosby, 1990, ch 6, p 59.

14. Hackett RP: The significance of arytenoid cartilage movement. In Robinson NE (ed); Current Therapy in Equine Medicine, 3rd ed. Philadelphia, Saunders, 1992, p 285.

15. Derksen FJ: Trachea and bronchi. In Traub-Dargatz JL, Brown CM (eds), Equine Endoscopy. St Louis, Mosby, 1990, ch 7, p 75.

16. Beech J: Technique of tracheobronchial aspiration in the horse. Equine Vet J 1981; 13:136.

17. Mansmann RA, Strouss AA: Evaluation of transtracheal aspiration in the horse. J Am Vet Med Assoc 1976; 169:631.

18. Beech J: Cytology of tracheobronchial aspirates in horses. Vet Pathol 1975; 12:157.

19. Larson VL, Busch RH: Equine tracheobronchial lavage: Comparison of lavage cytologic and pulmonary histopathologic findings. Am J Vet Res 1985; 46:144.

20. Sweeney CR, Humber KA, Roby KA: Cytologic findings of tracheobronchial aspirates from 66 thoroughbred racehorses. Am J Vet Res 1992; 53:1172.

21. Schatzmann U, Straub R, Gerber H: Bronchialsekretaspiration beim Pferd. Schweiz Arch Tierheilk 1972; 8:395.

22. Sweeney CR, Beech J, Koby KA: Bacterial isolates from tracheobronchial aspirates of healthy horses. Am J Vet Res 1985; 46:2562.

23. Derksen FJ, Brown CM, Sonea I, et al: Comparison of transtracheal aspirate and bronchoalveolar lavage cytology in 50 horses with chronic lung disease. Equine Vet J 1989; 21:23.

24. Nuytten J, Muylle E, Oyaert W, et al: Cytology, bacteriology, and phagocytic capacity of tracheobronchial aspirates in healthy horses and horses with chronic obstructive pulmonary disease. Zbl Vet Med A 1983; 30:114.

25. Whitwell KE, Greet TRC: Collection and evaluation of tracheobronchial washes in the horse. Equine Vet J 1984; 16:499.

26. Sweeney CR, Sweeney RW, Benson CE: Comparison of bacteria isolated from specimens obtained by use of endoscopic guarded tracheal swabbing and percutaneous tracheal aspiration in horses. J Am Vet Med Assoc 1989; 195:1225.

27. Wimberly N, Faling LJ, Bartlett JG: A fiberoptic bronchoscopy technique to obtain uncontaminated lower airway secretions for bacterial culture. Am Rev Respir Dis 1979; 119:337.

28. Wimberly NW, Bass JB, Boyd BW, et al: Use of a broncho-scopic protected catheter brush for the diagnosis of pulmonary infections. Chest 1982; 81:556.

29. Chastre J, Fagon J-Y, Soler P, et al: Diagnosis of nosocomial bacterial pneumonia in intubated patients undergoing ventilation: Comparison of the usefulness of bronchoalveolar lavage and the protected specimen brush. Am J Med 1988; 85:499.

30. Glanville AR, Marlin GE, Harnett BJS, et al: The use of fiberoptic bronchoscopy with sterile catheter in the diagnosis of pneumonia. Aust N Z J Med 1985; 15:309.

31. Lorch DG, John JF, Tomlinson JR, et al: Protected transbronchial needle aspiration and protected specimen brush in the diagnosis of pneumonia. Am Rev Respir Dis 1987; 136:565.

32. Darien BJ, Brown CM, Walker RD, et al: A tracheoscopic technique for obtaining uncontaminated lower airway secretions for bacterial culture in the horse. Equine Vet J 1990; 22:170.

33. Zink MC, Johnson JA: Cellular constituents of clinically normal foal bronchoalveolar lavage fluid during postnatal maturation. Am J Vet Res 1984; 45:893.

34. McKane SA, Canfield PJ, Rose RJ: Equine bronchoalveolar lavage cytology: Survey of thoroughbred racehorses in training. Aust Vet J 1993; 70:401.

35. Vrins A, Doucet M, Nunez-Ochoa L: A retrospective study of bronchoalveolar lavage cytology in horses with clinical findings of small airway disease. J Vet Med A 1991; 38:472.

36. Fogarty U: Evaluation of a bronchoalveolar lavage technique. Equine Vet J 1990; 22:174.

37. Winder NC, Grünig G, Hermann M, et al: Comparison of bronchoalveolar lavage and respiratory secretion cytology in horses with histologically diagnosed pulmonary disease. Schweiz Arch Tierheilk 1991; 133:123.

38. Rossier Y, Sweeney CR, Ziemer EL: Bronchoalveolar lavage fluid cytologic findings in horses with pneumonia or pleuropneumonia. J Am Vet Med Assoc 1991; 198:1001.

39. Sweeney CR, Rossier Y, Ziemer EL: Effects of lung site and fluid volume on results of bronchoalveolar lavage fluid analysis in horses. Am J Vet Res 1992; 53:1376.

40. Farrow CS: Radiography of the equine thorax: Anatomy and technique. Vet Radiol 1981; 22:62.

41. King GK, Martens RJ, McCall VH: Equine thoracic radiography: Part I. Air-gap rare earth radiography of the normal equine thorax. Compend Contin Educ Prac Vet 1981; 3:S278.

42. Lamb CR: Aspects of diagnostic imaging in equine pulmonary disease. Vet Ann 1989; 29:127.

43. Lamb CR, O'Callaghan MW: Diagnostic imaging of equine pulmonary disease. Compend Contin Educ Pract Vet 1989; 11:1110.

44. Martens RJ, Ruoff WW, Renshaw HW: Foal pneumonia: A practical approach to diagnosis and therapy. Compend Contin Educ Pract Vet 1982; 4:S361, and S374.

45. King GK: Equine thoracic radiography: Part II. Radiographic patterns of equine pulmonary and pleural diseases using air-gap rare earth radiology. Compend Contin Educ Pract Vet 1981; 3:S283.

46. O'Callaghan MW, Sanderson GN: Clinical bronchography in the horse: Development of a method using barium sulphate powder. Equine Vet J 1982; 14:282.

47. O'Callaghan MW, Goulden BR: Radiographic changes in the lungs of horses with exercise-induced epistaxis. N Z Vet J 1982; 30:117.

48. Rantanen NW: Diseases of the thorax. In Diagnostic ultrasound. Vet Clin North Am: Equine Pract 1986; 2:49.

49. Rantanen NW. Ultrasound appearance of normal lung borders and surrounding viscera in the horse. Vet Radiol 1981; 22:217.

50. Stadler P. Ultraschalluntersuchung des Thorax beim Pferd. Pferdeheilkunde 1990; 6:213.

51. Pipers FS, Reef VB: Thoracic ultrasound in the equine: A compilation of a decade of experience. *In* Proceedings of the 37th Annual Convention of the American Association of Equine Practitioners, 1991, p 351.

52. Raphel CF, Beech J: Pleuritis and pleural effusion in the horse. *In* Proceedings of the 27th Annual Convention of the American Association of Equine Practitioners, 1981, p 17.

53. Wagner AE, Bennett DG: Analysis of equine thoracic fluid. Vet Clin Pathol 1983; 11:13.

54. Cowell RL, Tyler RD, Clinkenbeard KD, et al: Collection and evaluation of equine peritoneal and pleural effusions. Vet Clin North Am: Equine Pract 1987; 3:543.

55. Mansmann RA, Bernard-Strother S: Pleuroscopy in horses. Mod Vet Prac 1985; 66:9.

56. Mackey VS, Wheat JD: Endoscopic examination of the equine thorax. Equine Vet J 1985; 17:140.

57. Raphel CF, Gunson DE: Percutaneous lung biopsy in the horse. Cornell Vet 1981; 71:439.

58. Willoughby RA, McDonell WN: Pulmonary function testing in horses. Vet Clin North Amer: Large Animal Pract; 1979; 1:171.

59. Spörri H, Leeman W: Zur Untersuchung der Lungenmechanik bei Grosstieren. Schweizer Archiv Tierheilk 1964; 106:699.

60. Woakes AJ, Butler PJ, Snow DH: The measurement of respiratory airflow in exercising horses. *In* Gillespie JR, Robinson NE (eds): Equine Exercise Physiology 2. Proceedings of the Second International Conference on Equine Exercise Physiology. Davis, CA, ICEEP Publication, 1987, p 194.

61. McDonell WN, Hall LW: Functional residual capacity in conscious and anesthetized horses. Brit J Anesthesiol 1974; 46:802.

62. Muylle E, Oyaert W: Lung function tests in obstructive pulmonary disease in horses. Equine Vet J 1973; 5:37.

63. Gallivan GJ, McDonell WN, Forrest JB: Comparative pulmonary mechanics in the horse and the cow. Res Vet Sci 1989; 46:322.

64. Garner HE, Rosborough JP, Amen JF, et al: Normal ventilation and acid base values in the laboratory pony. Cardiovasc Res Center Bull 1971; 9:160.

65. Derksen FJ, Robinson NE: Esophageal and intrapleural pressures in the healthy conscious pony. Amer J Vet Res 1980; 41:1756.

66. Speirs VC, Tschudi PR, Gerber H: Druck-und Strömungsverhältnisse in den oberen Luftwegen des Pferdes bei partiellen Obstruktionen. Schweiz Archiv Tierheilk 1981; 123:293.

67. Mansgeth G: Evaluation of tracheal pressure in the running horse. *In* Proceedings of the 4th Annual Meeting of the Association for Equine Sports Med, 1984, p 74.

68. Derksen FJ, Stick JA, Scott EA, et al: Effects of laryngeal hemiplegia and laryngoplasty on airway flow mechanics in exercising horses. Amer J Vet Res 1986; 47:16.

69. Holm K, Funkquist B, Obel N: Clinical method for evaluation of upper airway function. *In* Persson SGB, Lindholm A, Jeffcott LB (eds): Equine Exercise Physiology 3. Proceedings of the Third International Conference on Equine Exercise Physiology. Davis, CA, ICEEP Publications, 1991, p 449.

70. Funkquist B, Holm K, Karlsson A, et al: Studies on the intratracheal pressure in the exercising horse. J Vet Med A 1988; 35:424.

71. Holm K: Recording of intratracheal pressure in the horse under field conditions as a method for evaluation of upper airway resistance. J Vet Med A 1993; 40:516.

72. Williams JW, Pascoe JR, Meagher DM, et al: Effects of left recurrent laryngeal neurectomy, prosthetic laryngoplasty, and subtotal arytenoidectomy on upper airway pressure during maximal exertion. Vet Surg 1990; 19:136.

73. Nielan GJ, Rehder RS, Ducharme NG, et al: Measurement of tracheal static pressure in exercising horses. Vet Surg 1992; 21:423.

74. Young SS, Hall LW: A rapid, non-invasive method for measuring total respiratory impedence in the horse. Equine Vet J 1989; 21:99.

75. Hiedenstierna G, Nyman G, Kvart C, et al: Ventilation-perfusion relationships in the standing horse: An inert gas elimination study. Equine Vet J 1987; 19:514.

76. Amis TC, Pascoe JR, Hornof W, et al: Topographic distribution of pulmonary ventilation and perfusion in the horse. Am J Vet Res 1984; 45:1597.

77. O'Callaghan MW, Hornof WJ, Fisher PE, et al: Exercise-induced pulmonary hemorrhage in the horse: Results of a detailed clinical, post mortem and imaging study: VI. Ventilation/perfusion scintigraphy in horses with EIPH. Equine Vet J 1987; 19:423.

78. Rossdale PD: Some parameters of respiratory function in normal and abnormal foals with special reference to levels of PaO_2 during air and O_2 inhalation. Res Vet Sci 1970; 11:270.

79. Hörnicke H, Weber M, Schweiker W: Pulmonary ventilation in thoroughbred horses at maximal performance. *In* Gillespie JR, Robinson NE (eds), Equine Exercise Physiology 2. Proceedings of the Second International Conference on Equine Exercise Physiology. Davis, CA, ICEEP Publications, 1987, p 216.

80. Morris E: Application of clinical exercise testing for identification of respiratory fitness and disease in the equine athlete. Veterinary Clinics of North America: Equine Pract 1991; 7:383.

81. Rose RJ, Hodgson DR: Clinical exercise testing. *In* Hodgson DR, Rose RJ (eds), The Athletic Horse. Philadelphia, Saunders, 1994, p 245.

82. Holm-Roethlisberger K: Transtracheal Pressure Recording in the Exercising Horse. Doctoral Dissertation, Swedish University of Agricultural Sciences, Uppsala, 1995.

83. Williams JW, Meagher DM, Pascoe JR, et al: Upper airway function during maximal exercise in horses with obstructive upper airway lesions. Effect of surgical treatment. Vet Surg 1990; 19:142.

84. Lumsden JM, Derksen FJ, Stick JA: Evaluation of upper airway obstruction in exercising horses using flow-volume loops. Abstract ACVS 1992; Vet Surg 21:396.

85. Bayly WM, Schulz DE, Hodgson DR, et al: Ventilatory response to exercise in horses with exercise-induced hypoxemia. *In* Gillespie JR, Robinson NE (eds), Equine Exercise Physiology 2. Proceedings of the Second International Conference on Equine Exercise Physiology. Davis, CA. ICEEP publications, 1987, p 172.

86. Bayly WM, Grant BD, Modransky PD: Arterial blood gas tensions during exercise in a horse with laryngeal hemiplegia, before and after corrective surgery. Res Vet Sci 1984; 36:256.

87. Soma LR, Beech J, Gerber NH: Effects of cromolyn in horses with chronic obstructive pulmonary disease. Vet Res Comm 1987; 11:339.

88. Morris E: Dynamic evaluation of the equine upper respiratory tract. Vet Clin North Am Equine Prac 1991; 7:403.

89. Clarke AF: Nuclear imaging of the equine lung. Vet Annual 1988; 28:103.

90. Staddon GE, Weaver BMQ: Regional pulmonary perfusion in horses: A comparison between anesthetized and conscious animals. Res Vet Sci 1981; 30:44.

91. O'Callaghan MW, Hornof WM, Fisher PE, et al: Exercised-induced pulmonary hemorrhage in the horse: Results of a detailed clinical, post mortem, and imaging study. VII.

Ventilation and perfusion scintigraphy in horses with EIPH. Equine Vet J 1987; 12:423.

92. Amis TC, Pascoe JR, Hornof W, et al: Topographic distribution of pulmonary ventilation and perfusion in the horse. Am J Vet Res 1984; 45:1597.

93. O'Callaghan MW, Hornof WM, Fisher PE, et al: Ventilation imaging in the horse with 99mTechnetium-DTPA aerosol: Development of a method. Equine Vet J 1987; 19:19.

94. Clarke AF: A review of environmental and host factors in relation to equine respiratory disease. Equine Vet J 1987; 19:435.

95. Nelson R, Hampe DW: Measurement of tracheal mucous transport rate in the horse. Am J Vet Res 1983; 44:1165.

96. O'Callaghan MW: Nuclear imaging techniques for equine respiratory disease. Vet Clin North Am: Equine Pract 1991; 7:417.

The Nervous System

NERVOUS SYSTEM COMPONENTS

In broad terms the nervous system is divided topographically into central and peripheral components with superimposition of the autonomic system. Functionally, the nervous system is divided into sensory, central, and motor regions. The sensory section contains the afferent components, which, through a range of different receptors and sensory nerves and reflex arcs, are responsible for sensing the external and internal environment and transmitting the data to the central region for integration in the spinal cord and brain. Responses to the incoming data are executed through the motor, or efferent, system consisting of motor nerves, their endplates, and effector organs.

The motor system is subdivided into autonomic and somatic motor systems. The autonomic system comprises a system of opposing sympathetic and parasympathetic subdivisions that is dispersed throughout the nervous system and is responsible for the involuntary control of visceral function. This section of the system is not greatly involved in the general neurological examination. The somatic portion is also known as the voluntary motor system (contrasting with the involuntary system just mentioned), which, from a functional point of view, is considered to consist of an upper motor neuron (UMN) and a lower motor neuron (LMN). In reality both "neurons" consist of more than one component. The LMN consists of the motor neuron, its axon, and its terminal connections in the muscle. The LMN can be a ventral horn cell located in the spinal cord or the motor nerve cell of a cranial nerve located centrally. The UMN is the motor nerve cell in the cortex concerned with voluntary movement, and its impulses are transmitted through cranial or more distal spinal neurons. To initiate voluntary movement, the UMN, which is located in the brain, stimulates the LMN distributed in the brain stem and the ventral horn of the spinal cord, whose response is then transmitted to skeletal muscle of the head and body in the cranial and peripheral nerves, respectively, via the terminal axons. Each motor unit consists of the LMN and the muscle that it innervates. To facilitate evaluation, the central nervous system is also divided into sections:

- Brain
- C_1–C_5, upper cervical spinal cord segments
- C_6–T_2, spinal cord segments of the brachial enlargement
- T_3–L_3, thoracic and lumbar spinal cord segments
- L_4–S_2, spinal cord segments of the pelvic enlargement
- S_3–S_5, spinal cord segments supplying the rectum, anus, and bladder
- Co_1–Co_5, spinal cord segments supplying the tail

MANIFESTATIONS OF NERVOUS SYSTEM DISEASE

Although disease of the nervous system can result in higher body temperature, bacteremia, septicemia, pain, and involvement of adjacent organs, its dominant role in controlling various functions means that the major signs of disease will be an alteration or loss of function. Variation in function is therefore an important guide to the location of a lesion. Evaluating function requires an understanding of how the UMN and the LMN interact, as well as the ability to recognize the clinical signs associated with variation in function for each motor unit. Using this approach a lesion can be localized to a specific part of the system. This concept works best for solitary lesions, but often a process is distributed through the system either as a continuous lesion (diffuse) or as a series of focal lesions (multicentric). The LMN consists of a sensory component in an organ that communicates with the motor neuron in the local spinal cord and then communicates with an effector muscle via the axon. This is known as a *reflex arc*, whereby a sensory input can elicit an immediate response without traveling to the brain. There is a constant interaction between the LMN systems controlling opposing muscle groups (e.g., flexor and extensor muscles) that are, in normal circumstances, under the influence of the UMN, which in turn maintains an inhibitory control over the local reflex. Signs of UMN disease are related to loss of this inhibition, tending to cause increased activity in the end organ. This contrasts with a LMN lesion, which causes a reduction or loss of function seen generally as a loss of tone.

GENERAL PHYSICAL EXAMINATION

The objectives of an examination of the nervous system are first to establish whether there is any disease process present and then, if there is, to localize it in the nervous system. As stated, a thorough understanding of neuroanatomy and of the functional aspects of the nervous system is required. Although any systematic examination would be suitable, an initial objective should be to localize the lesion to one or more of the following regions, listed from cranial to caudal in accordance with the general overall progression of the examination:

- Cerebrum
- Brain stem
- Cerebellum
- Spinal cord
- Peripheral nerves and muscles

The cranial to caudal progression of the examination is based on the similar progression of neurological control from higher to lower.

Before a detailed and specific examination is made of the nervous system, a general clinical examination should be carried out, partly to detect the presence of disease in the other body systems and partly to detect the presence of disease that can produce secondary neurological signs. Hypoxia, anoxia, hypo-, and hyperglycemia, hepatopathy, uremia, hypocalcemia, hyper- and hypokalemia, acidosis, alkalosis, and hypo- and hyperthermia are often associated with neurological abnormalities. The following method for examination of the nervous system is drawn from published data.[1,2]

Head

Behavior

Abnormal behavior indicates malfunction of the cerebral cortex. A knowledge of normal behavior is necessary before one can identify abnormal behavior. Frequently recognized variations in behavior include head pressing, circling, licking, and changes in voice, appetite, and aggression. Aspects of normal behavior that the clinician must be familiar with include:

RESPONSE TO AN UPPER MOTOR NEURON LESION

- Reduced or absent voluntary movement (hyporeflexia, areflexia).
- Normal or exaggerated reflex response (hyperreflexia).
- Increased muscle tone (hypertonic), mild disuse atrophy
- Loss of proprioception and pain (hypoalgesia, analgesia)

RESPONSE TO A LOWER MOTOR NEURON

- Reduced or absent voluntary movement
- Reduced or absent reflex response
- Reduced (hypotonic) or absent muscle tone (atonic)
- Loss of proprioception and pain, severe muscle atrophy

- How horses react to people and other horses. Inability to maintain social rank may indicate illness or weakness. The development of aggression with a compulsion to attack is a sign of rabies.
- How horses relax when undisturbed.
- How much time is devoted to eating and sleeping.
- How often can one expect to see a horse lying down, and in which position it is most likely to be.
- Normal behavior of stallions and mares. Stallions are often more aggressive than mares and geldings, which must not be confused with development of aggression in an otherwise quiet individual. Aggression and a general cantankerous disposition are signs often associated with hormonal imbalance related to ovarian tumors or retained testicles.

Mental Status

Abnormalities in mental status indicate an involvement of the brain stem and lesser cerebral cortex. Mental status can be equated to an animal's state of awareness and reflects the functional capacity of the ascending reticular activating system in the brain stem as well as certain parts of the cerebral cortex. Normally, these systems respond to sensory inputs in the form of visual, tactile, auditory, olfactory, and gustatory stimuli. Mental status varies from normal through a series of minor stages of abnormality (stupor, depression, somnolence, delirium, lethargy, and depression) to coma and semicoma. Coma is present when there is no response to normal stimuli, and semicoma defines a state with no response to normal stimuli but with a response to excessive or noxious stimuli.

Head Posture and Coordination

Normal smooth coordinated movements of the head are under the control of the cerebrum, cerebellum, and vestibular system. Normal head motion involves various combinations of lateral flexion, rotation, and extension of the atlanto-occipital joint. An abnormal position may be due to pain from a fracture or infection. Vestibular lesions often cause a rotation characterized by head tilt with the poll deviated to one side but with the muzzle and neck remaining in the midline. Lesions of the cerebrum on the other hand may cause the horse to circle and show deviation of head and neck toward the side of the lesion, but the muzzle is not rotated around the poll. Cerebellar lesions interfere with normal coordination and fine control of movement, resulting in jerky movements during voluntary motion and a fine tremor when at rest, known as an intention tremor.

Head posture and coordination can be evaluated during normal activity. If some food is held beside the shoulder on either side, the horse will usually flex its head in order to take it in the mouth (prehend) (Fig. 4-1). The animal should be evaluated while at rest to detect tremors or abnormal head posture. The position of the poll in relation to the muzzle should be carefully evaluated.

Evaluation of Cranial Nerve Function

Localizing a lesion in the brain stem is facilitated by a close examination of the cranial nerves. As with the other components of the exam it is logical to proceed in a cranial to caudal direction.

EVALUATION OF SMELL (CRANIAL NERVE I, OLFACTORY NERVE). It is extremely difficult to evaluate smell in horses, and a deficit in this sense (anosmia) is consequently rarely reported. A crude assessment of smell can be made by noting how a horse smells such things as food, the clinician's hand, feces, or urine, the latter being a better test in stallions.

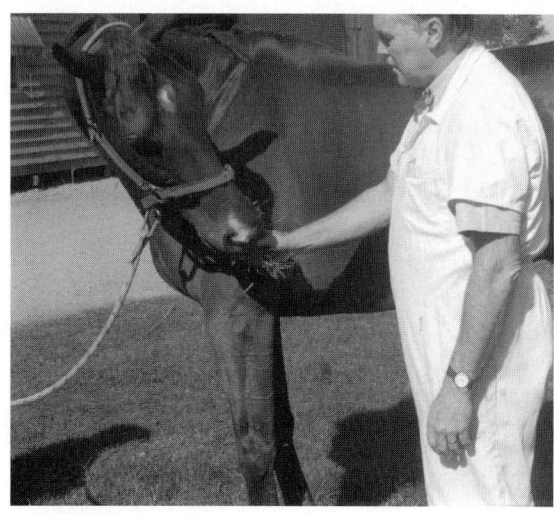

▶ FIGURE 4-1

Testing the ability to flex head and neck laterally by holding food adjacent to the shoulder.

EVALUATION OF VISION (CRANIAL NERVE II, OPTIC NERVE). Vision is tested by the menace reflex, in which a threatening gesture made toward the eye will usually elicit closure of the eyelid and sometimes withdrawal of the head (Fig. 4-2). Care should be taken to avoid causing air currents that can be sensed by the horse and that can result in a similar response. The reflex can be absent in depressed or excited horses and neonatal foals and can also become refractory if repeated too often. In the horse, as a result of almost complete crossover (decussation) at the optic chiasm, vision in one eye is controlled mainly in the contralateral cerebral hemisphere. The afferent pathway therefore involves first the retina, optic nerve, and optic chiasm, and then after decussation the contralateral optic tract, lateral geniculate nucleus, optic radiation, and occipital cortex. The efferent pathway involves the ipsilateral facial nerve nucleus, which provides a motor response that ends with closure of the eyelids. Lesions of the retina and optic nerve will therefore produce ipsilateral blindness, while

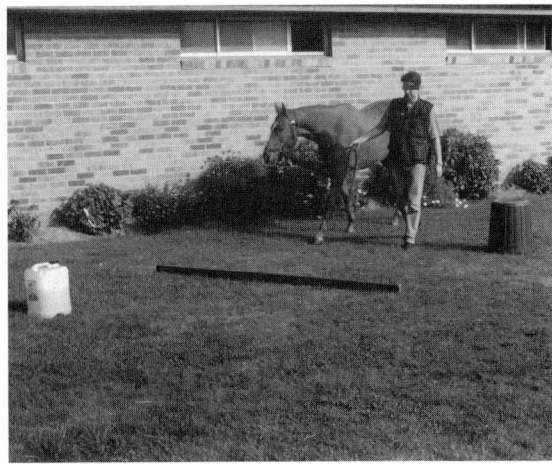

▶ FIGURE 4-3

Obstacle course to test for vision. Note that the attendant is allowing the horse to choose where it walks.

lesions located more centrally will cause contralateral blindness.

Tests for vision include the ability to follow a moving light or object and to negotiate an obstacle course (Fig. 4-3). Careful observation while the horse is eating or moving about, especially if in a strange environment, may allow blindness or poor vision to be detected. Unilateral blindness or poor vision are much harder to detect and may require blindfolding (Fig. 4-4).

EVALUATION OF PUPILLARY LIGHT REFLEX (CRANIAL NERVES 2, OPTIC NERVE, AND III, OCULOMOTOR NERVE). The size of the pupil depends on the balance between the constrictor muscles, innervated by parasympathetic fibers in the oculomotor nerves, and the dilator muscles, innervated by sympathetic fibers from the cranial cervical ganglion. The pupillary light reflex tests the function of the optic and oculomotor nerves simultaneously, whereby the neural impulses produced in response to a beam of light directed into the eye reach the brain through the optic nerve, are integrated in the pretectal region of the contralateral midbrain, and then bilaterally activate the parasympathetic component of the oculomotor nerves to make both pupils constrict. Constriction in the ipsilateral eye is known as the direct response, and constriction in the contralateral eye is the consensual response. The pathway for the response to a beam of light directed into one eye is shown in Figure 4-5. Before carrying out the test, each eye should be examined to ensure that there are no lesions, such as adhesions, that could mechanically interfere with

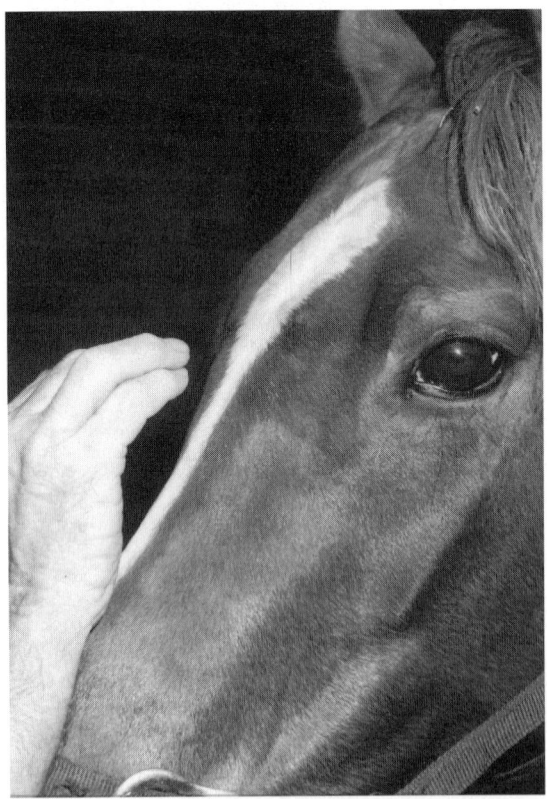

▶ FIGURE 4-2

The menace reflex. Fingers are directed quickly toward the eye, taking care to avoid contact or producing air currents.

constriction. The pupillary light reflex does not involve the visual cortex, and therefore the reflex can be positive in a horse with blindness resulting from damage to this region.

Malfunction of the sympathetic nerve supply to the eye produces a syndrome known as Horner's Syndrome consisting of pupillary constriction (miosis), drooping of the upper eyelid (ptosis), and protrusion of the nictitating membrane. There are also nonocular signs such as dilation of facial blood vessels, hyperemia of nasal and conjunctival mucosae, and sweating on the affected side of the head and neck.

EVALUATION OF EYE POSITION (CRANIAL NERVES III, OCULOMOTOR NERVE IV, TROCHLEA NERVE; AND VI, ABDUCENS NERVE).

Eye position is actively controlled by the four rectus muscles, the two oblique muscles, and the retractor bulbi muscles. The position can also be altered by space-occupying lesions within the orbit (abscess, neoplasia) that can produce deviation or displacement. The only eye muscles not innervated by the oculomotor nerve are the lateral rectus and retractor bulbi muscles, supplied by the abducens nerve (cranial nerve VI) and the dorsal oblique muscle, supplied by the trochlear nerve (cranial nerve IV).

The function of these muscles and nerves is evaluated by noting the positions of the eyes within the orbits and also the movement of each eye. Abnormal position is called strabismus, and abnormal movement is known as nystagmus. Before abnormal movement can be evaluated, normal eye movements must be understood. When a horse's head is elevated, the eyes tend to remain in the horizontal position and in doing so rotate ventrally in the orbits. Likewise, when the head moves to one side, the eyes shift rhythmically toward the new location in a series of small movements rather than staying in the middle of the orbit and moving with the head. This latter activity is normal vestibular nystagmus or the oculocephalic reflex and is the result of interplay between the centers controlling balance (vestibular nucleii) and the nerves responsible for eye movement. Examples of true strabismus are rare in horses, but when present the close anatomic association of nerves controlling eye movement usually means that all nerves are affected to some extent. Strabismus associated with damage to these nerves should be present regardless of head position, whereas eyes with nystagmus associated with vestibular damage can be moved and will respond to head movement.

ABILITY TO CHEW (CRANIAL NERVE V). The motor nerve fibers to the muscles of mastication are carried in the trigeminal nerve. Bilateral damage to this nerve reduces the effectiveness of chewing, whereas paralysis causes an inability to close the jaw. Atrophy of the masseter, temporal muscles, and the distal belly of the digastric muscle follows. Unilateral damage produces weak jaw tone and unilateral atrophy.

EVALUATION OF FACIAL CUTANEOUS SENSATION (CRANIAL NERVE V). The sensory nerve fibers from most of the head are carried in the mandibular, maxillary, and ophthalmic branches of the trigeminal nerve. Function of these sensory branches is tested by observing responses to stimulation. Movement of the eyelids, ear, and lips in response to gentle pricking tests the sensory branches as well as the motor component of the facial nerve, although conscious appreciation of the stimulus is not necessary. Each branch

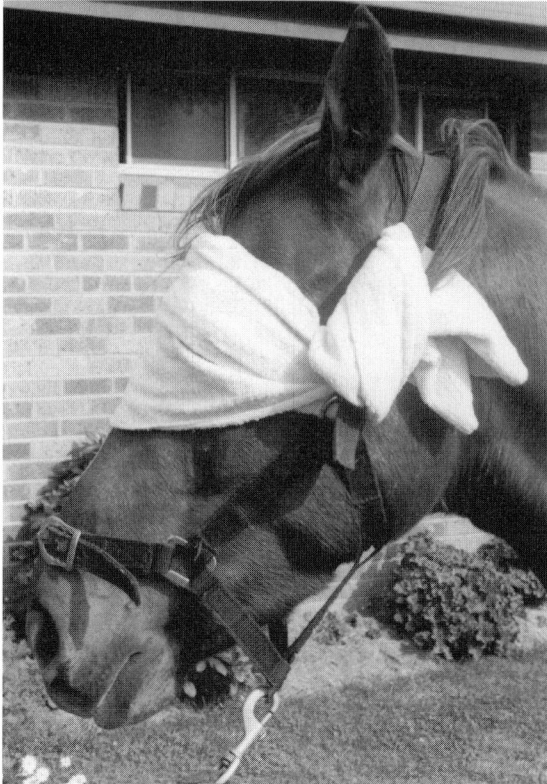

▶ FIGURE 4-4
A blindfold in place. Ensure that the eyes are adequately covered and that the horse cannot see through or around the edges of the blindfold.

can be tested by testing the area of distribution of each (Fig. 4-6).

EVALUATION OF FACIAL SYMMETRY AND MOVEMENT (CRANIAL NERVE VII). The muscles responsible for facial symmetry and expression are controlled by motor fibers in the facial nerve. First the head should be checked for loss of muscle tone, usually appreciated as a unilateral asymmetry involving the eyelid, ear or lips, and then the ability to move these structures in response to provocation tests. Facial paralysis is usually characterized by drooping of the ear and lips, incomplete elevation of the upper eyelid,

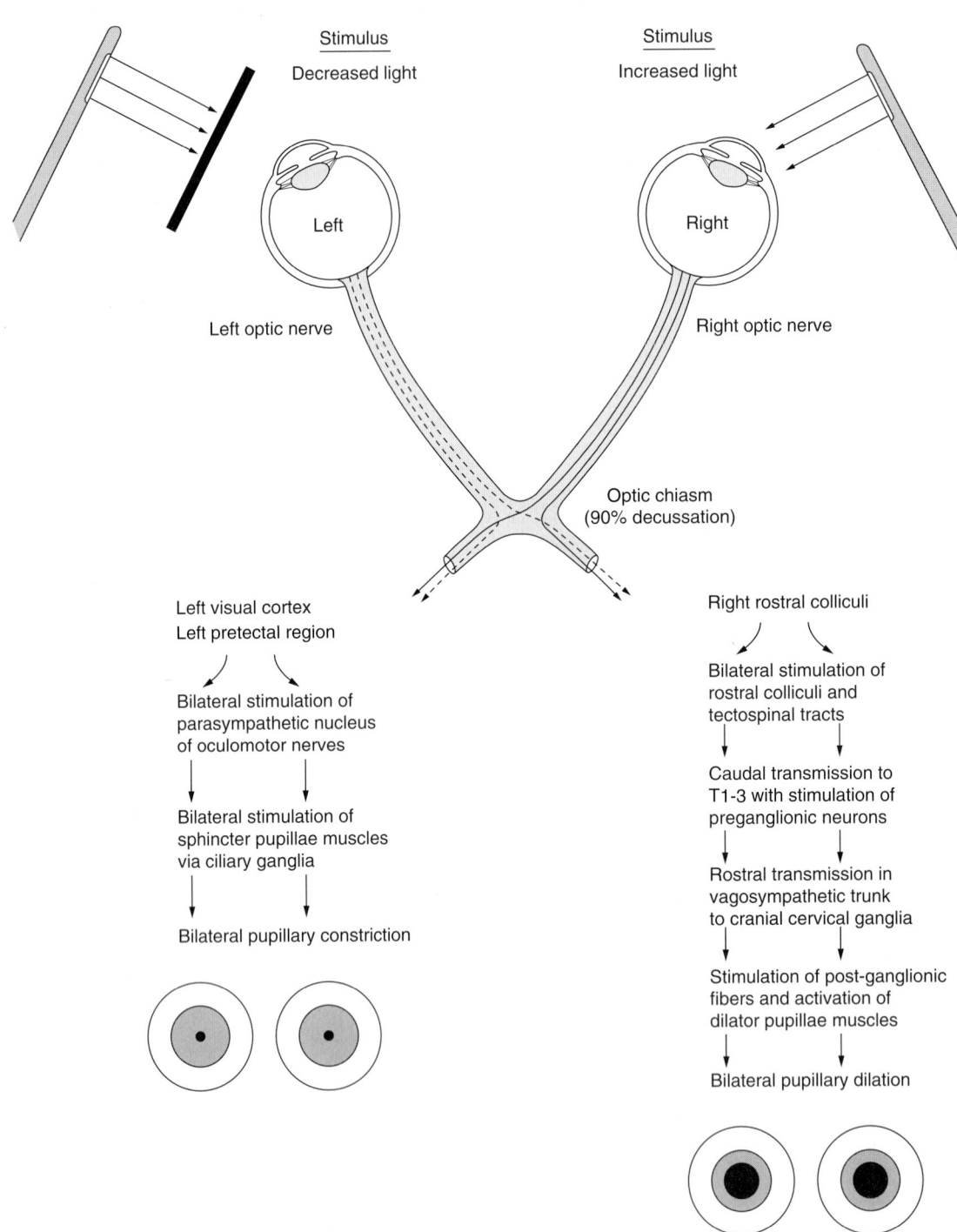

▶ **FIGURE 4-5**

Pathways involved in the pupillary light reflex.

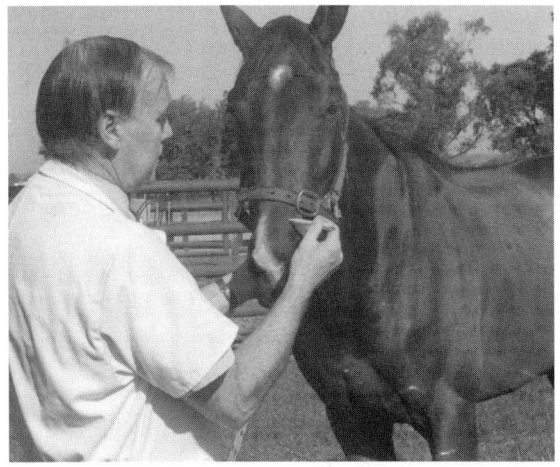

▶ **FIGURE 4-6**
Testing cutaneous sensation (cranial nerve V).

deviation of the muzzle to the unaffected side, and inability to open the nostril. The location of the nerve damage determines which structures are affected. A proximal lesion affects function of all structures innervated by the nerve, whereas a distal lesion involving the buccal branches will affect only the function of the lips.

EVALUATION OF HEARING (COCHLEAR OR AUDITORY BRANCH OF CRANIAL NERVE VIII). Unilateral hearing loss is difficult to detect, and for this reason clinically apparent deafness, which is rare, is usually bilateral. Otitis media-interna is the usual cause.

EVALUATION OF BALANCE (VESTIBULAR DIVISION OF CRANIAL NERVE VIII). This division of the 8th nerve provides the major input to the vestibular system, which is in turn responsible for balance and functions by controlling the orientation of the head, body, limbs, and eyes. Malfunction of the system is indicated by nystagmus, head tilt, limb weakness, and loss of balance.

Nystagmus refers to a rhythmic oscillation of the eye and occurs with the head in normal position (spontaneous nystagmus) or in different abnormal positions (positional nystagmus).[3] Movement may be horizontal, vertical, or rotary, with the nystagmus being described by the direction of the fast phase of movement. The direction of the fast phase can be used to help localize a lesion. For example, a peripheral lesion always produces nystagmus with the fast phase directed away from the side of the lesion. Some improvement in the clinical condition follows accommodation to vestibular disease, however this can be abolished or reduced by blindfolding.

When a head tilt is present, the head is rotated and flexed toward the side of the lesion, and the ipsilateral eye is deviated downward and the contralateral eye upward.[3] This is associated with a stumbling gait and circling toward the side of the lesion. Weakness of the ipsilateral limb and increased extensor tone of the contralateral limb occur as a result of loss of vestibulospinal tract control.

EVALUATION OF PREHENSION. Prehension, or the transfer of food into the mouth, involves a coordinated activity from the lips and jaws as well as central coordination from the basal nuclei that coordinate the motor activity of basic functions such as eating and drinking. Nigropallidal encephalomalacia, caused by yellow star thistle toxicity *(Centaurea solstitialis),* affects the basal nuclei and causes inability to prehend food or to masticate or move food to the back of the mouth. Malfunction of the facial nerve with paralysis of the lips renders prehension difficult, but a horse soon learns to move food into the mouth by pushing its head into the food and picking it up with the teeth, rather like a carnivore. In both these conditions swallowing is not affected and once food or water are in the mouth, normal swallowing can occur.

Abnormal or difficult prehension due to neurological disease should be differentiated from abnormality due to painful lesions such as fracture, lingual foreign body, or retropharyngeal abscess. Prehension can be assessed by hand-feeding the horse and by feeding it from a hard flat surface.

EVALUATION OF SWALLOWING (CRANIAL NERVES IX AND X). The glossopharyngeal and vagus nerves innervate the muscles that control swallowing. Normal swallowing involves the transport of food and water from the oropharynx to the esophagus without contamination of the larynx or nasopharynx. Malfunction of this process results in feed or water draining from the nose, the presence of food or water in the airway perhaps with aspiration into the lungs, and dribbling of saliva from the nose and mouth. There may be a total or partial inability to swallow. These abnormalities are easy to see. However, they should not be confused with esophageal obstruction or cleft soft palate, which may present with identical signs. Passage of a stomach tube will not only detect an obstruction but will also demonstrate an inability to swallow.

Endoscopy will both clarify palatal defects and help to evaluate esophageal patency. Contrast radiography may also be of use. Because of the extensive involvement of the vagus nerve in larynx, pharynx, and gastrointestinal tract function, abnormal function of this nerve is also associated with exercise intolerance.

The easiest and best way to detect swallowing abnormality is to observe the horse carefully while it is eating and drinking. Minor degrees of abnormality may go unobserved as a cough may not be stimulated, and there may be insufficient material to pass quickly to the external nares. This applies particularly if the horse is drinking from ground level when water can pass into the larynx and then out again without stimulating a significant cough reflex.

EVALUATION OF TONGUE FUNCTION (CRANIAL NERVE XII). The motor innervation to the tongue is from the hypoglossal nerve. Lesions of this nerve produce a loss of function of the tongue on the affected side. If the loss is unilateral, the tongue will deviate to the unaffected side and will be weak and eventually exhibit atrophy. If it is bilateral, the tongue cannot be drawn into the mouth. Painful lesions in the tongue (foreign body) can mimic the effects of paralysis. Weakness is easily detected by gently applying traction to the tongue (Fig. 4-7).

Gait and Posture

Lesions of the spinal cord, peripheral nervous system, muscles, and brain stem may cause abnormalities of gait and posture. The objectives of gait and postural analysis are to decide whether an abnormality exists and, if so, its localization. Lesions may be focal, diffuse, or multicentric, with clinical signs usually being caudal to the site of the lesion. Signs are usually bilaterally symmetrical, although some diseases are characterized by asymmetric involvement of the limbs.

Posture

The horse should be evaluated while at rest to note any postural abnormality. Horses standing with normal posture have the limbs positioned squarely beneath the body, although, when relaxed, a limb may be positioned with the fetlock in flexion and the hoof resting with the toe or cranial surface of the hoof touching the ground. Standing with limbs widely spaced may indicate weakness (paresis) or a lack of *proprioception* (ability to know the location in space of limbs).

Gait

The horse should be examined walking, trotting, being forced to move in a small circle, and backing. Other tests include walking across or up and down a hill or slope, negotiating an obstacle course, or being forced to walk in a wending path (see Chapter 5 for details on lameness examination). The abnormal gait should be localized to a limb(s) and described according to whether there is weakness, ataxia, spasticity, or dysmetria.

WEAKNESS, OR PARESIS. Weakness, or *paresis,* is characterized by signs such as dragging of the limbs with increased wear on the toe or cranial surface of the hoof, stumbling, falling down, and knuckling of the fetlock.

ATAXIA. *Ataxia* is the term used to describe loss of proprioception, or the ability to identify the spatial relationships between limbs. Signs caused by loss of proprioception include swaying movements, asymmetric foot placement, crossing of limbs, stepping on the opposite limbs, and circumduction of the outside limb when turning quickly.

SPASTICITY. *Spasticity* is characterized by stiff movements with little joint flexion and occurs when there is loss of upper motor neuron control over the lower motor neuron.

DYSMETRIA. Dysmetria is used to describe loss of control over the direction and range of limb movement and is characterized by overreaching,

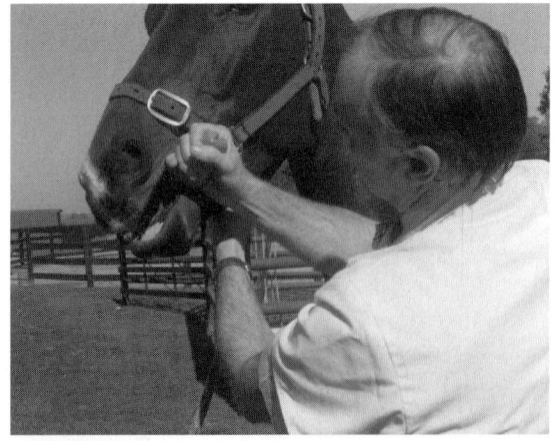

▶ **FIGURE 4-7**

Testing tongue tone. The horse's ability to retract the tongue is tested by pulling it gently from the mouth.

GRADING OF GAIT ABNORMALITY RELATED TO SPINAL CORD DISEASE

- *Grade 0 (normal).* No visible neurological abnormality
- *Grade 1.* Neurological abnormality barely detectable at a normal gait, but provoked by forcing the horse to back, turn, sway from side to side, and by extending the neck and applying pressure to the lumbar region
- *Grade 2.* Neurological abnormality detectable at normal gaits and greatly exaggerated by the provocation tests listed in 2
- *Grade 3.* Neurological deficits very obvious at normal gaits with a tendency to fall or stumble during the provocation tests
- *Grade 4.* Spontaneous stumbling and falling to the ground extending to complete paralysis

hypermetria (excessive movement), hypometria (decreased movement), and long or short stride.

To facilitate recording and comparison among animals or of the same animal at different stages, each limb can be graded individually using a scale of 0 to 4, as shown in the box.

Neck and Forelimbs

Examination and Palpation

Careful visual examination and palpation will detect asymmetry and muscle atrophy that may indicate neurological disease, obvious skeletal defects such as the congenital deformity seen often in Arabian horses, and localized sweating associated with damage to the sympathetic innervation.

Neck Mobility

Inability or reluctance to move the head and neck in any direction usually indicates a painful or mechanical lesion. Mobility can be tested by manual manipulation of the head and neck or by encouraging the horse to move its head and neck by tempting it with some feed, such as grass, held in the hand. It is particularly useful to hold the food on the left and right sides of the body in the region of the elbow joint (Fig. 4-1).

Neck and Forelimb Reflexes

CERVICAL RESPONSES. Stimulation of the skin on the lateral aspect of the neck, dorsal to the jugular groove, usually elicits contraction of the cutaneous muscle seen as twitching of the skin, contraction of the brachiocephalic muscle, and, when the test is performed in the cranial region, twitching of the ear. Sharp focal stimulation can be performed with a pin, needle, hemostats, or a ballpoint pen (Fig. 4-8).

CEREBRAL RESPONSES. Conscious appreciation of a stimulus in this region, applied as described, is under cerebral control, and awareness of the stimulus may be manifest by responses such as calling out, moving away, attempting to escape, head shaking, or biting.

SWAY REACTION. This test is made with the horse standing still and also walking, and it consists of attempting to push the horse sideways (Fig. 4-9). Evaluation involves assessing the horse's resistance to being pushed or pulled laterally, as well as checking to see whether the horse stumbles. The test is useful for detecting weakness and ataxia. The horse can be pushed at the shoulder and also pulled laterally with the halter.

RESISTANCE TO DORSAL PRESSURE ON THE WITHERS. Downward pressure on the withers in normal horses usually causes arching of the back (lordosis); (Fig. 4-10). However, when weakness is present, there may be an inability to resist with collapse of the forelimbs.

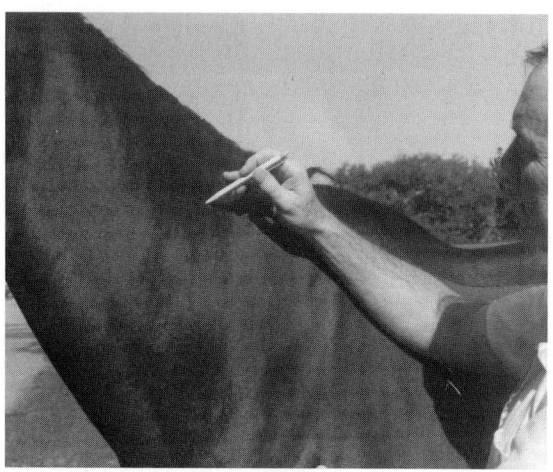

▶ **FIGURE 4-8**

Testing cervical cutaneous sensation.

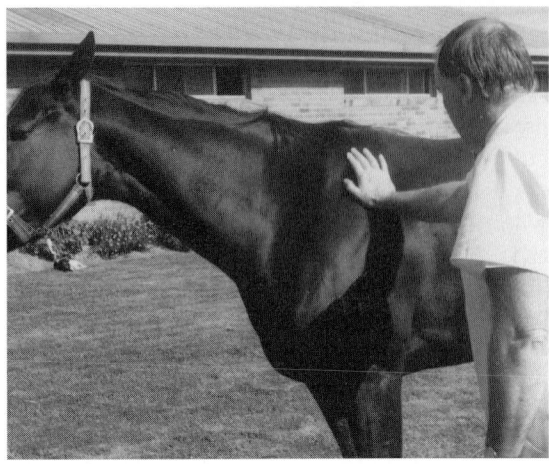

▶ FIGURE 4-9

Sway reaction, forelimb. Pressure is applied to the withers region, noting the ease with which the horse can be pushed or pulled, and the way in which equilibrium is reestablished.

THORACIC POSTURAL REACTIONS, THORACIC LIMB HOPPING. In smaller horses (foals and ponies), it may be possible to test some of the postural reactions commonly evaluated in cats and dogs, which are useful for detecting subtle defects:

- *Wheel-barrowing.* Both hind limbs are elevated and the animal is made to walk on the front limbs.
- *Sideways hopping.* Each forelimb is lifted in turn, and the horse is made to hop sideways on the other limb (Fig. 4–11).
- *Hemistanding,* or *hemiwalking.* Both left legs and then both right legs are lifted in turn,

and the horse is made to stand and then move sideways using the opposite limbs.

MANUAL POSITIONING OF A LIMB IN A CROSSED OR ABNORMAL POSITION. The objective with this test is evaluate the ability to sense that the limb is in an incorrect position and to then return it to a normal position (Fig. 4-12). This particularly evaluates proprioception.

Trunk and Hindlimbs

Palpation and Observation

The trunk and hindlimbs should be observed and palpated in order to detect abnormalities such as asymmetry, muscle atrophy, malformation, and localized sweating. Severe muscle atrophy on one side will produce lateral spinal curvature (scoliosis) with the convex side to the side of the lesion. Damage to spinal sympathetic tracts or peripheral fibers will produce localized sweating whose position can be of value in locating the lesion.

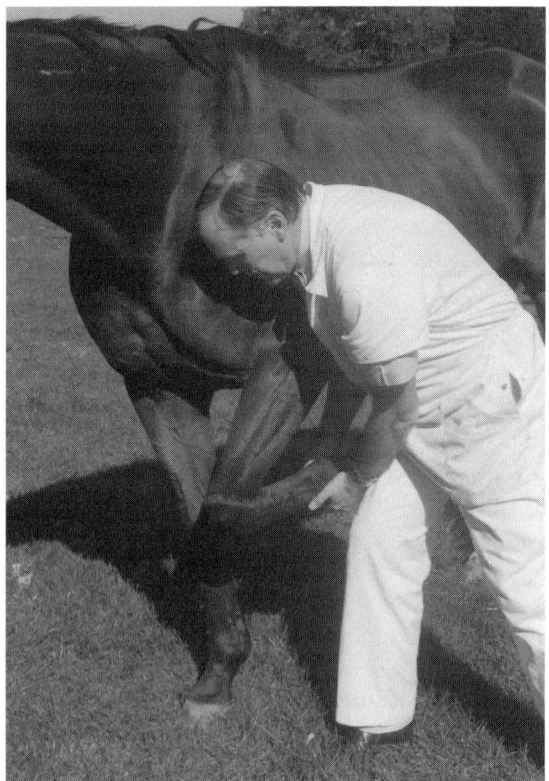

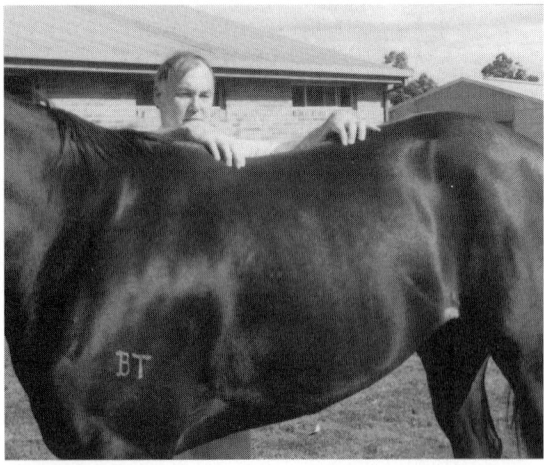

▶ FIGURE 4-10

Applying pressure to the withers to test back flexibility. Firm pressure usually induces the horse to lower, or ventroflex, its back.

▶ FIGURE 4-11

Sideways hopping. With one limb elevated the horse's ability to hop sideways on the other limb is tested by pushing it sideways, as shown.

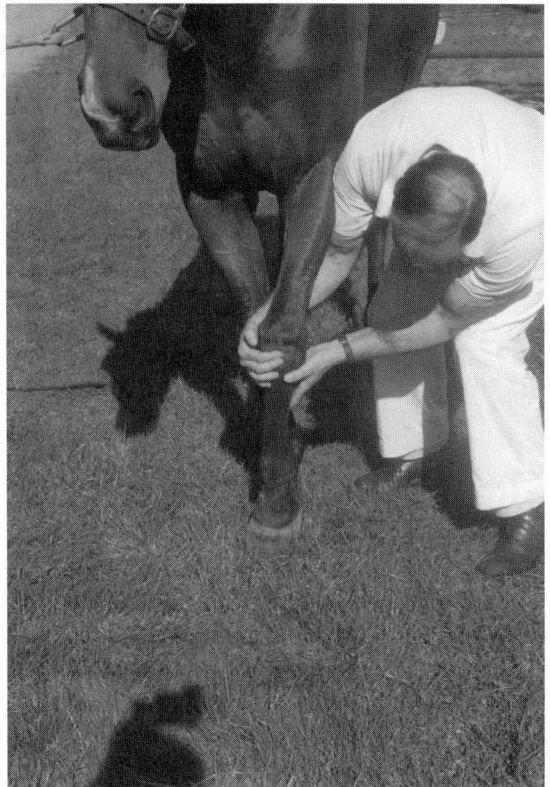

▶ FIGURE 4–12

Positioning limbs in a crossed position to test for proprioception.

Cutaneous Sensation

Cutaneous sensation is assessed using a needle, ballpoint pen, or a pair of hemostats, applied over the whole trunk (Fig. 4–13). Decreased sensation (hypalgesia, analgesia) caudal to a spinal lesion is a useful indication of the site of a lesion.

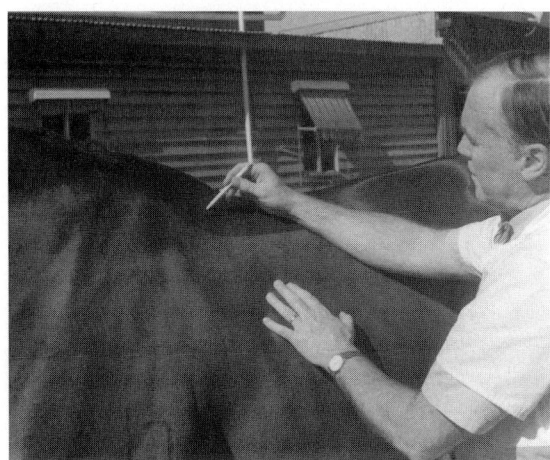

▶ FIGURE 4–13

Testing cutaneous sensation of the trunk region.

Trunk and Hindlimb Reflexes

THE PANNICULUS RESPONSE. This response is a reflex characterized by twitching of the tissues associated with contraction of the cutaneous trunci muscle following stimulation over the lateral aspects of the body. The sensory component of this reflex is carried to the spinal cord in the dorsal branches of the spinal nerves at the level of the stimulus, before traveling cranially to the C_8-T_1 region, where the lower motor neurons of the lateral thoracic nerves are located.

SWAY REACTION. This reaction is tested by pushing against the pelvis or by pulling the tail laterally while the horse is standing or walking (Fig. 4–14). Weakness and ataxia are most apparent during these maneuvers if the examiner is able to move the horse very easily away from its intended path or to cause it to trip and show marked overabduction and crossing of the legs.

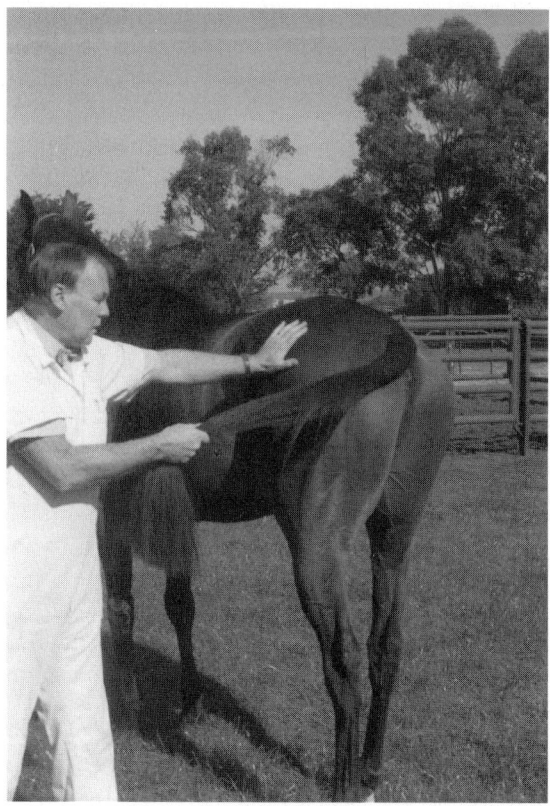

▶ FIGURE 4–14

Sway reaction, hind limbs. Pressure is exerted by pushing against the hip region or by pulling by the tail, noting the ease with which the horse can be pushed or pulled, and the way in which equilibrium is reestablished.

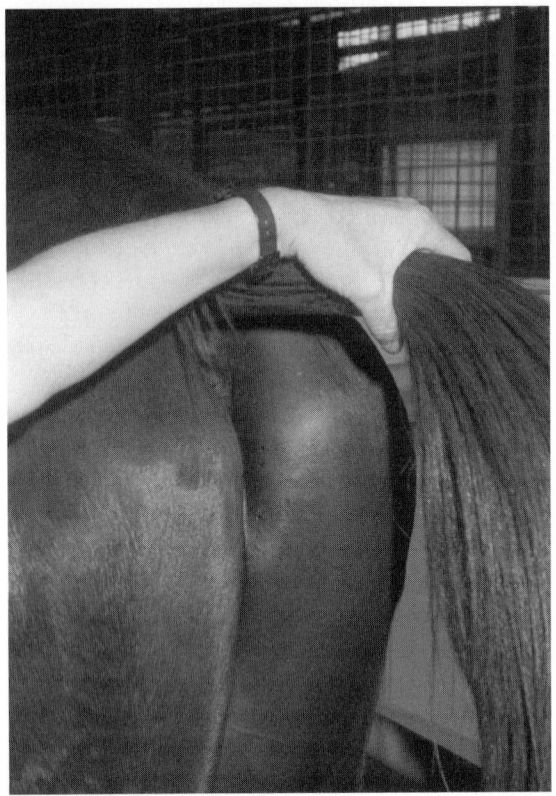

FIGURE 4–15
Testing tail tone.

PELVIC LIMB POSTURAL REACTIONS. These tests are the same as described for the thoracic limb and are interpreted in the same way.

Tail and Anus

In this section are the sacral and coccygeal parts of the spinal cord, associated nerves, and the structures innervated by the nerves.

Tail Tone

Most horses have muscle tone that provides resistance to elevation of the tail, although moderate force will allow tail elevation in all but the most nervous or excited animals (Fig. 4–15). Absence of voluntary muscle tone or weakness usually indicate a lesion in the sacrococcygeal section of the cord. However, severe lesions located more proximally also can produce weakness. Although tail wringing is sometimes associated with neurological disease, it is often a normal activity for some horses.

Perineal Reflex

This reflex is tested by gently pricking the skin of the perineum with a pin or a ballpoint pen and noting the response consisting of contraction of the anal sphincter and clamping down of the tail (Fig. 4–16). It is important to evaluate both the sensory and motor components of the reflex. The sensory innervation is through the perineal branches of the pudendal nerve (S_1–S_3), motor innervation to the anal sphincter is through the caudal rectal branch of the pudendal nerve, and tail flexion is mediated by spinal nerves associated with segments S_1–C_{10}.

Recumbent Horses

Recumbency in horses is a serious problem, and, although some examinations are precluded, certain spinal reflexes that cannot be evaluated when the horse is standing can be assessed in the recumbent horse. When the horse is recumbent, the ability to localize a lesion is even more important than usual because there is an urgent need to make a diagnosis and carry out treatment or euthanasia, decisions for which require precise anatomical location of the lesion.

Forelimb Flexor Reflex

This reflex is controlled by spinal cord segments C_6–T_2.

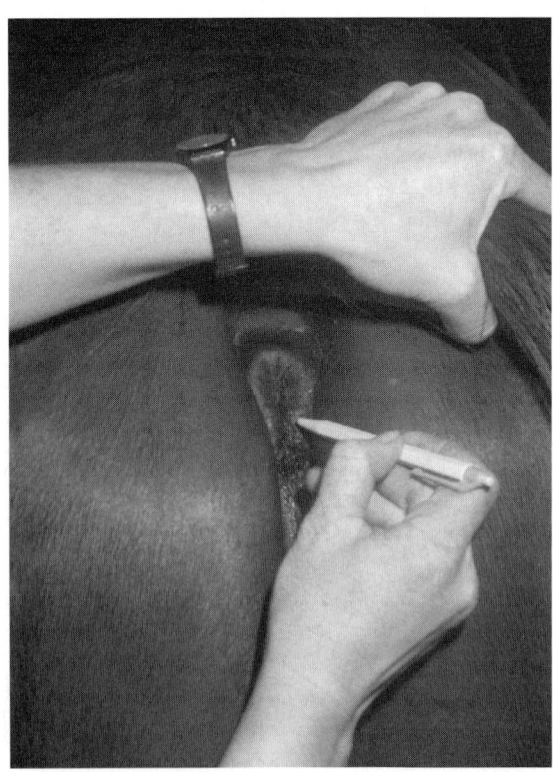

FIGURE 4–16
Testing the perineal reflex.

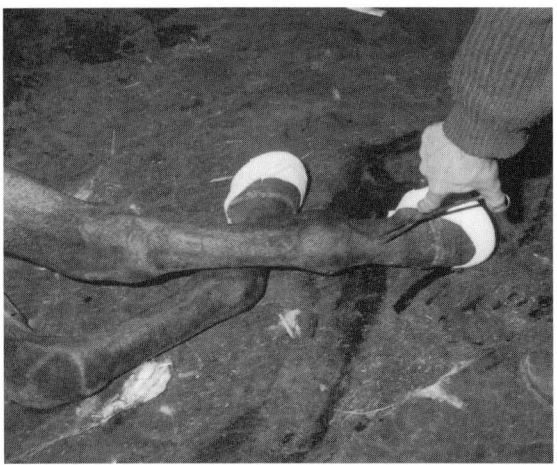

- *Stimulus.* With the limb extended the skin of the distal limb is stimulated by squeezing it with forceps (Fig. 4–17).
- *Response.* Withdrawal of the limb consisting of flexion of all joints.

Conscious perception involves afferent fibers in the median and ulnar nerve and ascending sensory pathways in the cervical cord and brain stem. Lesions cranial to C_6 allow release from UMN control leading to exaggeration of the reflex and maybe also to an exaggeration of the extensor reflex.

Biceps and Triceps Reflexes

These reflexes (spinal cord segments C_7-T_1) are usually difficult to evoke and often require the exageration of an UMN lesion before a positive response can be obtained.

- *Stimulus.* With the limb supported parallel to the ground and in slight flexion, the tendon of the biceps or triceps muscle is tapped with a neurological hammer. The biceps tendon is located cranial to its origin with the scapula (Fig. 4–18), and the triceps tendon proximal to its insertion on the olecranon (Fig. 4–19).
- *Response.* A positive response is seen as a sharp contraction of the associated muscle (i.e., slight extension of the elbow for the triceps reflex and slight extension of the shoulder and flexion of the elbow for the biceps reflex).

Hindlimb Flexor Reflex

This reflex has a sensory component, (sciatic nerve) and a motor component (spinal cord segments L_5-S_3).

- *Stimulus.* With the limb extended the skin of the distal limb is squeezed with forceps as described for the forelimb.
- *Response.* Withdrawal of the limb consisting of joint flexion.

The sensory component depends on where the stimulation occurs, being femoral for skin of the medial thigh region, peroneal for skin over the dorsal tarsus and metatarsus, and tibial for skin on the plantar aspect of the metatarsus.

Patellar Reflex

This reflex has a sensory component, (femoral nerve) and a motor component, (spinal cord segments L_4-L_5).

- *Stimulus.* With the limb parallel to the ground and slightly flexed, the middle patel-

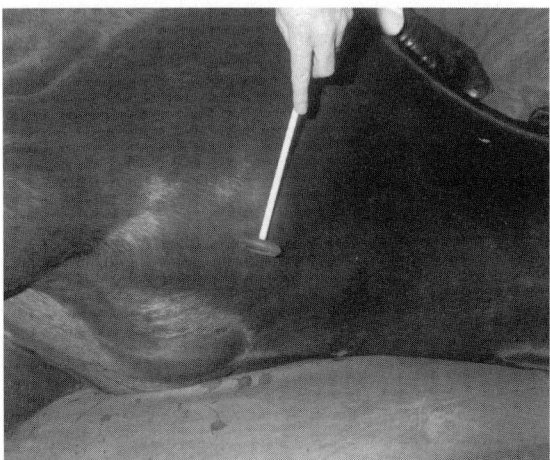

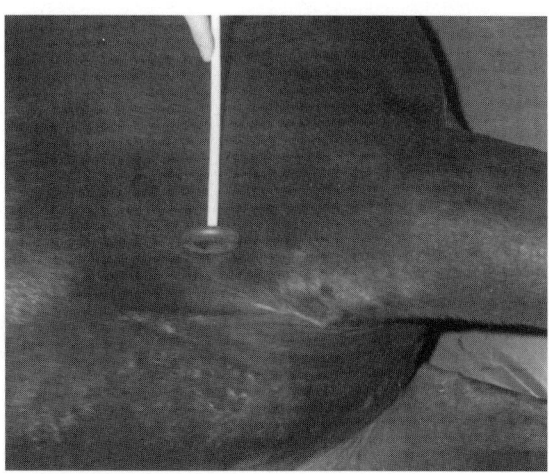

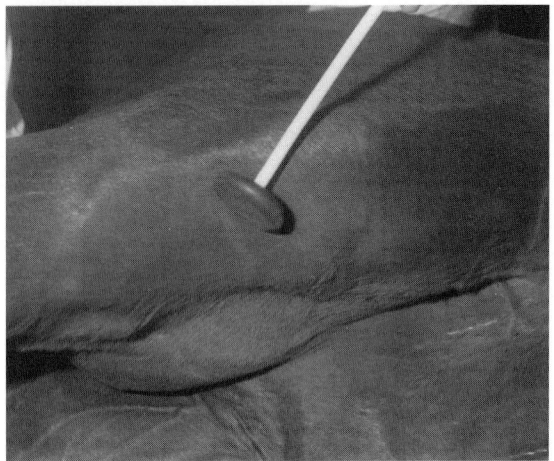

▶ FIGURE 4–20
Patellar reflex in the recumbent horse.

lar ligament is tapped with a neurological hammer (Fig. 4–20).

- *Response*. The quadriceps group of muscle contract and produce a sudden extension of the knee and limb.

Interpretation of a Horse's Ability to Move Its Head, Neck and Limbs When Recumbent

There are a number of assumptions that are usually true that can be made regarding correlation of the site of the lesion with a horse's ability to perform certain movements:

- If the horse can lift only its head, the lesion is in the cranial cervical region.
- If the horse can raise its head and neck, the lesion is in the caudal cervical region.
- If the horse cannot rise into a sitting position (''dog-sitting'' position), the lesion is in the cervical cord.
- If the thoracic limb is functional, the lesion is caudal to T_2.
- If the deficit is in the trunk or hind limbs, the lesion is located between T_2 and S_2.
- Localized sweating indicates a lesion in the descending sympathetic tracts.

Response to Skin Prick (Panniculus Reflex)

Skin stimulation by pricking with a pin or squeezing with a forceps elicits the contraction of cutaneous trunci muscles whose sensory branches lie in the dorsal branch of segmental nerves of the thoracolumbar cord at the level of stimulation. The response passes cranially to C_8-T_3 where the LMN cell bodies of lateral thoracic nerves are stimulated, producing contraction of the muscles. Hence, interruption of the cranial flow of sensory stimulation by a lesion will produce loss of the muscle response when the stimulus is made at, or caudal to, the site of the lesion.

SPECIAL EXAMINATION PROCEDURES

Collection and Examination of Cerebrospinal Fluid

Collection of cerebrospinal fluid (CSF) is a relatively simple procedure and can provide very useful information.[4] A sample can be collected from either atlanto-occipital or lumbosacral sites, the choice of which is dictated by the suspected lesion and its location. Usually, CSF obtained from the atlanto-occipital site is indicated for intracranial lesions and CSF from the lumbosacral site for more distal lesions. The advantage of lumbosacral collection is that it can be done in the standing horse, carries very little risk, and will usually be useful for diagnosing both central and distal lesions.

Procedure

Collection of fluid from the atlanto-occipital space is usually done with the horse in lateral

---

Materials for Collecting Cerebrospinal Fluid

- Spinal needle and stilette (Beckton Dickinson & Co. Franklin Lakes, NJ)
  For atlanto-occipital collection: 18-gauge, 9 cm (3.5")
  For lumbosacral collection: 18–20 gauge, 9 cm (3.5") for ponies and foals; 18-gauge, 15 cm (6") for most adults
- Hair clippers, #40 clipper head
- Scalpel blade (#12)
- Manometer
- Sample containers for cytology and bacteriology

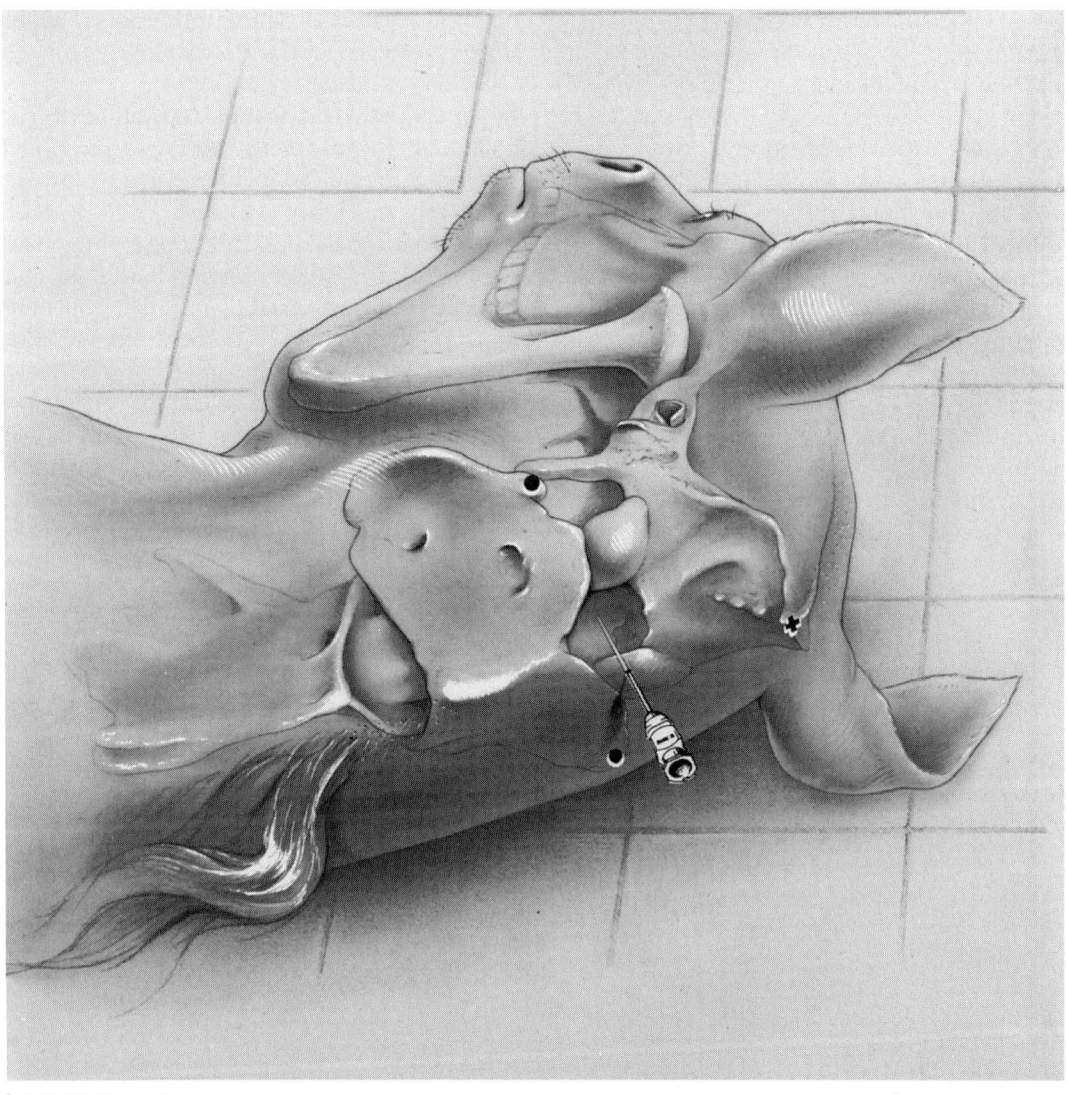

▶ **FIGURE 4-21**
Collection of cerebrospinal fluid from the atlanto-occipital space. The spinal needle is in place and the stilette removed. The landmarks used are the cranial borders of the atlas and the median eminence of the nuchal crest. (From deLahunta A: Veterinary Neuroanatomy and Clinical Neurology, 2nd ed, Philadelphia, Saunders, 1983, p 44. Reprinted with permission.)

recumbency under general anesthesia. If a horse is already recumbent because of disease, general anesthesia may not be required, but analgesia and excellent restraint are necessary. Collection from the lumbosacral space is usually done with the horse standing with appropriate sedation and restraint.

ATLANTO-OCCIPITAL COLLECTION. With the horse under general anesthesia and in lateral recumbency, an area 6 × 6 inches (15 × 15 cm) centered over the atlanto-occipital space is clipped and prepared for sterile puncture. The head is positioned so that it is at right angles to

the neck, and the nose is elevated to make the head parallel with the ground. The landmarks and the relevant anatomy are shown in Figure 4-21. The needle with stilette is inserted vertically in the midline on a line joining the cranial points of the wings of the atlas. Penetration of the dorsal atlanto-occipital membrane and dura mater is usually at a depth of about 5 to 7 cm (2-3″) indicated by a "popping" sensation and loss of resistance. Care should be taken to avoid sudden overpenetration by supporting the hand when advancing the needle. When the above signs are perceived or the depth is judged to be sufficient, the stilette should be removed. A successful ir sertion is indicated by the appearance of cerebrospinal fluid (CSF) at the hub of the needle. If no fluid is seen, the needle is rotated 90°, which often causes CSF to appear. If CSF is not obtained, the stilette is replaced and the needle advanced or redirected as indicated. The CSF pressure can be measured by attaching a manometer to the needle before any fluid is removed.

The most common problems are inserting the needle off the midline, thus missing the space, and directing it too far cranially or caudally, thus hitting the occipit or atlas, respectively. These errors can be minimized by giving attention to landmarks and positioning of the head and neck. If it is thought that the needle has been misdirected, it should be withdrawn and redirected, and it is important not to attempt correction by manipulating the position of the horse while the needle is inserted.

LUMBOSACRAL COLLECTION. Lumbosacral collection is made with the horse restrained in stocks. Sedation is recommended only when absolutely necessary, because such medication will often cause the horse to stand asymmetrically, with most of its weight on one hind limb, which makes collection difficult. Although collection is possible in laterally recumbent horses, similar difficulty with lack of symmetry makes the procedure more difficult. If collection is made in the recumbent horse, the upper pelvic limb should be elevated to ensure that the region is symmetrical, and both pelvic limbs can be advanced to enlarge the lumbosacral space and to tighten the interar-

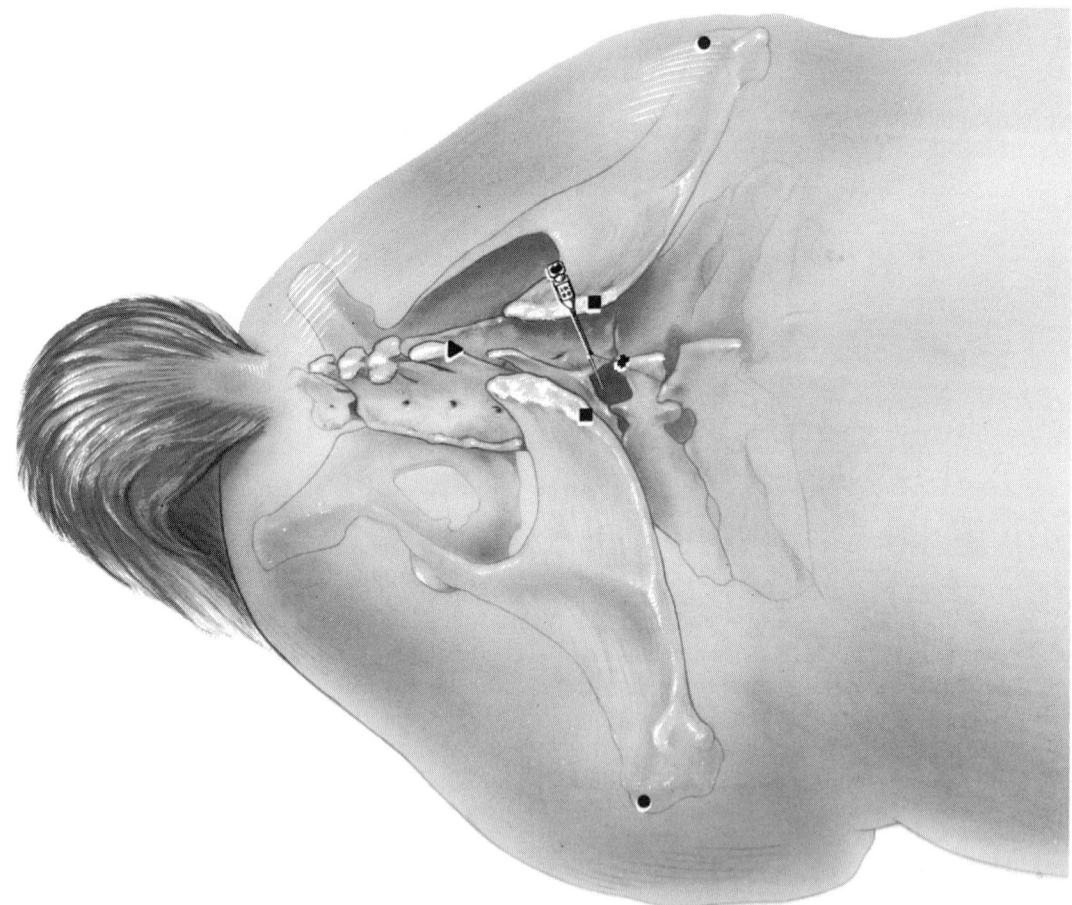

A

▶ **FIGURE 4-22**

Collection of cerebrospinal fluid from the lumbosacral space **A.** The spinal needle is in place and the stilette removed. The landmarks are the caudal borders of each tuber coxae, the caudal edge of the spine at L6, the cranial edge of the spine of the second sacral vertebra, and the cranial edge of each tuber sacrale. (From deLahunta A: Veterinary Neuroanatomy and Clinical Neurology, 2nd ed, Philadelphia, Saunders, 1983, p 42. Reprinted with permission.)

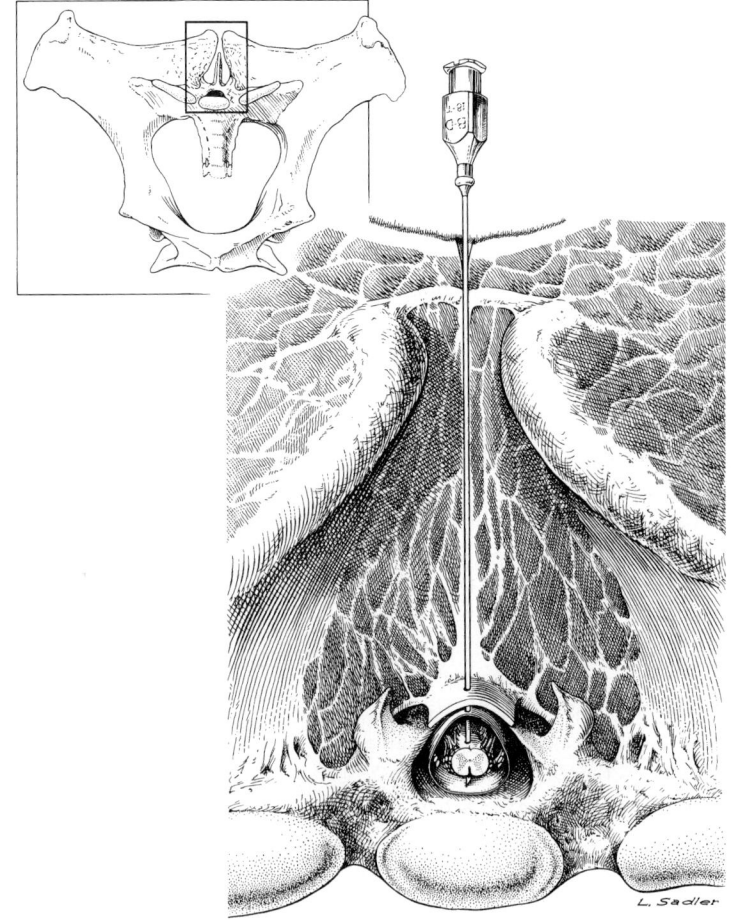

B

▶ **FIGURE 4–22** *Continued*

B. Transverse section demonstrating passage of the needle through all tissues, including the conus medullaris, to reach the ventral subarachnoid space. (From deLahunta A: Veterinary Neuroanatomy and Clinical Neurology, 2nd ed. Philadelphia, Saunders, 1983, p 43. Reprinted with permission.)

cuate ligament and meninges, thus improving perception of penetration.

The site for insertion of the needle in the midline is shown in Figure 4–22. There are different ways to locate the correct position:

1. Intersection of the midline and an imaginary line between the caudal borders of the tuber coxae.
2. Palpation per rectum of the ventral lumbosacral eminence that lies approximately beneath the correct location. This method is useful in obese horses in which normal landmarks are not so easily located.
3. Palpation of the dorsal lumbar and sacral spines in the midline. In the lumbosacral region a depression is usually easily palpated. However, it should be remembered that L_6 and S_1 are shorter than the adja-

cent L_5 and S_2, respectively, and that S_1 is usually not palpable. Therefore, as palpation proceeds caudally, the first depression is usually over L_6 and the correct location will lie caudal to this.

Location of the correct point for insertion is relatively easy if one remembers that there is considerable variation between horses and also that one should use all available landmarks as guides.

The horse is positioned so that the rear legs are symmetrically positioned and carrying equal weight. The selected site is clipped, prepared for sterile puncture, and injected with local anesthetic solution. A stab incision is made with a scalpel blade, and the spinal needle, with stilette, is inserted vertically. A 15-cm needle is long enough for all but the very largest horses.

Advancement of the needle is usually not resented and there is little resistance. As with the atlanto-occipital collection there is usually a sensation of sudden reduction in resistance as the interarcuate ligament is penetrated at a depth of about 11 to 12 cm (4.5-5″). Although a few horses react violently, penetration usually is accompanied by only slight movement of the tail, localized muscle twitch, or slight flexion of the hind limbs. The dura mater and arachnoid are usually penetrated simultaneously with the interarcuate ligament, although sometimes the needle must be advanced a little further. Again, it is important to rest the hand controlling the needle on the horse so as to avoid sudden overpenetration should the horse move without warning.

If CSF is not obtained, the needle can be advanced to the floor of the vertebral canal (passing through the dorsal dura mater and subarachnoid space, the conus medullaris, and ventral subarachnoid space and dura mater) and then, while rotating it, slowly withdrawn a millimeter at a time. Manual occlusion of both jugular veins (Queckenstedt's maneuver) increases intraspinal pressure and improves the chances of obtaining an adequate volume of CSF. **Gentle suction** can be used to obtain CSF, but this should be done very carefully so as to avoid producing bleeding. If the needle touches bone before CSF is obtained, the clinician must decide whether it is the floor of the canal or whether the needle has missed the lumbosacral space and has impinged on the sacrum or the dorsum of L_6.

PREPARATION OF SAMPLE. Cerebrospinal fluid should be examined as soon as possible. Otherwise, it should be diluted with an equal volume of alcohol added to preserve cells. The sample is collected into suitable containers and submitted for cytological and, if indicated, for bacteriological evaluation (Appendix C5).

Results

Cerebrospinal fluid is formed by secretion and filtration, mostly by the ventricular choroid plexuses, and flows from the lateral apertures of the fourth ventricle and then either over the cerebral hemispheres or caudally around the spinal cord, to exit through the dural reflections of the spinal nerve roots—hence the tendency for cranial lesions to be better diagnosed in an atlanto-occipital collection and caudal lesions in a lumbosacral collection. Anatomic and functional bar-

riers exist between blood and CSF, blood and brain, and CSF-brain compartments. Normal values are presented for adults in Tables 4-1 and 4-2, and for foals in Table 4-3.

Some disease categories and expected findings are as follows:

- *Infectious diseases.* Increased neutrophils with bacterial infections, small mononuclear cells with viral infections, eosinophils with protozoal and helminth infections
- *Necrosis and chronic infections.* Increased macrophages or large mononuclear cells
- *Trauma.* Xanthochromia and increased protein, erythrocytes, neutrophils without toxic change, and macrophages
- *Toxin damage* (e.g., leukoencephalomalacia from mouldy corn poisoning). Increased protein, mononuclear cells

▶ TABLE 4-1

**EQUINE CEREBROSPINAL FLUID (CSF):
REFERENCE VALUES OF NORMAL HORSES (N = 24)
AND PONIES (N = 21) FOR FLUID COLLECTED FROM
THE ATLANTO-OCCIPITAL (AO) AND LUMBOSACRAL
(LS) SPACES**

Variable	Mean	Standard Deviation
Opening pressure (mm of H2O)	308.80	75.15
CSF withdrawn (ml)	14.93	4.07
Closing pressure (mm of H2O)	223.58	74.46
White blood cells (No./μl)	1.41	1.74
Red blood cells (No./μl)	195.16	511.96
Protein (mg/dl) Horses	37.23	28.41
Ponies	60.48	20.45
LS-AO differences	−0.46	13.07
Glucose (mg/dl) AO	48.00	9.92
LS	55.13	8.22
(CSF/Serum %) AO	51.65	8.77
LS	58.38	9.48
Sodium (mEq/L)	144.58	1.86
Potassium (mEq/L)	2.95	0.05
Chloride (mEq/L)	109.22	6.90
Calcium (mg/dl)	4.18	0.87
Phosphorus (mg/dl)	0.83	0.20
Creatine phosphokinase (IU)	1.08	3.13
Aspartate transaminase (SF units)	30.74	6.31
Lactic dehydrogenase (IU)	1.51	1.75
Alkaline phosphatase (IU)	0.83	0.95
Urea nitrogen (md/gl)	11.82	3.26
Cholesterol (mg/dl)	4.76	5.72

Note: Electrolytes measured only for horses. Except where indicated all other values are the combined data from horses and ponies and AO and LS collection sites. (Source: Mayhew IG, Whitlock RH, Tasker JB: Equine cerebrospinal fluid: Reference values of normal horses. Am J Vet Res 1977;3:1271. Reprinted with permission)

▶ TABLE 4–2

ELECTROPHORETIC VALUES OF CEREBROSPINAL FLUID

		GLOBULIN (MG/100 ML)			
TOTAL PROTEIN (MG/100 ML)	ALBUMIN (MG/100 ML)	ALPHA$_1$	ALPHA$_2$	BETA	THETA
40.1	15.3	5.2	6.7	5.8	5.7
±3.1	±1.2	±0.9	±0.4	±0.6	±0.8

(Data drawn from Kirk GR, Neate S, McClure RC, et al: Electrophoretic pattern of equine cerebrospinal fluid. Am J Vet Res 1974;35:1263.)

COMPLICATIONS. Contamination with blood can occur, giving the CSF a reddish tinge. The following characteristics can be used to help determine when blood is present as a contaminant or when there has been pathological bleeding into the CSF:

- With minor contamination, the blood is not homogenously mixed, swirls in the sample, and usually decreases as more CSF is withdrawn.
- A heavily contaminated sample may clot; samples with preexisting bleeding will not.
- Centrifugation of a contaminated sample will yield a clear supernatant, whereas in cases of bleeding it will be xanthochromic.

▶ TABLE 4–3

BIOCHEMICAL CONSTITUENTS OF CEREBROSPINAL FLUID IN FULL TERM (GROUP A, N = 21) AND PREMATURE (GROUP B, N = 16) PONY FOALS (MEAN ± SD).

Parameter	Group A	Group B
Total protein (g/liter)	1.38 ± 0.5(20)	1.78 ± 0.86(17)
Creatine kinase (IU/liter)	15.2 ± 9.2(14)	5.29 ± 2.56(18)
Aspartate aminotransferase (IU/liter)	16.6 ± 7.6(16)	15.8 ± 6.6(17)
Lactate dehydrogenase (IU/liter)	23.2 ± 10.7(16)	34.0 ± 16.8(7)
Gammaglutamyl transferase (IU/liter)	1.50 ± 1.5(7)	2.73 ± 1.5(8)
Sodium (mmol/liter)	142.6 ± 28(8)	145.5 ± 3.3(7)
Potassium (mmol/liter)	3.6 ± 2.1(8)	3.7 ± 1.1(7)
Chloride (mmol/liter)	109 ± 3.4(7)	116 ± 12.5(12)

( ) Number of samples examined. (Source: Rossdale PD, Cash RSG, Leadon DP, et al: Biochemical constituents of cerebrospinal fluid in premature and full term foals. Equine Vet J 1982; 14:134. Reprinted with permission.)

Tentorial herniation can follow the removal of fluid when there is obstruction cranial to the site of collection. The presence of abnormally high pressure that falls suddenly (25–50%) after the removal of a few milliliters is indicative of this possibility. If pressure does not fall excessively, a volume of 30 to 40 mL can be collected.

Radiology of the Nervous System

Radiological examination of the nervous system can be extremely useful to localize and characterize injury related to trauma (vertebral fracture, vertebral dislocation), infection (vertebral abscess and osteomyelitis), and malformation (congenital, cervical spinal cord compression syndrome, or "wobbler syndrome"). There also is an occasional need to evaluate the head for trauma (skull fracture), infection (middle and inner ear infection with involvement of the tympanic bulla, and malformation, congenital hydrocephalus and atlanto-occipital malformation). The procedures and findings are described in detail elsewhere.[6]

Acceptable-quality radiographs of the head and proximal cervical spine can be obtained with high-speed film and a mobile X-ray unit. However, if high-quality radiographs or radiographs of the caudal cervical spine and caudal to this, or needed, and if the patient is large, general anesthesia, a high-output machine, and considerable expertise are necessary. The identification of space-occupying lesions is facilitated by myelography. In any case plain (noncontrast) radiographs should be taken first to define osseous integrity and the need for contrast techniques. The existence of lesions that are demonstrable only when the neck is placed in a stressed position (dynamic lesions), namely, the "wobbler syndrome," should be understood and appropriate techniques known.

Plain Radiography

Plain radiography is either carried out as a single diagnostic procedure or as a preliminary to contrast radiography. As stated, a portable machine often is satisfactory for head and proximal cervical radiography. Rare earth screens are recommended for all regions, and a grid is required for caudal cervical vertebrae and structures caudal to them.

PROCEDURE. When the procedure is carried out in the standing horse care must be taken, as always, to avoid unnecessary exposure to personnel and to minimize moving the patient or the radiographic equipment. This is done by ensuring stability of the X-ray machine, tranquilizing the horse when necessary, and holding the X-ray plate in a cassette holder or placing it in a stand. In the anesthetized animal the problem of exposure of personnel is still very important, but, because the patient is recumbent and the cassette is placed beneath the structures to be examined, it is more easily controlled. Under routine circumstances

Materials for Plain Radiography of the Head and Spine

▶ X-ray machine

High-output machine provides best quality radiographs and is necessary for caudal cervical spine and regions caudal to it.

Portable machine may be useful for radiographs of head and proximal cervical spine.

▶ X-ray film
▶ Rare earth screens
▶ Grids, especially for caudal cervical spine and caudally
▶ Cassette holders or stands
▶ Chemical restraint (see Chapter 1 Chemical Restraint of the Adult Horse)

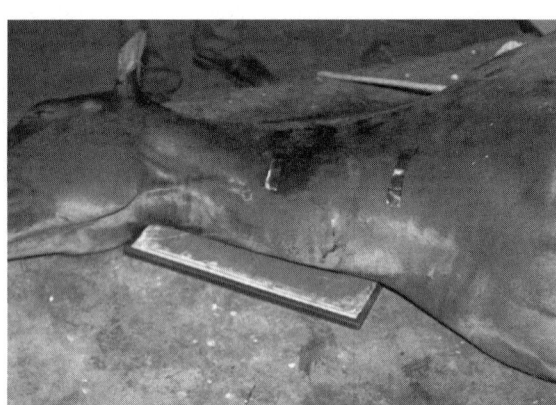

A

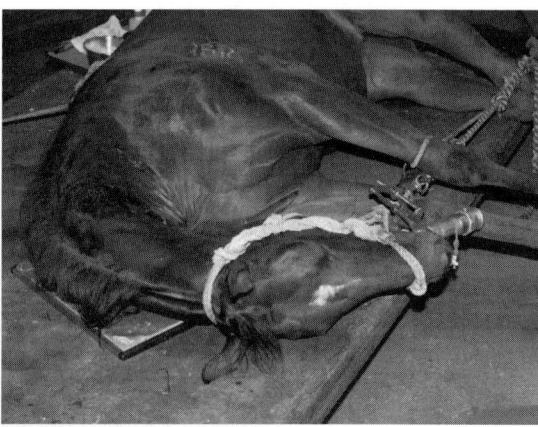

B

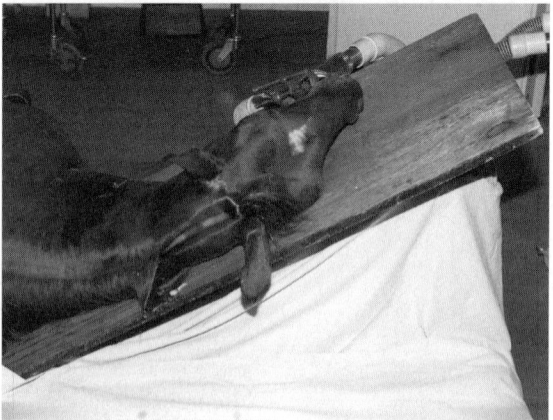

C

▶ **FIGURE 4-23**

Radiological examination of the cervical spine. **A.** Neck positioned in a neutral position. **B.** Neck positioned in a flexed position. **C.** Head and neck elevated to ensure caudal flow of the contrast media.

only lateral views are taken, but on certain occasions other projections, especially dorsoventral views, are necessary. Large cassettes and lead markers placed on the skin over the spine facilitate the identification of individual vertebrae.

When the head is radiographed, a rope halter should be used to avoid the superimposition of metal buckles from a headstall over a region of interest. Left and right projections are often useful to determine which side a lesion is on, as the image is smaller and clearer when it is closest to the plate. If the horse is recumbent, the neck should be raised a little to ensure that the spine and plate are parallel and that a true lateral radiograph can be obtained. Positioning for stressed views is demonstrated in Figure 4–23.

RESULTS. The ability to interpret spinal and head radiographs requires knowledge of normal structures and dimensions.[6] In addition to recognizing fractures, osteomyelitis, neoplasia, and congenital malformation, identifying lesions associated with "wobbler syndrome" is important. With respect to the latter entity a nomenclature describing the dimensions of the cervical vertebrae has been developed (Fig. 4–24), with special emphasis being given to the minimum sagittal diameter (MSD) of the vertebral foramen in plain radiographs (Table 4–4). An example of plain radiography showing a normal cervical spine is found in Figure 4–25.

Contrast Radiography (Myelography)

Contrast radiography is used to detect space-occupying lesions that are causing pressure on nervous tissue. Contrast radiography of the spine usually implies myelography. However, intraosse-

▶ **TABLE 4–4**

REFERENCE VALUES FOR THE MINIMUM SAGGITAL DIAMETER (MEAN ± 1SD) OF THE CERVICAL VERTEBRAL FORAMEN IN NORMAL HORSES

CERVICAL VERTEBRAE	MINIMUM SAGGITAL DIAMETER (MM)	
	>320 KG	<320 KG
C2	26.7 ± 2.3	23.8 ± 1.5
C3	22.2 ± 1.8	19.8 ± 0.9
C4	21.3 ± 1.8	18.7 ± 1.0
C5	22.5 ± 1.8	19.7 ± 1.2
C6	24.1 ± 2.5	21.1 ± 1.5
C7	27.4 ± 2.6	22.9 ± 1.6

Radiographs taken with a focal-film distance of 90cm, and with the cassette placed against the neck of the horse. (Data drawn from Mayhew IG, Whitlock R, de Lahunta A: Spinal cord disease in the horse. Cornell Vet 1978; 68 (Suppl 6): 44.)

ous venography is another technique that has received some attention, although it has not gained a regular place in diagnostic radiology.[7]

PROCEDURE. Owners should be warned of the chances of reaction to the procedure, and prophylactic use of nonsteroidal antiinflammatory drugs or corticosteroids is indicated. The procedure is carried out with the horse in lateral recumbency and usually under general anesthesia. Myelography is sometimes possible in the standing horse, but this is not recommended. Recumbent, unanesthetized horses can be investigated, but appropriate restraint must be in place to prevent movement.

Metrizamide has been used extensively as the contrast material, but it has the disadvantage that it should be filtered through a 0.22-μm filter to ensure sterility. Recently, other water-soluble,

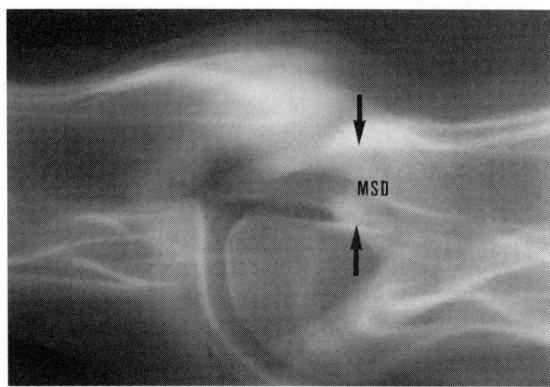

▶ **FIGURE 4–24**

Lateral radiograph of the cervical spine demonstrating the minimum saggital diameter (MSD).

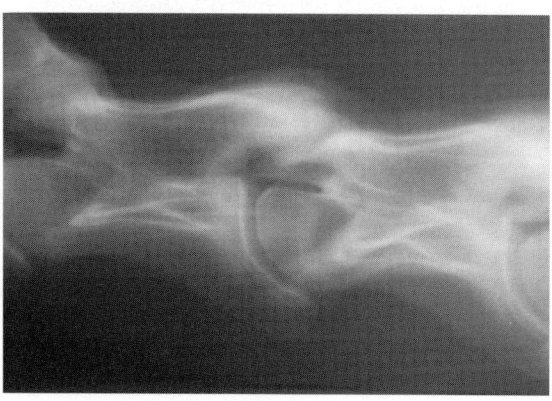

▶ **FIGURE 4–25**

Lateral radiograph of a normal cervical spine.

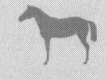

Materials for Myelography of the Spinal Column

▸ Spinal needles as for CSF collection
▸ Radiographic contrast material
Sterile - iohexol (Omnipaque, Winthrop Pharmaceuticals, New York, NY), iopamidol (Niopam 300, Merck) Nonsterile - metrizamide (Metrizamide, Accurate Chemical Company, Hicksville, NY)
▸ Syringe (60 ml)
▸ Antiinflammatory drug (e.g., phenylbutazone)

less irritant and nonionic agents such as iopamidol (370 mgI/mL) and iohexol (350 mgI/mL) have been introduced and are now in regular use.

To ensure that contrast material does not flow rostrally, the horse's head and neck should be placed on an incline of about 30° so as to elevate the nose and head. The procedure for inserting the needle is identical to that described for CSF collection. After inserting the needle, approximately 40 to 50 ml of CSF is removed, and an equivalent volume of the contrast material is slowly injected over 5 minutes. To encourage caudal flow, the bevel of the needle can be directed caudally. Alternatively, a needle can be placed in the lumbosacral space and CSF allowed to exit during injection of contrast material through the atlanto-occipital space. The head and neck are kept elevated for 5 minutes after injection before they are lowered and radiography completed. To evaluate the "wobbler syndrome" radiographs are taken with the neck in neutral, extended, and flexed positions. Care must be taken not to overflex the neck, especially in smaller animals. The need for a full range of positions, including dorsoventral and oblique projections, is dictated by the suspected lesion.

RESULTS. The evaluation of the "wobbler syndrome" relies especially on the flexed and extended views. In the neutral view in normal horses the dorsal column of contrast material is significantly wider and more regular than the ventral one, which also narrows slightly at each intervertebral junction. In the flexed view the ventral column gets narrower and the dorsal column is unchanged. During extension the dorsal column narrows somewhat, especially in the caudal region of the neck. Guidelines to interpretation are as follows:

- Failure of contrast material to pass a specific site is indicative of obstruction and spinal cord compression.
- Focal narrowing of the ventral dye column with the neck in any position is probably not significant.
- Narrowing of the dorsal dye column in the flexed view indicates a compressive lesion.
- Narrowing of the dorsal column in the extended view is probably not significant.

Some examples of a myelogram are shown in Figure 4-26.

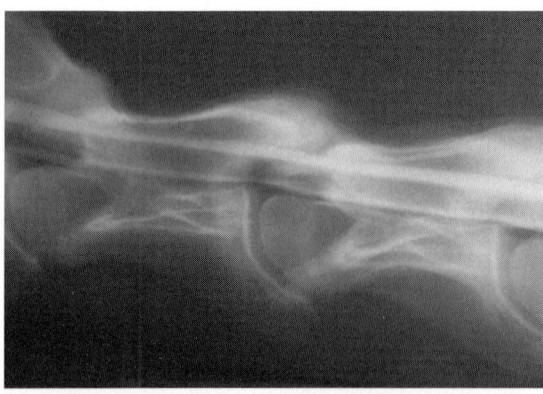
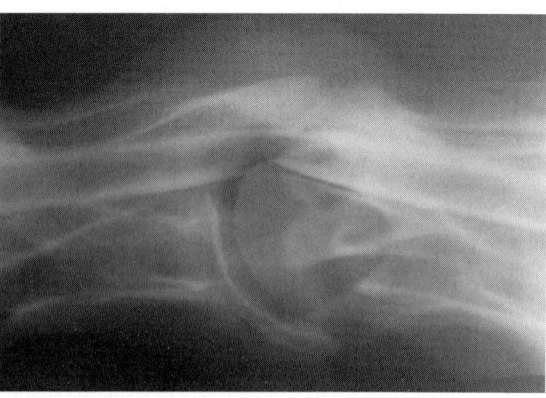

A   B

▸ **FIGURE 4-26**

Contrast myelography. **A.** Normal. Note the dorsal and ventral dye columns. **B.** Abnormal. Demonstration of a compressive lesion produced by flexion. Note the decrease in the width of the dye columns.

COMPLICATIONS. Complications do occur and can be very serious.[8] Overflexion can cause loss of both contrast columns and also cause an exacerbation of signs. The main complication is stimulation of the nervous system (tremors and seizures). This problem has been minimized with the use of iohexol and iopamidol.

Computed Tomography

Computed tomography (CT) requires specialized and expensive equipment that is available only in a few centers worldwide. Furthermore, the usual design dictates that only the head and proximal cervical region of anesthetized horses can be imaged. Consequently, although the technique has been described for horses, it has not been utilized to any significant extent in equine diagnosis.[9,10] The special advantage conferred by CT is the ability to produce a three dimensional view of a region in a series of slices. This has special value in interpretation of cervical stenotic myelopathy, and other spinal cord compressive syndromes where there is a need to establish if the cord is undergoing compression. The added advantage of combining myelography with CT in evaluation of CSM has also been demonstrated.[11] Diagnosis of pituitary tumors[12,13] and a brain abscess[14] has also been reported.

Electrodiagnosis

Changes in cellular electrical activity associated with neurological disease can be recorded in different ways. Electromyography (EMG), auditory brain stem evoked response testing (ABR), nerve conduction studies (NCS), and electroencephalography (EEG) are all useful in improving the accuracy of diagnosis. This topic has been reviewed elsewhere, and the information presented here is mainly drawn from that publication.[15]

Electromyography

Needle EMG is the recording of muscle cell electrical activity by means of an electrode inserted into the muscle. The NCS consists of stimulating a peripheral nerve with electrical current and recording the response in the muscle(s) supplied by the nerve or in other parts of the same nerve. A graphic and auditory record of the electrical response can be made. The results of such studies provide data concerning the functional status of the nerves, myoneural

---

Materials for Electromyography

- Electromyograph (including stimulator capable of 150 V for 0.1 to 3.0-msec at 100 Hz, amplication device, cathode ray oscilloscope, loudspeaker; optional equipment includes reel-to-reel tape recorder, computer, printer).

- Needle electrodes (usually monopolar and bipolar)

---

junctions, and muscles involved in the various motor units present in the neuromuscular system.

PROCEDURE.

Needle Electromyography. The examination is carried out whenever possible in the standing, sedated horse. General anesthesia, if necessary, precludes certain measurements but can also enhance interpretation under some conditions. A complete EMG examination includes the major extrinsic muscles of the hind and forelimbs, paravertebral muscles between L_6 and C_1, and, when indicated, the muscles of the face, esophagus, larynx, pectoral region, and external anal sphincter. Reference, ground, and exploring electrodes are usually used. The reference and ground electrodes often are combined into one concentric electrode, with the reference electrode consisting of the outer needle section and the ground being a central wire. The concentric electrode is inserted into the subcutaneous tissue over a bony prominence close by the site for evaluation, and the monopolar electrode is inserted into the muscle being investigated. (Three bipolar electrodes can also be used, in which case the ground electrode is inserted over the bony prominence, and the reference electrode between the ground electrode and the exploring electrode.)

After inserting the concentric electrode, the exploring electrode is inserted quickly into the muscle and held until the patient is relaxed, at which stage insertional and resting activity can be evaluated. In smaller muscles, at least four different regions and depths and, in larger muscles at least six, should be examined. Examination can be carried out during relaxation, contraction, or after nerve stimulation.

Results. After insertion of the exploring electrode in normal muscle there is a brief period of *insertional activity* characterized by high-amplitude, moderate- to high-frequency waves that may be related to nerve stimulation, nerve injury, or depolarization in adjacent muscle. Insertional activity ceases rapidly and is followed by a period of electrical silence, termed *resting activity.* Resting activity can be interrupted by the appearance of end-plate noise and end-plate spikes, seen as rippling of the baseline and high-amplitude spikes, respectively. These are normal findings resulting from the insertion process. Motor unit action potentials (MUAPs) are seen after insertion and result from voluntary or reflex muscle contraction. They are the sum of a number of single-fiber potentials in the same motor unit and appear as one, two, three, and occasionally more wave deflections. Their amplitude is less important than their duration and number.

Abnormal activity after insertion includes prolonged or decreased insertional activity, polyphasic motor unit action potentials, neuropathic motor unit action potentials, fibrillation potentials, positive sharp waves, fasciculation potentials, and complex repetitive discharges versus myotonic potentials. In horses EMG has been used for conditions such as CSM[7] and protozoal myelitis, brachial plexus injury, and suprascapular nerve injury.[15]

Nerve Conduction Studies. Nerve conduction studies are used to measure the velocity of conduction along large myelinated nerves. The tests are conducted with the patient under general anesthesia. A knowledge of the anatomy of each nerve and of the muscles innervated are required. The method involves the insertion of stimulating monopolar electrodes adjacent to a nerve and of other recording electrodes in the muscle to record the evoked motor unit action potential. Studies of the median and radial nerves have been conducted.[16,17]

Results. When a nerve with sensory and motor fibers is stimulated, two potentials are observed. The first is the *direct evoked muscle action potential* (M wave), which is the result of transmission of the impulse down the motor fiber to the muscle, which then responds. The second response is the *reflex evoked muscle action potential* (H wave), which follows the retrograde transmission of the impulse through the sensory fibers to the CNS and then back through the motor nerves to the muscle. The M-wave, which is used most commonly, is usually bi- or triphasic and is larger than the H wave. The time lapse between stimulation, passage of the stimulus down the motor nerve, and the response is known as the *latency.* When two stimulating electrodes, a known distance apart, are used, the nerve conduction velocity can be calculated by relating the difference between the electrodes to the difference between the two latencies. Such data are available for the radial and median nerves in the horse (normal values, 60–80 m/s).[16,17] Because of its more complex route, the reflex evoked muscle action potential is useful to evaluate the sensory and central parts of the reflex.

Auditory Brainstem Response Testing

Auditory brain stem response testing involves evaluating the potentials generated by the eighth cranial nerve and its projections in response to an acoustic stimulus.[18,19]

PROCEDURE. The procedure can be carried out with the patient awake, with or without sedation, and under general anesthesia. The ear phones are inserted into the external ear canals and stabilized with the wax ear plugs, which provide acoustic isolation from external noise. The exploring, reference, and ground electrodes are inserted subcutaneously at the back of the pinna, in the dorsal midline behind the ear, and dorsolaterally high on the same side of the neck as the ear under investigation, respectively. The electrodes are connected through the amplifier to the electromyograph. The stimulus is in the form of a click, delivered by a square-wave generator that produces 20 clicks per second. Testing is

---

Materials for Auditory Brainstem Response Testing

‣ Electromyograph and amplifier
‣ Insert earphones with hearing aid receivers (frequency response, 100–6000Hz)
‣ Wax ear plugs
‣ Platinum needle electrodes

Materials for Electroencephalography

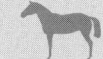

▶ Electroencephalogram, including facilities for adequate high- and low-noise filtration, variable paper speed (15, 30, and 60 mm/s), printer, and amplifier with variable gain

▶ Cathode ray oscilloscope and computer (not essential)

▶ Platinum monopolar needle electrodes

usually performed over a 70-dB range, between 30 and 90 dB. Further details, see available references.[15]

RESULTS. Five peaks or waves can be related to certain anatomical regions at each level of sound within 10 ms of stimulus. Wave i, and possibly part of wave ii, originates from the bipolar neurons of the eighth cranial nerve, whereas waves iii to v are associated with more diffuse activity in the region of the medulla and pons, ipsilateral, and contralateral to the side of stimulus. Knowing the origins of the abnormal wave helps to locate the lesion in a variety of cases, including head tilt and middle- and inner-ear infections, as well as more diffuse conditions in the brain stem.

Electroencephalography

Electroencephalography involves recording the electrical activity related to the cerebral cortex. It can be used to localize cerebral lesions, although experience in horses is limited.[15,20]

PROCEDURE. Horses are placed in stocks when suitable. For horses prone to seizures or poor temperament, sedation or anesthesia are used. Care should be taken to avoid altering the seizure threshold with acetylpromazine, and the effects of this and other drugs on cerebral activity should be understood.[20] To detect EEG artefacts, a ground and two EEG electrodes are attached to the neck. External stimuli should be reduced by turning off lights and reducing noise. Recordings can be obtained with a five-point bipolar system arranged in the right and left occipital, right and left frontal, and vertex positions. These sites are located approximately along two lines that run

diagonally from the base of each ear to the opposite eyeball. The occipital sites are located about 1 inch from the ear, the frontal sites about 1.5 inches from the zygomatic arch, and the vertex is located where the lines bisect.

RESULTS. The bipolar system allows recordings to be made of each of the possible electrode pairs, thereby allowing comparison between left and right occipital regions, left and right frontal regions, and left and right sides. In the normal alert horse findings are characterized by a low-voltage, high-frequency dominant wave (8–15 µV, 18–30 Hz) carrying a series of higher-voltage, slower-frequency (10–40 µV, 5–19 Hz) waves. Details of waveform such as symmetry, shape, frequency, and amplitude are important, and variations of these components can indicate disease. Although there are no particular changes that are pathognomonic for any specific condition, findings are generally useful to differentiate between general and localized lesions and irritative and degenerative processes.[15]

R E F E R E N C E S

1. Mayhew IG: Large Animal Neurology. A Handbook for Veterinary Clinicians. Philadelphia, Lea & Febiger, 1989.
2. Blythe L: Neurologic examination of the horse. *In* Neurologic Diseases. Vet Clin North Amer: Equine Pract 1987; 3:255.
3. Watrous BJ: Head tilt in horses. *In* Neurologic Diseases. Vet Clin North Amer: Equine Pract 1987; 3:363.
4. Mayhew IG: Collection of cerebrospinal fluid from the horse. Cornell Vet 1975; 65:500.
5. Mayhew IG, Beal CR: Techniques of analysis of cerebrospinal fluid. Vet Clin North Am: Small Anim Pract 1980; 10:155.
6. Butler JA, Colles CM, Dyson SJ, et al: The spine. *In* Clinical Radiology of the Horse. Oxford, Blackwell, 1993, ch 9, p 355.
7. Mayhew IG, Whitlock R, de Lahunta A: Spinal cord disease in the horse. Cornell Vet 1978; 68 Suppl 6:44.
8. Hubbell J, Reed S, Myer C, et al: Sequelae of myelography in the horse. Equine Vet J 1988; 20:438.
9. Barbee DD, Allen JR: Computed tomography in the horse: General principles and clinical application. *In* Proceedings of the 32nd Annual Convention of the American Association of Equine Practitioners, 1986, p. 483.
10. Barbee D, Allen J, Gavin P: Computed tomography in horses: Technique. Vet Radiol 1987; 28:144.
11. Moore BR, Holbrook TC, Stefanacci JD, et al: Contrast-enhanced computed tomography in six horses with cervical stenotic myelography. Equine Vet J 1992; 24:197.
12. Allen J: Diagnosis of pituitary tumors by computed tomography. Part 1. Compend Contin Ed 1988a; 10:1103.
13. Allen J: Diagnosis of pituitary tumors by computed tomography. Part 11. Compend Contin Ed 1988b; 10: 1196.

14. Allen J, Barbee D, Boulton C, Major M, et al: Brain abscess in a horse: Diagnosis by computed tomography and successful surgical treatment. Equine Vet J 1987; 19:552.

15. Andrews FM, Fenner WR: Indication and use of electrodiagnostic aids in neurologic diseases. *In* Neurologic Disease. Vet Clin North Am: Equine Pract 1987; 3:293.

16. Henry RW, Diesem CD, Wiechers MD: Evaluation of equine radial and median nerve conduction velocities. Am J Vet Res 1979; 40:1406.

17. Henry RW, Diesem CD: Proximal equine radial and median motor nerve conduction velocity. Am J Vet Res 1981; 42:1819.

18. Marshall AE, Byers TD, Whitlock RH, et al: Brain stem auditory-evoked response in the diagnosis of inner ear injury in the horse. J Am Vet Med Assoc 1978; 178:282.

19. Marshall AE: Brainstem auditory-evoked response in the nonanesthetized horse and pony. Am J Vet Res 1985; 46:1445.

20. Mysinger PW, Redding RW, Vaughan JT, et al: Electroencephalographic patterns of clinically normal, sedated, and tranquilized newborn foals and adult horses. Am J Vet Res 1985; 46:35.

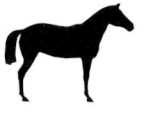

The Musculoskeletal System

5

COMPONENTS

The musculoskeletal (MS) system consists of hard- and soft-tissue structures, but, because of their anatomical integration into a functional unit, the division between them is not a distinct one. In general, the *hard tissue* includes the appendicular and axial skeleton with associated articular cartilages, and the *soft tissue* components include tendons, ligaments, muscles, bursae, synovial structures, and associated nerves. Although evaluation of the nervous system has been described in Chapter 4, it is relevant to the MS system because of the importance of diagnostic anesthesia to evaluate lameness and because lameness is the main sign of several specific nerve injuries.

MANIFESTATIONS OF DISEASE

The MS system is vital for body support and mobility, activities that require normal neuromuscular function. The most frequent sign of disease in the MS system is an abnormality of gait or stance. Other signs include soft- or hard-tissue swelling, localized pain, muscle atrophy, discharge from a sinus or fistula, and systemic signs such as pyrexia, mental depression, and loss of body condition.

EVALUATION OF LAMENESS

Definition of Lameness

For an excellent review of lameness and its diagnosis, the reader is referred to Adams' Lameness in Horses.[1] Lameness can be defined as an abnormality of gait. Under normal circumstances this applies to painful lesions, but it is not clear where gait abnormalities characterized by incoordination, specific nerve defects, or joint stiffness not associated with pain can be placed. It is probably preferable to include all gait abnormalities under the single definition as this can be done without loss of usefulness. In addition to a classification based on severity, lameness is often divided into *swinging leg* or *supporting leg* lameness. In a swinging leg lameness, when the leg is being advanced, it is usually swung forward in an arc outside the normal line (circumducted). A supporting leg (or weightbearing) lameness is apparent during the weightbearing phase of the stride and is characterized by abnormal body and head movements as the horse attempts to redistribute its weight. The supposed value of the classification is that problems in the upper limb tend to produce a swinging leg lameness, and lower limb problems tend to cause a supporting leg lameness. Although this is often so, frequently it is not, and, to complicate matters, both types often coexist (mixed lameness). Therefore, from

GRADING OF LAMENESS ACCORDING TO SEVERITY

- *Grade 1.* Lameness is seen when the horse is trotting but not while walking.
- *Grade 2.* Lameness is seen at the walk, but no obvious head movement is present.
- *Grade 3.* Lameness is obvious at the walk and obvious head movement is present.
- *Grade 4.* The horse cannot bear weight on the affected limb.

a diagnostic point of view, the value of the classification is limited, although, for descriptive purposes, such as in reports and case records, it is quite useful.

Visual Examination at Rest

The first part of the examination is a careful visual appraisal with the horse at rest and before palpation or manipulation. This exam evaluates conformation and will detect abnormal swelling, muscle atrophy, deformity, presence of a fistula or sinus, wounds, scars, and abnormal stance such as resting the front of a hoof on the ground (pointing). Many horses have old lesions that are unrelated to the problem under investigation, but all abnormalities should be noted and then considered in the context of the presenting problem and the other findings.

Visual Examination during Exercise

Gait during Exercise

After the visual examination is completed, the horse should be examined while it is moving. It should be remembered that horses are used for many different purposes and that many lamenesses are associated with a particular type of use and may be evident only while the horse is undergoing that activity. This applies particularly to trotters and pacers, jumpers, and dressage horses. Although many lamenesses can be seen while the horse is walking or trotting, it is often necessary to have the horse moving faster and to observe it while it is performing its normal work. For horses accustomed to working in a lunging ring, a fast canter can be achieved, but galloping

requires the wider expanse and safety of a racecourse or similar area, with a rider in the saddle. In most circumstances, regardless of the type of horse and the problem, the initial examination will be carried out at a walk and, if necessary, a trot. Next, if necessary, a faster gait is used or the horse is made to perform the activity with which the lameness is associated. Because some problems are evident only when the horse is performing a specific task, such as pacing around a bend at high speed or jumping over an obstacle, the preliminary steps are often neglected. This procedure is not usually recommended, but when it does occur it should be undertaken in the knowledge that a full examination has not been carried out, that such neglect has been based on information obtained from the person with the horse, and that the ultimate responsibility for any subsequent errors of judgment rests with the clinician. Pain will often cause a horse to break from its normal gait, seen most often in trotters and pacers where it is defined as "breaking" or "losing its gear" and also in dressage horses.

The usual routine is to examine the horse as it moves away from, toward, and across the examiner. Forelimb lameness is usually best seen from the front and side, and hindlimb lamenesses are best seen from the rear and the side.

Surface for Lameness Examination

The examination can be conducted on hard or soft surfaces. Conditions that cause supporting leg lameness tend to be more obvious on a hard surface because of the increased concussion, whereas swinging leg lamenesses tend to be more obvious when the horse has to lift its feet out of soft ground, such as sand. Horses with sensitive soles often improve when working on soft ground and worsen when working on stoney or gravel surfaces. The sounds heard when the horse is on a hard surface are also of assistance, there being a louder sound when the normal leg contacts the ground than when the lame leg does.

Head Movements in Lame Horses

The manner in which the horse moves its head is an important diagnostic aid, and, as a result of this, the person leading the horse should not hold the lead in such a way as to restrict head movement. Usually the lead is allowed to hang rather loosely, but care is necessary to maintain control of the horse. The correct way to hold the lead is demonstrated in Figure 5-1.

Head movements are useful in localizing the problem to front or hind limb and to left or right side. This applies especially to the fore limbs. Some important guidelines for interpreting head movements are listed in the box.

In cases of bilateral lameness, when head movement is minimal or absent, the horse compensates for the pain by reducing the support phase for both limbs, thus producing a gait best described as a shuffle. However, if one limb is more painful than the other, the horse will elect to reduce bearing weight on it to a greater extent than on the less painful limb, thereby producing a gait in between the extremes of unilateral and symmetrical bilateral lameness. Care should also be taken in the trotting horse not to confuse a forelimb lameness with lameness of the opposite hind limb. There is a tendency to do this because in the trot both limbs of the diagonal (left fore-right hind or right fore-left hind) bear weight simultaneously and, as explained, the head is lowered in response to lameness of either limb.

HEAD MOVEMENTS IN LAME HORSES

- *Forelimb lameness.* The horse's head is lowered when the sound leg is placed on the ground (conversely, the head is raised when the lame leg is placed on the ground).
- *Hindlimb lameness.* The horse's head is lowered when the lame leg contacts the ground and vice versa (note that this is the opposite situation to that seen in the forelimb).
- *Bilateral lameness.* Nodding of the head is absent when equal weight is placed on equally painful limbs (see comment in text about asymetrical forelimb lameness).

Vertical Displacement of the Tuber Coxae

When a horse is moving there is an associated movement of the hind quarters, specifically the gluteal musculature and tuber coxae. Hindlimb lameness usually alters this movement, and the resulting asymmetry between the left and right sides is relatively easy to see, although correct identification of the affected limb is much more difficult. The literature contains numerous explanations of the diagnostic significance of variation, but they are confusing and often conflict. It has been demonstrated that *the best criterion for identifying the lame hindlimb with a painful lesion, regardless of site and type of lesion, is increased vertical displacement of the tuber coxae compared with the opposite limb.*[2] Experienced clinicians can easily identify this parameter, but, for others, adhesive tape markers placed on the tuber coxae make it a little easier (Fig. 5-2). The height of the tuber coxae on the affected side is greatest when the limb contacts the ground, thereafter sinking gradually until just before the next weightbearing phase when it rapidly elevates to its high point.[2] In situations where there is mechanical interference with flexion of the hindlimb there is a tendency for the toe to contact the ground when the leg is advanced, causing the horse to respond by circumducting the limb as well as elevating the quarters. An example of this is intermittent

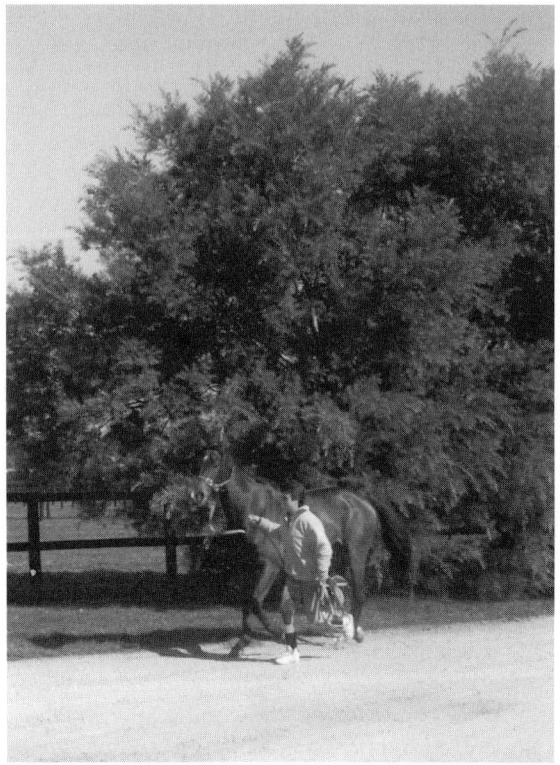

▶ FIGURE 5–1

Lameness examination. Hold lead loosely so that head movements are not restricted.

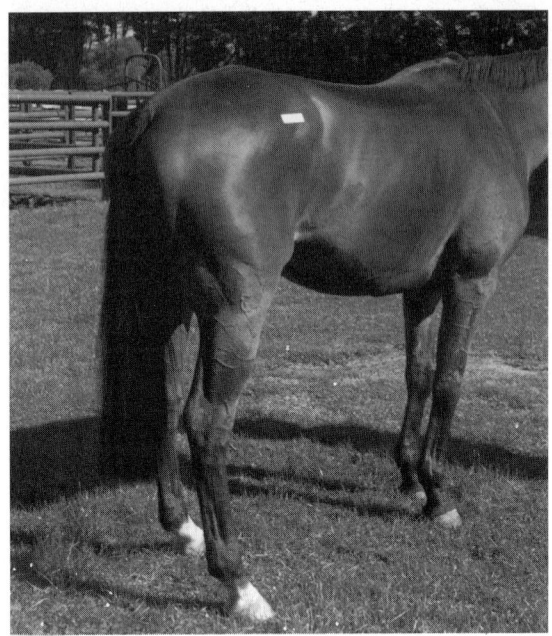

▶ FIGURE 5-2
White markers placed on tubers coxae to help detect vertical movement of the pelvis.

patellar fixation, a problem especially seen in pacing and trotting horses, where the hip elevation is often known as "hiking."

Gluteal Rise

The height of the croup, or gluteal musculature, during exercise is also used to detect hindlimb lameness, and the term *gluteal rise* describes this upward movement. It is likely that measuring displacement of the tuber coxae and observing upward movement of the croup are assessing much the same activity, although increase in muscle mass during contraction may also be a factor. The duration of the rise is less when painful lesions are present, caused by the need to shorten the time of weightbearing. Although the croup on the affected side is raised at the commencement of the stride, vertical displacement of the tuber coxae is easier to detect and shows greater disparity between normal and affected limbs.

Normal Gait

Lameness diagnosis requires a knowledge of the normal gaits, which are classed as *natural* or *artificial* (learned). The main natural gaits are the walk, trot, canter, and gallop (a canter is defined as a collected gallop). Artificial gaits are the running walk, amble, rack (broken amble or singlefoot), and pace, which can also, depending on the individual, be natural. The traditional saddle horse is expected to exhibit the natural gaits. Specialized selections of gaits are seen in the five-gaited horses and Tennessee Walking Horses. While dressage horses are required to perform numerous different movements, these do not constitute a separate gait.

Although a detailed study of the different gaits is not required here, a summary of the common gaits is presented, with notation for the left fore, right fore, left hind, and right hind foot (LF, RF, LH, and RH respectively):[3]

- *Walk.* The walk is a lateral four-beat gait, with the feet contacting the ground at regular intervals in the order LH, LF, RH, RF. There is no period of suspension (all feet off the ground), and at least two feet are always on the ground.

- *Trot.* The trot is a two-beat gait with diagonal feet contacting the ground simultaneously in the order LH-RF, RH-LF. A period of suspension is often present.

- *Canter.* The canter is a three-beat gait, with pairing of one set of diagonal limbs. Ground contact is in the order of LH, RH-LF, RF or RH, LH-RF, LF. A short period of suspension is present. The single limbs are known as the lead limbs and carry the most weight. The horse will change the lead as necessary to avoid fatigue. By using appropriate aids the rider can stimulate the horse to change leads. Sometimes a four-beat canter occurs when the paired diagonal limbs do not land exactly together, (e.g., LH, RH, LF, RF).

- *Gallop.* The gallop is an extended four-beat gait with the same lead system as described for the canter. The order of ground contact is LH, RH, LF, RF with a period of suspension. The horse will change the lead to avoid fatigue as well as when turning. When turning to the right, the horse will lead with the RF leg and the LF when turning to the left. Change of leads occurs during the period of suspension, although, sometimes, the fore and hindlimbs do not change at the same time. Unwillingness to use the appropriate lead or to change as directed by the rider may indicate pain.

- *Pace.* The pace is a lateral two-beat gait with ground contact occurring in the order

LH-LF, RH-RF with a period of suspension. The pace is faster than the trot and slower than a gallop.

- *Flatfoot Walk.* This gait is the natural walk of the Tennessee Walking horse. It is similar to the walk but faster.
- *Running Walk.* This is the fast walk of the Tennessee Walking Horse. It is similar to the walk and flatfoot walk, and it is characterized by a gliding motion.
- *Fox Trot.* This is similar to the trot except that the hindlimb in each diagonal pair contacts the ground slightly before the forelimb.
- *Rack.* This is a walk characterized by exaggerated limb movement.
- *Amble.* The amble is a slow, walking speed pace, with the hindlimb contacting the ground just before the forelimb on the same side. Unlike the pace, it exhibits no period of suspension.

PHASE OF STRIDE. There are cranial and caudal phases to the stride. The cranial phase is that part of the stride in front of the footprint of the opposite foot, and the caudal phase is that part behind it. Lengthening of one is compensated for by shortening of the other. The phases of the stride have little application to routine lameness diagnosis.

ARC OF FLIGHT. The arc of flight is the curve the foot makes in a vertical plane as it is advanced during the swing phase of the stride. It is viewed from the lateral side. The main cause of alteration is a reduction in joint flexion (e.g., painful joint lesions or patellar fixation) that produces a lower arc with a tendency for the toe of the hoof to catch or drag on the ground. A hoof with a long toe alters the arc by increasing the height of the caudal section and decreasing the height of the cranial section. The reverse is seen when the toe is short.

PATH OF FLIGHT. The path of flight describes the line taken by the hoof during the swing phase. Ideally this is a straight line, but it can be curved inward or outward. An inward curve increases the possibility of contact between a hoof and the medial side of the opposite limb, which can result in fracture of the second metacarpal bone as well as other trauma.

WAY OF LANDING. The hoof is usually placed on the ground with heel contact occurring first. Painful lesions are capable of altering this se-quence, with pain in the toe region (e.g., abscess, foreign body penetration) tending to exaggerate the normal sequence, and pain in the heel region (e.g., navicular syndrome) tending to cause a toe first landing. Pain located in the lateral or medial regions (e.g., abscess, fracture) tend to cause increased loading of the medial and lateral sides of the hoof, respectively. Toe first landing oftens cause a horse to stumble and even fall. Observation of the manner of landing will assist in localizing the lesion.

Examination of Specific Regions

Both forelimbs and hindlimbs and the back should be examined systematically. Because most problems are located in the lower limb, examination of the limbs should begin at the hoof and then proceed proximally. The examination consists of a series of palpation and manipulation procedures designed to detect abnormalities, including pain, crepitus, elevated skin temperature, and swelling. Now is the time to evaluate anything detected in the visual examination. The exact procedure is a matter of personal preference and will vary with the skill and experience of the examiner. The significance of some findings can often be solved by comparison with the opposite limb, especially to evaluate suspected elevation of surface temperature. Skin or hoof temperature is checked with the palm or back of the hand. The back of the hand appears to be more sensitive, but it may not be appropriate for all anatomical regions because of the surface contour.

Examination of the Forelimb

Hoof

VISUAL. Hoof shape is related partly to individual variation and partly to the way in which the farrier has trimmed or shod the hoof, and also to abnormal growth resulting from chronic, painful lesions. The foot is inspected for conformation, heel height, space between heels, growth rings, cracks in the wall, discharge from the coronary band or sole, and improper shoeing.

PALPATION. Regions to palpate include the coronary band, lateral cartilages, frog, and sole. Abnormalities of the coronary band include pain (laminitis, abscess), increased temperature (laminitis, abscess), swelling (abscess, scar), discharge (abscess), loss of firmness, and downward deviation of the skin (distal displacement of the third phalanx within the hoof due to laminitis, known as a "sinker"). The lateral cartilages should be palpated while the horse is bearing weight and also when its foot is elevated. The lateral cartilages should be soft and pliable in young horses. They become stiffer with age ("side bone"), and, when fractured or undergoing ossification as a result of inflammation, they are often painful.

HOOF PICK. The hoof pick is used to remove debris from the sole and frog region, which otherwise obscures the hoof proper and precludes examination (Fig. 5-3). The hoof knife should not be used for this purpose.

HOOF KNIFE. The hoof knife is an indispensible instrument for foot examination. It is used to pare away excess sole, to explore suspicious cracks or defects in the sole or bearing surface of the hoof walls, and to remove sole or frog tissue overlying a localized region of pain such as an abscess or bruise (Fig. 5-4). Although bruises can be caused by the horse standing on a stone or similar object, especially when the ground surface is hard, the commonest cause of bruising is the shoe. Shoes should be positioned so that they contact the hoof wall and a small part of the sole adjacent to the white line. When the contact extends too far onto the sole (incorrect shoeing technique, convex soles), pain and bruising result. Correct shoeing ensures that the ends of the shoe (heel) curve inward and contact the wall and the bars of the hoof. If a shoe is left on the horse for too long, or, sometimes, because of poor shoeing technique, the ends contact the sole

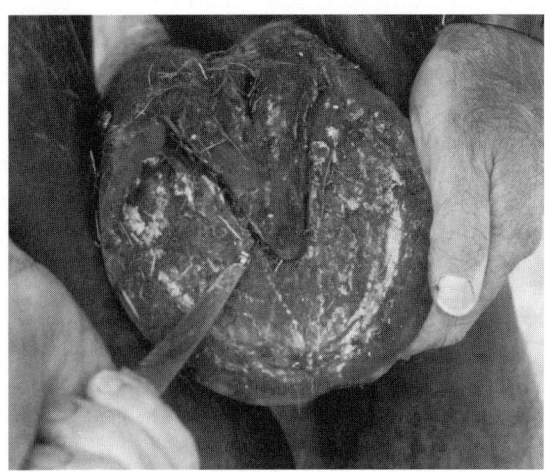

▶ **FIGURE 5-4**
Hoof knife used to remove excess horn or to pare it away while searching for deep lesions such as abscesses or hematomata.

in the angle between the wall and the bar of the hoof and produce a bruise.

HAMMER. Striking the hoof with a hammer can help localize a painful region (abscess, laminitis, fracture) or, by eliciting a hollow sound, can indicate a region where the hoof wall has separated from the underlying structures (chronic laminitis, healing abscess). The sole can be struck only when the foot is elevated, but the wall is usually struck when the hoof is bearing weight.

HOOF TESTERS. Hoof testers are indispensable for detecting pain, and they are extremely useful for indicating the exact site of the pain so that overlying tissue can be removed to relieve pressure (bruise) or establish drainage (abscess). Excessive pressure is painful and will cause a false-positive reaction. They should be applied systematically over the hoof as indicated (Fig. 5-5).

THE BOARD TEST. The board test is an effective method of extending the distal interphalangeal joint, and it is common in Europe. It is particularly useful in cases of navicular syndrome, where it increases tension in the deep flexor tendon and increases the compressive load on the navicular bone and its bursa. The test is conducted with a 6-foot-long board (6″ wide, 1″ thick), as shown in Fig. 5-6. The exact dimensions are not important except that the board should be thick enough to resist bending and be long enough to allow it to be elevated safely and easily. The board is placed on the ground with one end adjacent and lateral to the leg to be tested, and the other end extending directly out in front

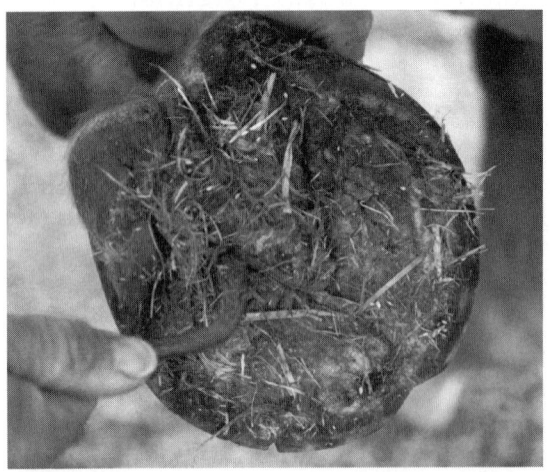

▶ **FIGURE 5-3**
Hoof pick used to remove dirt, stones, and debris from the sole and frog regions.

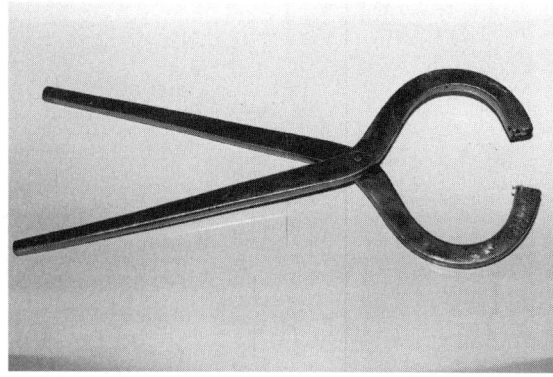

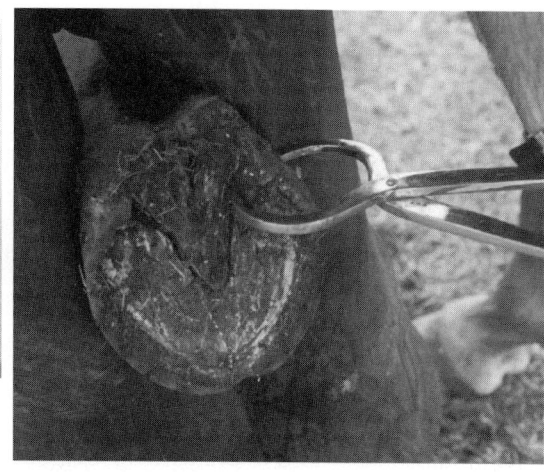

A

B

▶ **FIGURE 5-5**

Hoof testers. **A.** An example of a hoof tester. **B.** Using hoof tester to locate a painful focus by squeezing the hoof systematically.

of the horse. The limb to be tested is picked up and, after the board has been pushed under the horse, it is placed on the board at the same time as the opposite limb is picked up. The board is slowly elevated to a 45° angle while the examiner is observing the horse for signs of pain. Both limbs are tested. A negative test occurs when the horse stands squarely on the board without showing any inclination to jump off. The test is positive if the horse attempts to counteract the applied load by rocking back on its forelimb or by jumping off the board. The test also stresses the interphalangeal and fetlock joints, and pain in these regions will

also produce a positive result. A simple, but crude, form of the test consists of elevating the toe with a metal clip attached to the shoe, or by placing a wedge or similar object under the toe. These variations lack the precise control of the board test. Medial or lateral stress can be applied by varying the placement of the board or clips.

Pastern

VISUAL. The main visual alterations detected in this region include enlargement of the proximal interphalangeal joint ("ringbone" or arthritis) dorsally, laterally, and medially, scars from wounds, and caudal enlargement related to lesions of the distal sesamoidean ligaments and the deep flexor tendon.

PALPATION AND MANIPULATION. Palpation and manipulation verify pain in the region and detect the crepitus associated with fracture of the first and second phalanges. Care is required to evaluate old scars because they are often associated with a painful neuroma of one of the digital nerves as they run along the dorsolateral (medial) border of the deep flexor tendon.

Fetlock

VISUAL. Thickening and distension of the joint capsule and flexor tendon sheath are the most common visual signs. Thickening of the capsule is a chronic process caused by fibrosis (arthritis, proliferative synovitis). Distension of the capsule is caused by effusion (chronic arthritis, acute trauma), blood (trauma, fracture of the third metacarpal or metatarsal bone or the first pha-

▶ **FIGURE 5-6**

Board test to detect pain caused by extending the distal limb.

lanx) or exudate (septic arthritis). Capsular thickening is seen mainly on the dorsal aspect of the joint as an obvious bulging, whereas increased fluid causes distension of the medial and lateral palmar (plantar) pouches of the capsule between the third metacarpal or metatarsal bone and suspensory ligament just proximal to the sesamoid bones. Thickening and distension of the flexor tendon sheath are seen on the caudal aspect, mainly proximal and distal to the joint, where the sheath is not confined by the annular ligament.

PALPATION AND MANIPULATION. Palpation and manipulation are used to evaluate the degree of thickening in the capsule and the sheath, the presence of pain, and the existence of fibrotic or osseous masses within the synovial cavities. The apex and base of each sesamoid bone is palpated to check for pain where the suspensory ligament inserts and the distal sesamoidean ligaments originate.

FETLOCK FLEXION TEST. The flexion test is an integral part of lameness evaluation and is used for detecting reduced range of movement (capsule fibrosis) and pain. The joint can usually be flexed to an angle of about 90° (Fig. 5-7). When flexing the joint the first thing to note is whether or not full flexion is possible or painful. Full flexion is then maintained for 30 to 60 s (varies with preference, *but be consistent*). As the flexion is completed, the horse is made to lead off at a trot, and the flexion test is adjudged negative (no lameness) or positive (lameness or increased lameness). Note that flexion of the fetlock joint also involves flexion of the proximal and distal interphalangeal joints, which must be considered when interpreting the test. An attempt can be made to flex mainly the fetlock joint, but this is difficult.

Metacarpus

VISUAL. Visible lesions in this region include osseous swellings involving the proximal aspects of metacarpal or metatarsal 2 and 4 ("splints"), and the dorsal aspect of metacarpal 3 (metacarpal periostitis or "sore shins"), and soft-tissue swelling involving the flexor tendons and suspensory ligaments.

PALPATION AND MANIPULATION. Palpation is carried out with the limb bearing weight and

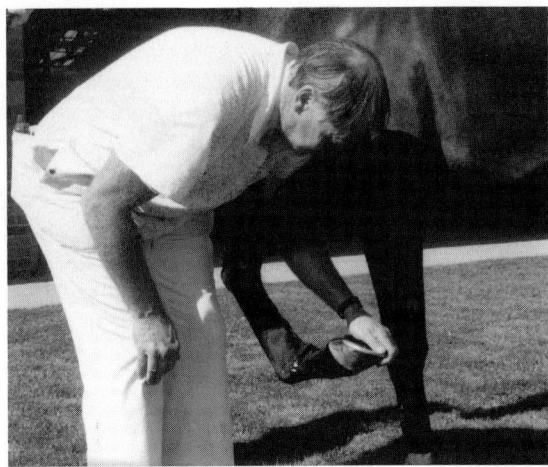

▶ **FIGURE 5-7**
Flexion of the metacarpophalangeal and interphalangeal joints.

then with it elevated. When it is elevated, the soft tissues are not under tension, and they can be examined more thoroughly. Osseous swellings should be firmly palpated to check whether they are painful. A pain response indicates that active inflammation (periostitis) or fracture (metacarpal 2 or 4) are probably present. The full length of the flexor tendons and interosseous ligament should be carefully palpated. The accessory ligament of the deep flexor tendon (inferior check ligament) can be palpated best, with the limb elevated, by pressing a thumb in between the suspensory ligament and deep flexor tendon immediately below the carpus on medial and lateral aspects.

Carpus

VISUAL. Thickening of the carpal joint capsule and distension of the joint cavity, as well as distension of the extensor tendon sheaths, are seen on the cranial aspect of the joint. Distension of the carpal sheath is seen where it protrudes proximal and distal to the carpal canal on the caudal aspect of the joint. Distinct fluid-filled swellings on the dorsal aspect (bursae) may arise, or be separate, from a tendon sheath or a carpal joint.

PALPATION AND MANIPULATION. Palpation involves careful examination of the dorsal aspect to detect swelling, effusion, and pain. The examination is begun with the limb weightbearing and is completed with it elevated. When the limb is elevated, the fingers can be inserted into the depressions between the carpal bones where the extent of thickening and swelling are best judged. The carpal sheath region can be examined in a similar fashion. The most common lesions are fracture of the small bones of the joint. Lesions of the flexor and extensor tendon sheaths occur less frequently.

CARPAL FLEXION TEST. The joint is flexed for 30 to 60 s by elevating the metacarpal region so that it contacts the forearm (Fig. 5–8A). More severe flexion is obtained by pulling the limb slightly laterally so that the hoof and metacarpus come to lie lateral to the radius (Fig. 5–8B). Flexion is judged positive if it is painful or if it produces, or exacerbates, lameness. Another use for flexion is to ascertain whether flexion reduces or abolishes the arterial pulse distal to the carpus (carpal tunnel syndrome).

Upper Forearm (Radius, Elbow, Humerus, Shoulder)

VISUAL. With the much greater soft-tissue cover in this region, lesions are not so apparent. Visible signs include atrophy of the supra- and infraspinatus muscles ("sweeney") as a result of damage to the suprascapular nerve, fluid-filled swelling over the olecranon process (olecranon bursitis), and swelling of the shoulder joint (arthritis).

PALPATION AND MANIPULATION. Although palpation of the elbow and shoulder joints is difficult, the procedure is still useful. The medial and lateral aspects of the elbow can be palpated to evaluate the collateral ligaments. Manipulation of the olecranon will usually detect the pain or

mobility of a fracture. The collateral ligaments can also be assessed by adducting or abducting the elevated limb. Special care should be given to firm palpation of the region of the shoulder joint, where problems such as arthritis, bicipital bursitis, and fracture of the scapular and humerus in the region of the bicipital groove occur.

FLEXION, EXTENSION, AND ABDUCTION TESTS OF THE UPPER FOREARM. Some methods for stressing the upper forelimb are demonstrated in Figure 5–9. A test is positive if the horse exhibits pain or if lameness is induced or exacerbated. It is apparent that it is difficult to examine a specific joint when using these stress tests. Elevation of the limb flexes the elbow joint and increases the tension in the triceps muscles, producing a positive test when there is a fracture of the olecranon process or an elbow joint lesion is present. Extension of the shoulder is claimed to be induced by flexion of the elbow with the distal limb relaxed, rather than extended, and flexion by simultaneous caudal retraction of the limb and forward pressure to the olecranon. Caudal retraction of the limb is often used to demonstrate pain in the region of the biceps structures dorsal to the shoulder joint, but obviously this activity will also increase tension in structures that resist elbow extension.

Examination of the Hindlimb

Examination of the limb distal to the tarsus is similar to that for the forelimb distal to the carpus

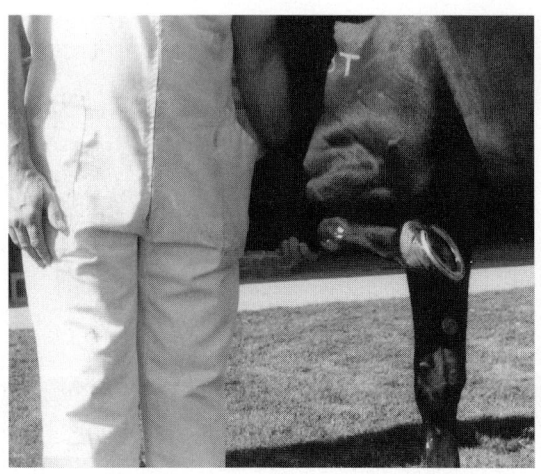
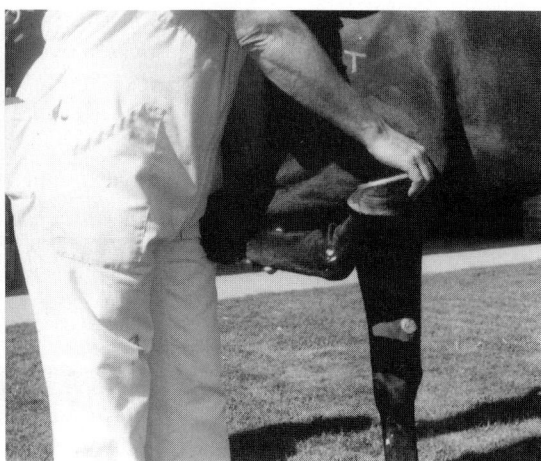

▶ **FIGURE 5–8**
Flexion of the carpal joint. **A.** Normal flexion. **B.** Extreme flexion.

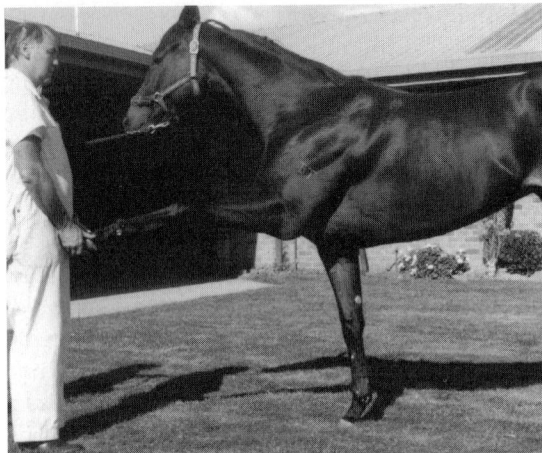

A

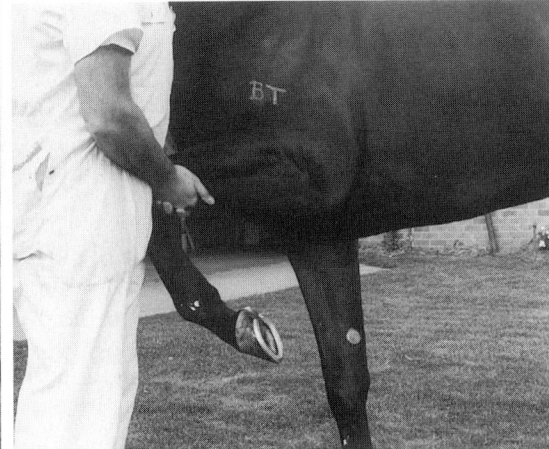

B

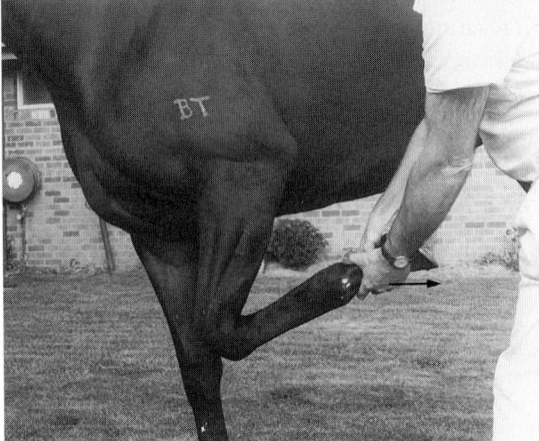

C

▶ **FIGURE 5-9**

Applying stress to upper limb. **A.** Shoulder extension. **B.** Elbow flexion. **C.** Elbow extension.

although the fetlock flexion test is different (Fig. 5–10).

Tarsus (Hock)

VISUAL. The hock is examined for signs that include distension of the talocrural joint capsule ("bog" spavin), osseous enlargement located over the small joints on the dorsomedial aspect ("bone" spavin), fluid-filled swelling over the proximal aspect of the tuber calcis ("capped" hock or bursitis), displacement of the superficial digital flexor tendon from its normal position over the tuber calcis, and distension of the extensor tendon sheaths.

PALPATION AND MANIPULATION. Palpation is directed particularly toward assessing the extent of swelling and the presence of pain. Pain is usually not present with joint distension unless sepsis is present. Firm palpation of the swelling of bone spavin will often elicit a pain response, particularly in early cases. Dislocation of the superficial flexor tendon is characterized by the

ability to displace the tendon manually, either medially or laterally off the tuber calcis.

FLEXION AND EXTENSION OF THE TARSUS. The hock flexion test is so useful in the diagnosis

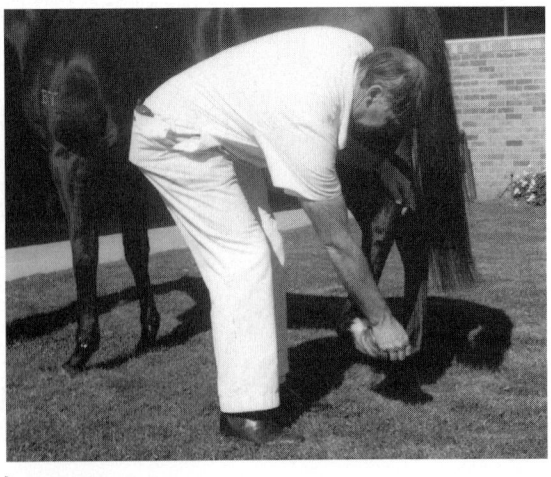

▶ **FIGURE 5-10**

Flexion of the metatarsophalangeal joint.

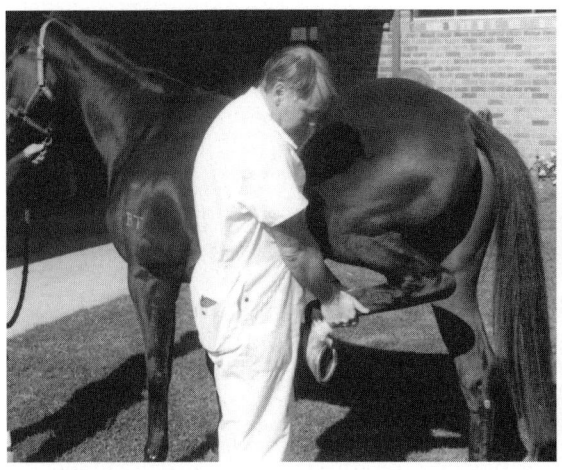
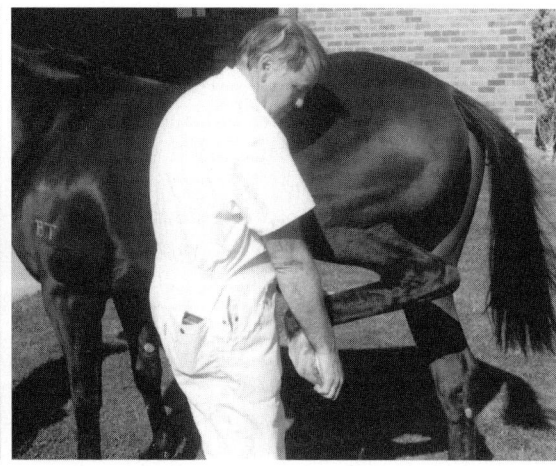

A

B

▶ **FIGURE 5-11**

Spavin test. The spavin test without **A.** and with **B.** flexion of the metatarsophalangeal joint.

of bone spavin that the test is often termed "the spavin test." The test is demonstrated in Figure 5-11. The reciprocal apparatus, which coordinates flexion and extension in the hindlimb, ensures that all joints flex and extend together. Therefore, flexion of the hock also results in flexion of the fetlock, stifle, and hip, which must be considered when interpreting the test results. Nevertheless, the high incidence of spavin means that a positive hock flexion test is often diagnostic for spavin. It is preferable to hold the limb above the fetlock, as demonstrated in the figure, so that fetlock flexion is minimized.

Loss of integrity of the reciprocal apparatus also helps diagnose the site of injury. Disruption of the dorsal (peroneus tertius muscle) or caudal

(superficial flexor tendon) component removes the reciprocal flexion-extension of the stifle and hock, making it possible to extend the hock when the stifle is flexed, and flex the hock when the stifle is flexed. The test is demonstrated in Figure 5-12.

Stifle

VISUAL. The stifle is evaluated for evidence of distension of the femoropatellar joint capsule and atrophy of muscles of the thigh region. Minor distension of the femoropatellar joint is difficult to see, but significant distension is obvious when viewed from the side. The position of the patella should also be noted as a check for patella luxation.

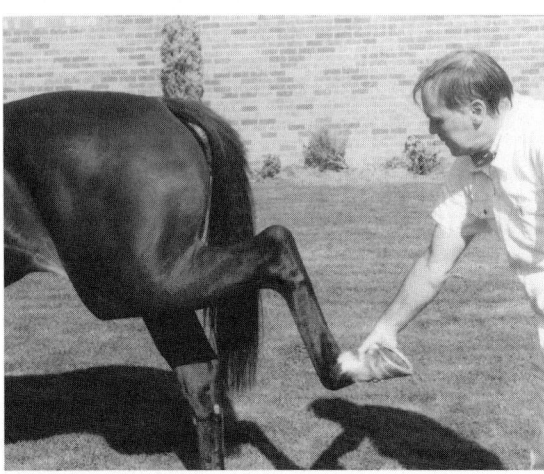
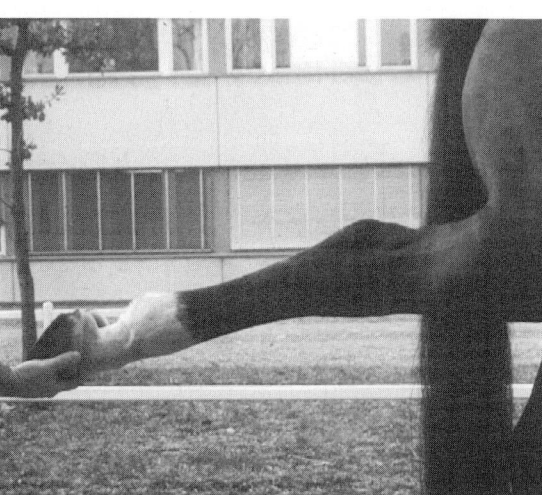

A

B

▶ **FIGURE 5-12**

Testing the integrity of reciprocal apparatus. **A.** Normal. Note that the hock cannot be extended while the stifle is flexed. **B.** Rupture of perineus tertius. Note that the hock is extended while the stifle has remained flexed.

PALPATION AND MANIPULATION. The femoropatellar joint capsule is palpated on either side of the middle patellar ligament where the pouch bulges between this ligament and the medial and lateral patellar ligaments. Distension of the joint and thickening of the capsule can be palpated. Comparison with the opposite limb is made whenever necessary. The normal position of the patellar in the femoral trochlea should be noted, as should the presence of pain and increased mobility. It should not be possible to luxate the patella.

PATELLAR DISPLACEMENT TEST. When the horse desires to fix the limb in extension, the medial patellar ligament and the accessory cartilage can be made to hook over the proximal part of the large medial femoral condyle. This process is normally under voluntary muscular control, but in horses with poorly developed musculature, especially in those with upright hindlimb conformation, the fixation can activate spontaneously and produce either a temporary inability to flex the leg at the beginning of the stride or a complete fixation in extension. In horses with this tendency it is often possible to produce fixation manually, using the patellar displacement test. The test is made with the limb in extension and consists of grasping the patella between the thumb and fingers, pulling it laterally, and then making the horse take a few steps (Fig. 5–13). With a negative result the horse is able to flex the stifle normally. With a positive result there is either a momentary or total inability to flex the limb, seen

as a delay in flexion or dragging the toe, respectively. A false positive is more likely in small horses, and a false negative is more likely in large strong animals.

TEST OF THE CRUCIATE LIGAMENTS. In small animals cranial or posterior displacement of the proximal tibia relative to the distal femur is known as a drawer sign and is useful to test the integrity of the cruciate ligaments. The size of a horse makes it virtually impossible to perform an identical test, the closest being when the horse is in lateral recumbency under general anesthesia. In standing horses the test is conducted by pulling or pushing the proximal tibia sharply in a caudal direction, with the clinician standing behind or in front of the limb, respectively. The limb is released after each movement, and allowed to rebound. The test is repeated 10 to 20 times, noting any crepitus, pain reaction, or unusual joint mobility. The horse is then trotted and observed for lameness or exacerbation of an existing lameness. The test is useful only for advanced cases.

TEST OF THE MEDIAL AND LATERAL COLLATERAL LIGAMENTS. The medial collateral ligament is associated with the medial meniscus and is more likely to be injured than the lateral ligament. The medial ligament is tested by holding the metatarsus and applying medial pressure to the proximal tibial with the shoulder (Fig. 5–14A). If the ligament is elongated or ruptured, simultaneous palpation will detect the separation of the tibia and femur on the medial aspect. The lateral ligament is tested by placing both hands around the stifle region and pulling laterally (Fig. 5–14B). Both tests can also be repeated a number of times and the horse trotted to check for induced or exacerbated lameness.

Muscles of Proximal Limb

VISUAL. The region is examined for signs of atrophy (femoral nerve injury), swelling (hematoma, abscess), and distortion or puckering of skin surface (underlying fibrosis).

PALPATION AND MANIPULATION. These muscles should be palpated firmly. In acute cases tears and hematomata are palpable, and, in chronic cases, fibrosis and bone also are palpable. The most common sites of injury are the semimembranous and semitendinosis muscles on the caudal aspect of the thigh.

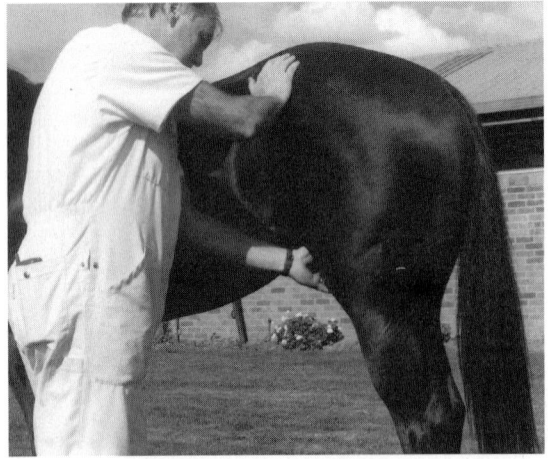

▶ **FIGURE 5-13**

Patellar fixation testing. This test is conducted by pulling the patella laterally with the limb extended.

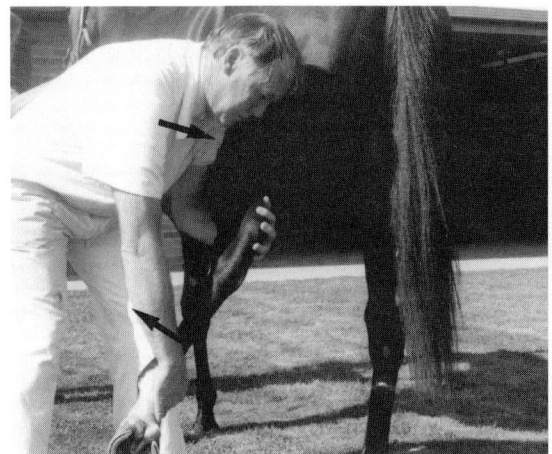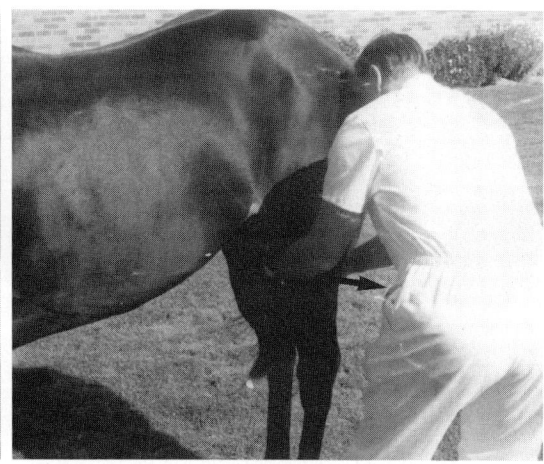

A

B

▶ FIGURE 5-14

Applying stress to collateral ligaments of the femorotibial joint (stifle). **A.** Medial collateral ligament. **B.** Lateral collateral ligament.

The Hip

VISUAL. Chronic pain in the hip (arthritis, fracture) causes disuse atrophy, which is readily apparent. Coxofemoral luxation in horses is usually in a craniodorsal direction, producing an apparent shortening of the limb and a stifle-out, hock-in, toe-out stance. If the round ligament is ruptured, the stance is similar, but there is no limb shortening.

PALPATION AND MANIPULATION. Palpation of the greater trochanter (Fig. 5-15) is useful for detecting crepitus (fracture, arthritis) and displacement (luxation). Displacement can be assessed by comparing the distance from the trochanter to the tuber ischiadicum and the tuber sacrale, using the opposite side for comparison.

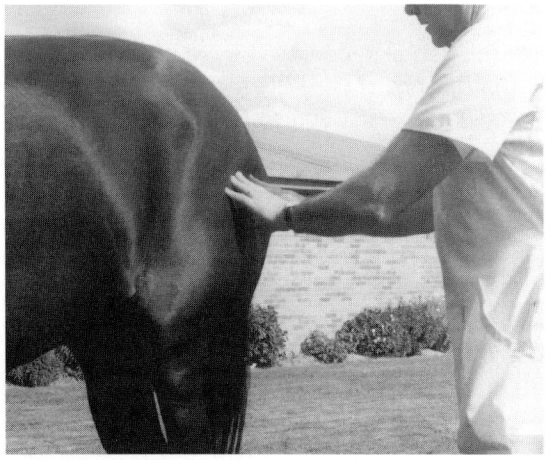

▶ FIGURE 5-15

Palpation of the greater trochanter.

When a craniodorsal luxation is present, the limb cannot be rotated inwardly. Rupture of the round ligament with luxation allows rotation without crepitus.

Examination of the Back and Pelvis

Examining the back is a particularly difficult task because of the size of the patient and the inability to see and palpate most of the structures. Although any horse can be afflicted with a back problem, show jumpers, dressage horses, and pacers and trotters are especially predisposed. The signs with which horses with a back problem present are many and include reluctance or inability to perform normal activity, loss of performance, refusal to accept weightbearing from the saddle or rider, muscle atrophy, asymmetry of musculature, rotation of the pelvis, and uneven heights of the tubers sacrale.[4]

VISUAL. The full length of the back is examined from either side as well as from above. Signs that are seen include disuse atrophy of the musculature (pain), deviation or loss of height of the wither, (fracture of the thoracic dorsal spinous processes), localized nodules (folliculitis, insect bites), hair loss (pressure from saddle, fungal infection), unequal heights of the tubers sacrale and tubers coxae (sacroiliac subluxation), ventral displacement of the tuber coxae or "dropped hip" (fracture). The sacral and coxal tubers are best evaluated from behind with the horse standing squarely on even ground. The sacral tubers are

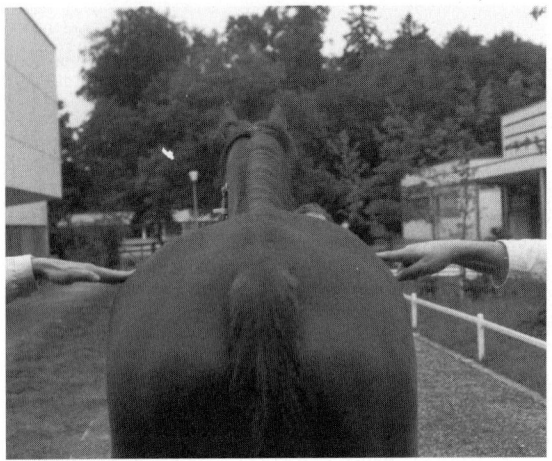

FIGURE 5–16

Assessing the relative heights of the left and right tuber coxae.
The right tuber coxae is higher than the left. The right tuber
sacrale is also higher and muscle atrophy of the left gluteal
mass is evident.

compared directly, but for the coxal tubers it is an
advantage to have a person stand on either side of
the horse and place a finger on the tuber coxae
(Fig. 5–16).

PALPATION AND MANIPULATION. The back
should be firmly palpated with the fingers to
discover any pain or hypersensitivity. This is done
along the midline, to evaluate the tip of each
spinous process and the associated dorsal spinous ligament and, lateral to the midline, to
evaluate the musculature. The wither is checked
for fracture by attempting to pull it laterally,
which produces pain in an acute fracture and
crepitus in a chronic fracture. The sacral tubers
and surrounding musculature are palpated to
detect pain in cases of subluxation.

TESTS OF BACK MOBILITY. Most horses respond to firm, localized, digital pressure in the
dorsal musculature of the thoracolumbar region
by ventroflexion of the back and to similar
pressure in the croup region by dorsiflexion. A
more sensitive way to produce the same response
is to run a pen, or similar instrument, along the
back either side of the midline. Lateral flexion can
be produced by running the pen directly away
from the midline or along the back well away from
the midline. Free, relaxed movement is indicative
of absence of pain. An excessive response, even
to the extent where the horse falls to the ground,
is sometimes present. Although this is often taken
to indicate pain, some type of hypersensitivity
cannot be excluded as many horses with this

response are otherwise clinically normal. Back
rigidity, reluctance to flex, and lack of flexion indicate pain.

RECTAL EXAMINATION. A rectal examination
(see Chapter 11, Per Rectum Palpation of the
Abdomen) is an important part of back examination. Specific examination of the sublumbar
region for evidence of swelling (myositis, vertebral fracture with hematoma), abnormality of the
aorta or its branches (thrombosis), and enlargement of lymph nodes (neoplasia) should be made.
The pelvis is checked for symmetry (fracture) and
special attention is given to the region over the
acetabulae, the ilial shafts, and the ventral surface
of the sacrum (subluxation).

Diagnostic Anesthesia ("Nerve Blocks")

Local anesthesia is a most important part of
lameness evaluation. The principle behind its use
is that once a painful lesion has been desensitized,
lameness and pain response to palpation or manipulation resolve partially or completely, thereby
proving that the site of pain lies in the desensitized
region that can then be further evaluated by other
methods as required, usually by radiography. The
following description of diagnostic anesthesia is
based largely on the author's experience, and for
further information the reader is referred to other
texts.[1,5,6] The local anesthetic can be delivered in
several different ways:

- Local infiltration in a specific region
- Linear deposition proximal to a suspected
  lesion (field block), used in lameness for
  depositing anesthetic solution around a limb
  (ring block)
- Perineural deposition (nerve block)
- Intrasynovial deposition in joints, tendon
  sheaths, and bursae

The procedure usually commences in the distal
limb and moves systematically up the leg until the
anesthesia abolishes pain. There are two reasons
for this distal-to-proximal progression. The first is
that because the source of lameness is much more
likely to be in the distal portion of the limb,
considerable time is saved by identifying the site
of the problem earlier and avoiding unnecessary
testing. The second reason is that if perineural
anesthesia (the usual form of anesthesia) is begun
unsuccessfully in the upper limb, injection of any
distal sites must be delayed because all structures

distal to the site of the first injection(s) will already be desensitized. Exceptions to this pattern can be made when intrasynovial or infiltration techniques are used because they desensitize only specific sites rather than all distal structures.

Choice of Anesthetic Agent

Traditionally, lidocaine has been used most frequently for diagnostic anesthesia. However, mepivacaine is now used more often because it is less irritant to tissues.[7] Its effect is of longer duration.[8] Local anesthetics interfere with interpretation of scintigraphy and in this respect mepivacaine should be used when scintigraphy is scheduled within 2 to 3 days.

The onset of action is usually within 5 minutes, although full anesthesia may require 10 to 15 minutes. A delayed effect beyond this period can indicate that the agent has diffused into the surrounding tissue and has anesthetized structures other than those expected. The duration of effect is about 30 minutes for lidocaine and 120 minutes for mepivacaine. Adrenalin prolongs the duration but serves no useful purpose in diagnostic anesthesia.

Preparation and General Procedure

Optimal skin preparation for intrasynovial injection includes removing hair and a routine skin scrub with an antiseptic and 70% alcohol. The catastrophic effects of septic synovitis, especially septic arthritis, dictate that all possible care be taken, although in a busy practice a less strict

---

Materials for Diagnostic Anesthesia

- Local anesthetic (unopened bottle for intrasynovial injection)
    Mepivacaine 2% (Carbocaine-V, Winthrop Laboratories, New York, NY)
    Lidocaine 2% (Xylocaine, Astra Pharmaceutical Products, Worcester, MA)
- Sterile syringes and needles (not Luer-Lok)
- Sterile gloves for intrasynovial injection
- Hair clippers (#40 clipper head)
- Antiseptic (e.g., Betadine, Hibiclens)
- 70% alcohol

---

protocol is often used. Such thorough preparation is unnecessary for the other forms of local anesthesia, where the usual methods include simply wiping the region with a swab moistened with 70% alcohol or clipping the hair and then rubbing the site with a swab moistened with 70% alcohol. Identifying the exact site for injection almost always involves palpation of the site, and, for this reason, the hands should be gloved for intrasynovial injection and at least washed with antiseptic for the other injections.

The horse should be adequately restrained so as to avoid injury to the clinician. This applies particularly to injection in the hindlimbs. A competent horse handler is required and a lip twitch is necessary for some horses. Some horses are unsafe to inject and the procedure should be avoided, or curtailed, when the danger is too great. The position where the clinician should stand for maximum safety is to some extent a matter of personal preference. The positions preferred by the author are apparent in the figures demonstrating the different injections.

Horses will often react to injection by pulling the limb away. For this reason, it is usual to insert the needle first and to release it immediately. If it is attached to the syringe, movement of the horse during needle insertion will usually result in the needle being pulled out of the horse because the syringe cannot be released as quickly or as easily as the needle alone. This is more important for intrasynovial injection because a pain reaction is seen more often. Luer-Lok attachments should be avoided because they prevent the rapid removal of the syringe from the needle if it is thought that the horse is going to pull away.

Evaluation of Local Anesthesia

Anesthetic solutions are not always deposited where expected. Therefore, before the results of the test can be evaluated, it should be ascertained whether the anesthetic has desensitized the expected region distal to the injection site. Confirmation that an intrasynovial injection will be correctly completed relies on ensuring that synovial fluid can be aspirated through the needle before injection. This is not possible with the other techniques, and confirmation depends on observing cutaneous desensitization in the region innervated by the sensory nerve(s) being blocked. It is common practice to use a hypodermic needle to test whether skin sensation is present. However, not only is it an unreliable test of deep sensation, but also its repeated use is resented by the patient. It is preferable to use a blunt object, such as a ballpoint pen, and at first to apply gentle and then firmer pressure to the skin until it is evident that desensitization has been achieved. Some clinicians use the hoof tester to squeeze the hoof or skin fold. There are numerous reasons for failing to achieve anesthesia:

- Inaccurate deposition
- Inadequate volume of anesthetic
- Presence of aberrant nerve fibers
- Presence of fibrous tissue
- More than one source of pain
- Painful lesion is not associated with region injected

Complications of Local Anesthesia

There are few complications to correctly performed local anesthesia, but they do occur and include:

- Excessive tissue reaction
- Breakage of needles
- Infection (cellulitis, septic synovitis)
- Loss of hair pigmentation and skin necrosis when using anesthetic solutions containing adrenalin

Anesthesia of the Forelimb

The procedures for anesthetizing the different regions of the forelimb are described in the following paragraphs and proceed from distal to proximal.

PALMAR DIGITAL NERVES. These nerves are blocked more frequently than any others. The lateral and medial palmar digital nerves are usually blocked in the mid pastern region (Fig. 5-17). If the block is carried out too far proximally, the other branches of the palmar digital nerves (dorsal, intermediate) can be inadvertently blocked. The procedure is usually done bilaterally, although, to identify the exact site of a lesion, it is often done as a unilateral procedure, or as a bilateral procedure by injecting the medial and lateral sites about 15 to 30 minutes apart. Because of the nature of the problems that occur in the forelimb, anesthesia of both limbs is usually carried out.

Procedure 1. Injection immediately above the lateral cartilages provides maximal insurance that only the palmar branches are blocked. The medial and lateral palmar digital nerves course along the medial and lateral borders, respectively,

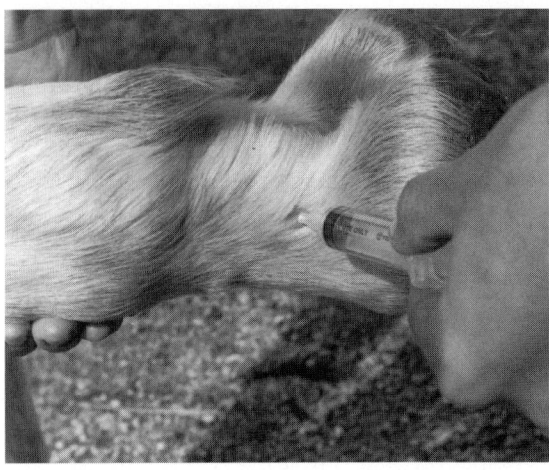

▶ **FIGURE 5-17**

Palmar digital nerve block. The location and angle of insertion of the needle are demonstrated for anesthesia of the lateral palmar digital nerve.

Materials for Palmar Digital Nerve Block

▶ Anesthetic (2 mL)
▶ Needle (22–25 gauge, 15 mm [⅝″])

---

of the superficial digital flexor tendon above, and of the deep flexor tendon below, the proximal interphalangeal joint. The nerves lie caudal to the corresponding artery and vein. The injection is done with the limb elevated. The appropriate site is identified by palpating the border of the tendon. The ligament of the ergot is often recommended as a landmark, but this is useful only for indicating the level of the injection, and identifying the correct site in a dorsal-palmar direction still relies on locating the tendon.

Another way to make the injection is for the clinician to hold the limb between his or her knees and to insert the needle from behind the tendon, directing it to lie adjacent to the medial and lateral borders. This technique is useful when a helper is not available to hold the limb.

Region Desensitized. The heels and caudal one-third to one-half of the hoof and coronary band are desensitized. Inadvertent block of the dorsal branches will desensitize the dorsal regions. The dorsal coronary band should always be checked to ensure this has not happened before the effects of the block on the lameness are evaluated.

Procedure 2 (Ramus Pulvinus). A method, claimed to restrict desensitization to within the region bounded by the lateral cartilages is described.[9] This block is used in order to provide more specific evaluation of the navicular bone and its associated structures and involves blocking that branch (pulvinus ramus) of the palmar digital nerve that passes medial to the cartilage.

Procedure. Medial and lateral injections are carried out with the foot elevated. The sites for injection are located axial to the lateral cartilages immediately caudal to the deep flexor tendon. The needle is directed distally along the medial surface of the cartilage, for about 30 mm, and at right angles to the solar surface.

Region Desensitized. When correctly carried out, desensitization is confined to the deep structures in the vicinity of the navicular bone and associated structures, including the frog, heels, caudal region of distal interphalangeal joint, lateral cartilages, and wings of the third phalanx. The skin between the heels is not anesthetized unless some anesthetic is deposited subcutaneously during insertion or withdrawal of the needle.

DISTAL INTERPHALANGEAL JOINT. The distal interphalangeal joint is anesthetized not only for conditions that involve the joint specifically, such as fractures and arthritis, but also because its anesthesia is often positive in the navicular syndrome. Two injection sites are described.

Procedure 1 (Dorsal Approach). The injection is made preferably with the horse standing on the limb. Weightbearing ensures that the joint

 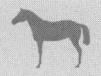
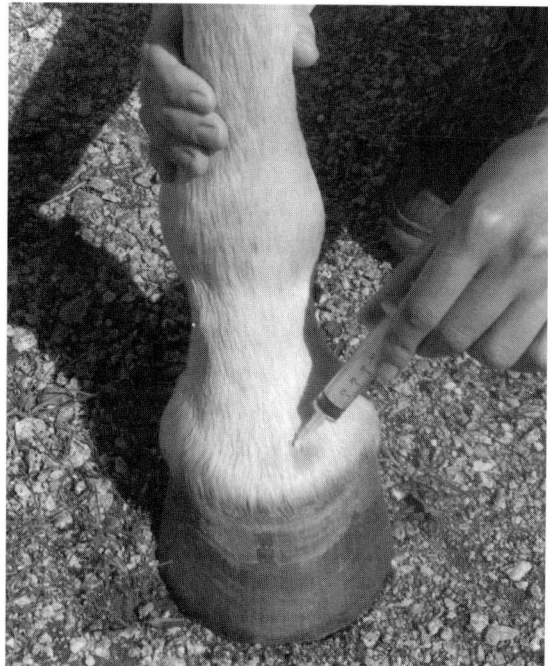

▶ **FIGURE 5–18**
Anesthesia of the distal interphalangeal joint.

fluid is under pressure and will flow readily from the needle when the joint cavity is entered. This is important because the clinician does not perceive clearly when the needle enters the joint. The site for injection is 1.5 cm medial or lateral to the midline and 2.0 cm proximal to the rim of the hoof (Fig. 5–18). The needle is directed slightly caudally and axially just off the vertical. Variations include increasing the distance from the midline and the coronary band, which necessitates directing the needle more obliquely toward the midline.

Procedure 2 (Palmar Approach). With the limb preferably weightbearing the needle is inserted in the palmar midline, 0.5 cm proximal to the fossa above the heels, and directed toward a point midway between the toe and the coronary band.

Region Desensitized. The initial desensitization is presumed, logically, to be limited to the joint itself, but diffusion of solution into surrounding tissues complicates interpretation of any delayed response. A response within 10 to 15 minutes is generally taken to be positive for an intraarticular lesion, and a delayed response after 20 to 30 minutes is the result of extraarticular lesions such as navicular syndrome.

Complications. In addition to the possibility of infection, calcification of the extensor tendon,

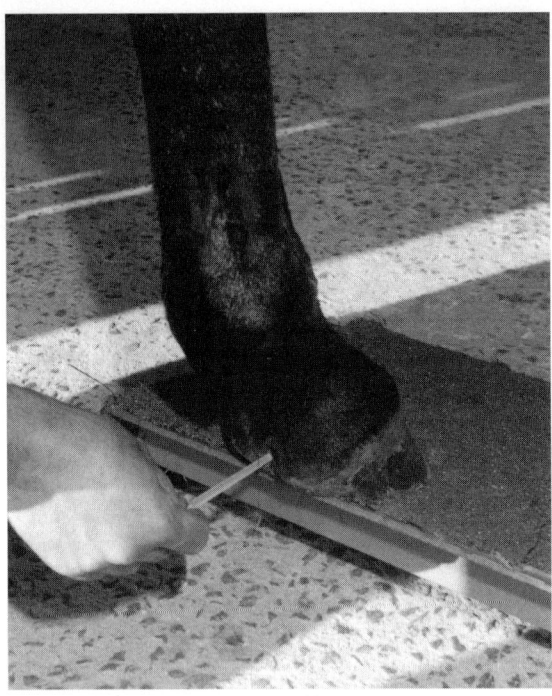

▶ **FIGURE 5–19**
Anesthesia of the navicular bursa.

thought to be associated with needle trauma, has
been reported.[10] The exact cause is not known,
but, presumably, inaccurate and rough insertion of the needle would be a contributing factor.
The complication has not been observed by the
author. Use of the palmar approach will avoid
the problem. With the palmar approach it is
possible to enter accidentally the navicular bursa
if the needle is directed too far distally.

NAVICULAR BURSA

Procedure 1. The injection is made from the
palmar aspect with the limb weightbearing. It is
an advantage to place the horses hoof on a block
of wood. A bleb of local anesthetic is deposited
subcutaneously (26-gauge, 1-inch needle) at the
injection site in the midline in the base of the
interdigital fossa. The 20-gauge needle is then
inserted through the anesthetized region and
directed dorsally and horizontally until bone is
encountered (Fig. 5–19). The needle passes
through the deep flexor tendon and impinges on
the palmar surface of the navicular bone. The
needle is withdrawn slightly before injection. The
use of radiographic guidance is recommended
whenever possible to ensure that the bursa is
entered.

Procedure 2. The bursa can also be injected
from the lateral aspect. The needle is inserted just
proximal to the lateral cartilage and directed
distomedially between the deep flexor tendon and
the second phalanx.

Regions Desensitized. In addition to the
bursa, there is evidence to suggest that the
anesthetic solution diffuses into the distal interphalangeal joint and sheath of the deep flexor
tendon, thus complicating interpretation of the
results. In addition, many horses that exhibit signs
of navicular syndrome respond to anesthesia of
the distal interphalangeal joint. In view of these
observations and of the complications, many

clinicians prefer to inject the joint rather than the
bursa, when navicular syndrome is suspected.

Complications. The major complication has
traditionally been septic bursitis. Why this should
be so is not known. However, it is probably
related to the difficulty of adequately preparing
the injection site in the interdigital fossa and the
high frequency of injection of corticosteroids in
earlier times. The technique is not easy and entry
into the distal interphalangeal joint is not an
uncommon occurrence. Radiographic guidance
ensures accurate bursal puncture.

PROXIMAL INTERPHALANGEAL JOINT. Anesthesia of the proximal interphalangeal joint is an
uncommon procedure.

Procedure. The injection is made with the
limb bearing weight or elevated. The usual site for
injection is located about 1.5 cm medial or lateral

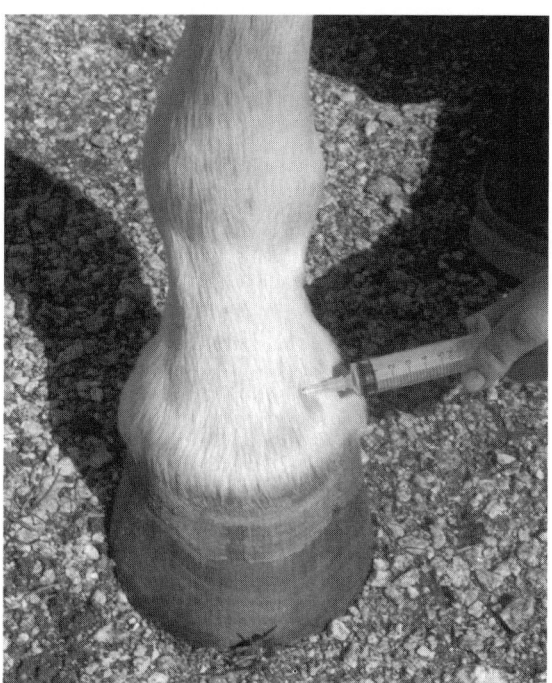

▶ **FIGURE 5–20**

Anesthesia of the proximal interphalangeal joint.

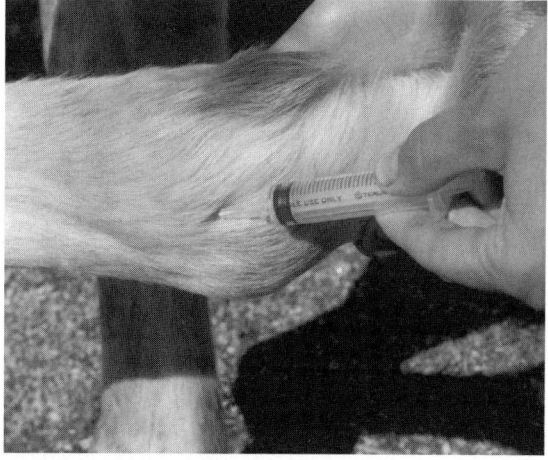

▶ **FIGURE 5–21**

Anesthesia of the palmar digital nerves at the level of the proximal sesamoids (abaxial sesamoid nerve block). The site for injection over the lateral nerve is demonstrated.

to the dorsal midline, adjacent to the edges of the extensor tendon, on a line about 1.0 cm distal to a line joining the medial and lateral distal eminences of the proximal phalanx. The needle is directed axially beneath the tendon, at right angles to the long axis of the pastern. Alternatively, the injection can be in the midline with the needle directed caudally and downward so that it can enter the curved joint space. Similarly, the needle can be inserted from the palmar aspect, passing through the deep flexor tendon and its sheath (see Fig. 5–20).

PALMAR DIGITAL NERVES AT THE LEVEL OF THE PROXIMAL SESAMOIDS (ABAXIAL SESA-MOID BLOCK). The palmar nerves divide at the level of the proximal sesamoids, and injection at this site will anesthetize all branches. It is easy to carry out because the nerves can be palpated.

Procedure. The injection is made with the foot elevated. The nerve(s) can be palpated lying immediately caudal to the digital artery by rolling the structures beneath the thumb or finger. The needle is directly proximally at an angle of about 25° to the skin surface (Fig. 5–21).

Region Desensitized. With the exception of a dorsally located, V-shaped region extending distally from the fetlock sometimes as far as the coronet, all structures distal to the site of injection are anesthetized. The sesamoids and the fetlock joint are not affected.

FETLOCK JOINT. Anesthesia of the fetlock joint can be accomplished by three methods.

Procedure 1. Approach to the palmar pouch. This is the traditional method, and it can be carried out with the limb elevated or weightbearing. Weightbearing tends to cause the pouch to bulge and therefore increases the accuracy of insertion. Elevating the limb and flexing the joint are safer in unruly horses, and this method is

---

Materials for Palmar Digital Nerves Anesthesia at the Level of the Proximal Sesamoids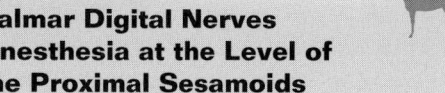

▶ Anesthetic (3–5 mL)
▶ Needle (26 gauge, 25 mm [1″])

Materials for Fetlock Joint Anesthesia

▶ Anesthetic (10 mL)
▶ Needle (21 gauge, 25 mm [1″])

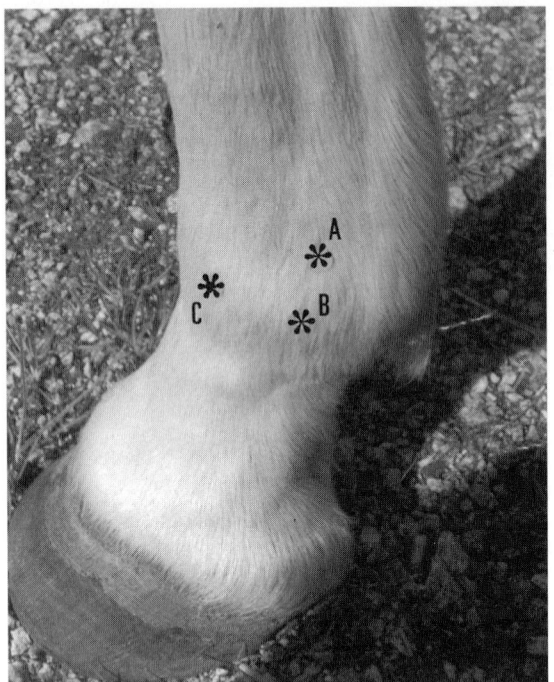

▶ FIGURE 5-22

Anesthesia of the metacarpophalangeal joint. Three different sites are demonstrated. **A.** Site for injection into the lateral volar pouch. **B.** Site for injection from the lateral aspect, passing through the lateral ligaments. The needle is directed horizontally and medially. **C.** Site for injection from the dorsolateral (medial) aspect. The needle passes horizontally and medially, behind the extensor tendons.

favored by the author. Flexion also displaces the sesamoid palmarly from metacarpal 3 and makes it easier to insert the needle into the joint. When there is excessive joint fluid present, the task is much easier, regardless of technique. Each palmar pouch extends proximally from the level of the apex of the ipsilateral sesamoid bone, bounded dorsally by the palmar border of the metacarpal 3 and palmarly by the suspensory ligament. Ease of approach from the lateral side dictates that the lateral pouch be used, although a medial approach is equally possible. The site for insertion is within the above borders, just proximal to the apex of the sesamoid, with the needle directed horizontally or slightly downward (Fig. 5-22A).

Procedure 2. The second site is located distal to that just described, with the needle penetrating the joint through the lateral collateral sesamoidean ligament (Fig. 5-22B). When the limb is weightbearing, a needle cannot be inserted into the joint at this site. Therefore, the limb must be elevated and the joint must be flexed. Flexion displaces the sesamoid caudally and opens a space

between it and metacarpal 3. With the limb elevated and slightly flexed, the needle is inserted about half way down the space that can be palpated between the sesamoid and metacarpal 3.

Procedure 3. The needle is inserted into the dorsal part of the joint from a dorsolateral (usually) or dorsomedial approach, usually with the limb weightbearing. The needle is inserted lateral to the border of the common extensor tendon, about 1.5 cm proximal to the joint surface, and directed horizontally, and palmaromedially to enter the joint palmar to the extensor tendon (Fig. 5-22C).

DORSAL ASPECT OF FETLOCK AND PASTERN. As explained, the palmar nerves do not innervate the dorsal pastern or fetlock. To anesthetize this region, the palmar metacarpal nerves must be blocked by depositing anesthetic solution where the nerves emerge at the end of the small metacarpal bones or by carrying out a ring block around the pastern or immediately proximal to the fetlock.

Ring Block. A ring block can be carried out at any level desired. As described, its prime purpose is to block the metacarpal nerves. However, it is sometimes also useful for those cases when the presence of aberrant nerve fibers is suspected or when standard blocking procedures have, for some reason, failed to produce desensitization. Ring blocks are usually done in conjunction with, depending on the level of the block, anesthesia of the palmar digital or palmar nerves. The method consists of infiltrating anesthetic solution subcutaneously around the limb. The disadvantage is that it requires more solution than the specific blocks.

Metacarpal Nerves. The metacarpal nerves are usually blocked as part of the four-point blocks described in the following sections.

LOW FOUR-POINT BLOCK (MEDIAL AND LATERAL PALMAR AND PALMAR METACARPAL NERVES). This combination of blocks follows an unsuccessful block of structures distal to the fetlock joint.

Procedure.

• *Palmar nerves.* The medial and lateral palmar nerves course distally between the deep flexor tendon and the suspensory ligaments, lying adjacent to the edge of the tendon. The injections are made at the level of the distal ends of the small metacarpal bones,

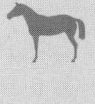
with the limb elevated or weightbearing. To anesthetize the lateral nerve, the needle is inserted from the lateral side and directed horizontally or obliquely (Fig. 5–23). The needle must go deeper than the subcutaneous fascia, otherwise the anesthetic solution is seen as a subcutaneous bleb and the block will be unsuccessful. The medial nerve is usually anesthetized, similarly, from the medial side. Medial and lateral nerves can also be anesthetized from the lateral side with the one injection by using a slightly longer needle, which, after the solution has been deposited adjacent to the lateral nerve, is then passed medially, dorsal to the deep flexor tendon, so that its tip lies adjacent to the medial nerve.

• *Palmar metacarpal nerves.* The lateral and medial metacarpal nerves emerge from

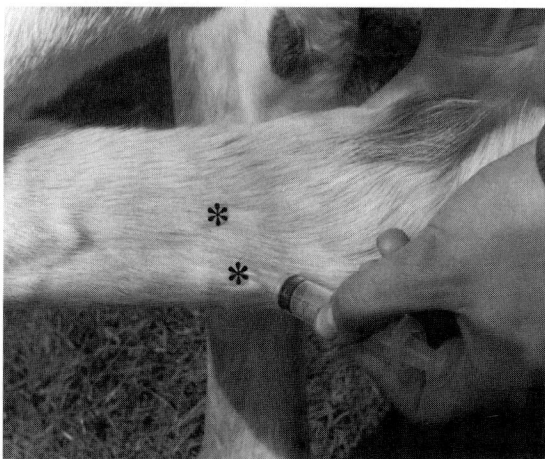

▶ FIGURE 5-23

Low four-point nerve block. This block includes the medial and lateral palmar nerves plus the medial and lateral metacarpal nerves. The sites for injection of the lateral nerves are demonstrated. The precise angle of insertion for anesthesia of the palmar nerves is not important, but to anesthetize the metacarpal nerves the needle must be directed dorsomedially, beneath the end (the "button") of the small metacarpal bones.

beneath the distal ends of the small metacarpal bones. The injections are made with the limb elevated or weightbearing and consists of depositing the anesthetic solution just beneath the distal ends of the bones (Fig. 5–23).

Region Desensitized. The blocks desensitize all deep structures distal to the injection sites. The medial cutaneous antibrachial nerves may provide some sensation to the dorsum of the fetlock region, which is unlikely to affect the ability to reduce or eliminate lameness but will interfere with using skin tests to check if the anesthesia has effectively blocked sensation.

Complications. In the horse that suddenly pulls its leg away, the possibility of needle breakage is increased when the medial and lateral palmar nerves are being blocked with the one injection. For this reason the method is not recommended.

HIGH FOUR-POINT BLOCK (MEDIAL AND LATERAL PALMAR AND PALMAR METACARPAL NERVES). Anesthesia of these nerves is useful to localize lesions of the metacarpal region. The blocks are carried out above the palmar communicating branch of the palmar nerves and below the carpus.

Procedure.

• *Palmar nerves.* The procedure is similar to that for the same nerves in the low four-point block (Fig. 5–24). Here again, the nerves lie adjacent to the dorsolateral and dorsomedial surfaces of the deep flexor tendon, except that they lie beneath a thick subcarpal fascia. The injection is made with the limb elevated or weightbearing, ensur-

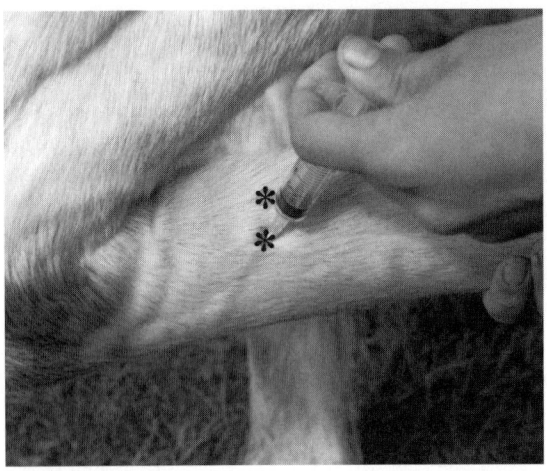

▶ FIGURE 5-24

High four-point nerve block. This block includes the medial and lateral palmar nerves plus the medial and lateral metacarpal nerves. The sites for injection of the lateral nerves are demonstrated. The precise angle of insertion for anesthesia of the palmar nerves is not important, but to anesthetize the metacarpal nerves the needle must be directed dorsoproximally, passing between the suspensory ligament and the axial surface of the small metacarpal bones.

ing that the solution is deposited beneath the fascia. A subcutaneous bleb indicates that the solution lies superficial to the fascia. The injection can be made from medial and lateral sides or from the lateral side only, as described. When using the single injection method, anesthetic solution is injected first over the lateral nerve and, then the needle is directed medially between the suspensory ligament and the deep flexor tendon so that solution can be deposited over the medial palmar nerve. For this method a 36-mm needle is required. Aspiration should be carried out to avoid accidental injection into the palmar artery.

• *Palmar metacarpal nerves.* These nerves run parallel and axial to the second and fourth metacarpal bones. Separate injections are required for each nerve. The needle is inserted immediately axial to the small metacarpal bone, with the limb elevated. It is then directed dorsoaxially between the axial surface of the bone and the suspensory ligament (Fig. 5-24). Solution is deposited adjacent to the third metacarpal.

Region Desensitized. In addition to the structures desensitized by the low four-point block, the high four-point block desensitizes the deep structures of the metacarpal region distal to

the level of injection site. The origin of the suspensory ligament is not affected.

SUSPENSORY LIGAMENT. The caudal metacarpal region and the origin of the suspensory ligament are often the source of pain in performance horses. This region can be desensitized by perineural anesthesia of the lateral palmar nerve or by direct infiltration. The lateral palmar nerve is blocked proximal to where its deep branch provides innervation to the origin of the suspensory ligament and divides to form the medial and lateral metacarpal nerves.

Lateral Palmar Nerve at the Level of the Accessory Carpal Bone. This method allows an approximate assessment, with a single injection, of the proximocaudal aspect of the metacarpus.

Procedure. The site for injection is midway between the distal border of the accessory carpal bone and the proximal aspect of the fourth metacarpal bone, on the palmar border of the accessoriometacarpal ligament (Fig. 5-25). The needle must penetrate the 3-mm-thick flexor retinaculum in order for the anesthetic solution to contact the nerve.

Region Desensitized. The origin of the suspensory ligament and the caudal metacarpus, as well as those distal structures innervated by the lateral palmar nerve and medial and lateral metacarpal nerves, are desensitized. Logically, by including the medial palmar nerve, all deep structures distal to the carpus can be desensitized.

Infiltration of the Origin of the Suspensory Ligament:

Procedure. Injections are made with the limb elevated. The sites for injection are medial and lateral high in the metacarpal region. The needle passes between the suspensory ligament and the inferior check ligament (accessory ligament of the deep digital flexor tendon) to end adjacent to the origin of the suspensory ligament.

Materials for Lateral Palmar Nerve Anesthesia at the Level of the Accessory Carpal Bone

---

▶ Anesthetic (5 mL)

▶ Needle (20 gauge, 25 mm [1″])

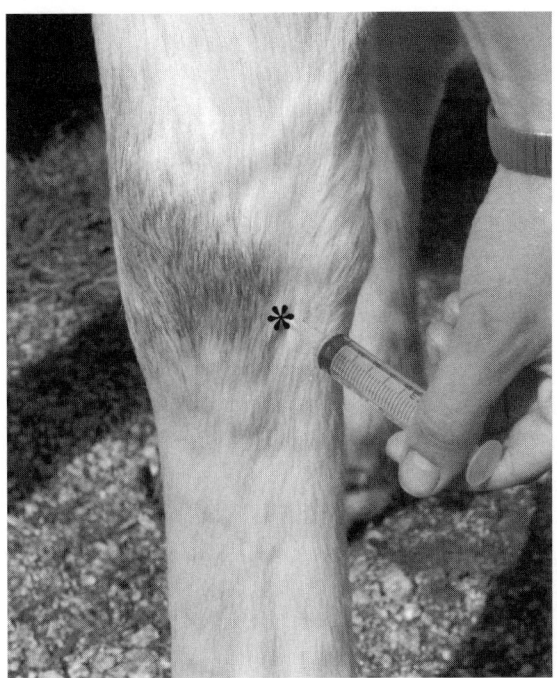

▶ **FIGURE 5-25**
Lateral palmar nerve at the level of the accessory carpal bone.

**Materials for
Suspensory Ligament
Infiltration**

▶ Anesthetic (5 mL/site)
▶ Needle (21 gauge, 25 mm [1"])

Region Desensitized. Only the deep structures in the vicinity of the injection should be desensitized.

Complications. Because the needle passes through thick fascia sudden movement of the horse during injections in this region are more likely to result in a broken needle than with injections in other sites. The reason for this is the shear forces acting on the needle as the fascia, skin, and underlying tendons and suspensory ligament move independently. It is for this reason that, when there is an option, it is safer to inject when the limb is elevated and, therefore, under better control.

As a result of the close proximity of the medial and lateral distopalmar pouches of the carpometacarpal joint to the sites of proximal injection, accidental anesthesia of the middle and carpometacarpal joints occurs in a proportion of

---

**Materials for
Carpal Joints Anesthesia**

▶ Anesthetic (10 mL/joint)
▶ Needle (20 gauge, 25 mm [1"])

---

cases.[11] Therefore, these nerve blocks must be interpreted with caution, and separate anesthesia of the joints is sometimes indicated to clarify a diagnosis.

CARPAL JOINTS. Anesthesia of the three joints in the carpus can be blocked with injections of the proximal and the middle joints. The proximal carpal joint is a separate cavity, and the middle and distal carpal joints always communicate. Caudolateral approaches are also described and claimed to cause less cartilaginous trauma, increase safety for the clinician, and eliminate the need to elevate the limb.

Procedure 1. The injection is made with the limb elevated and the carpus in flexion, making the joint spaces visible and easily palpable. The injections can be made medial or lateral to the extensor carpi radialis (ECR) tendon, but, because of its ease, the lateral approach is preferred (Fig. 5-26A). Care is taken to avoid the sheath of the common digital extensor, which lies lateral to the tendon of the ECR. To avoid injuring the joint cartilages the needle should be inserted parallel to the joint surfaces.

Procedure 2. The carpal joints can also be blocked from palmarolateral approaches, with the limb weightbearing. The proximal joint can be injected by inserting a needle into the palmarolateral pouch just proximal to the articulation between the radius and the accessory carpal bone or, where a horizontal line through the joint between the radius and the ulnar carpal bone meets the dorsal aspect of the accessory carpal bone (Fig. 5-26B). The middle carpal joint is injected distal to this site, where the palmar reflection of the capsule bulges palmarolaterally behind the ulnar and fourth carpal bones.

DESENSITIZATION FROM THE DISTAL RADIUS TO THE FOOT (MEDIAN, ULNAR, AND MUSCULOCUTANEOUS NERVES). This set of blocks is not often necessary but is useful to differentiate between an upper- and a lower-limb problem.

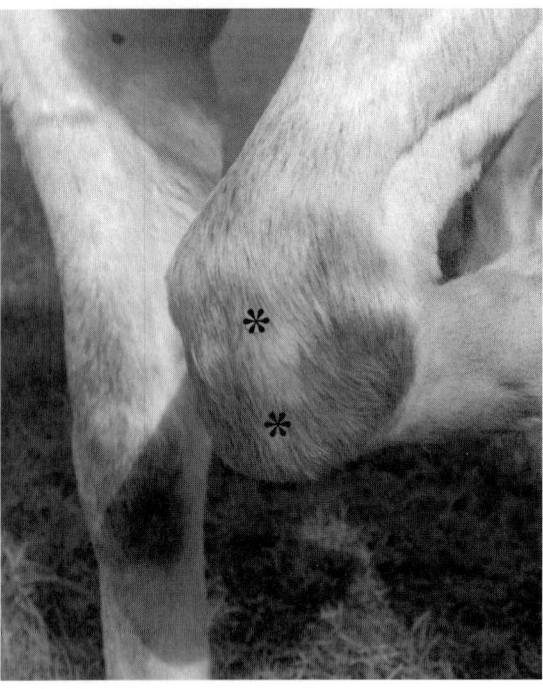
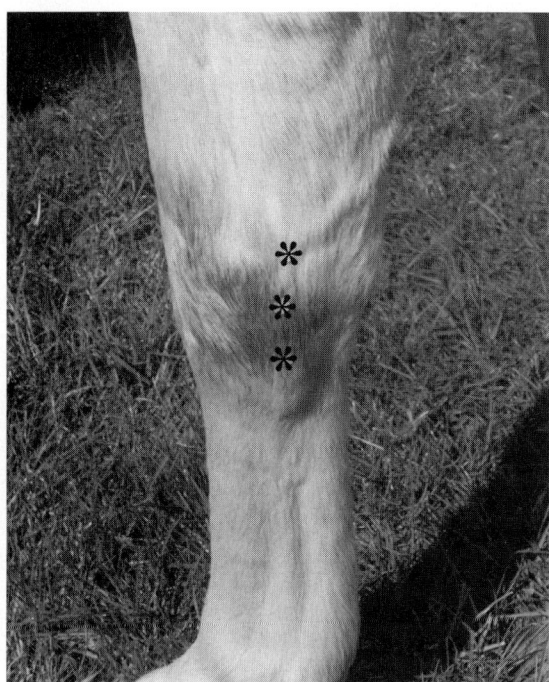

A

B

▶ FIGURE 5–26

Anesthesia of the carpal joint. **A.** The sites for injection of the radiocarpal (proximal marker) and intercarpal (distal marker) are shown. **B.** The sites for injection into the caudal aspects of the joints are indicated. The two proximal markers show sites for access to the radiocarpal joint, and the distal marker indicates the location of the intercarpal joint.

> **Materials to Desensitize from the Distal Radius to the Foot**
>
> ▶ Median nerve
>   Anesthetic (10 mL)
>   Needle (20 gauge, 36 mm [1.5"])
>
> ▶ Ulnar nerve
>   Anesthetic (10 mL)
>   Needle (20 gauge, 25 mm [1.0"])
>
> ▶ Medial cutaneous antibrachial nerve
>   Anesthetic (5 mL/site)
>   Needle (22 gauge, 25 mm [1.0"])

Median Nerve. The nerve is blocked approximately 10 cm proximal to the chestnut, using a medial or caudomedial approach (Fig. 5–27).

- *Medial approach.* The needle is inserted at the distal border of the pectoralis descendens muscles. It is directed slightly proximally and in a caudolateral direction to pass caudal to the radius and cranial to the flexor carpi radialis muscle. The anesthetic solution is deposited when the needle is in-

serted to the hub, just adjacent to the caudomedial border of the radius.

- *Caudomedial approach.* The needle is inserted caudal to the flexor carpi radialis muscle in the groove between this muscle and the flexor carpi ulnaris muscle. The direction is cranial and slightly lateral, the cleft between the muscles being easily detected by gently moving the hub of the needle a short distance up and down.

Ulnar Nerve. The needle is inserted between the flexor carpi ulnaris and the ulnaris lateralis muscles, on the caudal aspect of the forearm about 10 cm proximal to the accessory carpal bone. The needle must penetrate the subcutaneous fascia. To avoid accidental injection beneath the nerve, it is advisable to also inject some solution as the needle is withdrawn (Fig. 5–28).

Medial Cutaneous Antibrachial Nerve. This nerve can be blocked proximally or distally.

- *Proximal approach.* Using the proximal approach the nerve is blocked before it bifurcates. The site of injection is craniomedially in the proximal forearm, where the nerve can be palpated as it crosses the lacertus fibrosis (Fig. 5–29A).

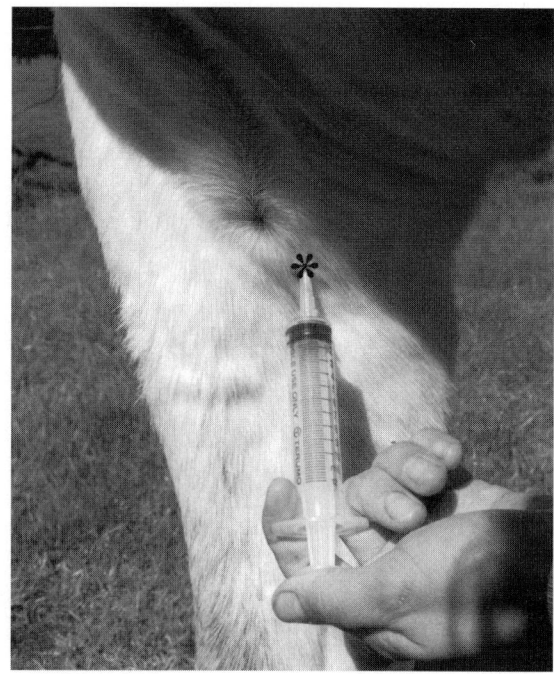

A

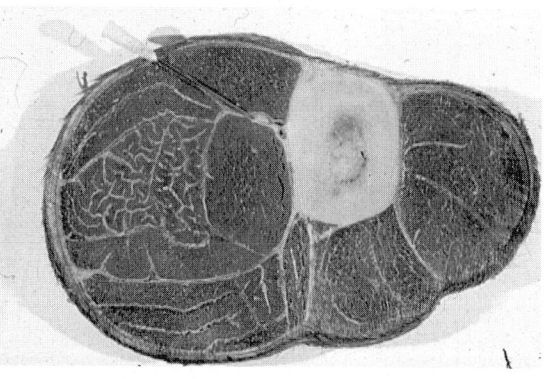

B

▶ **FIGURE 5-27**

Median nerve. The nerve can be approached cranial or caudal to the flexor carpi radialis muscle. **A.** Cranial approach to the median nerve is demonstrated. **B.** Cross section of the limb in the proximal radial region, indicating the path of a needle inserted caudal to the flexor carpi radialis muscle.

- *Distal approach.* After branching, the nerve passes distally on the medial aspect of the forearm in close association with the cephalic and accessory cephalic veins. The

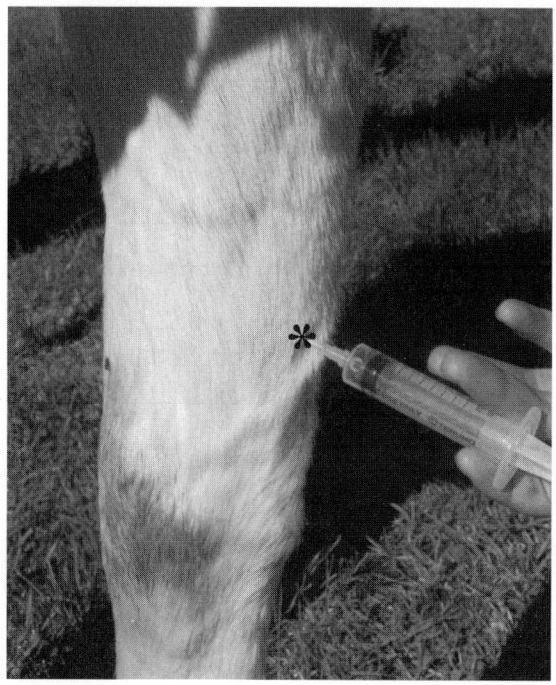

▶ **FIGURE 5-28**

Anesthesia of the ulnar nerve.

branches are blocked midway between the elbow and the carpus, where the veins are visible and the nerves can usually be palpated. To combat variation in position, the anesthetic is deposited cranial and caudal to both of the veins, using 5 mL for each injection (Fig. 5-29B).

Region Desensitized. The carpus and all structures distal to it are desensitized. There is little use in blocking these nerves individually. Anesthesia of the median nerve alone has a similar effect to a block of the medial and lateral palmar nerves. Anesthesia of the ulnar nerve alone desensitizes part of the lateral aspect of the limb and has some effect on the structures in the region of the origin of the suspensory ligament.

Complications. Puncture of the median artery or vein often occurs because of their close proximity to the median nerve. This is not serious but necessitates withdrawing the needle slightly before injecting the anesthetic. Occasionally there will be some loss of motor control to muscles in the proximal limb, which is disturbing for the horse. The horse should be confined and not exercised until the effect has resolved.

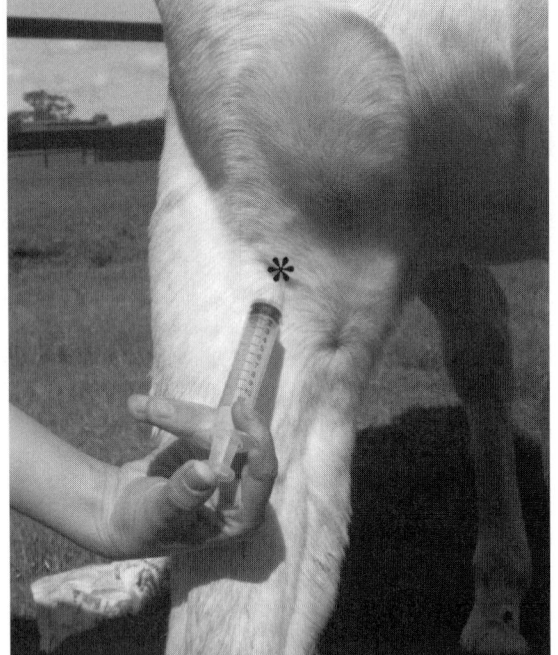

A

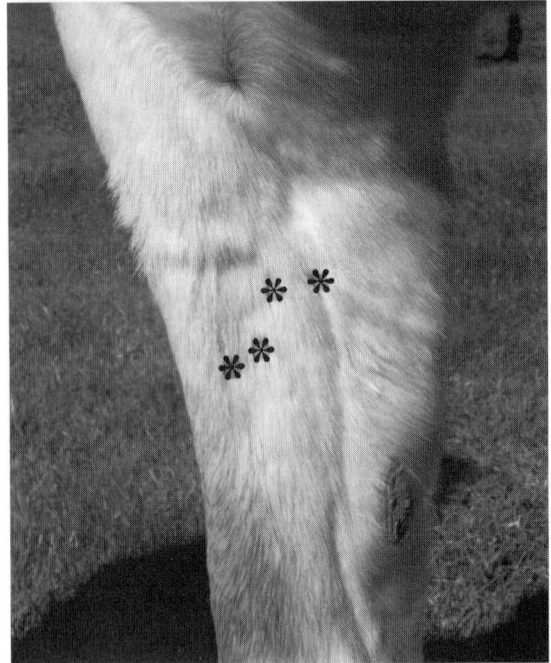

B

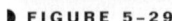

▶ FIGURE 5–29

Medial cutaneous antibrachial nerve. **A.** Proximal approach. The injection is made where the nerve crosses the lacertus fibrosis. **B.** Distal approach. Branches of the nerve are blocked cranial and caudal to the cephalic and accessory cephalic veins in the mid-radius region.

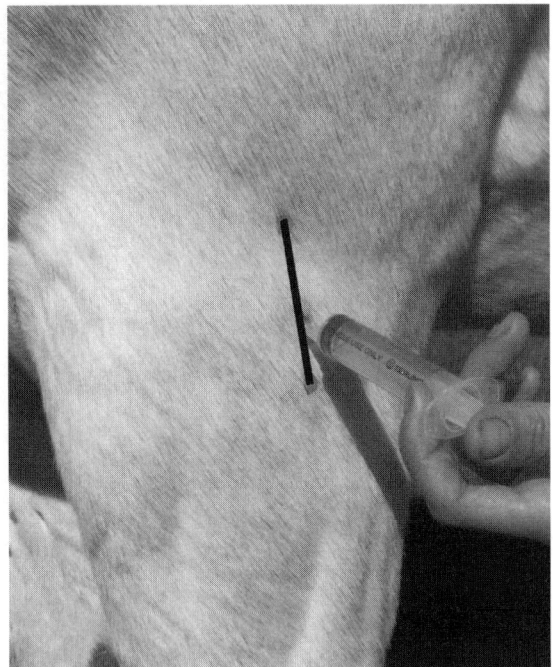

A

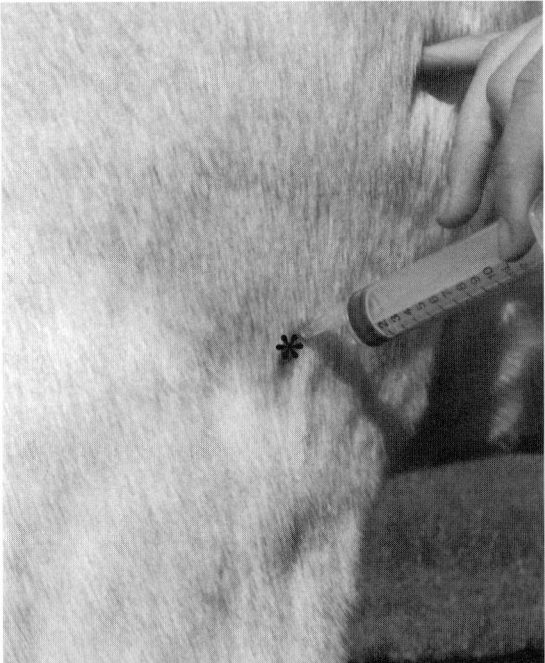

B

▶ FIGURE 5–30

Anesthesia of the elbow joint. **A.** Lateral approach. The sites for injection are cranial or caudal to the lateral collateral ligament (black strip) and approximately two thirds distal from its proximal attachment to the lateral humeral epicondyle. **B.** Caudolateral approach. The site for injection is located in the depression between the caudal aspect of the lateral humeral epicondyle and the cranial border of the olecranon.

CUBITAL (ELBOW) JOINT. The elbow is not often the source of pain, and, consequently, anesthesia is relatively infrequently required.

Procedure 1. The elbow is injected from the lateral side with the limb weightbearing. The injection sites are cranial or caudal to the lateral collateral ligament, and two thirds of the way, distally, from its attachments to the lateral humeral epicondyle and the lateral radial tuberosity (Fig. 5–30A). At the caudal site the injection is actually into the bursa of the ulnaris lateralis tendon, which communicates with the joint.

Procedure 2. The second approach is also from the lateral side, with the limb weightbearing. The needle is inserted into the pouch of the humeroradial joint, which is located in the depression between the cranial border of the olecranon and the caudal border of the lateral epicondyle of the humerus (Fig. 5–30B).

SHOULDER JOINT

Procedure. The site for injection is located in the depression between the cranial and caudal eminences of the lateral tuberosity of the humerus. The injection is made with the limb weightbearing. The eminences are palpated with the thumb and second finger, and the first finger is used to locate the depression. The needle is then inserted horizontally in a caudomedial direc-

tion at an angle of 45° to the long axis of the body (Fig. 5–31).

Complications. There are no major complications. The most common cause of failure to locate the joint is by increasing the angle of insertion so that the needle passes across in front of the joint. This has occurred if the needle penetrates deeply without contacting bone or cartilage. Contact with the humerus or scapula is corrected by adjusting the end of the needle up or down so as to enter the joint space.

BICIPITAL BURSA. The bicipital bursa lies beneath the tendon of the biceps brachii muscle as it passes over the bicipital groove.

Procedure. The needle is inserted just cranial to the deltoid tuberosity and 3 cm distal to

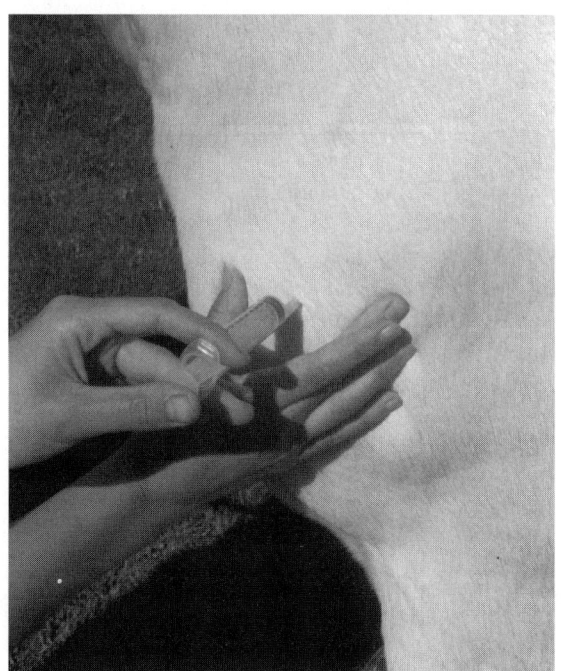

▶ **FIGURE 5–31**

Anesthesia of the shoulder joint. The site for injection lies between the cranial and caudal eminences of the lateral tuberosity of the humerus, which are indicated by the thumb and second finger.

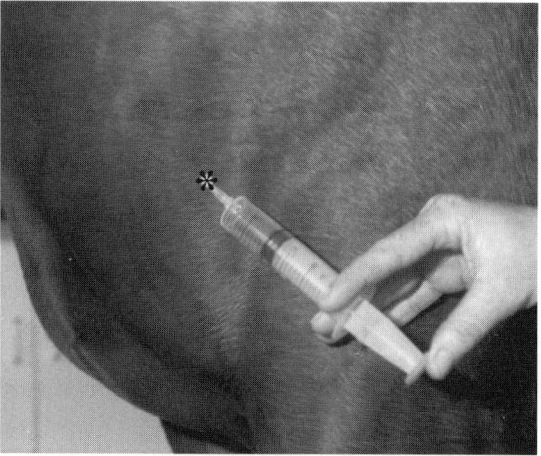

▶ **FIGURE 5–32**

Anesthesia of the bicipital bursa. The site for injection is cranial to the deltoid tuberosity and approximately 3 cm distal to the cranial prominence of the lateral tuberosity of the humerus. Note the angle at which the needle should be inserted.

the cranial prominence of the lateral tuberosity of the humerus. It is important to remember to aim the needle in a proximal and medial direction toward the cranial edge of the humerus beneath the biceps tendon (Fig. 5-32).

Complications. Failure to locate the bursa is a common problem, which is rectified most easily by directing the needle toward the cranial edge of the humerus, as described.

MISCELLANEOUS SYNOVIAL STRUCTURES IN THE FORELIMB. There are a number of synovial structures that occasionally require injection of diagnostic anesthetic, of medications, or of radiographic contrast materials. Normally, the structures contain little synovia, and it is often difficult to ensure that a needle will enter the synovial cavity. Fortunately, effusions usually accompany disease and make puncture much easier. Synovial structures in the forelimb that have not been described separately include:

- Digital synovial sheath
  (metacarpophalangeal joint)
- Tendon sheaths in the vicinity of the carpus
    Carpal synovial sheath
    Extensor carpi obliquus tendon
    Extensor carpi radialis tendon
    Common digital extensor tendon
    Lateral digital extensor tendon
    Ulnaris lateralis tendon
- Olecranon bursa

Procedure. An anatomy textbook should be consulted when necessary. However, injection is usually made into a prominent distension of the synovial structure.

Anesthesia of the Hindlimb

Anesthesia of the hindlimb is more difficult than the forelimb because of the increased danger of being injured. It is imperative that a competent horse handler be available to provide assistance and that heroic efforts to inject a horse are not

---

**Materials for
Anesthesia of
Miscellaneous Synovial
Structures in the Forelimb**

▸ Anesthetic (5–10 mL)
▸ Needle (21 gauge, 36 mm [1.5″])

---

indulged in. Although the distal limb can be injected when it is weightbearing, the author prefers to have the limb elevated by a helper. The danger varies greatly with the size and type of horse in question. Injecting a highly strung thoroughbred is far more dangerous than a standardbred much used to harness and manipulation around the hind limbs.

DISTAL HINDLIMB. Anesthesia of the hindlimb distal to the hock is similar to the equivalent region in the forelimb. The main difference is the presence of nerves that innervate the dorsal parts of the limb. The most significant of these are the medial and lateral dorsal metatarsal nerves (branches of the deep peroneal nerve), which extend as far distally as the fetlock and pastern region and provide deep innervation. The other nerves are the two terminal dorsal and lateral branches of the superficial peroneal nerves (descending distally to the fetlock), the terminal branch of the caudal cutaneous sural nerve (descending dorsolaterally as far as the fetlock), and the terminal branch of the saphenous nerve (which descends on the medial side of the metatarsus), which provide superficial innervation.

Anesthesia of the joints (fetlock, distal and proximal interphalangeal joints), navicular bursa, and the plantar, plantar metatarsal, and plantar digital nerves is identical with anesthesia in their counterparts in the forelimb.

Lateral and Medial Dorsal Metatarsal Nerves. The lateral dorsal metatarsal nerve passes distally, dorsal to the dorsal metatarsal 3 artery, which lies in the groove between metatarsals 3 and 4 and then runs distally to the dorsolateral fetlock and pastern, with innervation extending as far distal as the laminar corium. The medial dorsal metatarsal nerve emerges in the proximal metatarsal region from beneath the medial edge of the long digital extensor tendon. It runs distally between the tendon and metatarsal 2, to end on the medial aspect of the limb as does its lateral counterpart on the lateral side.

To anesthetize all the deep structures in the distal limb, these nerves should be blocked at the desired level in combination with the other nerve blocks (medial and lateral plantar metatarsal and plantar nerves), constituting a *high* or *low six-point block*. It is not usual to block the nerves providing superficial innervation. However, if necessary, they are best anesthetized with a ring

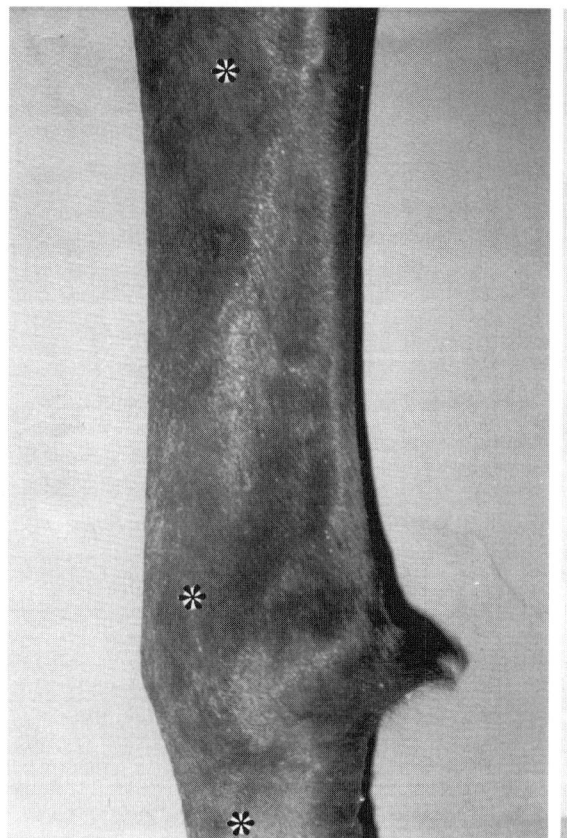
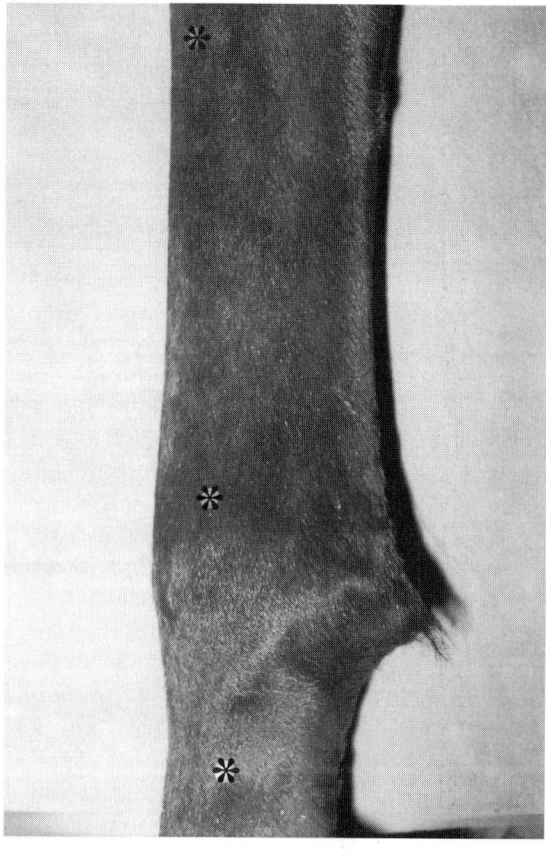

A   B

▶ **FIGURE 5-33**

Anesthesia of the dorsal metatarsal nerves. (These nerves are usually blocked at the same time as the plantar metatarsal and plantar nerves, as part of a six-point block.) **A.** Injection sites to block the lateral dorsal metatarsal nerve at three different levels. **B.** Injection sites to block the medial dorsal metatarsal nerve at three different levels.

block extending around the medial, dorsal, and lateral aspects of the limb.

- *Lateral dorsal metatarsal nerve.* In the proximal metatarsus the lateral nerve is blocked by depositing 5 mL of anesthetic solution subcutaneously, midway between the junction of metatarsals 3 and 4 and the lateral border of the lateral extensor tendon (Fig. 5–33A). Further distally, the dorsal landmark is the long extensor tendon. At the level of the fetlock the anesthetic is deposited subcutaneously on the dorsolateral aspect of the joint. In the midpastern region the nerve is located just lateral to the extensor branch of the suspensory ligament. The choice of injection site is governed by the level at which anesthesia is required.
- *Medial dorsal metatarsal nerve.* The medial nerve runs from the medial edge of the long extensor tendon obliquely over the dorsomedial aspect of the metatarsus, to termi-

nate in similar fashion to the lateral nerve. In the proximal metatarsus, the nerve is blocked by injecting anesthetic solution adjacent to the long extensor tendon (Fig. 5–33B). In the distal metatarsus, the site is on the medial aspect of metatarsal 3. The midpastern site is just medial to the extensor branch of the suspensory ligament.

Regions Desensitized. As stated, desensitization is limited mainly to the deeper structures distal to the level of injection. This may well resolve the lameness, but evaluation of anesthesia is impossible because of the presence of the superficial innervation of the dorsal and dorsolateral and dorsomedial regions. Hence, testing the effectiveness of anesthesia is limited to the caudal aspects of the limb. Complete desensitization requires a ring block. However, this is seldom needed.

Complications. The main complication is the inability to evaluate completely the effectiveness of the anesthesia and the variation in response related to the number of injections required.

TARSUS. Although there are four synovial cavities in the tarsus, full anesthesia requires only three injections because of intercommunication. The tarsocrural and proximal intertarsal spaces communicate in all cases, and the simple injection into the tarsocrural joint ensures that the proximal intertarsal joint also is anesthetized. Although there is communication between the distal intertarsal and tarsometatarsal joints (8% to 9%, increasing to 24% with increased injection pressure), they must be injected separately to ensure anesthesia.[12]

These joints are usually injected with the limb bearing weight. In most cases, especially when the horse is unruly, it is also advisable to have someone pick up and hold the ipsilateral forelimb to reduce the chances of getting kicked. Occasionally, when there is an indication that the chances of being kicked are increased, the limb to be injected must be picked up and held. In these cases the holder should pick up the limb as described and, standing close to the horse's flank, bring it forward so that the holder is medial to the limb. The clinician, also standing in front of the limb, can then proceed with the injection with little chance of being injured.

Procedures.

- *Talocrural joint.* The injection can be made with the clinician standing on the same side of the horse as the limb to be injected (preferred by the author) or on the opposite side. When injecting from the same side, the clinician usually stands slightly in front of the limb and facing backward. The site for injection is on the dorsomedial aspect, just medial or lateral to the cranial branch of the medial saphenous vein and distal to the medial malleolus of the tibia (Fig. 5–34A). When joint effusion is present, the plantarolateral pouch, which becomes visible between the lateral malleolus and the calcaneous, can also be injected.

- *Distal intertarsal joint.* The site is on the medial side of the joint, between the combined first and second tarsal bones and the third and central tarsal bones (Fig. 5–34B). This site can be difficult to enter because of exostoses associated with joint disease, difficulty in locating the correct location, and because the medial site is usually reached by standing on the opposite side of the horse and reaching across beneath it. Ways to locate the correct site for insertion include:

  Palpation: The gap between the bones used as landmarks can sometimes be palpated.

  The point at which an imaginary line from the distal tubercle of the tibial tarsal bone and the space between the second and third metatarsal bones crosses the distal border of the cunean tendon.

  Approximately 1.0 cm proximal to the space between the second and third metatarsal bones and then 1.5 dorsally.

Materials for Tarsus Anesthesia

▶ Talocrural joint
   Anesthetic (20 mL)
   Needle (20 gauge, 25 mm [1"])

▶ Distal intertarsal joint
   Anesthetic (5 mL)
   Needle (22 gauge, 25 mm [1"])

▶ Tarsometatarsal joint
   Anesthetic (5 mL)
   Needle (20 gauge, 25 mm [1"])

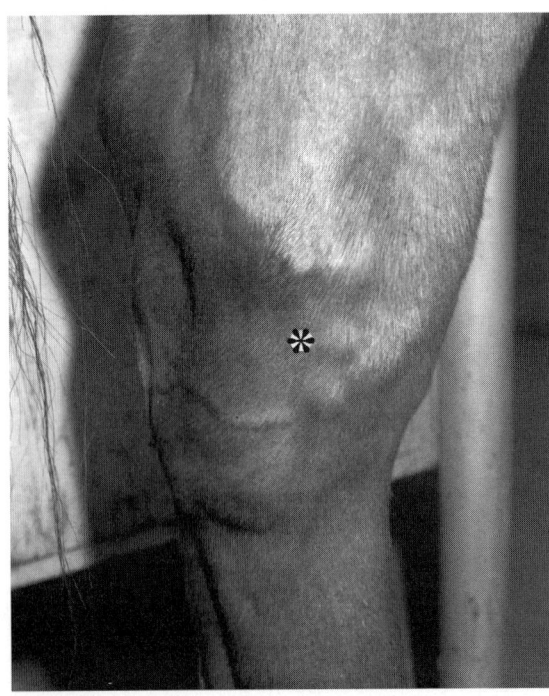

A

▶ **FIGURE 5–34**
Anesthesia of the tarsus. **A.** Talocrural joint.

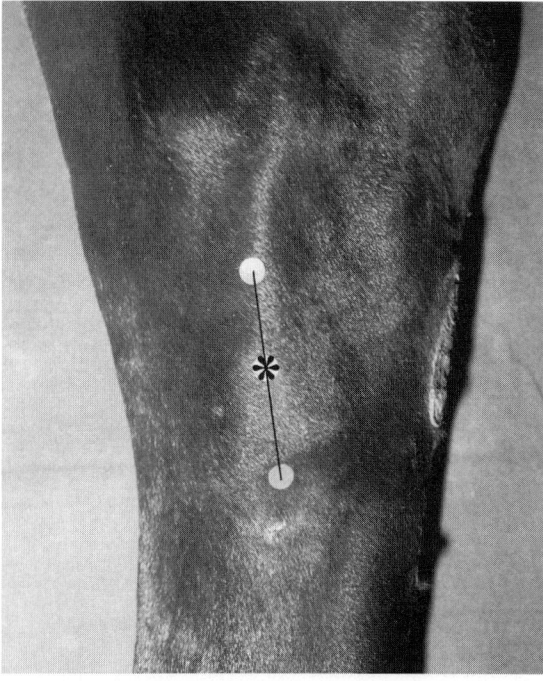

B

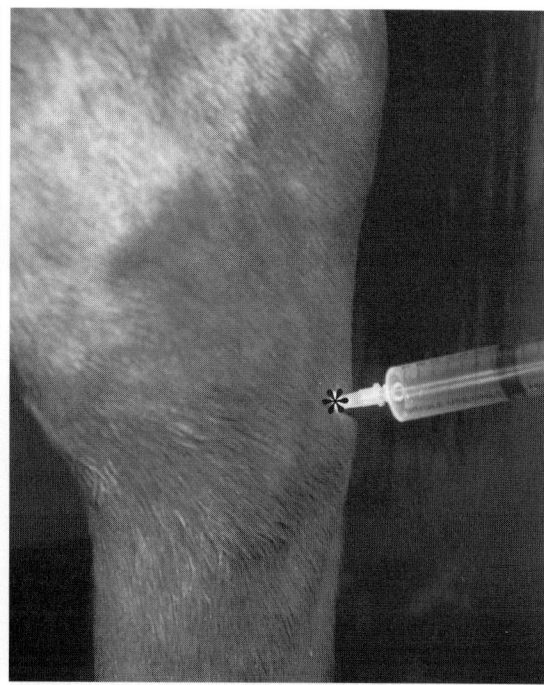

C

▶ **FIGURE 5–34** *Continued*

B. Distal intertarsal joint. One way of finding the site for injection (marker) is to visualize where an imaginary line between the distal tubercle of the tibial tarsal bone and the junction between the second and third metatarsal bones crosses the distal border of the cunean tendon. **C.** Tarsometatarsal joint. Site for injection is just proximal to the head of the fourth metatarsal bone and from the plantarolateral aspect. The angle of injection is critical to successful injection.

- *Tarsometatarsal joint.* This joint is approached over the head of the fourth metatarsal bone from the plantarolateral aspect of the limb. The proximal limits of the bone are easily palpated, and the needle is inserted approximately 1.0 cm proximal to this and directed dorsomedially and slightly distally so as to run along the joint surfaces of the fourth metatarsal and fourth tarsal bones (Fig. 5–34C).

THE CUNEAN BURSA. The bursa lies on the medial side of the joint beneath the cunean tendon (medial branch of the cranial tibial tendon).

Procedure. The bursa can be reached by inserting the needle through the cunean tendon or by directing it beneath the distal border of the tendon (Fig. 5–35). Successful injection is indi-

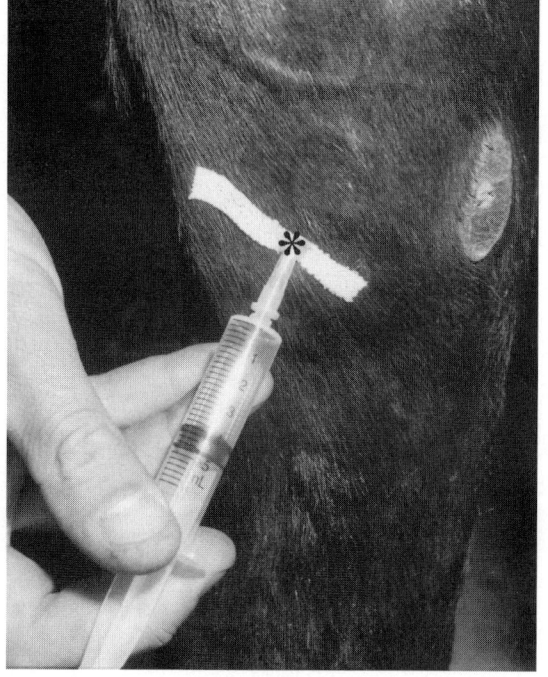

▶ **FIGURE 5–35**

Anesthesia of the cunean bursa.

**Materials for
Cunean Bursa Anesthesia**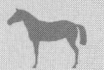

▶ Anesthetic (5 mL)

▶ Needle (22 gauge, 25 mm [1″])

cated by a bulging of the bursa above and below the tendon.

DESENSITIZATION OF THE TARSUS AND DISTAL LIMB (DEEP AND SUPERFICIAL PERONEAL NERVES AND TIBIAL NERVE).

These blocks are used to localize a lesion to the upper or lower limb or when the other more specific blocks are for some reason inappropriate or cannot be adequately completed. To ensure reliable results, the author prefers larger volumes of anesthetic than is usually described in other texts.

Deep and Superficial Peroneal Nerves. Both nerves are blocked at the same site, but at different depths.

Procedure. The site for injection is on the lateral aspect of the limb, about 10 cm above the point of the hock, in the groove between the long and lateral digital extensor muscles (Fig. 5–36A). The superficial branch is blocked first, by depositing 15 mL of anesthetic solution subcutaneously, in and adjacent to the described site. This injection also facilitates insertion of the larger needle for anesthesia of the deep branch. The larger needle is then inserted through the same site and directed medially, and slightly caudally, between the two muscle bellies. The deep branch lies close to the tibia where 15 ml of solution should be deposited. A common variation is to use the same needle for both injections, making the injection over the superficial branch during insertion or during withdrawal after the deep injection.

Tibial Nerve. The tibial nerve is usually blocked at the same time as the peroneal nerves.

Procedure. The site for injection is on the medial side of the limb, 10 cm proximal to the point of the hock, just caudal to the deep

---

Materials for Peroneal Nerve Anesthesia (Deep and Superficial Branches)

- Superficial branch
  Anesthetic (15 mL)
  Needle (22 gauge, 25 mm [1″])

- Deep branch
  Anesthetic (15 mL)
  Needle (20 gauge, 36 mm [1.5″])

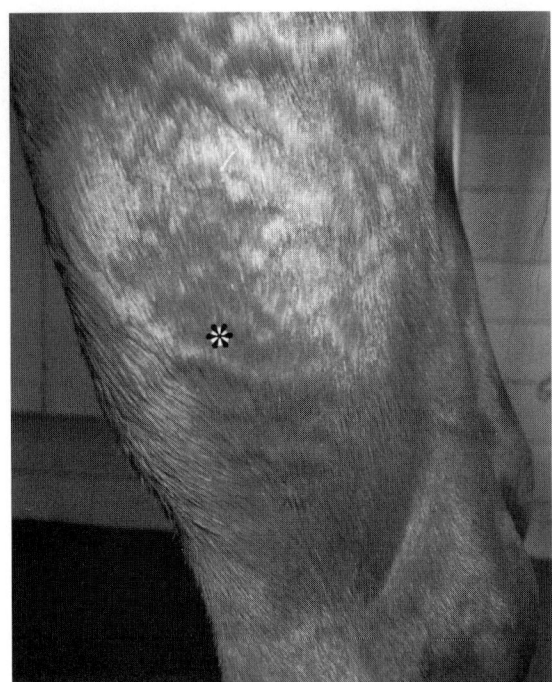

A

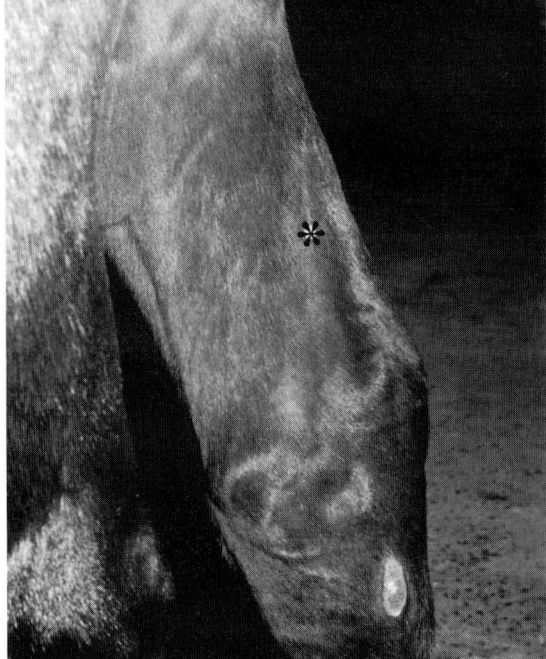

B

▶ **FIGURE 5–36**

Anesthesia of the tarsal region. **A.** Deep and superficial branches of the peroneal nerve. **B.** Tibial nerve.

flexor tendon (Fig. 5–36B). At this site, the nerve can be palpated as a 0.5-cm-thick structure, lying caudal to the deep flexor tendon. The author prefers to stand beside the opposite leg. However, this is a matter of preference, and it also depends on the temperament of the horse.

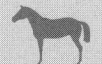

Materials for Tibial Nerve Anesthesia

▸ Anesthetic (20 mL)
▸ Needle (25 gauge, 25 mm [1″]; 20 gauge, 36 mm [1.5″])

A bleb of anesthetic is deposited subcutaneously with the small needle, then 20 mL of solution is infiltrated around the region of the nerve with the larger needle.

Region Desensitized. This set of injections blocks the deep structures distal to, and including, the hock. As described, the superficial sensation is variably affected.

Complications. Interference with motor nerve function sometimes occurs, which is alarming for the horse. If this occurs, the horse should not be exercised and should be placed in a stall until the effects wear off. The results of the block are not always as desired. This is usually related to poor technique, especially the use of an insufficient volume of anesthetic.

GENUAL (STIFLE) JOINT. The stifle joint is composed of three synovial cavities: the femoropatellar, and the medial and lateral femorotibial joints. The femoropatellar joint communicates with the medial femorotibial joint in all cases and with the lateral femorotibial in about 20% of cases.[13] Although anesthesia of the femoropatellar and lateral femorotibial joints would, therefore, anesthetize all joints on most occasions, absolute certainty requires that each joint be injected separately. These injections are made with the limb bearing weight.

Materials for Genual (Stifle) Joint Anesthesia

▸ Femoropatellar joint
  Anesthetic (30 mL)
  Needle (20 gauge, 50 mm [2″])
▸ Femorotibial joints (medial and lateral)
  Anesthetic (20 mL)
  Needle (20 gauge, 25 mm [1″])

Procedure

• *Femoropatellar joint.*
  Method 1. The site for injection is between the middle and medial or middle and lateral patellar ligaments, just distal to the apex of the patella (Fig. 5–37A). The needle is directed caudally and horizontally until it contacts the surface of the femur or, caudoproximally beneath the patella. Unless a copious effusion exists, it is often difficult to aspirate joint fluid to entry into the joint.
  Method 2. The joint can also be approached from the caudolateral aspect, with the advantage that joint fluid can nearly always be obtained for evaluation or to indicate that the joint has been penetrated.[14] This site is located caudal to the lateral ridge of the femoral trochlea and the lateral patellar ligament and approximately 5 cm proximal to the lateral condyle of the tibia.

• *Medial femorotibial joint.* The site for injection is between the medial patellar and the medial collateral (femorotibial) ligaments, just proximal to the tibia (Fig. 5–37B).

• *Lateral femorotibial joint.* The site for injection lies just proximal to the tibial plateau, between the lateral patellar and the lateral collateral (femorotibial) ligaments, either side of the tendon of the long digital ex-

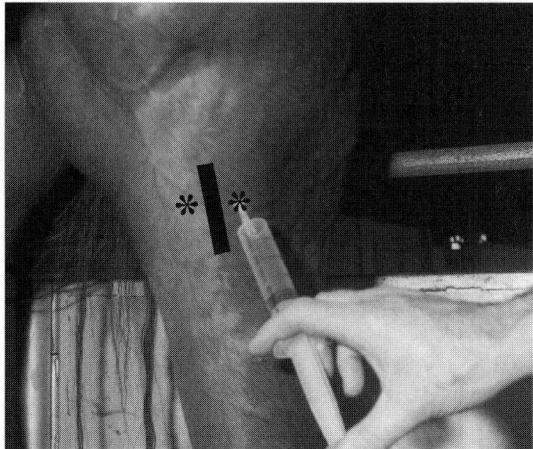

A

▸ **FIGURE 5–37**
Anesthesia of the stifle. **A.** Femoropatellar joint. The site for injection is medial or lateral to the middle patellar ligament. The needle can be directed horizontally until it touches the femur or, as shown, caudoproximally beneath the patella. (A lateral approach is described in the text.)

Illustration continued on following page

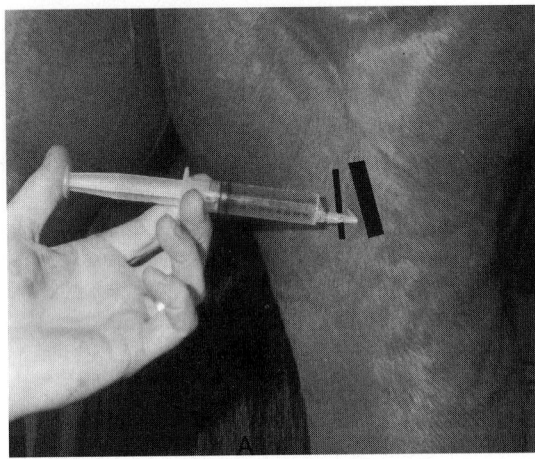

B

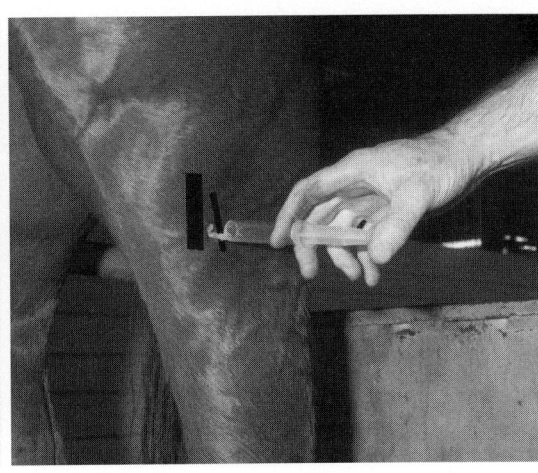

C

▶ **FIGURE 5-37** *Continued*

B. Medial femorotibial joint. The site for injection is between the medial collateral (femorotibial) and the medial patellar ligaments (thick line), just proximal to the tibial plateau. **C.** Lateral femorotibial joint. The site is between the lateral collateral (femorotibial) and the lateral patellar ligaments (thick line), just proximal to the tibial plateau and cranial or caudal to the tendon of the long digital extensor.

tensor (LDE) that bisects this space (Fig. 5-37C). Penetration caudal to the LDE tendon results in entry into the diverticulum of the joint capsule that lies beneath the tendon.

COXOFEMORAL (HIP) JOINT. Injection of the hip joint is difficult to achieve consistently because of its depth and the volume of muscle around it. As the needle must penetrate this muscle, there is a danger that movement of the horse will bend or break the needle. To maximize the chances of successful joint puncture and minimize the chances of damage to the needle, the horse should be restrained in stocks and be standing squarely with its weight distributed equally.

Procedure. The horse should be restrained and standing symmetrically, as stated. The site for insertion is the notch between the greater and lesser trochanters (Fig. 5-38). The greater tro-

chanter is the most lateral osseous structure in the region of the proximal femur, and it is usually palpable in all but the most heavily muscled horses. As this is an important landmark, it is unwise to continue with the procedure if it cannot be located. The lesser trochanter lies just caudal to the greater trochanter, separated by a notch that is usually not palpable. The site for injection is through this notch, which is located midway between the trochanters and about 1 cm distally. The skin and subcutaneous tissues are first anesthetized with 5 mL of anesthetic deposited with a

Materials for Coxofemoral (Hip) Joint Anesthesia

▶ Anesthetic (15 mL)
▶ Needle (16–18 gauge, 15–20 cm [6″–8″]), 20 gauge, 36 mm [1.5″])
▶ Scalpel blade (#12)

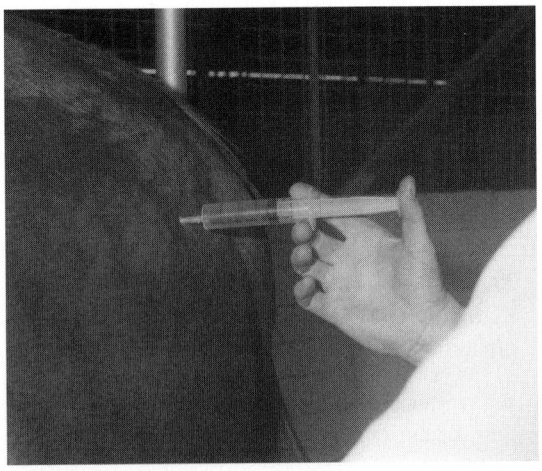

▶ **FIGURE 5-38**

Anesthesia of the coxofemoral joint. The site for injection is through the knotch between the greater and lesser trochanters. The angle of insertion, as indicated, is important.

20-gauge, 36-mm (1.5″) needle. To facilitate insertion and control of the larger needle, a small stab incision is made through the skin with a size 12 scalpel blade. The large needle is then inserted horizontally and craniomedially at 45° to the long axis of the horse. As the joint is entered, the clinician can feel the needle penetrating the thick joint capsule. After synovia has been obtained, the injection can be made.

Complications.   Failure to locate the joint is a not uncommon difficulty. The most significant complication is breakage and loss of the distal part of the needle. Caudal misdirection of the needle can result in contact with the sciatic nerve, producing an immediate and violent response. It cannot be stressed too much that the horse must be tractable, standing squarely, and that the landmarks must be identified before an attempt to inject this joint is made.

TROCHANTERIC BURSA.   Inflammation of the trochanteric bursa is a problem found mostly in pacing and trotting horses. The bursa lies between the tendon of the middle gluteal muscle and the cranial part of the greater trochanter.

Procedure.   The bursa can be reached by inserting the needle through the middle gluteal muscle from directly over the trochanter or, usually, by inserting the needle distal to the trochanter and directing it proximally beneath the muscle (Fig. 5–39). The site for the distal approach is approximately 5 cm distal to the palpable cranial part of the trochanter. The needle is directed proximally so that it slides across the lateral surface of the trochanter.

MISCELLANEOUS SYNOVIAL STRUCTURES IN THE HINDLIMB.   There are other synovial structures that occasionally require injection of diagnostic anesthetic medications, or radiographic contrast materials. Normally they contain little synovia, and it is often difficult to ensure that a needle will enter the synovial cavity. Fortunately, effusions usually accompany disease and make puncture much easier. Synovial structures in the hindlimb that have not been described separately include:

- Digital synovial sheath (metatarsophalangeal joint)
- Tendon sheaths in the vicinity of the tarsus
    Tarsal synovial sheath
    Long digital flexor muscle
    Long digital extensor muscle
    Lateral digital extensor muscle
- Bursae at the calcaneal tuber
    Between the tendons of the superficial digital flexor muscle and the calcaneal tendon of the gastrocnemius muscles
    Between the calcaneal tuber and the tendon of the superficial digital flexor muscle (usually communicates with the above)

Procedure.   An anatomy text should be consulted when necessary. However injection is usually made into a prominent distension of the synovial structure.

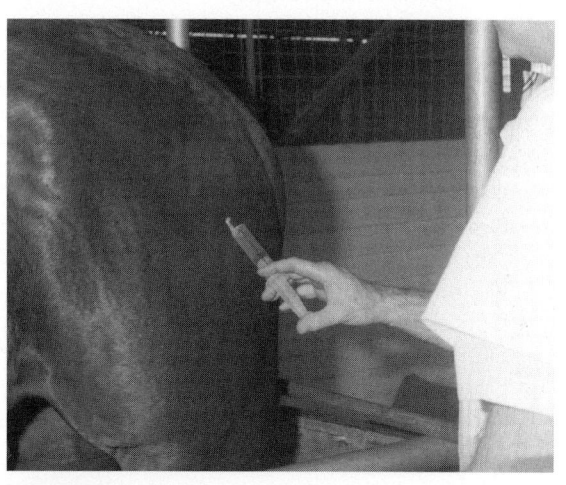

▶ **FIGURE 5–39**
Anesthesia of the trochanteric bursa. The site for injection is approximately 5 cm distal to the cranial border of the trochanter. The correct angle of insertion is indicated.

Materials for Trochanteric Bursa Anesthesia

▸ Anesthetic (10 mL)
▸ Needle (18 gauge, 7.5 cm [3″])

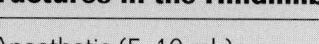

Materials for Anesthesia of Miscellaneous Synovial Structures in the Hindlimb

▸ Anesthetic (5–10 mL)
▸ Needle (21 gauge, 36 mm [1.5″])

SPECIAL EXAMINATION PROCEDURES

Radiology

The equine clinician involved in evaluating the musculoskeletal system frequently needs to use radiological techniques. In many cases the clinician will be responsible for the exposures and will use a portable unit. To image the axial and proximal skeleton and in situations where special skills are required, a specialist radiologist with appropriate equipment is required. Therefore, some clinicians must have the skills required to make, develop, and interpret the exposures, whereas others are responsible only for imparting the results to the client and providing some interpretation. In all situations, the clinician must decide which region should be exposed and what type and number of exposures are necessary. To do this a knowledge of current acceptable methodology is required. Excellent descriptions of radiology of the equine musculoskeletal system are available, and the reader is referred to these for detailed information.[15,16]

Equipment

Exposure factors vary with the radiologist and the type of accessory apparatus used, and, therefore, accurate recommendations cannot be provided. The reader is referred to the literature for an example of an exposure guide used in one institution.[15]

Terminology of Radiographic Exposures

The terminology used to identify the various radiographic views is described elsewhere.[17] Briefly, the view is described by a directional system according to the point at which the beam enters and then leaves the limb, thus producing a two-part term (i.e., dorso-palmar, latero-medial). For oblique views, the orientation relative to the front or back of the limb is placed first in each two-part combination (i.e., *dorso*lateral-*palmaro*medial oblique). For oblique views in the horizontal plane, the angle relative to the long axis of the horse is also included when it differs from 45°. For oblique views in the vertical plane, the angle is measured relative to the ground surface. Proximal to the antibrachiocarpal (radiocarpal) and tarsocrural joints the terms *cranial* and *caudal* are used. Distal to these points it is *dorsal* and *palmar* (forelimb)

Materials for Plain Radiography of the Musculoskeletal System

▶ X-ray machine
  A high-output machine provides the best-quality radiographs and is necessary for axial (exception proximal cervical spine) and proximal appendicular skeletons.
  A portable machine is useful for radiographs of the head, proximal cervical spine, and lower limbs.

▶ X-ray film

▶ Screens (rare earth or calcium tungstate)

▶ Grids for head, trunk, upper limbs (above carpus and tarsus), and some hoof exposures

▶ Cassette holders or stands, hoof blocks

▶ Protective gloves, gowns

▶ Film markers

▶ Sedative drugs (see Chapter 1. Chemical Restraint of the Adult Horse)

or *plantar* (hindlimb). For some sites, the beam is directed distally from above to produce a tangential view (e.g., the dorsoproximal-dorsodistal oblique for the carpus).

The abbreviations used to describe the terms included in the view descriptions are: dorsal, D; cranial, Cr; palmar, Pa; plantar, Pl; caudal, Ca; proximal, Pr; distal, Di; lateral, L; medial, M; oblique, O. Hence,

- Dorsopalmar, DPa
- Lateromedial, LM
- Flexed lateromedial, flexed LM
- Dorsolateral-palmaromedial oblique at 45°, DL-PaMO or D45° L-PaMO
- Dorsolateral-palmaromedial oblique at 60°, D 60° L-PaMO
- Dorsomedial-palmarolateral oblique, DM-PaLO
- Dorsoproximal-dorsodistal oblique, DPr-DDiO
- Palmaroproximal-palmarodistal oblique, PaPr-PaDiO

Plain Radiography

For most regions a minimum number of views are regarded as necessary for a routine radiological examination. Frequently, extra views are required to detect lesions in unusual sites. The need for a complete set will vary with the situation, but the clinician should be aware of the fact that failure to carry out a full series constitutes an incomplete examination.

FOOT. The foot should be prepared by removing the shoes, cleaning the sole, and removing flakes of horn, and packing the sole to eliminate air shadows that otherwise appear in the radiographs and confuse interpretation (Fig. 5–40). A common packing material is Play Doh (3M, Minnesota, USA).

Distal Phalanx (Fig. 5–40)

- LM. This view is taken with the foot elevated and resting flat on a block of wood.
- DPa views with horizontal beam
  DPr-PaDiO ("upright pedal"). Toe on ground, sole vertical, beam centered on coronet
  DPa "standing." Sole horizontal, beam centered on mid-dorsum of hoof wall

- DPa view with angled beam
  D65° Pr-PaDiO ("high coronary"). Sole flat, standing on cassette
- Pa45° Pr-PaDiO. Sole flat on ground, standing on cassette, beam centered between bulbs of heels
- Other oblique views
  Flexed D35°-60° M-PaL, D35°-60°L-PaM. Toe on ground, sole vertical

Hoof. The hoof can be imaged with similar views to those just described, but the exposures should be reduced. Hoof radiology is usually done to detect separation of hoof wall and third phalanx, such as is seen with laminitis and abscessation.

NAVICULAR BONE. Good radiographs of the navicular bone require especially good technique and specific projections. Shoes must be removed, and the sole cleaned and packed. It is important that in the radiograph the navicular bone is projected so that it does not overlie the structures of the distal interphalangeal joint. This is achieved by using a special stand, the design varying according to whether it is used for one or a number of views (Fig. 5–41).

- LM view. Sole flat, resting on a raised wooden block. Beam centered on the end of the navicular bone.
- DPr-PaDiO view ("upright pedal"). Hoof on block with surface angle of 55°, beam horizontal and centered 1 cm proximal to the coronet

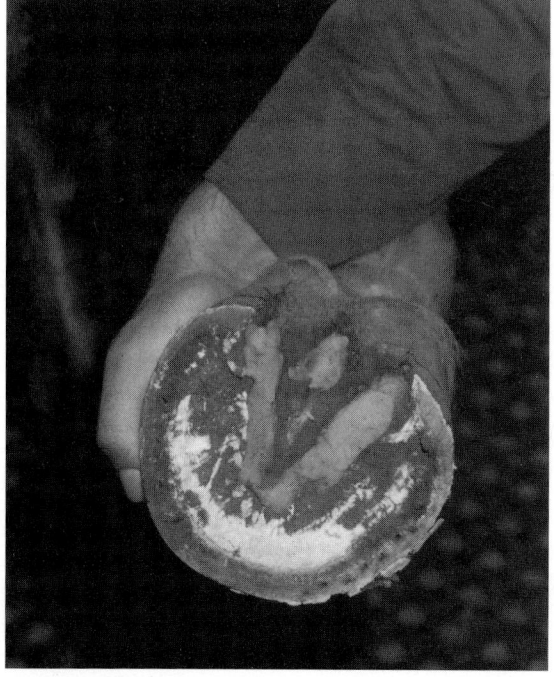

▶ FIGURE 5-40
Packing crevices of the foot with Play Doh prior to radiography to eliminate shadows in the radiograph.

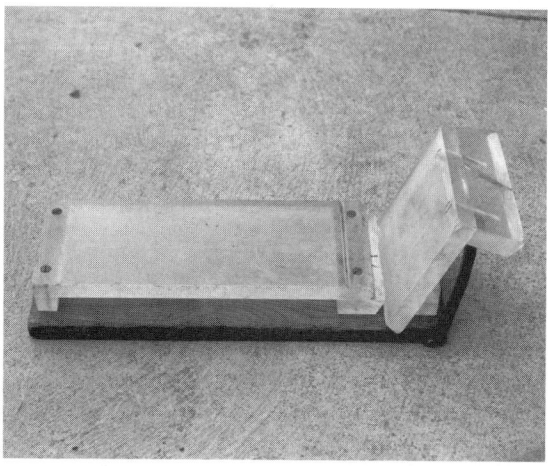

▶ FIGURE 5-41
Navicular block. An example of one type of device used to help position the hoof and phalanges for special radiographic exposures, especially for imaging the navicular bone.

- D60° Pr-PaDiO view ("high coronary"). Sole flat on ground, standing on cassette, beam at 60° and centered 2 cm proximal to coronet
- Pa45°Pr-PaDiO ("tangential"). Sole flat on ground, standing on cassette, beam at 45° and centered between bulbs of heels

In hindlimbs positioning for the DPl views is difficult and plantarodorsal (PlD) views are appropriate. This involves placing the cassette in front of the hoof.

PROXIMAL AND MIDDLE PHALANGES. These radiographs are usually taken with the limb bearing weight. In addition to the usual DPa, LM, DM-PaLO and DL-PaMO, additional oblique views are often necessary to detect linear fracture lines.

- DPa
- LM
- Flexed LM
- DM-PaLO
- DL-PaMO

METACARPO(TARSO)PHALANGEAL JOINT
Standard Views. The four standard views are taken with the limb bearing weight and with the beam horizontal

- DPa(DPl)
- LM
- D45°M-PaLO (D45° M-PILO)
- D45°L-PaMO (D45° L-PIMO)

Additional Views

- To image the abaxial surface of the proximal sesamoids, the LM view is modified by aiming the beam at a 45° angle from proximal to distal (e.g., Pr45°L-DiMO to image the medial sesamoid in a forelimb).
- Other DM-PaLO (DM-PILO) and DL-PaMO (DL-PIMO) views
- To visualize the articular surface of the third metacarpal better, the angle at which the beam crosses the joint can be varied by altering the angle of the fetlock and/or the angle of the beam relative to the ground. These views are termed DPr-PaDiO or DDi-PaPrO views. For the DDi-PaPrO views the hoof should be placed on a block with joint extended.
- To view the articular surfaces of the proximal sesamoids and the sagittal ridge of the

third metacarpal bone, the LM view is made with the joint flexed (i.e., flexed LM).

METACARPUS(TARSUS)
Standard Views

- DPa (DPl)
- DL-PaMO (DL-PIMO)
- DM-PaLO (DM-PILO)
- LM

Additional Views. The distal articular surface of the third metacarpal(tarsal) bone can be imaged with DPr-PaDiO or DDi-PaPrO views, as explained.

CARPUS
Standard Views. The standard views, with the exception of the flexed LM, are conducted with the limb bearing weight.

- DPa
- LM
- Flexed LM. Metacarpus horizontal (less if flexion is painful)
- D45°L-PaMO
- D45°M-PaLO

Additional Views. Additional oblique views are often necessary to locate lesions not visible on the two 45° oblique views, such as chip fractures "around the corner" from the silhouetted surface. Lesions such as slab fractures or sclerosis, involving the dorsal surfaces or the adjacent bodies of the bones are best imaged with DPr-DDi tangential views ("skyline").

- Additional DM-PaLO and DL-PaMO views
- D80°, 55°, or 30°Pr-DDi (to image radius, proximal row of carpal bones, or distal row of carpal bones, respectively). Carpus flexed, metacarpus horizontal, plate horizontal under metacarpus and extending dorsally beyond the level of the carpus (Fig. 5-42).

RADIUS. The radius is examined using the traditional four views.
Standard Views

- CrCa
- LM
- Cr45°L-CaM
- Cr45°M-CaL

Additional Views. These include oblique views as necessary.

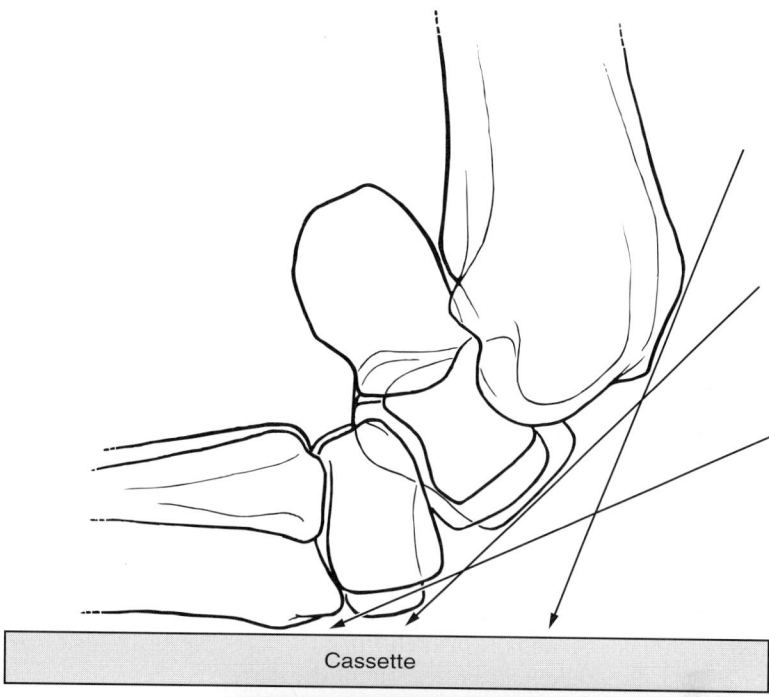

A

B

▶ **FIGURE 5–42**

Carpal tangential ("skyline") view. **A.** Diagram demonstrating how to position the carpus and cassette and how to direct the radiographic beam to image the different rows of bones in the carpus. **B.** An example of a carpal "skyline" view showing a fracture of the radial facet of the third carpal bone.

CUBITAL (ELBOW) JOINT. The cubital joint is usually radiographed with the horse bearing weight, although protraction of the limb is occasionally useful. The ML view is preferred over the LM because the musculature and thorax prevent the cassette from being positioned proximally.

Standard Views

- ML. The limb to be radiographed is placed cranial to the other (may be held in protracted position), the cassette is lateral to joint, and the X-ray machine is on the opposite side of the horse.
- CrCa. The cassette is placed behind the ulna (position of cassette and/or angle of beam can be varied slightly to suit regional

anatomy) or limb can be protracted by hand and plate placed along caudal surface of forearm.

Additional Views. Additional oblique views are taken as necessary.

SCAPULOHUMERAL JOINT (ALSO SCAPULA AND HUMERUS). A radiograph in the region of the joint also allows the distal scapula and proximal humerus to be evaluated. The distal humerus is imaged by centering the beam more distally. The proximal scapula is very difficult to image, although the spine is sometimes visible on oblique views. Inability to carry out a full range of projections, for anatomical reasons, means that results are sometimes incomplete. The shoulder region can be radiographed with the horse standing, but better quality radiographs are obtainable under general anesthesia. In either case the limb must be protracted to bring the structures as far cranially as possible. If general anesthesia is used, the limb to be radiographed is closest to the ground for the ML view.

Standard Views

- ML-limb protracted, cassette lateral to joint, beam centered over estimated site of greater tubercle of humerus.
- CrM-CaLO-limb protracted, cassette caudolateral to joint
- CaL-CrMO-useful if horse is anesthetized

Additional Views. Additional oblique views are taken as necessary.

TARSUS. The standard views are taken with the limb bearing weight and the beam horizontal. The horse's tail should be held or tied out of the way. Otherwise, it hangs down over the tarsus and interferes with accurate positioning of the cassette.

Standard Views

- LM
- DPl
- D35° L-PIMO
- D35° M-PILO. Alternatively, a Pl35°L-DMO view is often used to avoid directing the beam under the horse

Additional Views

- Flexed LM. The metatarsus is horizontal (for visualizing the proximal parts of the trochlear ridges of the talus, coracoid process of the calcaneus, and caudal tibia).
- Pr10°L-DiMO. The small joints slope distally in a lateral-to-medial direction; and angling the beam downward slightly will allow the joints to be visualized without overlapping.
- Flexed DPl. The metatarsus is horizontal, the cassette horizontal beneath the metatarsus and extending caudally beyond the calcaneus, the beam is perpendicular to the cassette and is centered on the dorsum of the calcaneus for visualizing the calcaneal tuber and sustentaculum tali (Fig. 5–43). The terminology is DPl because the reference is to the calcaneus itself, rather than to the limb, in which case it would be CaPr-CaDi.

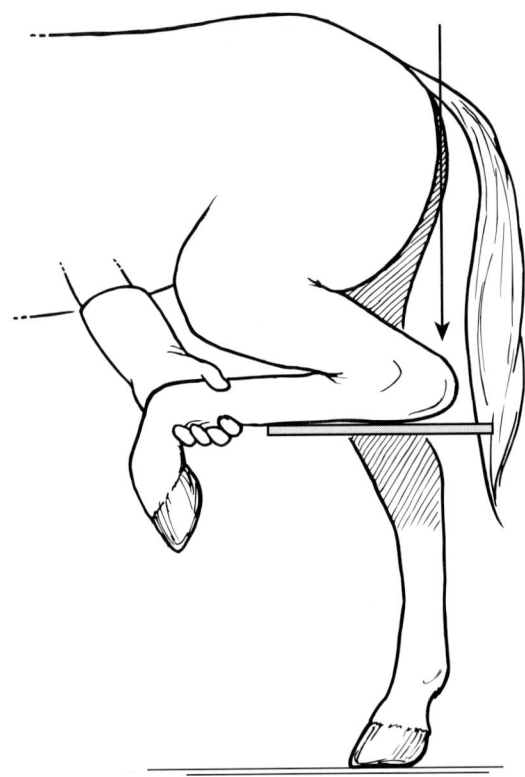

▶ **FIGURE 5-43**

Tarsal tangential ("skyline") view showing how to position the tarsus and cassette and to direct the radiographic beam to image the sustentaculum tarsi.

GENUAL (STIFLE) JOINT. The standard views can be made with the limb bearing weight, although general anesthesia is often necessary. The angle of the tibial plateau should be considered when choosing the correct angle for the beam. Radiographs of this joint also image the distal femur and the proximal tibia and fibula.

Standard Views

- LM
- CaCr. Positioning is easier than for CrCa.

Additional Views

- Ca30°L-CrMO. Preferred by some as positioning is easier, and this position avoids some overlapping of images. The beam should be centered on the femorotibial joint and angled slightly downward.
- CrPr-CrDiO. For imaging the patella and femoral trochlea and intertrochlear groove. The limb is elevated and extended caudally, the tibia is horizontal, the cassette is held horizontally under the cranial tibia and extending forward beyond the level of the

patella. The beam is perpendicular and directed onto the patella from directly above the joint.

TIBIA.   The tibia can be imaged in the standing horse with the limb bearing weight. The proximal and distal parts of the tibia appear in radiographs of the stifle and tarsus, respectively.

Standard Views

- LM
- CrCa (alternately, CaCr)
- CrL-CaMO
- CrM-CaLO

Additional Views.   Additional oblique views are taken as necessary to locate lesions such as spiral fractures.

FEMUR AND PELVIS.   The distal femur is visualized in radiographs of the stifle. Radiographs of the pelvis and of most of the femur require general anesthesia, with occasional exceptions for foals and ponies. High-output equipment and a specialized facility are necessary.

Standard Views.   The ventrodorsal view is the normal projection as lateral views are rarely useful. In the VD view, the horse is recumbent, the hindlimbs flexed and abducted. Several overlapping views are necessary to image the entire region.

Contrast Radiography

The main application of plain radiology is to evaluate hard tissues. Contrast radiology adds the ability to investigate a variety of soft-tissue structures that contain a lumen, or opening, into which the contrast agent can be injected or infused. Positive contrast techniques use a radioopaque material to detect the presence and extent of abnormal cavities or tracts, the extent of normal cavities, presence of space-occupying lesions within a cavity, and variation or deformation in the contours of the walls of a cavity. Negative contrast techniques, which use a radiolucent gas, can also outline cavities, but their main value lies in providing visualization of a structure lying within the structure being distended. Negative contrast is not used often in equine radiology. Double-contrast radiography, using a combination of positive and negative techniques, is also possible, whereby the positive contrast material coats the surfaces of internal structures, thus enhancing the contrast between them and the air.

Contrast radiography is used in joints (arthrography), tendon sheaths (tenography), and draining tracts (fistulography). The reader is referred to the literature for more details of the methodology and results.[15,18]

MATERIALS.   Room air and carbon dioxide are used as negative-contrast agents although, because carbon dioxide is absorbed faster and provides no chance of gas embolism, it is preferred. Positive-contrast agents containing aqueous organic iodine have been extensively used. They include ionic and nonionic agents. Some examples of ionic materials are meglumine iothalamate (Conray; Mallinckrodt, Inc., Diagnostic Products Division, St Louis, MO), sodium and meglumine diatrizoate (Hypaque; Winthrop Laboratories, New York, NY; Renografin; E R Squibb & Sons, Inc., Princeton, NJ). Some examples of nonionic agents are metrizamide (Amipaque; Winthrop Laboratories, New York, NY), iopamidol (Isovue; E R Squibb & Sons, Inc., Princeton, NJ), and iohexol (Omnipaque; Winthrop Laboratories, New York, NY).

ARTHROGRAPHY

Procedure.   The procedure is conducted in sterile fashion, as described for joint anesthesia. After removal of hair from the puncture site and surgical preparation of the skin, a needle is inserted with a gloved hand. A sample of synovia is obtained for analysis, and the joint is then distended with an equal volume of the material of choice. Iohexol has been shown to be superior for arthrography.[19] Exposure factors are increased by 10 to 20 kVp to maximize the definition of the contrast material. The joint is gently flexed to ensure dispersal of the agent, and radiographic exposures are made within 5 minutes, for ionic agents, and 10 minutes for nonionic agents. The concentration of contrast material in the synovial fluid decreases rapidly, and later exposures will not be effective.

If a double-contrast method is to be used, as much synovia as possible is removed, and the gas is then injected first, to distend the joint, followed by a volume of the positive contrast material equal to 10% of the volume of the gas.

Complications.   With proper precautions, the effects of using a nonionic agent are no more than those for arthrocentesis alone.[19] Bubbles, which interfere with interpretation, may form if the gas is injected last, and if the joint is manipulated too vigorously.

TENOGRAPHY AND TENDONOGRAPHY.
Tenography is the use of contrast radiography to outline a tendon sheath and its contents, and tendonography refers to peritendinous injection of contrast to outline a tendon in a region where no sheath exists.

Procedure for Negative Contrast Tenography and Tendonography. The examination is best done under general anesthesia and with a tourniquet applied to localize gas to the region of interest.[20,21] After surgical preparation of the injection site, the gas is injected in sterile fashion into the tendon sheath. Where more than one tendon is enclosed in the sheath, gas is injected between the tendons to increase separation and enhance visualization.

Procedure for Positive-Contrast Tenography. This procedure is carried out in the conscious horse. The injection site is clipped and prepared for sterile puncture. The tendon sheath is distended with an appropriate volume of contrast agent.[22,23] The anatomy and volumes of tendon sheaths and bursae of the distal limbs have been described.[24]

Results. Tenography is helpful in detecting adhesions, distension, tendon disruption, and abnormal communication between a sheath and adjacent cavities. Tendonography is also useful in cases of tendinitis for detecting adhesions and disruption.

FISTULOGRAPHY. Fistulography is the term used to describe a contrast radiographic procedure conducted on a fistula, an abnormal communication between a hollow internal organ and the exterior or another organ. The most frequent indications are to investigate penetrating wounds of the navicular bursa, flexor tendon sheaths, joints, miscellaneous wound tracts, and other sheaths and bursae.

Procedure. Fistulography should always be preceded by routine radiography to establish the status of structures in the region. The most useful results are obtained when the fistula is well filled with the liquid contrast material. To ensure good distension of the tract, backflow of material can be prevented by using a cuffed Foley catheter or any other tight-fitting catheter. The catheter, which has been prefilled with the agent to avoid injection of air, is inserted into the tract and the cuff inflated. Contrast is injected until resistance is perceived on the syringe plunger, at which stage a radiograph is taken. Further injection and

radiographs are carried out as indicated. Care must be taken to avoid rupturing the structure by excessive injection pressure or by too forceful manipulation of the catheter.

Results. Part of the tract is usually well outlined. However, full visualization is not always possible. Repeated injections and manipulation of the limb may be necessary to improve penetration of the contrast agent. Foreign bodies may be visualized as a region of decreased density (a "filling defect") within the mass of contrast material. In cases when it is suspected that a synovial cavity has been penetrated, it is often more rewarding to inject the cavity with contrast material (or saline) and observe outflow from the fistula. In such a case, the injection should be through a prepared site away from the contaminated opening of the fistula. An example of the use of contrast radiography is demonstrated in Figure 5-44.

Ultrasonography

The reader is referred to Appendix B for information concerning the physics of ultrasound and some details of equipment.

Skin Preparation

The horse should be adequately restrained to avoid damaging the expensive equipment. The examination is usually carried out with minimum restraint, although, in certain horses, sedation and the use of stocks are necessary. Care is necessary to ensure that the holder is attending to the horse, and not watching the monitor. The skin overlying the region to be investigated is prepared as described in Appendix B. Acoustic coupling gel is applied to the skin and the probe and also to the standoff if one is used. A standoff is usually used when imaging the flexor tendons or other superficial structures.

Tendons and Ligaments

Ultrasonography has become virtually indispensible in the diagnosis and management of tendon and ligament injuries.[25]

PALMAR (PLANTAR) ASPECTS OF THE METACARPAL (TARSAL) AND PHALANGEAL REGIONS

Procedure. A systematic procedure was developed to examine this region, and record results.[25] A strip of skin approximately 2 cm wide on the palmar (plantar) aspect of the limb overlying

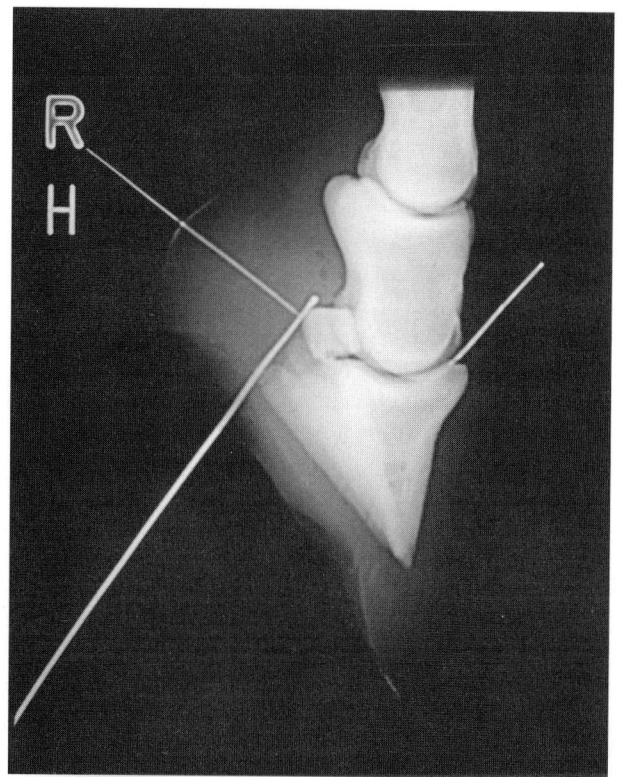

A

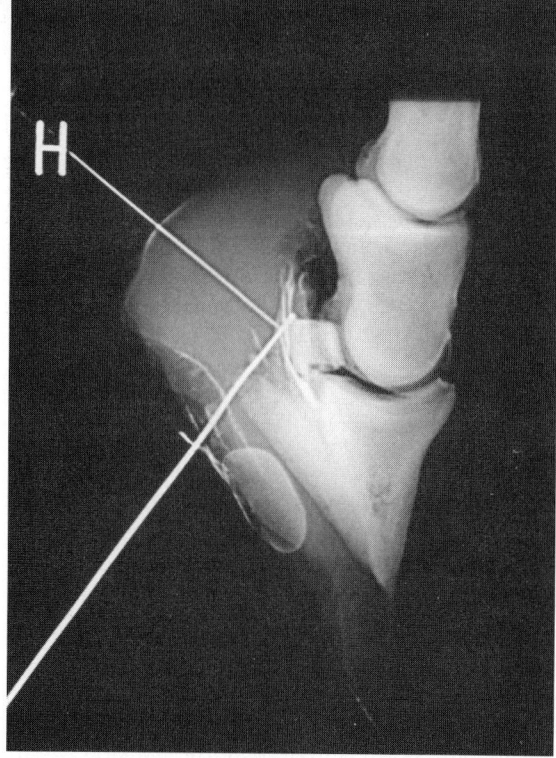

B

▶ **FIGURE 5-44**

Example of contrast radiography to investigate a penetrating wound of the sole. **A.** Hypodermic needles have been placed in the distal interphalangeal joint (DIJ) and navicular bursa and a probe inserted into the wound. **B.** Radiograph taken after injection of air into the DIJ (and removal of the needle) and radio-opaque contrast material into the bursa. Note that the air has remained in the joint and that the radio-opaque material outlines the bursa and the tract of the wound, but has not entered the DIJ.

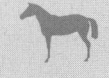

Materials for Tendon and Ligament Ultrasonography

▸ Ultrasound machine

▸ Scanhead with transducer(s) (7.5 and sometimes 5.0 MHz, linear array [preferred] or sector)

▸ "Standoff" (built-in or separate)

▸ Hair clippers (#40 clipper head)

▸ Safety razor

▸ Ultrasound coupling gel

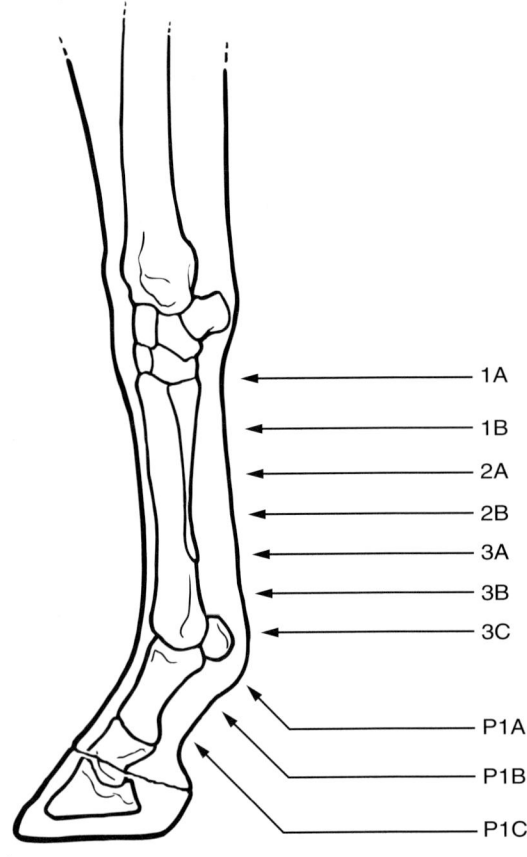

1A
1B
2A
2B
3A
3B
3C

P1A
P1B
P1C

▸ **FIGURE 5-45**

Diagram showing division of forelimb into zones to help identify the levels at which ultrasonograms are recorded.

the tendons is clipped, shaved, and smeared with gel. The examination should be conducted with the horse standing squarely and with weight equally distributed, in order to avoid the variation in size and echogenicity caused by variation in the tendon load. The scan begins in the proximal region and extends distally, with horizontal and longitudinal sections of each region being produced by changing the orientation of the scanhead. The long axis of the beam of ultrasound should be perpendicular to the structure being imaged, in order to obtain maximum-quality images.

To help identify the site of a lesion, in order to facilitate description and reexamination, two systems are used. In the first, the limb is divided into sections each with a thickness of approximately two forefingers,[25] and in the second the site is defined by its distance from the accessory carpal bone.[26] The author prefers the latter system. For transverse scans there are seven sections in the metacarpus, nine in the tarsus and metatarsus, and three to five for the phalangeal regions. For longitudinal scans the corresponding numbers are three, four, and one. The scheme is shown in Figure 5-45. Ultrasonography of the soft tissues of the palmar metacarpal region is shown in Figure 5-46.

The branches of the suspensory ligament can be imaged from the palmar or plantar surfaces by angling the scanhead laterally or medially or by placing it directly over each branch. Subtle changes in the angle of the scanhead can often be used to improve the definition of each structure. In the pastern region, the branches of the superfi-

cial digital flexor tendon are imaged by rotating the scanhead medially or laterally through 45°.

Lesions are localized according to the system of choice and then recorded on film with appropriate labeling. Whenever possible, it is recommended that the opposite limb be examined for comparison, as well as to check for bilateral lesions.

Results. Interpretation of a scan requires knowledge of the regional anatomy and the appearance of normal and abnormal structures. The former is available in anatomy texts and clinical publications,[27] and the learner is advised to obtain a limb and study the cross-sectional anatomy. The latter comes from experience and study of published data.[25,26,28-31]

Some examples of normal structures are shown in Figures 5-47 to 5-51. The useful portion of the ultrasonogram lies between the skin and the palmar surfaces of the third metacarpal bone, the proximal sesamoids, and the phalanges. The skin and subcutaneous tissues are seen as an hyper-

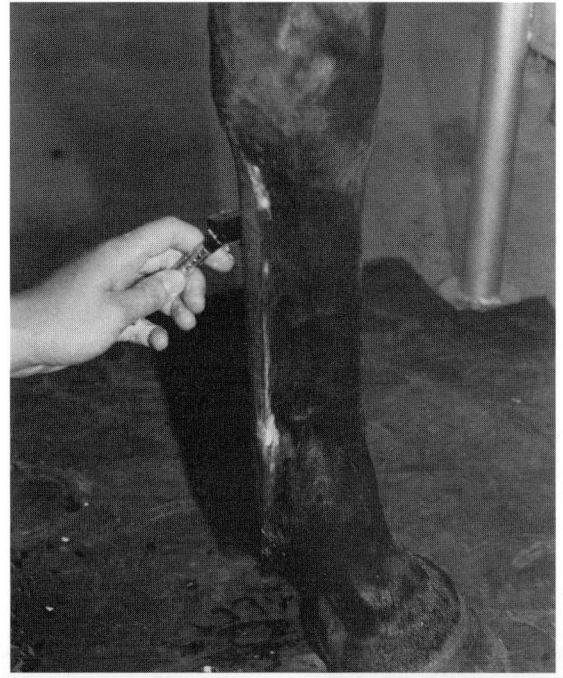

A

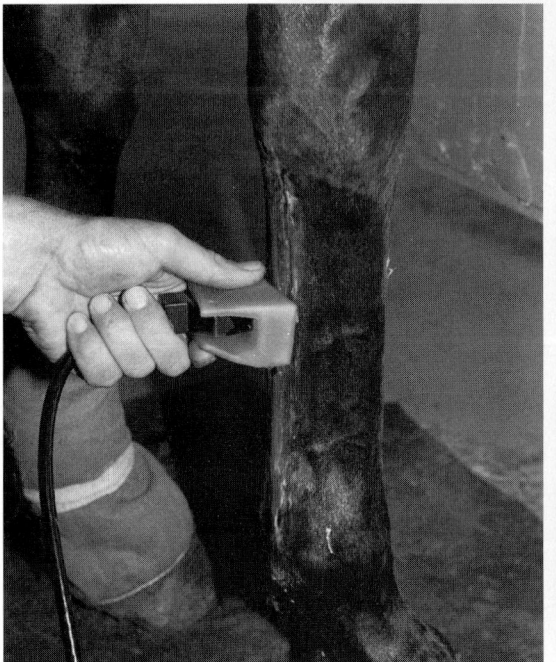

B

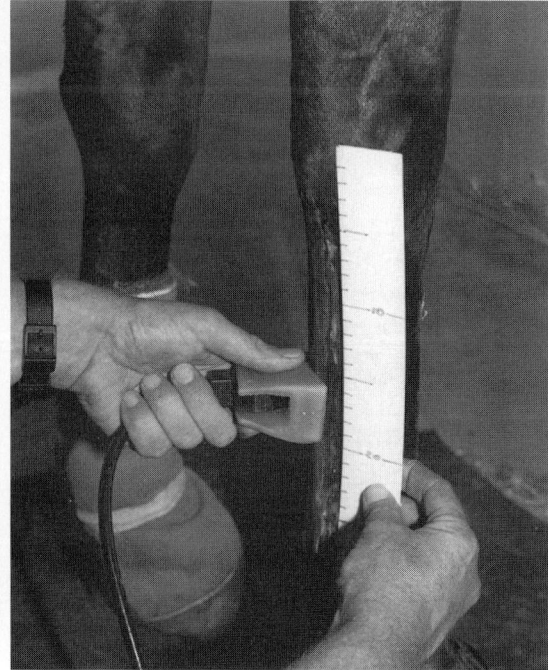

C

▶ **FIGURE 5-46**

Ultrasonography of the palmar soft tissues of the metacarpal region. **A.** Clipping the hair. **B.** Transducer and standoff being applied. **C.** Measuring distance of lesion from the accessory carpal bone.

echogenic line and a slightly less echoic space, respectively. The longitudinal arrangement of fibers in tendons and ligaments is in evidence, seen as a series of dots in cross section and striations in longitudinal section. The suspensory ligament, because of its muscle content, has a more mottled appearance. The accessory ligament of the deep digital flexor tendon (inferior check ligament) is often the most echogenic of these structures, followed by the deep digital flexor tendon and then the superficial digital

Text continued on page 150

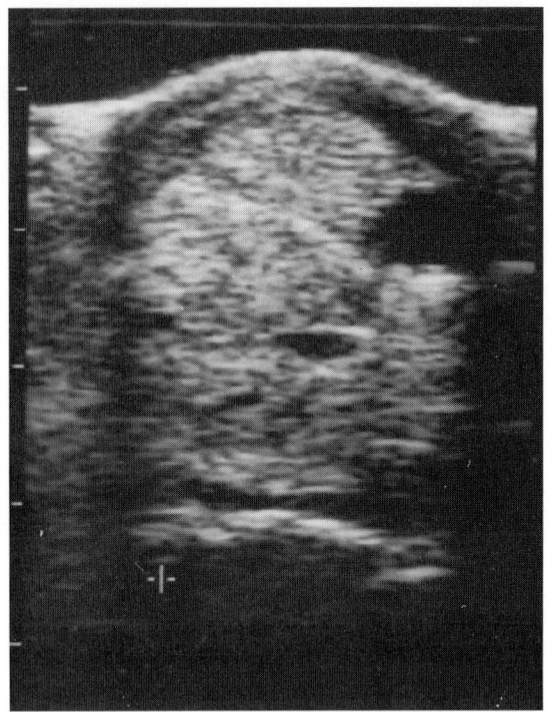

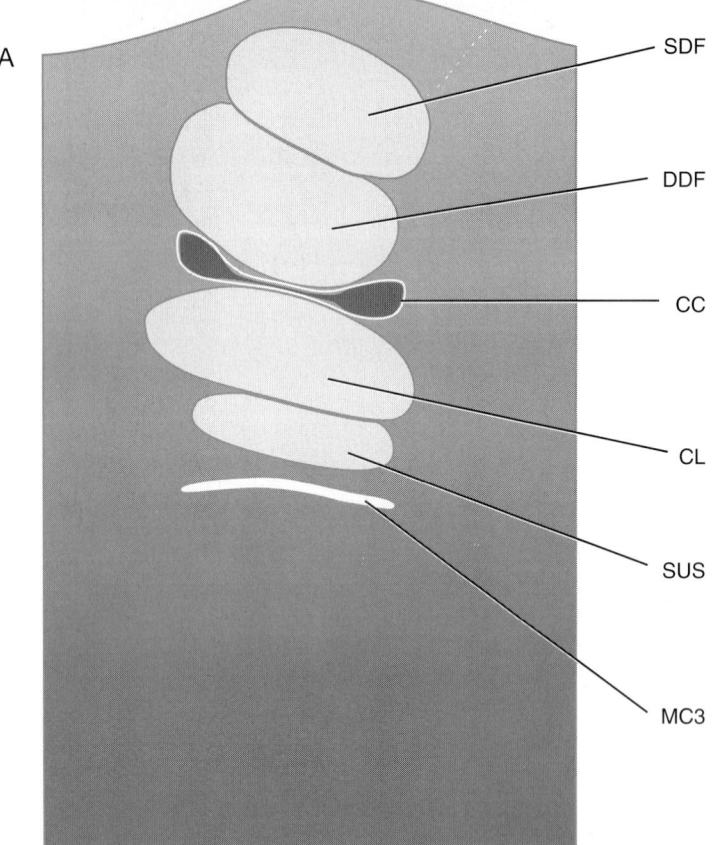

A

SDF

DDF

CC

CL

SUS

MC3

▶ FIGURE 5-47

Transverse ultrasonograms of the palmar metacarpal flexor tendons and associated ligaments
made with a 7.5-MHz linear array transducer and
standoff pad. The superficial digital flexor tendon is
seen just below the skin surface as a relatively less
echogenic band. The deep digital flexor tendon is
more echogenic. The accessory (inferior) check
ligament is also relatively hyperechoic and lies on
the dorsal surface of the deep digital flexor tendon.
The suspensory ligament lies on the hyperechoic
surface of the third metacarpal bone. *Abbreviations:* SDF, superficial digital flexor; DDF, deep
digital flexor; CC, carpal canal; CL, check ligament;
SUS, suspensory ligament; V, palmar vessel;
MC3, third metacarpal bone; DS, digital sheath;
SES, proximal sesamoids; IS, intersesamoidean
ligament. **A.** Transverse image acquired from zone
1A. The superficial digital flexor and deep digital
flexor (DDF) tendons are similarly sized elliptical
structures. Fluid is present in the carpal canal
between the check ligament and deep digital flexor
tendon. The origin of the suspensory ligament lies
adjacent to the third metacarpal bone. (Courtesy
R. H. Wrigley.)

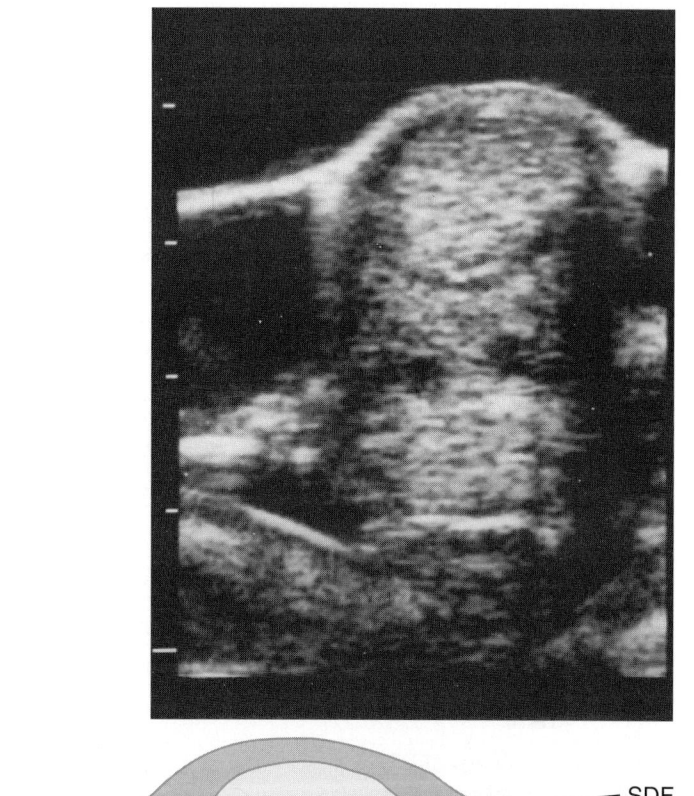

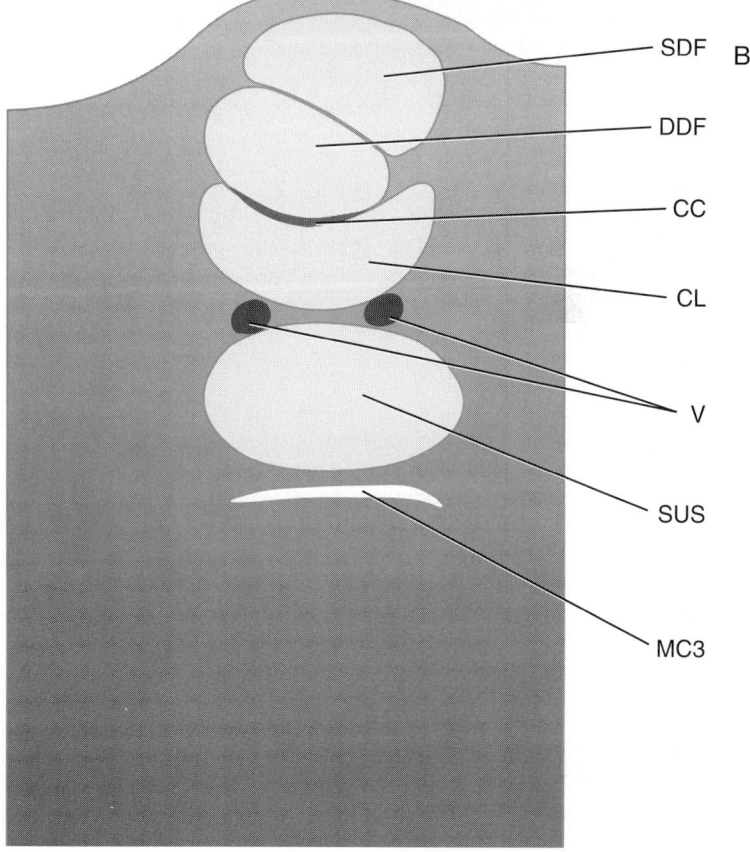

SDF B

DDF

CC

CL

V

SUS

MC3

▶ **FIGURE 5–47** *Continued*

B. Transverse image acquired from zone 1B. At this level the check ligament has become crescent-shaped as it approaches the dorsal surface of the deep digital flexor tendon. A small amount of fluid is detected in the carpal canal. The lateral and medial palmar vessels lie between the check ligament and the suspensory ligament. (Courtesy R. H. Wrigley.)

Illustration continued on following page

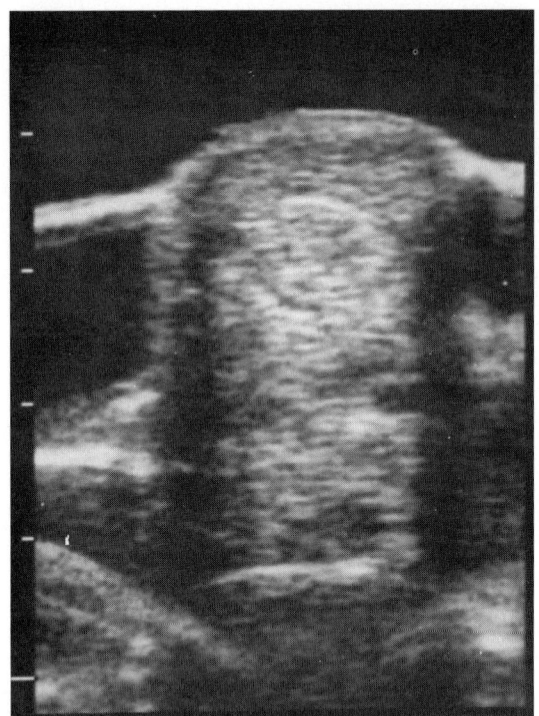

C

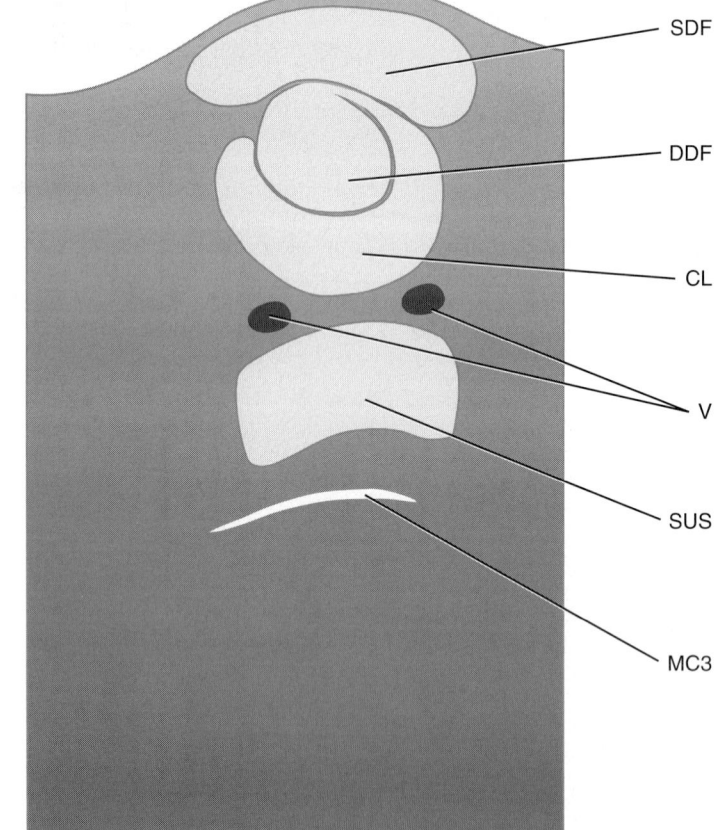

SDF

DDF

CL

V

SUS

MC3

▶ FIGURE 5-47 *Continued*

C. Transverse image acquired of zone 2A. The more echogenic check ligament blends into the dorsal surface of the deep digital flexor tendon. The prominent palmar vessels are evident. The body of the suspensory ligament has separated from the surface of the third metacarpal bone. (Courtesy R. H. Wrigley.)

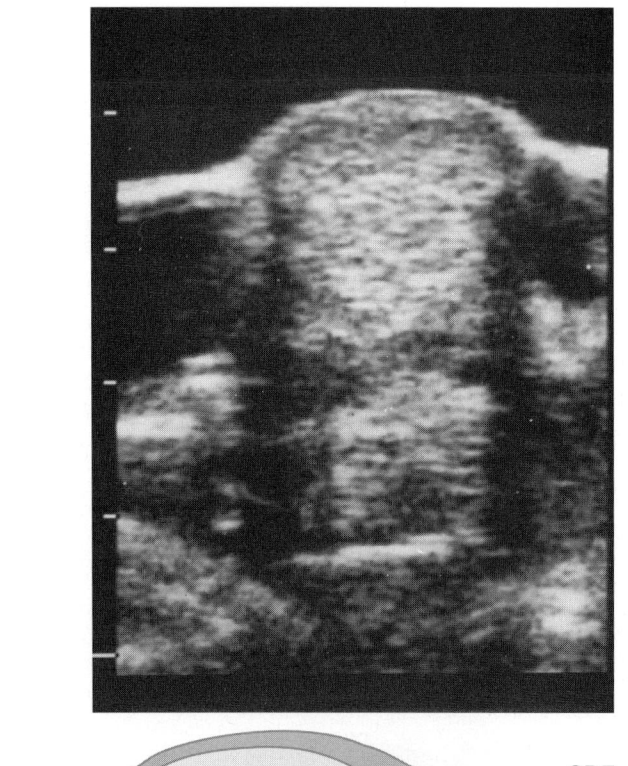

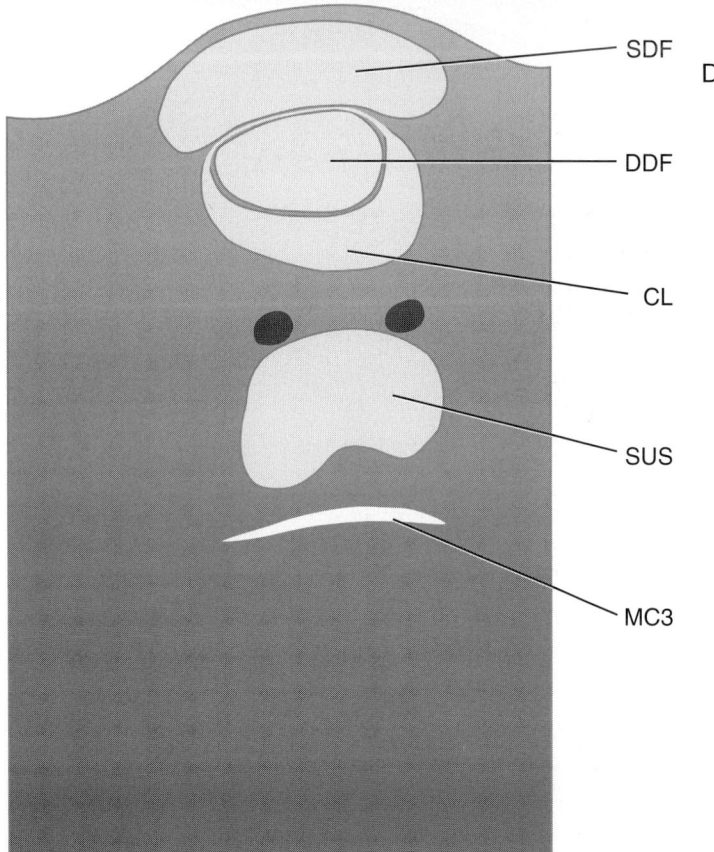

SDF

D

DDF

CL

SUS

MC3

▶ **FIGURE 5-47** *Continued*

D. Transverse image acquired from zone 2B. The more hypoechoic superficial digital flexor (SDF) tendon has become more straplike in shape. The check ligament is thinner. The suspensory ligament begins to divide into two branches. (Courtesy R. H. Wrigley.)

Illustration continued on following page

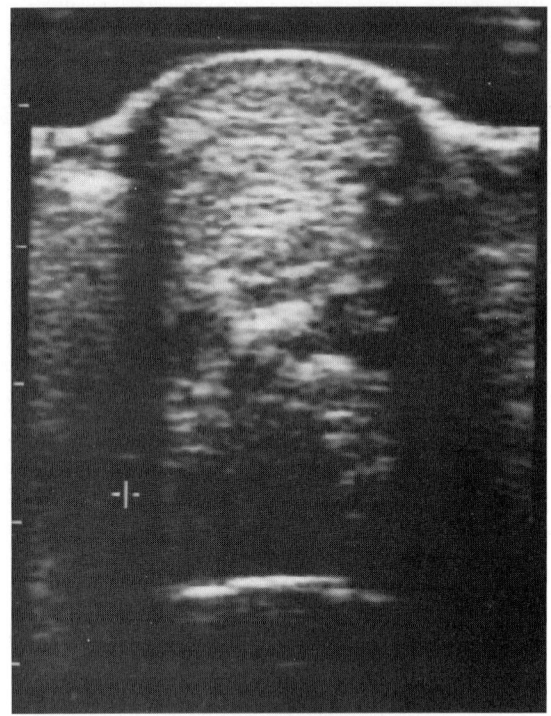

E

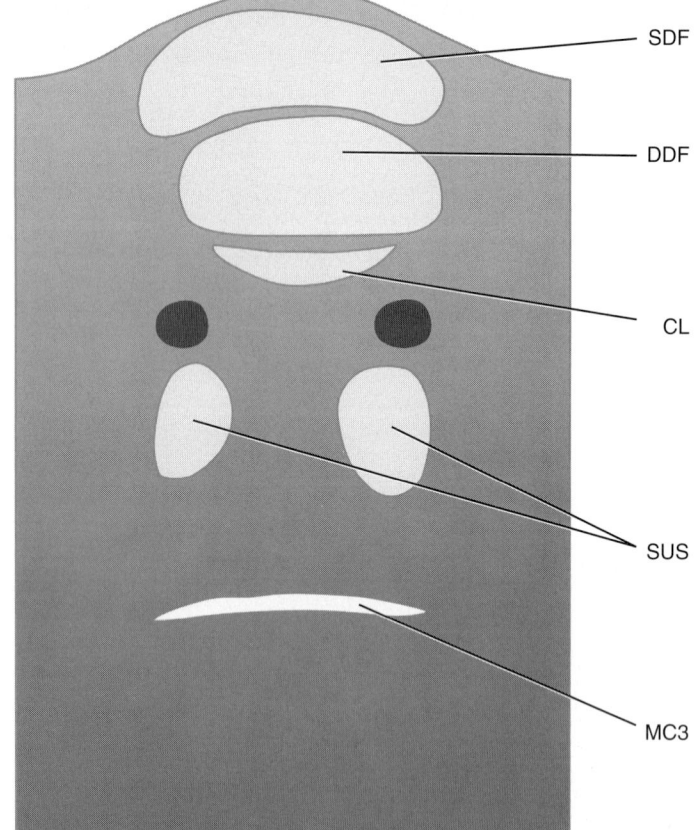

SDF

DDF

CL

SUS

MC3

▶ **FIGURE 5-47** *Continued*

E. Transverse image acquired from zone 3A. The check ligament is now very thin. The suspensory ligament has divided into two branches. (Courtesy R. H. Wrigley.)

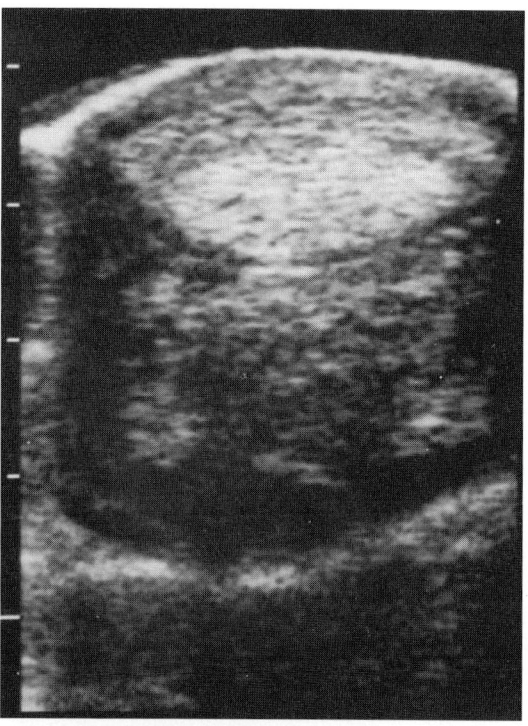

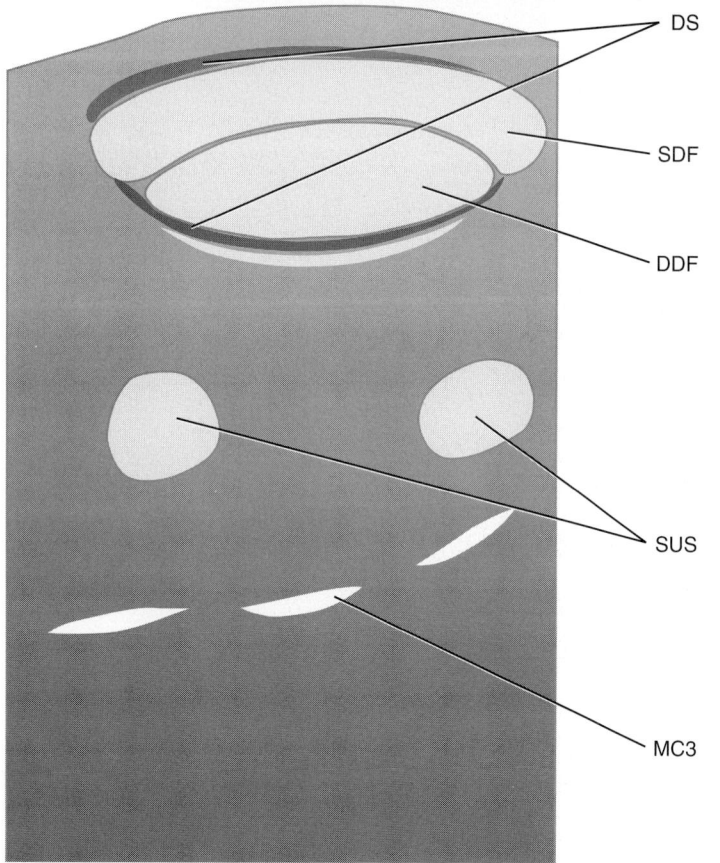

F

DS

SDF

DDF

SUS

MC3

▶ **FIGURE 5–47** *Continued*

F. Transverse image acquired from zone 3B. The strap-shaped superficial digital flexor tendon and the digital sheath now surround the deep digital flexor tendon. The relatively hypoechoic region between the DDF, the third metacarpal bone (MC3), and the branches of the suspensory ligament (SUS) is due to echoes from the connective tissue in the region of the volar pouches of the fetlock joint. (Courtesy R. H. Wrigley.)

Illustration continued on following page

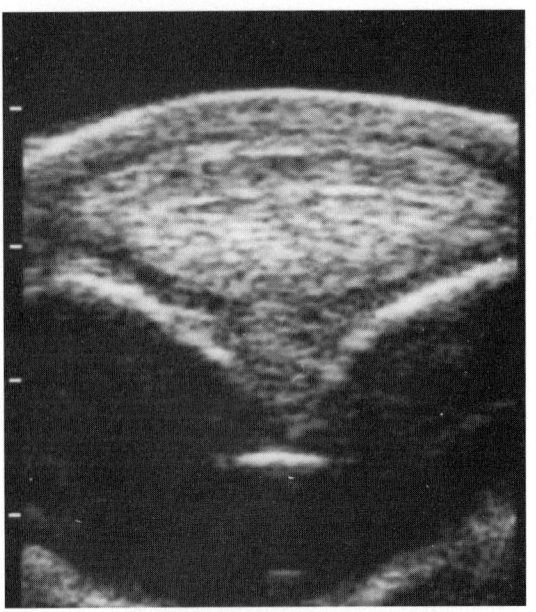

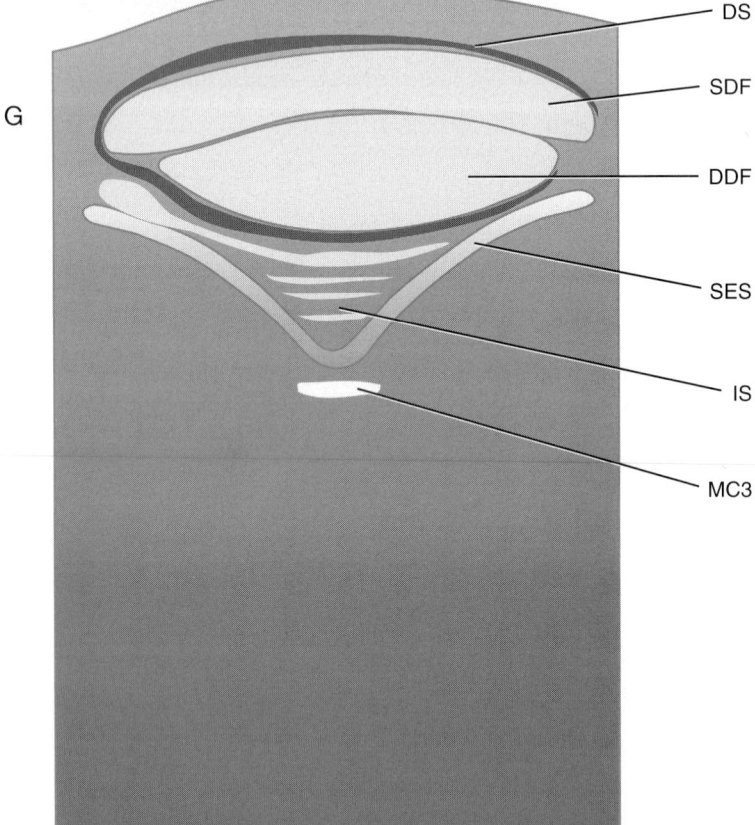

G

DS

SDF

DDF

SES

IS

MC3

▶ **FIGURE 5-47** *Continued*
G. Transverse image acquired from zone 3C. The superficial digital flexor and deep digital flexor tendons lie on the palmar surface of the sesamoids (SES). The palmar aspect of the digital synovial sheath lies on the surface of the superficial digital flexor tendon. The annular ligament of the fetlock lies below the skin/subcutaneous tissues. The intersesamoidean ligament (IS) runs between the sesamoids just palmar to the fetlock joint *(arrows).* (Courtesy R. H. Wrigley.)

flexor tendon. In the pastern region the straight and oblique distal sesamoidean ligaments, the deep digital flexor tendon, and the superficial digital flexor tendon before and after its bifurcation can be imaged.

Injury to tendons and ligaments ranges from complete rupture with loss of all fibers, through lessor disruption with loss of some fibers and focal accumulation of blood and tissue fluid, to slight injury with little fiber loss and presence of some

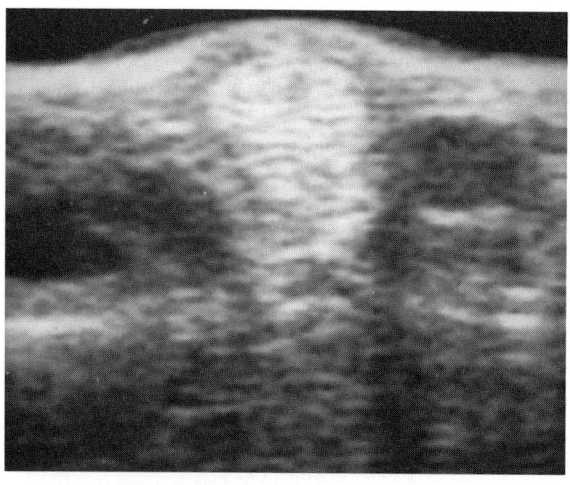

A

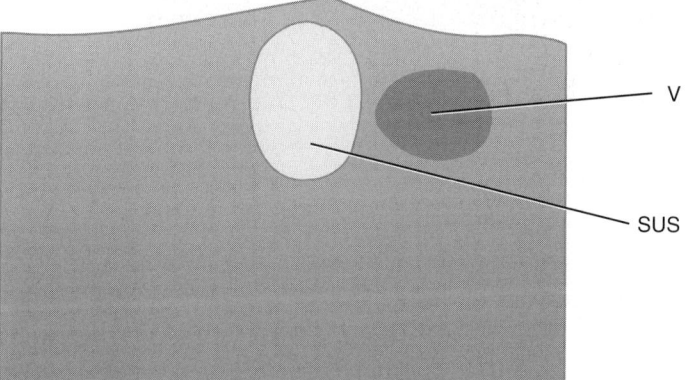

V

SUS

► **FIGURE 5-48**

Transverse ultrasonograms made by placing the transducer directly over the suspensory ligament branch, just proximal to the fetlock at zone 3. *Abbreviations:* SUS, suspensory ligament branch; V, vessels; SES, Proximal sesamoid. **A.** The suspensory ligament branch *(SUS)* proximal to the fetlock was better visualized adjacent to the palmar vessels (V). (Courtesy R. H. Wrigley.)

Illustration continued on following page

edema with enlargement. When there is loss or separation of fibers, the resulting space, which contains fluid and blood, is seen as a hypoechoic region, known as a "core" lesion. Subsequently, as healing proceeds with the production of granulation tissue and ultimately mature fibrous tissue, there is a gradual increase in echogenicity in the region of the core. In longitudinal scans, the core often extends over a considerable tendon length.

The normal, mottled appearance of the suspensory ligament is sometimes confused with fiber disruption and edema accumulation. In such cases, diagnosis must then be confirmed by clinical evaluation of signs such as pain and swelling, as well as by reexamination. Enthesiophytes and avulsion fractures in the region of origin of the suspensory ligament and elsewhere are seen as discontinuities and fragments in the outline of the bone. Some examples of the types of lesions seen are presented in Figure 5-52.

Thickening in the palmar or plantar region of the fetlock joint often is associated with lesions of the flexor tendons, digital sheath, and annular ligament. Ultrasonography is useful in determining what lesion(s) is present.[32]

Complications. Complications include cutaneous sensitivity to the coupling gel and skin infection through wounds produced by shaving. Shaving must be done carefully to avoid injuring the thin skin in the region, and the limb should be washed and dried after the procedure is completed. Poor-quality images related to inadequate patient preparation, transducer selection, unsuitable control panel settings, and poor scanning technique, are avoidable complications.[33]

OTHER TENDONS AND LIGAMENTS. Other specific tendons and ligaments that can be imaged include the bicipital tendon and bursa;[28,34] the common calcaneal tendon[28,35] (superficial digital flexor and gastrocnemius tendons) and associated bursae; peroneus tertius,[36] virtually all accessible extensor and flexor tendons and their sheaths, and periarticular ligaments.

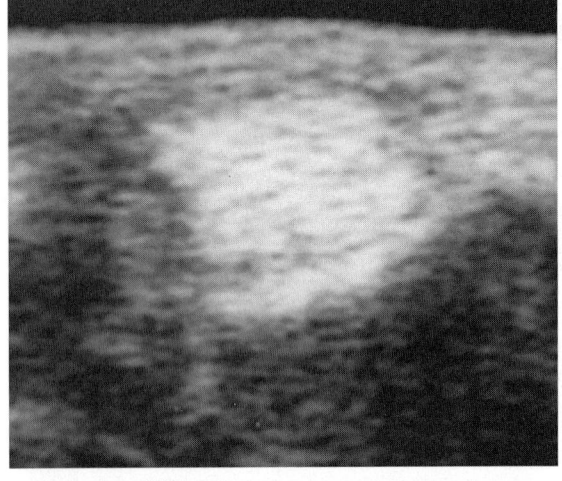

B

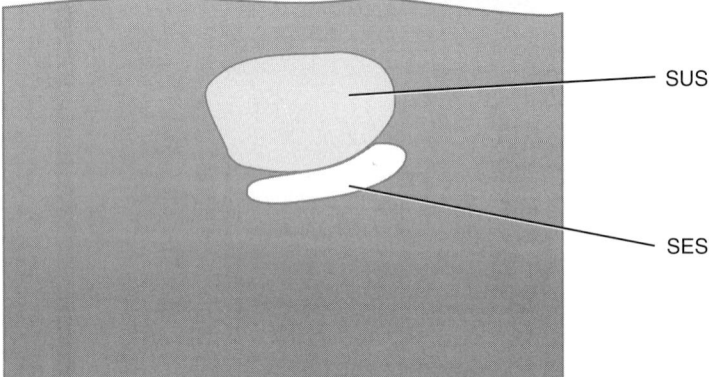

SUS

SES

▶ **FIGURE 5–48** *Continued*
B. The image was acquired at the level of the sesamoid. The suspensory ligament branch is attached to the sesamoid *(SES)*. (Courtesy R. H. Wrigley.)

Muscle

Ultrasonography of muscle is indicated to diagnose and characterize lesions such as abscesses, hematomata, neoplasia, and fibrosis. Transducers with lower frequencies than those used for tendons are necessary to image the deeper structures. The normal image consists of a regular pattern produced by the hypoechogenic muscle fibers and the hyperechogenic fascia. Abscesses (Fig. 5-53) and hematomata can be difficult to differentiate because both begin with a fluid-filled cavity, produce a loss of normal muscle image, and subsequently produce focal hyperechoic regions as fibrin clots form and organization begins.

Bones and Joints

The surface of bone appears as a hyperechoic line in the image, which, in most routine ultrasonography, marks the extent of the useful image and is not of great interest. In certain cases, variations in profile and the presence of defects and hyperechoic foci indicate new bone produc-

tion and fractures, respectively. Lesions of the origin of the suspensory ligament have already been mentioned. Fractures of ribs, which are difficult or impossible to image radiographically, and of the pelvis can often be detected, reducing the need for general anesthesia.[37]

Some intraarticular chip fractures involving regions not visible in standard radiographic views, such as the trochlear ridges in the tarsus and stifle, can be imaged with ultrasonography. The full extent of such lesions is not always apparent, although some details of their localization and size are provided.

Muscle Biopsy

The indications for muscle biopsy include evaluation of primary (e.g., myositis) or secondary (e.g., neurogenic) muscle disease, performance testing, and research into muscle metabolism associated with disease or performance. Open or percutaneous needle biopsy techniques are possible. The open technique, used to collect a sample to investigate contractile proper-

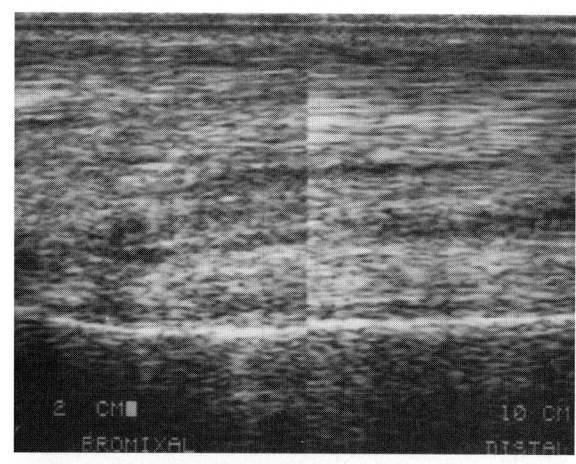

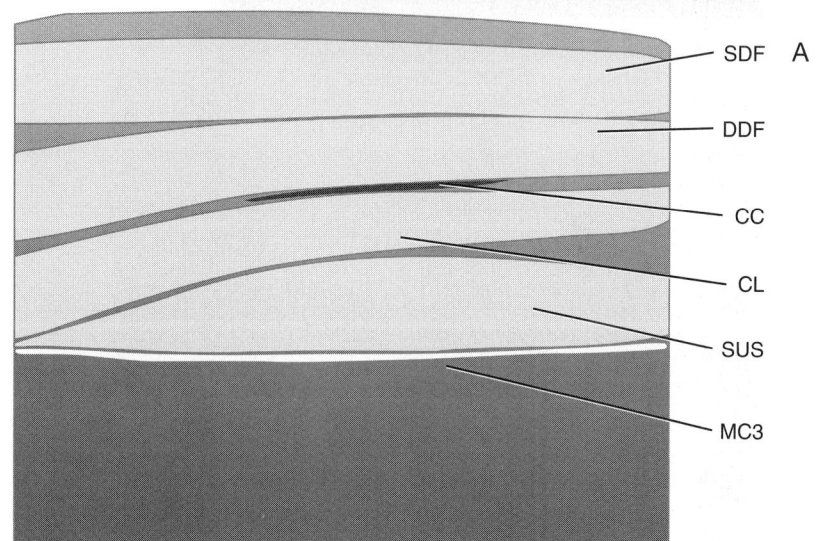

SDF A

DDF

CC

CL

SUS

MC3

▶ **FIGURE 5-49**

Longitudinal ultrasonograms of the palmar metacarpal flexor tendons and associated ligaments, made with a 7.5-MHz linear array transducer. Tendon and ligament fiber alignment is best evaluated on longitudinal scanning. *Abbreviations:* SDF, superficial digital flexor tendon; CC, carpal canal; DDF, deep digital flexor tendon; CL, check ligament; SUS, suspensory ligament MC3, metacarpal three; SES, proximal sesamoid. **A.** Dual stored images of zone 1A to 2A. The more hypoechoic superficial digital flexor tendon is just under the skin. Fluid is present in the carpal canal between the deep digital flexor tendon and the accessory (inferior) check ligament. The suspensory ligament arises from the proximal end of the third metacarpal bone and runs along the echogenic bony surface. (Courtesy R. H. Wrigley.)

Illustration continued on following page

ties, is rarely necessary and will not be described. The advantages of needle biopsy are its ease, safety, and lack of significant tissue trauma.

Materials for Percutaneous Needle Biopsy of Muscle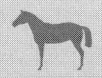

- Biopsy needle (Stille-Eschmann)
- Local anesthetic (2% lidocaine)
- Scalpel blade (#10)
- Syringe (5 mL, needle, 25 gauge, 25 mm [1"])
- Surgical scrub solution (e.g., Betadine)
- 70% alcohol

Percutaneous Muscle Biopsy

Procedure.   Any muscle can be sampled, but to avoid variation between muscles and between different sites in the same muscle, a standardized procedure has been developed.[38] Except for cases when biopsy of a specific muscle is required, the middle gluteal muscle is usually used. A 2.5-cm^2 area of skin is clipped, shaved, and prepared for a sterile procedure. One milliliter of local anesthetic is infiltrated subcutaneously and into the muscle fascia in the middle of the prepared field. The solution is not injected into the muscle. A 1-cm incision is made through the skin and also the fascia if it is thick. The biopsy apparatus consists of an outer needle, an inner cutting cylinder, and a stylette. The needle containing the cutting cylinder is pushed through the incision and into the muscle. The cutting cylinder is partially withdrawn to expose the side window of

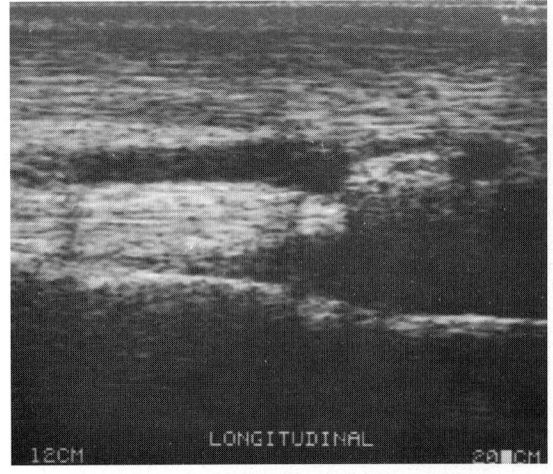

B

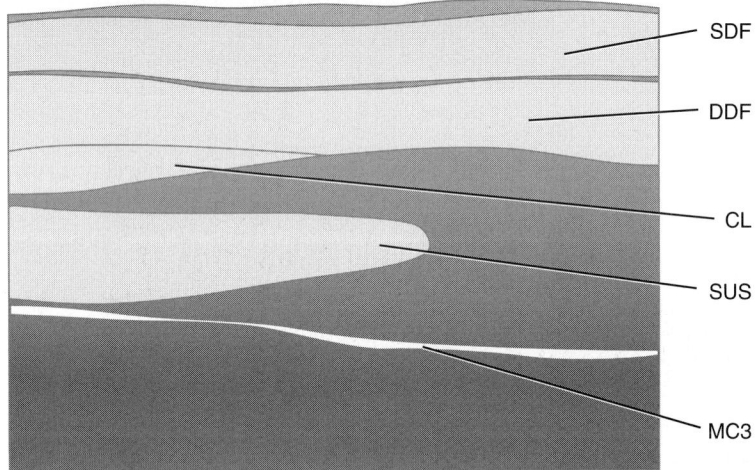

SDF

DDF

CL

SUS

MC3

▶ **FIGURE 5–49** *Continued*
B. Dual stored images of zone 2B to 3A. The check ligament blends into the dorsal surface of the deep digital flexor tendon, ending midway down the image. Likewise the suspensory ligament appears to end because of the formation of the two branches. (Courtesy R. H. Wrigley.)

the needle, which is then pressed against the muscle. This allows a small piece of muscle to intrude through the window and into the needle lumen, which is then cut off by fully inserting the cutting cylinder. This is repeated a number of times to obtain up to 200 mg of muscle. The needle is then withdrawn and the stilette is used to push the sample out from the needle. The wound can be sutured, but this is not necessary when only a small incision is made.

Preparation of Samples. The samples are usually then prepared for histochemical, biochemical, and ultrastructural studies as required. Samples for histochemical analysis are mounted as a transverse section and frozen immediately in liquid nitrogen. After cutting, sections are stained to identify its twitch type, oxidative capacity, and glycolytic ability. For biochemical analysis, blood and connective tissue are removed and the specimen frozen in liquid nitrogen for later preparation. For ultrastructural studies, a few muscle fi-

bers are dissected from the sample and placed in a fixative.

Results. The reader is referred to the literature for a detailed description of the results of studies using muscle biopsies.[39]

Analysis of Synovial Fluid

Collection and analysis of synovial fluid is a common clinical procedure.[40] The main indication is usually to differentiate between a nonseptic and a septic condition. The procedure is conducted most frequently on joints and to a lesser extent on tendon sheaths and bursae. The type of evaluation required depends on the condition suspected, and, therefore, full sterile collection and evaluation are not necessary for all samples.

Procedure. Samples should always be collected under sterile conditions to avoid iatrogenic infection. When a bacteriological evaluation is necessary and accidental contamination must be

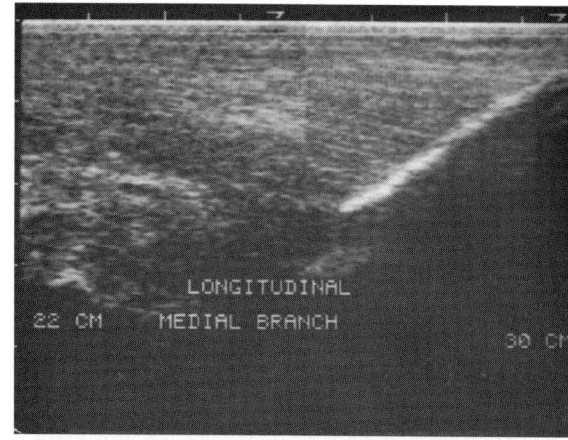

C

SES

▶ **FIGURE 5–49** *Continued*

C. Dual stored longitudinal ultrasono-grams of zone 3 made by placing the transducer on the surface of the suspensory ligament branch. The longitudinal alignment of the ligament fibers is seen at the insertion into the abaxial surface of the sesamoid bone. (Courtesy R. H. Wrigley.)

Materials to Collect Synovial Fluid

▶ Syringe (10 mL)
▶ Needle (size depends on the depth of the structure being investigated. See section on Lameness, Local anesthesia)
▶ Hair clippers #40 clipper head
▶ Surgical scrub solution
▶ 70% alcohol
▶ Collection tubes

---

avoided, a full sterile procedure with caps, masks, gowns, and drapes is often indicated. Collection is usually done with the horse standing, although general anesthesia is necessary when the patient is uncooperative and when a full sterile procedure is conducted.

The preparation of the site and the size of the needle are as described for local anesthesia of the synovial cavities (see Diagnostic Anesthesia). The procedure for a full sterile collection is described in Appendix C. So that the first part of the aspirate can be used for bacteriology, with virtually no chance of accidental contamination, the syringe should be attached to the needle during insertion. After inserting the needle, with the syringe attached, the sample is gently aspirated and the syringe removed and capped. A fresh syringe is attached to the needle, and more fluid is collected for the remaining measurements.

Management of Samples. The management of samples for bacteriology is described in Appendix C. The way in which the sample is handled depends on the type of organisms expected and the delay before processing. If a delay is expected, a suitable transport medium is used.

Assessments that can be made on the remaining sample include appearance, volume, clot formation, protein, viscosity, hyaluronate, quality of mucinous precipitate, cytology, enzymes, and particle analysis. A routine evaluation of a sample would include assessment of appearance, volume, clot formation, protein, viscosity, and cytology. The sample is evaluated for appearance and vol-

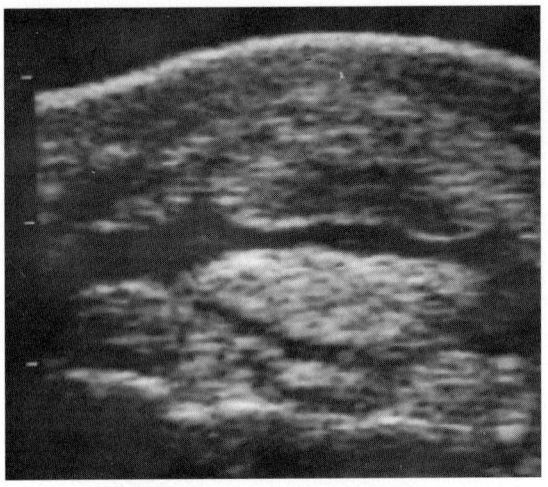

A

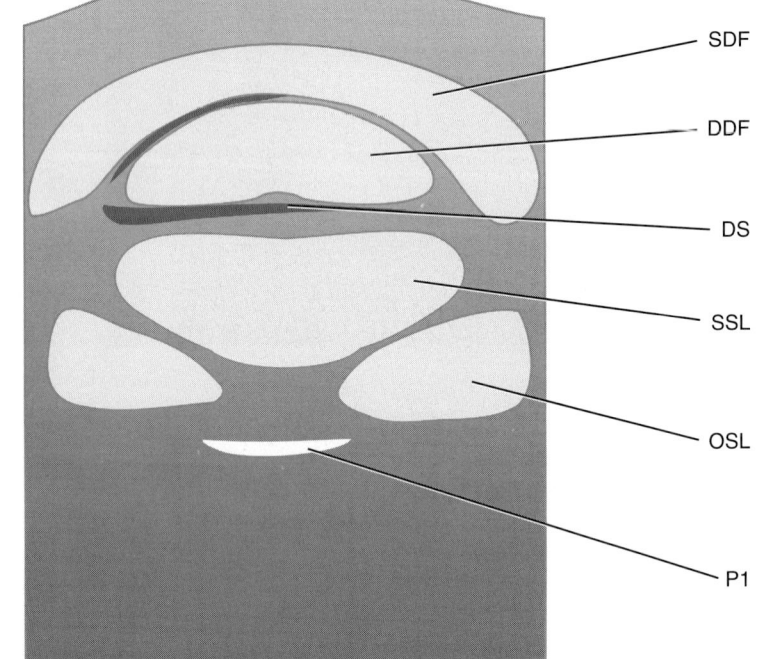

SDF

DDF

DS

SSL

OSL

P1

▶ **FIGURE 5-50**

Transverse ultrasonograms of the pastern region, produced with a 7.5-MHz linear array transducer. *Abbreviations:* SDF, superficial digital flexor tendon; DDF, deep digital flexor tendon; DS, digital synovial sheath; SSL, straight (middle) distal sesamoidean ligament; OSL, oblique distal sesamoidean ligament; P1, first phalanx. **A.** Image acquired just below the ergot. The superficial digital flexor tendon has become a thin band overlying the deep digital flexor tendon. Fluid is frequently detected in the digital synovial sheath at this level. The straight (middle) distal sesamoidean and oblique distal sesamoidean ligaments lie adjacent to the surface of the first phalanx. (Courtesy R. H. Wrigley.)

ume during collection. Ability to clot is checked on fluid placed in a plain Vacutainer tube (red top). Viscosity, protein, and hematological values are measured on fluid placed in a Vacutainer tube containing EDTA (violet top). Although viscosity can be measured, it can also be estimated very simply by placing a few drops of fluid between the thumb and first finger and then noting how long the fluid will string out as the digits are separated. The mucin clot test is conducted on the EDTA sample as soon as possible.[40]

Results. Some reference values for the parameters commonly used to evaluate synovial fluid are presented in Table 5-1, using joint fluid as an example. The reader is referred to the literature for further data on reference values.[41-49] As a general rule, synovial fluid in cases of sepsis is characterized by elevated total nucleated cell counts, protein concentration, and proportion of neutrophils; tendency to clot; turbidity; reduced viscosity and quality of mucinous precipitate; and variable presence of bacteria. Bacteria are not always visible in a smear and often fail to grow in culture because of the presence of antibiotics in the synovia and of sequestration of bacteria in the synovial membrane.

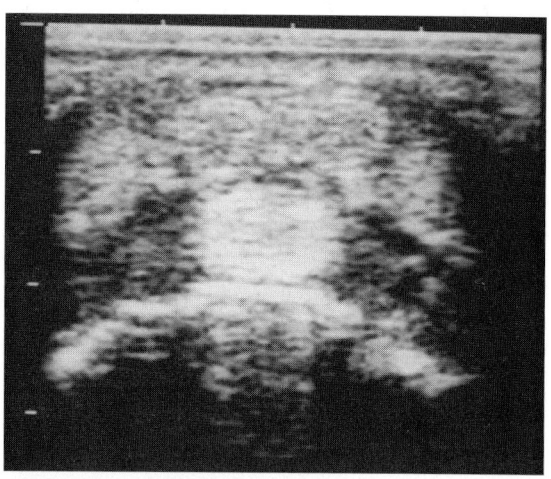

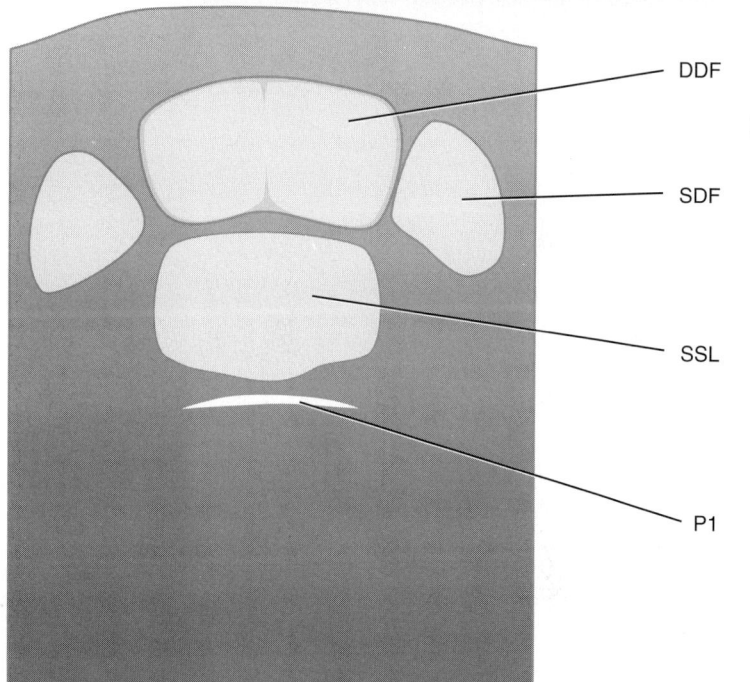

B

DDF

SDF

SSL

P1

▶ **FIGURE 5-50** *Continued*

B. Image acquired midway along the first phalanx. The superficial digital flexor tendon has divided into two branches. The deep digital flexor tendon often appears almost as two distinct bundles. The straight sesamoidean ligament remains at this level. (Courtesy R. H. Wrigley.)

Illustration continued on following page

▶ **TABLE 5-1**

REFERENCE VALUES FOR SYNOVIAL FLUID

Parameter	Value
Color	Yellow-amber
Clarity	Clear
Viscosity	Finger test (strand of 3–5 cm)
Tendency to clot	None
Mucinous precipitate	Normal precipitate is thick
Total protein (g/L)	8.0 ± 2.0
Erythrocytes	Rare
Total nucleated cells ($\times 10^9$/L)	<0.5
Neutrophils	8%
Mononuclear cells	92%

Synovial Membrane Biopsy

In many cases of septic synovitis it is impossible to isolate bacteria from a sample of the synovial fluid. Although not always rewarding, a biopsy of the synovial membrane can be taken to increase the chances of identifying bacteria. This is especially important if it is necessary to change antibiotic therapy when treatment is unsuccessful. The biopsy is usually made under direct arthroscopic control, which requires general anesthesia.

Procedure. The horse is placed under general anesthesia and positioned for arthroscopic surgery.[50] After inserting the arthroscope and

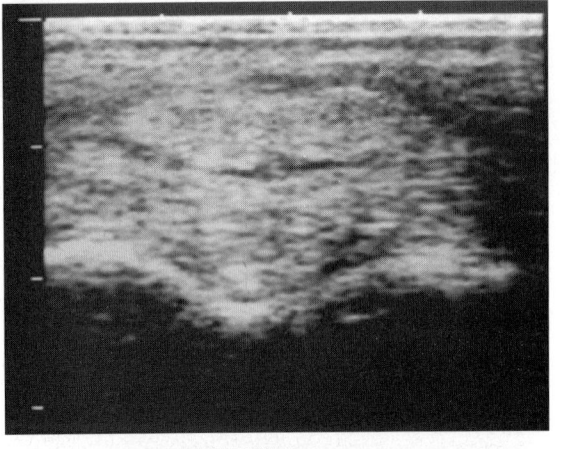

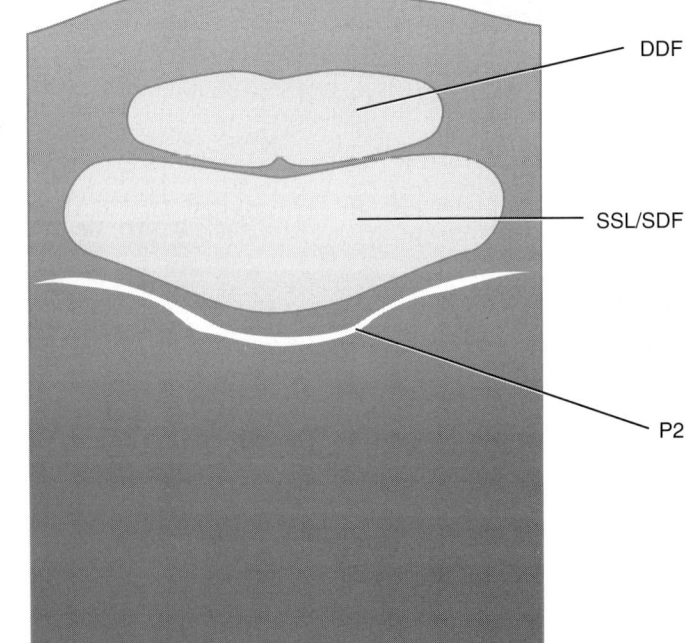

C

DDF

SSL/SDF

P2

▶ **FIGURE 5-50** *Continued*

C. Image acquired at the pastern just proximal to the bulbs of the heel. Dorsal to the deep digital tendon, the straight distal sesamoidean ligament, the branches of the superficial digital flexor tendon, and the capsule of the first interphalangeal joint have coalesced as these structures insert on the second phalanx. (Courtesy R. H. Wrigley.)

choosing the biopsy site, the biopsy forceps (e.g., Ferris-Smith rongeurs from Scanlan) are inserted through a second portal and a specimen(s) removed. Portals for arthroscope and instrument are specific for each anatomical region.[50] The sample is then submitted for culture and, if necessary, histological examination.

Scintigraphy

There are many occasions when the cause of lameness cannot be located by the traditional physical and radiographic examinations. Although this is sometimes due to inexperience and lack of patient cooperation, this most often happens because the exact site of pain in the limbs cannot be located by diagnostic anesthesia or because it lies deep within the tissues of the upper body, where anesthesia, manipulation, and palpation are useless. Scintigraphy was introduced for lameness evaluation in 1977,[51] and since then its value as an imaging technique in difficult cases has been confirmed. Scintigraphy consists of the intravenous injection of a gamma-ray–emitting radiopharmaceutical whose activity during distribution throughout the body is detected by a sodium iodide crystal mounted in a gamma camera or a small, manual scintillation or point-counting device. The radiopharmaceutical consists of a radionuclide bound to a tissue tracer. The radionuclide commonly used is [99m]Technetium, which is bound to a diphos-

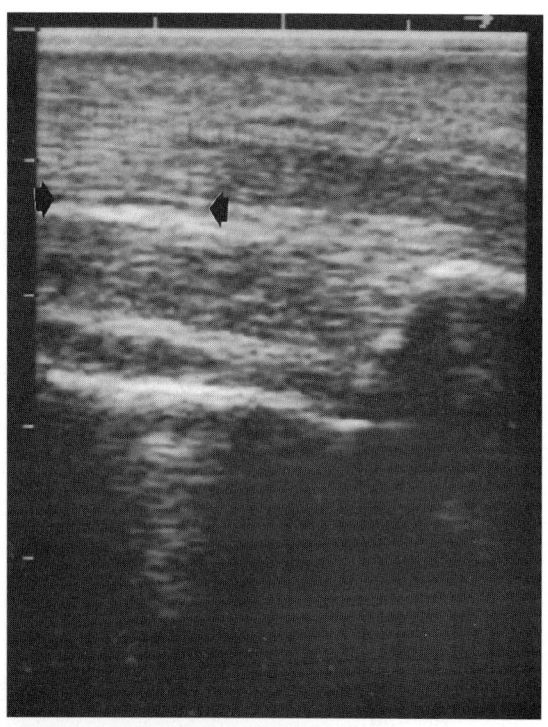

A

DDF

DS

SSL

P2

P1

► **FIGURE 5-51**

Longitudinal ultrasonograms of the pastern, produced with a 7.5-MHz linear array transducer. *Abbreviations:* P1, first phalanx; P2, second phalanx; SSL, straight (middle) sesamoidean ligament; DDF, deep digital flexor tendon; SDF, superficial digital flexor tendon; DS, digital sheath. **A.** Midline scan demonstrates the palmar surface of the first phalanx and the proximal eminence of the second phalanx. The straight distal sesamoidean ligament inserts onto the proximal eminence of the second phalanx. The deep digital flexor tendon runs superficial to the sesamoidean ligament and the second phalanx. A small volume of fluid *(arrows)* is normally present in the digital sheath. Thick subcutaneous tissue and the annular ligament of the pastern lie below the skin. (Courtesy R. H. Wrigley.)

Illustration continued on following page

phonate, such as methyldiphosphonate (^{99m}Tc-MDP). Technetium has a half-life of 6 hours, and, via the carrier to which it is bound, it is exchanged with phosphate in bone. In broad terms there are three phases in the distribution process:

- *Phase 1.* Occurs in the first 30 seconds after injection when the agent is still in the large vessels.
- *Phase 2.* The material leaves the vessels to enter the extracellular compartment and soft tissues, and, eventually, the bone.

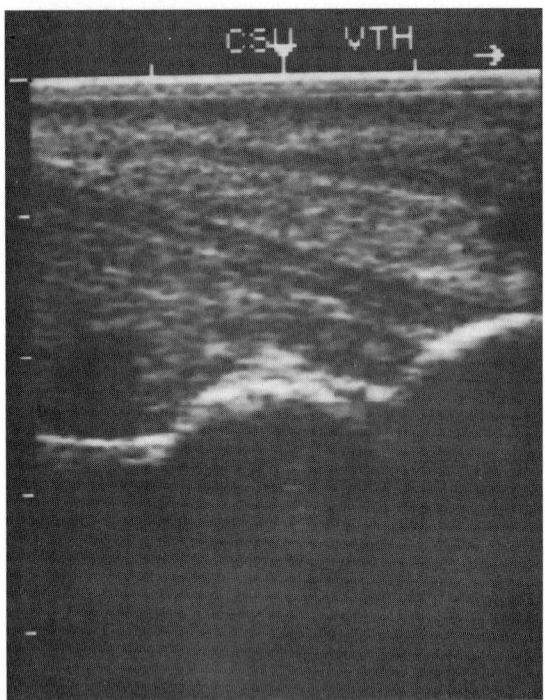

B

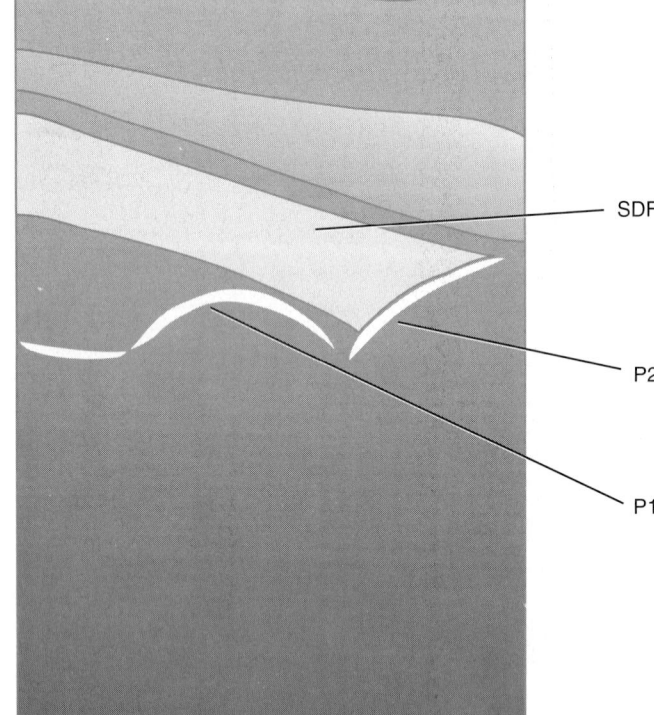

SDF

P2

P1

▶ **FIGURE 5–51** *Continued*

B. Oblique scan centered over the medial branch of the superficial digital flexor tendon demonstrates the medial palmar aspect of the condyle of the first phalanx and the overlying superficial digital flexor tendon inserting on the proximal eminence of the second phalanx. (Courtesy R. H. Wrigley.)

• *Phase 3.* The agent has entered the skeleton and been cleared from the soft tissues.

Although Phase 2 scintigrams can be useful under some circumstances, it is the Phase 3 scans that are mainly used to diagnose lameness. The extent of bone uptake, and hence the extent of gamma ray emission, depends on the blood flow and metabolic activity of bone. Because bone tissue is

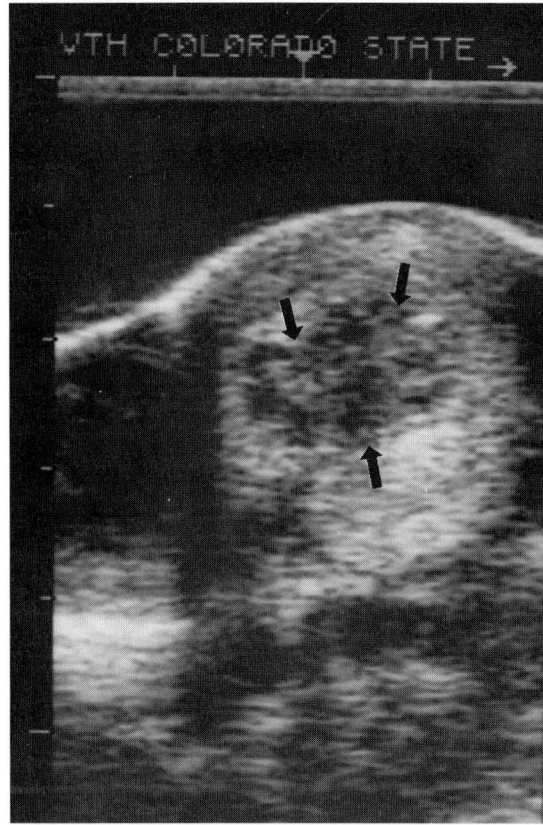

A

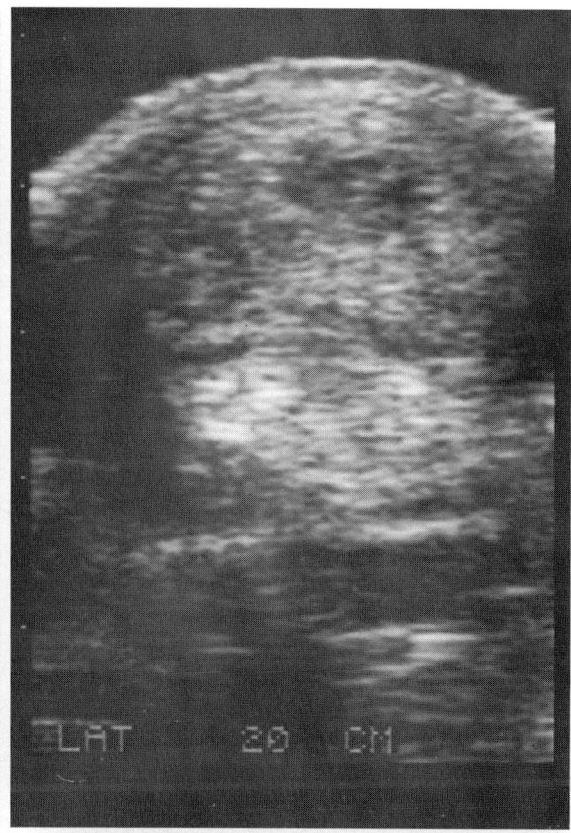

B

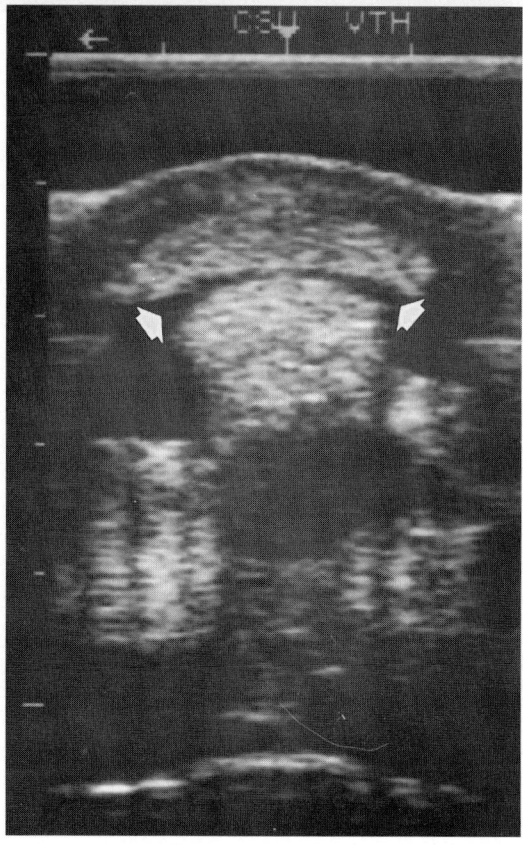

C

▶ **FIGURE 5-52**

Ultrasonograms, produced with a 7.5-MHz linear array transducer and standoff, of some tendon lesions. **A.** Tendinitis, "core" lesion. Transverse ultrasonogram made 20 cm distal to the accessory carpal bone. There is a large area (10 cm long) of focal tendinitis in the superficial digital flexor tendon. (Courtesy R. H. Wrigley.) **B.** Follow-up examination of the lesion in 5-52A 7 months later. The superficial digital flexor tendon remains enlarged. However, the focal lesion now contains echogenic fibers indicating progression of a healing response. (Courtesy R. H. Wrigley.) **C.** Tenosynovitis with distension of the digital sheath. Transverse ultrasonogram of the metatarsal region made 38 cm distal to the calcaneal tuber. Normal flexor tendons and an effusion of the digital sheath (arrows) can be seen. (Courtesy R. H. Wrigley.)

Illustration continued on following page

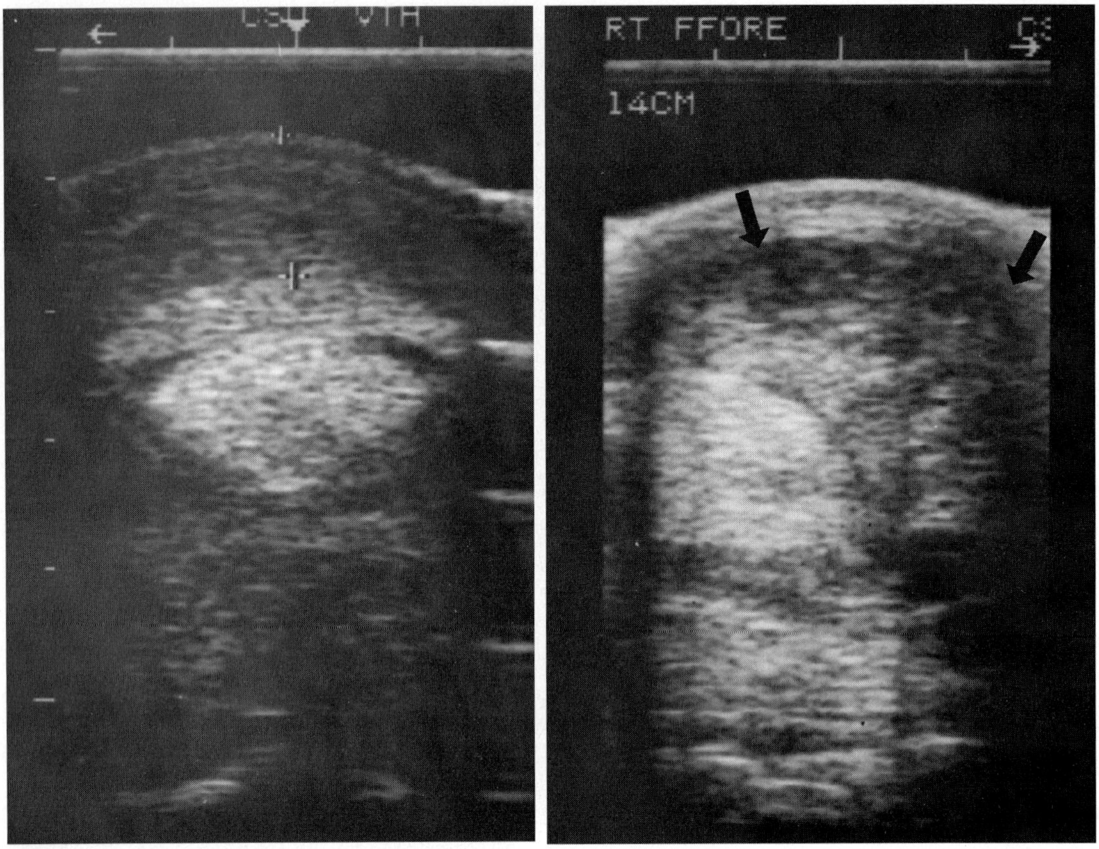

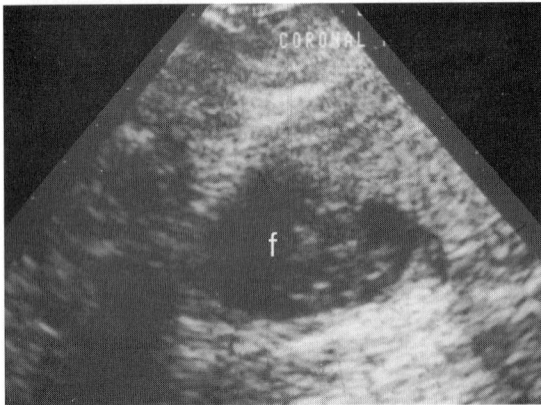

D   E

▶ FIGURE 5-52 *Continued*

D. Tenosynovitis with thickening of the peritendinous tissues and the digital sheath. Transverse ultrasonogram of the metatarsal region made 41 cm distal to the calcaneal tuber, just proximal to the fetlock joint. The thickening in this region (distance between calipers is 1.1 cm) is due to thickened peritendinous tissues and the digital sheath. Tendons are normal. (Courtesy R. H. Wrigley.) **E.** Diffuse tendinitis. Transverse ultrasonogram of the metacarpal region made 14 cm distal to the accessory carpal bone. The superficial digital flexor tendon is enlarged and has a patchy hypoechoic appearance (18 cm long) *(arrows)* indicating diffuse tendinitis. (Courtesy R. H. Wrigley.)

undergoing modeling and remodeling, consisting of bone resorption and deposition, each specific bone has a certain background activity that varies normally with age and physical activity. Abnormal activity as a result of injury is superimposed on

▶ FIGURE 5-53

Dorsal ultrasonogram of the shoulder region made with a 3-MHz sector transducer. There is a cavity filled with echogenic fluid (F) in the musculature adjacent to the shoulder. An ultrasound-guided needle biopsy obtained a purulent exudate from which *Corynebacterium tuberculosis* was cultured. (Courtesy R. H. Wrigley.)

Materials for Skeletal Scintigraphy

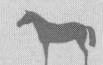

▶ Radiopharmaceutical (^{99m}Tc methyl diphosphonate)

▶ Gamma camera or manual scintillation detector

▶ Computer software

▶ Disposable gloves

▶ Syringe shield

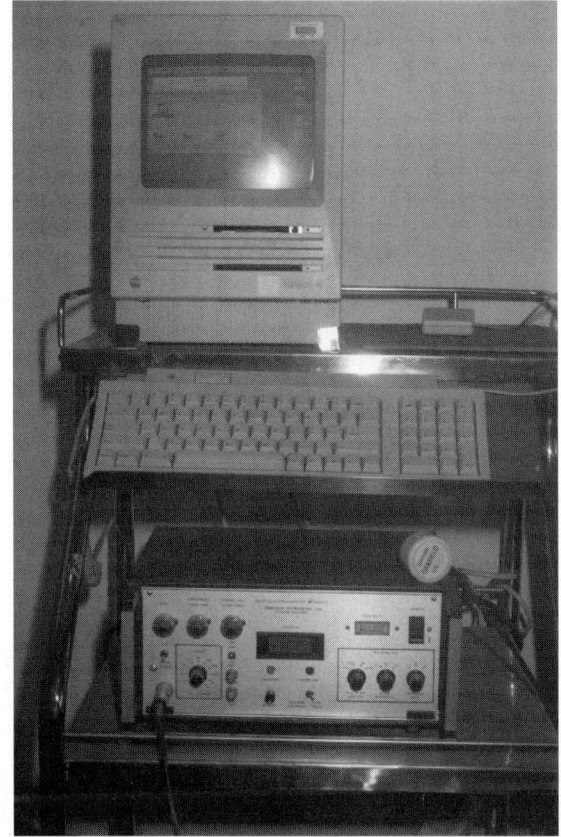

A

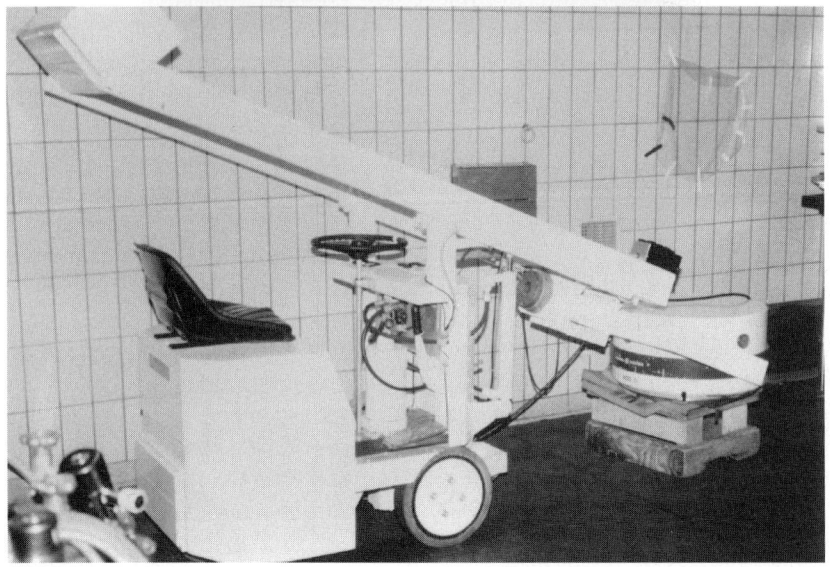

B

▶ **FIGURE 5–54**

Scintigraphy. **A.** Scintillation counter. **B.** Gamma camera mounted on a mobile cart. (University of Bern.)

this normal, but variable, state with the consequence that interpretation requires considerable experience and detailed knowledge of normal activity. Scintigraphy has also been shown to be a valuable diagnostic tool in muscle injury.

The small scintillation devices are hand-held, and the larger gamma camera is mounted to a gantry or some form of transport to render it more mobile (Fig. 5–54). The use of the radionuclide is under the control of the appropriate regulatory body for ionizing radiation. The 6-hour half-life of Technetium means that, after an overnight stay in a special designated stall, the patient can be examined further or discharged from the hospital, and bedding can be removed.

Procedure. The patient should be adequately hydrated. As the anesthetics used for diagnostic anesthesia interfere with interpretation, there must be a delay between anesthesia and scintigraphy of at least 3 days,[52] although this can be shortened when mepivacaine is used.[53] The dose rate of the radiopharmaceutical ranges from 2 to 8 MBq/kg for manual scintillation and gamma camera acquisition, respectively.[52] It is administered intravenously, and gloves must be worn and a syringe shield used. Imaging is carried out 30 minutes later for a Phase 2 scan or 2 to 3 hours later for a Phase 3 scan. All imaging is carried out with the horse adequately restrained, either standing under sedation or under general anesthesia. For horses with an appropriate temperament imaging of the lower limb is conducted with the horse standing and sedated if necessary. General anesthesia is often required to examine the upper limb and trunk and for all sites in uncooperative horses that cannot be examined standing. Although many scans are conducted to improve the chances of evaluating a lesion already located by radiography, in many cases radiography will be used after scintigraphy has identified a region of increased activity.

Data acquisition continues until a specified number of counts has been detected. Depending on the equipment, the data are processed and portrayed in scintigram form or as a series of histograms comparing left and right symmetry. The exact techniques vary with equipment and institution and will not be described here.

Results. It should be remembered that scintigraphy identifies sites where there is increased radioactivity as a result of increased blood flow, increased metabolic activity of bone, or both, and sites where activity is reduced because of a decrease in the afore-mentioned parameters, such as when bone infarction is present. Although there are many situations where scintigraphy is indicated, some of the specific clinical conditions that can be better defined with the added information obtained from a bone scan are as follows:

• *"Stress" or incomplete fractures.* Fractures occurring in the proximal long bones[54] and

the third metacarpal bone[55] are often not visible on radiograph in the early stages, and identification of the site by radiograph is always difficult and often impossible. Stress fractures tend to have a specific location for each bone, according to the prevailing mechanical loads. Similar fractures can also involve the small bones of the carpus and tarsus.

• *Navicular syndrome.* This is a puzzling syndrome in which scintigraphy is very useful in helping to decide whether observed osseous changes are active and the cause of pain, or whether there is soft-tissue involvement of the navicular bursa and deep flexor tendon.

• *Pedal osteitis.* Inflammation of the third phalanx is a common problem, and scintigraphy can indicate increased bone activity before radiographic changes develop, as well as define the state of activity of the radiographic changes usually taken as indicating pedal osteitis.

• *Arthritis.* Septic and traumatic arthritis show increased activity as a result of increased blood flow and also later as a result of increased bone activity.

• *Vertebral column.* Performance horses are frequently disabled from pain associated with arthrosis of the spinal articulations and overcrowding or impingement of the dorsal spinous processes. The syndrome is often difficult to diagnose, and the significance of radiographic changes is often unknown. Scintigraphy, by identifying bone activity, is useful in establishing the clinical significance of radiographic changes.

• *Sites of attachment of ligaments and tendons onto bone.* Injury to these sites results initially in soft-tissue inflammation and, eventually, in a focal region of bone production that can be seen in a radiograph if the site of injury can be identified. Scintigraphy can both identify such sites before bone is produced and evaluate the state of activity of preexisting bone seen in a radiograph.

It is stressed that interpreting bone scans is open to abuse, most frequently by identifying incorrectly all regions of increased activity, the so-called "hotspots," as regions of pathology. The reader is referred to the literature for more information on scintigraphy.[52,56]

Noninvasive Locomotion Analysis

Although unassisted visual examination is of vital importance in gait and lameness evaluation, the human eye is limited in what it can see and its ability to detect events occurring when the horse is moving rapidly. Fortunately, numerous technologies can be applied to gait analysis and can supplement the information obtained by a routine clinical examination. To date, such technologies have been restricted mainly to the research laboratory because of the cost of the equipment, the difficulty in attaining the necessary expertise, and the time required to develop different methods and establish the databases. The reader is directed to recent reviews for more information.[57-59]

Biomechanical Analysis

FORCES GENERATED BY HOOF–GROUND CONTACT. The force generated when the hoof contacts the ground, the ground reaction force (GRF), can be measured with force plates, shoes, and mats, and, depending on instrumentation, the GRF can be separated into vertical, horizontal, and longitudinal components. To allow easier comparison, results can be normalized to a specific body mass and duration of the stance phase. Force plates must be concealed and installed in a strong housing. They have the disadvantage that the hoof must contact the plate correctly, an event that occurs about 50% of the time during the walk and less often as velocity increases. By using interconnecting plates it is sometimes possible to have two or more limbs striking the system at the same time.

Although some value has been shown for lameness evaluation[60,61] there are restrictions to its use in a clinical situation. Instrumented shoes circumvent the main problem of the force plate by allowing a recording to be made during successive footfalls. After overcoming earlier problems, the force shoe is now developed sufficiently for it to be applied to lameness and gait evaluation.[62,63]

A pressure-sensitive mat allows recordings to be made for all four limbs and provides additional information on the distance between limb placements. The force mat was introduced as the Kaegi Equine Gait Analysis System[64], and later modified as the Equine Gait Analysis System. The system consists of a series of sensors embedded in parallel lines within a measurement zone, over which a rubber mat is placed. The procedure consists of running the horse directly over the mat until the required number of strides have been recorded, the data then being processed by computer. Early work has focused on lesions of the lower limb, such as navicular syndrome.[65]

ACCELEROMETERS. Accelerometers are recording devices that measure acceleration and deceleration of the specific part of the limb or trunk to which they are attached. Depending on their complexity, data can be obtained for more than one axis, and this information can then be used to derive the forces producing the changes in velocity. Presently, their application for lameness and gait evaluation is limited.

ELECTROGONIOMETRY. Electrogoniometry measures the change in joint angle by using a potentiometer placed over the axis of rotation of the joint. The equipment is inexpensive, and the signal can be recorded with an onboard recorder or transmitted by radiotelemetry to a stationary receiver (Fig. 5-55). The method can be applied

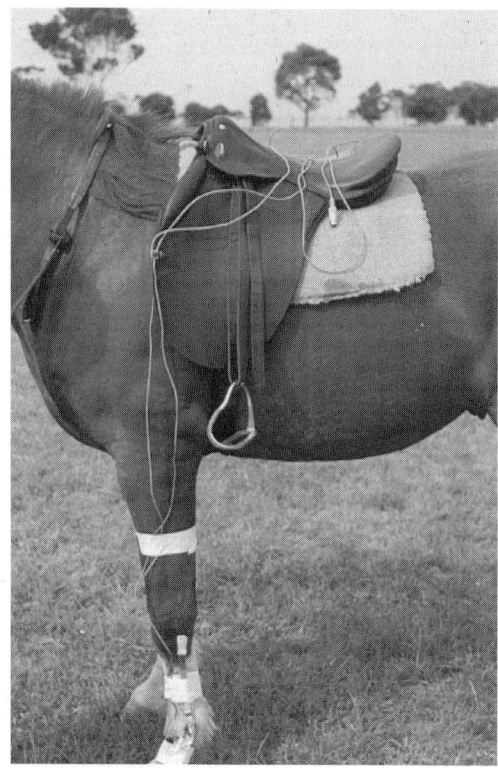

▶ **FIGURE 5-55**

Electrogoniometer mounted on the horse's fetlock. The leads that run up along the leg are connected to the recording and telemetric apparatus carried by the rider.

to single or multiple joints and has some value in gait and lameness evaluation.[66–69]

High-Speed Cinematography and Videography

High-speed cinematography and, more recently, videography, facilitate the study of the kinematic variables of gait by recording the activity for later analysis. Cinematography has received most attention, and its advantages and disadvantages are a matter of record.[70] The procedure has improved with experience and the introduction of more sophisticated analysis systems, such as Trackeye (Innovativ Vision AB, Linköping, Sweden).[71] Videography, which has several advantages, especially that of immediate playback, is being adapted to gait analysis and is likely to assume a greater role.[72]

Although the ability to record and analyze gait when the horse is in its usual training environment is very useful, the difficulty in achieving optimum position and orientation of the camera(s) limits the amount of quantitative information that can be obtained. Standardization of recording conditions is best achieved in a controlled environment or by using a treadmill.

OPTOELECTRONIC SYSTEMS. Automatic recording and analysis of angles and spatial positioning of specific body segments can be achieved by using technology that monitors body and limb displacement through skin markers. The markers are placed at specific locations and are classed as passive or active, depending on whether they are identified during use by reflecting or generating a signal, respectively. The CODA-3 (Movement Techniques Ltd, Loughborough, UK) and Selspot systems (Selcom AB, Sweden) have been applied to horses, and both require the attachment of light-emitting diodes (LED) to the limbs or body to act as markers. The Selspot system has been used to examine the walk in normal and lame horses[73,74] and to diagnose tarsitis.[75]

THERMOGRAPHY. Thermography is a noninvasive technique that measures and records the infrared radiation emitted from the body surface.[76] The pictorial record is known as a thermogram. The radiation is detected by contact or noncontact. Contact thermography employs liquid crystals embedded in a deformable base that is applied closely to the body surface. The crystals change shape and color according to the incident temperature. Noncontact thermography uses an infrared thermometer or camera to record the radiation. The thermometer measures temperature at a specific point or, with certain equipment, the temperature difference between two points, while the camera is a more complicated apparatus and uses a cathode ray tube to display a black-and-white image or, with appropriate circuitry, a colored image (Fig. 5–56). The infrared camera is the most versatile technology because contact between skin and instrument is unnecessary and because regions, rather than specific points, can be imaged and portrayed as a thermogram.

The temperature of the skin depends on many factors, including blood supply, tissue metabolism, length of haircoat, environmental temperature, drugs affecting the cardiovascular system, and external radiant energy. To control these extraneous factors, imaging should be carried out under cover and away from the sun and drafts, the horse should be restrained in stocks without additional chemical restraint, and an acclimatization period of about 20 minutes should be allowed. Excessively long hair will reduce heat loss and apparent skin temperature, and recently clipped regions will have a higher temperature. Imaging from different directions will ensure a more accurate identification of regions of high or low skin temperature.

Inflammation, as a result of tissue injury or disease, usually causes an increase in regional skin temperature, and, occasionally, a decrease is seen when blood supply is reduced by swelling or thrombosis. The objective of thermography is to detect these variations in temperature. Interpretation is based on differentiating the changes present as a result of tissue pathology from the normal background temperature. Although thermography has been shown to be useful in lesions of a number of soft and hard tissues, the interference from extraneous factors and inability to identify precisely lesions limit its clinical usefulness.[77–84]

Arthroscopy

Although the pain responsible for lameness can often be localized to a joint, the specific cause and its precise location cannot always be identified by clinical examination or by use of imaging techniques. In such cases arthroscopy can be very useful as a diagnostic tool. The technique is well described.[50]

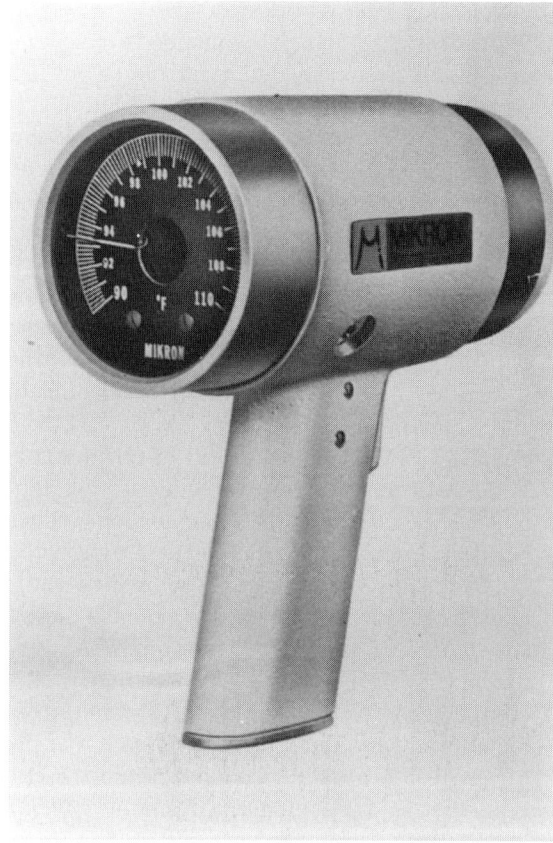

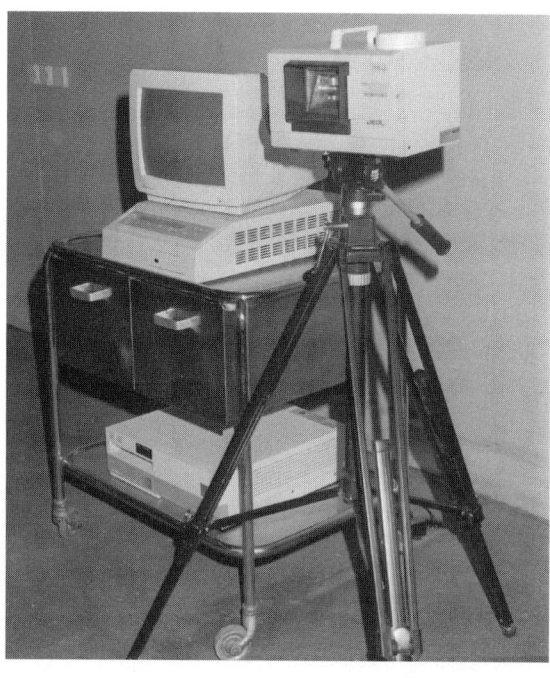

B

A

▶ **FIGURE 5–56**

Methods of detecting infrared radiation. **A.** Infrared thermometer. **B.** Infrared camera.

Bone Biopsy

Although cancellous bone is frequently collected from the tibia, sternum, or iliac crest to encourage osteogenesis during surgical repair of fractures, bone biopsy has been limited almost exclusively to research investigations. Recently, techniques and data suitable for clinical purposes have become available, and it is likely that bone biopsy will be carried out more often in clinical situations where information concerning bone metabolism is required, such as with osteochondrosis. Bone biopsy is an integral part of evaluation of metabolic bone disease in people, where the preferred site is the iliac crest, yielding a corticocancellous sample. To be useful, the site used must yield a corticocancellous sample suitable for histology and histomorphometry, and the procedure must be safe for both the horse and clinician, be conducted under local anesthesia, and carry minimal complications. It should be possible to locate the biopsy site accurately because there is considerable within- and between-bone variation in measured parameters. These requirements and the important need to collect a specimen without disrupting its architecture indicate that the iliac crest also is the favored site in horses. Collection from the 12th rib has been described but it is not suitable for routine use.[85] The iliac crest satisfies the above prerequisites and has been well described and validated, and a considerable body of reference data provided.[86-88] The biopsy can be made with a standard, hand-driven trephine, but a motor-driven device is preferable to minimize collection time and specimen damage. The sample can be collected for routine histology on demineralized sections or for quantitative histomorphometry after intravital labeling with bone-seeking fluorochromes.

Procedure. If bone labeling is required for routine histomorphometry, two oxytetracycline labels are given 7 days apart, the biopsy being scheduled at least 2 to 4 days after the last label so that some mineralization can occur and thus prevent the label from being leached from the calcification front by materials used in the preparation processes. For research purposes, a combination of the different labels can be used and different labeling periods selected. The proce-

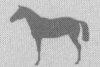

Materials for Iliac Crest Bone Biopsy

- Bone biopsy instrument (e.g., Custom-made drill bit and drill bit guide suitable for power use, and electric drill; or "Osteocore" [The Straumann Company, Cambridge, MA, USA])
- Lidocaine (2%)
- 20-mL syringe, 20-gauge, 25-mm needle
- Scalpel blade (#22)
- Container with 70% alcohol
- Fluorochrome
  Oxytetracycline (15 mg/kg in 500 mL 0.9% NaCl, IV)
  Chlortetracycline (10 mg/kg, IV)
  Fluorescein complexone (10 mg/kg dissolved in 60 mL of 3% NaOH and added to 500 mL 0.9% NaCl, IV)

dure described here is for the wing of the ilium.[86] The procedure is carried out in the restrained and sedated standing horse. An area 6 × 6 inches is clipped and prepared for sterile biopsy. It is centered just caudal to the tuber coxae. The site for insertion of the biopsy instrument is located by identifying the dorsal and ventral sections of the tuber coxae and then moving approximately two inches in a dorsocaudal direction. Local anesthetic is infiltrated at this site and along a line parallel to the fibers of the middle gluteal muscle (cranioventral-dorsocaudal), extending through all tissues down to the periosteum. A 1.5- to 2.0-inch incision is made through the skin and subcutaneous fascia. Scissors are used to dissect bluntly through the muscle and down onto the periosteum. To cut the biopsy without having the drill bit slide over the surface of the bone, the drill guide must first be inserted into the incision and seated onto the periosteum. This is done in different ways depending on the equipment used. If the guide is a separate instrument it is inserted into the incision first and then held firmly while the drill bit is inserted. With the Osteocore instrument, both sections are inserted as a unit. The drill bit is placed perpendicular to the bone and the biopsy is cut by activating the drill and pushing firmly. The passage of the bit through the proximal and distal cortex can be sensed, at

which time it is withdrawn while still rotating. The biopsy core, which is contained in the hollow drill bit, is then expelled manually or automatically, and placed in 70% alcohol for 24 hours. The sample is then embedded in a plastic medium, sectioned for light and fluorescent microscopy, and evaluated using a combination of manual and computer-assisted techniques to obtain directly measured and derived parameters.[87]

Results. The procedure yields a cylindrical specimen of cancellous bone with a cap of cortical bone on both ends. Only minor complications, in the form of superficial wound infection and hematoma, in less than 5% of cases were observed in the original report of this method.[86] There is little variation in values from samples taken in the vicinity of the standard biopsy site and between samples from the left and right sides.[87] This indicates that successive samples can be taken immediately from the same bone if there are any technical problems compromising use of the first sample and that a later biopsy of the contralateral side can be taken to monitor bone metabolism. It should be remembered that bone metabolism is altered by biopsy. The local effect is known as the regional acceleratory phenomenon (RAP), and the systemic effect as the systemic acceleratory phenomenon (SAP). A selection of parameters for young and older horses is presented in Table 5–2. A more extensive body of data is found in the original publication.[88]

New Imaging Techniques

Even more sophisticated imaging techniques are being introduced in veterinary medicine.[89] These include computed tomography, magnetic resonance imaging, single and dual photon absorptiometry, dual energy absorptiometry, quantitative computed tomography, and ultrasonic densitometry. These techniques all require extreme expertise, and most are very expensive to establish. In general, the tomographic techniques and magnetic resonance imaging allow tissue to be imaged in a series of slices, thus providing a three-dimensional picture that greatly enhances diagnosis. The size of the horse at present limits these investigations to the head, neck, and lower limbs, which are regions that can be inserted into the apparatus designed for people. Magnetic resonance imaging is particularly useful for soft-tissue investigation. The absorptiometric and densitometric techniques are useful to determine bone

▶ TABLE 5-2

MEASURED AND DERIVED HISTOMORPHOMETRIC PARAMETERS (MEAN ± SD) FOR CANCELLOUS BONE
IN YOUNG (4–8 MONTHS) AND OLDER (18–180 MONTHS) HORSES.

Parameter	Young Horses	Older Horses
Cancellous bone volume (%)	18.4 ± 4.0	20.5 ± 2.7
Osteoid surface (%)	28.0 ± 15.0	7.1 ± 8.7
Eroded surface (%)	8.4 ± 3.2	3.3 ± 2.0
Final erosion depth (μm)	33.9 ± 8.1	43.5 ± 8.9
Mean wall thickness, corrected value (μm)	32.9 ± 8.3	39.6 ± 3.5
Mean osteoid thickness, corrected value (μm)	6.8 ± 1.2	8.1 ± 0.8
Mineral apposition rate (μm/day)	1.9 ± 0.2	1.1 ± 0.2
Mineralizing surface (%)	16.5 ± 6.5	3.6 ± 2.9
Mineralization lag time (days)	6.8 ± 4.5	19.7 ± 22.3
Formative period (days)	34.8 ± 26.4	96.8 ± 112.2
Quiescent surfaces (%)	64.1 ± 16.1	90.0 ± 9.3
Quiescent period (days)	78.5 ± 38.2	3,349.0 ± 4,511.0
Resorption period (days)	10.1 ± 5.9	102.7 ± 121.6
Activation frequency (/year)	3.6 ± 1.9	0.3 ± 0.3
Remodelling period (days)	44.9 ± 31.3	199.5 ± 182.1

Source: (Data from Savage CJ, Tidd LC, Østblom LC, et al: Bone biopsy in the horse. 3. Normal histomorphometric data according to age and sex. J Vet Med 1991; A38: 793.)

density and the presence of microscopic regions of weakness.

R E F E R E N C E S

1. Stashak TS (ed): Adams' Lameness in Horses, 4th ed. Philadelphia, Lea & Febiger, 1987.
2. May SA, Wyn-Jones G: Identification of hindleg lameness. Equine Vet J 1987;19:185.
3. Adams OR: Natural and Artificial Gaits. In Stashak TS (ed), Adams' Lameness in Horses, 4th ed. Philadelphia, Lea & Febiger, 1987, Ch 13, p 834.
4. Jeffcott LB: Diagnosis of back problems in the horse. Contin Educat 1981; 3:134.
5. Goodman NL, Baker BK: Lameness diagnosis and treatment in the quarter horse. Vet Clin North Am: Equine Pract 1990; 6:85.
6. Schmotzer WB, Timm KI: Local anesthetic techniques for diagnosis of lameness. Vet Clin North Am: Equine Pract 1990; 6:705.
7. Specht TE, Nixon AJ, Moyer DJ: Equine synovia after an intraarticular injection of lidocaine or mepivacaine. Vet Surg 1988; 17:42.
8. Moore DC, Bridenbaugh DL, Bridenbauer PO, et al: Bupivacaine for peripheral nerve block: A comparison with mepivacaine, lidocaine, and tetracaine. Anesthesiology 1970; 32:461.
9. Keller H: Lahmheitsdiagnostik beim Pferd. Tieraerztl Prax 1976; 4:349.
10. Boening KJ: Komplikationen bei diagnostischen und chirurgischen Eingriffen am Hufgelenk des Pferdes. Praktische Tieraerzte 1980; 10:863.
11. Ford TS, Ross MW, Orsini PG: A comparison of methods for proximal palmar metacarpal analgesia in horses. Vet Surg 1989; 18:146.
12. Sack WO, Orsini PG: Distal intertarsal and tarsometatarsal joints in the horse. Communication and injection sites. J Am Vet Med Assoc 1991; 179:355.
13. Vacek JR, Ford TS, Honnas CM: Communication between the femoropatellar and medial and lateral femorotibial joints in horses. Am J Vet Res 1992; 53:1431.
14. Hendrickson DA, Nixon AJ: A lateral approach for synovial fluid aspiration and joint injection of the femoropatellar joint of the horse. Equine Vet J 1992; 24:399.
15. Butler JA, Colles CM, Dyson SJ, et al (eds). Clinical Radiology of the Horse. Oxford, Blackwell, 1993.
16. Park RD, Lebel JL: Equine radiology. In Stashak TS (ed): Adams' Lameness in Horses, 4th ed., Philadelphia, Saunders, 1987, ch 4, p 157.
17. Smallwood JE, Shively MJ, Rendano VT: A standardized nomenclature for radiographic projections used in veterinary medicine. Vet Radiol 1985; 26:2.
18. Lamb CR: Contrast radiography of equine joints, tendon sheaths, and draining tracts. Vet Clin North Am: Equine Pract 1991; 7:24.
19. Wright JD, Wood AKW: Arthrography of the equine tarsus: A comparison between iohexol and sodium and meglumine diatrizoate. Vet Radiol 1988; 29:191.
20. Verschooten F, de Moor A: Tendinitis in the horse: Its radiographic diagnosis with air tendograms. J Am Vet Radiol Soc 1978; 19:23.
21. Verschooten A, Picavet TM: Desmitis of the fetlock annular ligament in the horse. Equine Vet J 1986; 18:138.
22. Dik KJ, Merkens HW: Unilateral distension of the tarsal sheath in the horse: A report of 11 cases. Equine Vet J 1987; 19:307.
23. Hago BED, Vaughan LC: Use of contrast radiography in the investigation of tenosynovitis and bursitis in the horse. Equine Vet J 1986; 18:375.
24. Hago BED, Vaughan LC: Radiographic anatomy of tendon sheaths and bursae in the horse. Equine Vet J 1986; 18:102.
25. Genovese RL, Rantanen NW, Hauser ML, et al: Diagnostic ultrasonography of equine limbs. Vet Clin North Am: Large An Pract 1986; 2:145.
26. Steyn PF, McIlwraith CW, Rawcliff N: The ultrasonographic examination of the palmar metacarpal tendons and ligaments of the equine digit: A review. Equine Pract 1991; 13:24.

27. Hauser ML: Ultrasonic appearance and correlative anatomy of the soft tissues of the distal extremities in the horse. Vet Clin North Am: Equine Pract 1986; 2:127.

28. Smith RKW, Webbon PM: Diagnostic imaging in the athletic horse. Musculoskeletal ultrasonography. In Hodgson DR, Rose RJ (eds), The Athletic Horse. Philadelphia, Saunders, 1994, ch 14B, p 297.

29. McClellan PD, Colby J: Ultrasonic structure of the pastern. J Equine Vet Sci 1986; 6:99.

30. Dyson S: Ultrasonic examination of the metacarpal and metatarsal regions in the horse. Equine Vet Educat 1992; 4:139.

31. Reef VB, Martin BB, Elser A: Types of tendon and ligament injuries detected with diagnostic ultrasonography: Description and followup. In Proceedings of the 34th Annual Convention of the American Association of Equine Practitioners, 1988; p 245.

32. Dik KJ, van den Belt AJM, Keg PR: Ultrasonic evaluation of fetlock annular ligament constriction in the horse. Equine Vet J 1991; 23:149.

33. Neuwirth LA, Selcer BA, Mahaffey MB: Equine tendon ultrasonography: Common artifacts. Equine Vet Educat 1991; 3:149.

34. Bone A, Papageorges M, Grant BD: Ultrasonic evaluation and surgical treatment of humeral osteitis and bicipital tenosynovitis in a horse. J Am Vet Med Assoc 1992; 201:305.

35. Dyson SJ, Kidd L: Five cases of gastrocnemius tendinitis in the horse. Equine Vet J 1992; 24:351.

36. Dik KJ: Ultrasonography of the equine peroneus tertius muscle (abstract). Vet Radiol Ultrasound 1992; 33:126.

37. Reef VB: Diagnosis of pelvic fractures in horses using ultrasonography (abstract). Vet Radiol Ultrasound 1992; 33:121.

38. Snow DH, Guy PS: Percutaneous needle muscle biopsy in the horse. Equine Vet J 1976; 8:150.

39. Snow DH, Valberg SJ: Muscle anatomy, physiology and adaptations to exercise and training. In Hodgson DR, Rose RJ (eds), The Athletic Horse. Philadelphia, Saunders, 1994, ch 8, p 145.

40. McIlwraith CW: Disease of joints, tendons, ligaments, and related structures. In Stashak TS (ed), Adams' Lameness in Horses, 4th ed. Philadelphia, Lea & Febiger, 1987, ch 7, p 339.

41. Van Pelt RW: Properties of equine synovial fluid. J Am Vet Med Assoc 1962; 141:1051.

42. Hilbert BJ, Rowley G, Antonas KN: Hyaluronic acid concentration in synovial fluid from normal and arthritic joints of horses. Aust Vet J 1984; 61:22.

43. Van Pelt RW: Characteristics of normal equine tarsal synovial fluid. Can J Compend Med Vet Sci 1967; 31:342.

44. Van Pelt RW: Interpretation of synovial fluid findings in the horse. J Am Vet Med Assoc 1974; 165:91.

45. Korenek NL, Andrews FM, Maddux JM, et al: Determination of total protein concentration and viscosity of synovial fluid from the tibiotarsal joints of horses. Am J Vet Res 1992; 53:781.

46. Persson L: On the synovia in horses. Acta Vet Scand (suppl) 1971; 35:1.

47. Tew WP: Synovial fluid particle analysis in equine joint disease. Mod Vet Prac 1980; 61:993.

48. Tew WP, Hacket RP: Identification of cartilage wear fragments in synovial fluid from equine joints. Arthritis Rheum 1989; 24:1419.

49. Rose RJ, Paris R: Biochemical values in the serum and carpal synovial fluid of Thoroughbred horses in training. J Equine Med Surg 1979; 3:237.

50. McIlwraith CW: Diagnostic and Surgical Arthroscopy in the Horse, 2nd ed. Philadelphia, Lea & Febiger, 1990.

51. Ueltschi G: Bone and joint imaging with ^{99m}Tc-labelled phosphates as a new diagnostic aid in veterinary orthopedics. J Am Vet Radiol Soc 1977; 18:80.

52. Schramme MC, Webbon PM: Diagnostic imaging in the athletic horse: Scintigraphy. In Hodgson DR, Rose RJ (ed): The Athletic Horse. Philadelphia, Saunders, 1994, ch 14c, p 237.

53. Trout DR, Hornof WJ, Liskey CC, et al: The effects of regional perineural anesthesia on soft tissue and bone phase scintigraphy in the horse. Vet Radiol 1991; 32:140.

54. Mackey VS, Trout DR, Meagher DM, et al: Stress fractures of the humerus, radius, and tibia in horses: Clinical features and radiographic and/or scintigraphic appearance. Vet Radiol 1987; 28:26.

55. Koblik PD, Hornof WJ, Seeheman HJ: Scintigraphic appearance of stress-induced trauma of the dorsal cortex of the third metacarpal bone in racing Thoroughbred horses: 121 cases (1978–1986). J Am Vet Med Assoc 1988; 192:390.

56. Steckel RR: The role of scintigraphy in the lameness evaluation. Vet Clin North Am: Equine Pract 1991; 7:207.

57. Dalin G, Jeffcott LB: Biomechanics, gait and conformation. In Hodgson DR, Rose RJ (eds), The Athletic Horse, Philadelphia, Saunders, 1994, ch 3, p 27.

58. Leach D: Noninvasive technology for assessment of equine locomotion. Comp Contin Educ Pract 1987; 9:1124.

59. Clayton HM: Advances in motion analysis. Vet Clin North Am 1991; 7:365.

60. Goodship AE, Brown PN, MacFie HJH, et al: A quantitative force plate assessment of equine locomotor performance. In Snow DH, Persson SGB, Rose RJ (eds), Equine Exercise Physiology. Cambridge, MA, Burlington Press, 1982, p 263.

61. Merkens HW, Schramhardt HC, Hartman W, et al: The use of H(orse) INDEX: A method of analysing the ground reaction force patterns of lame and normal gaited horses at the walk. Equine Vet J 1988; 20:29.

62. Ratzlaff MH, Wilson PD, Hyde ML, et al: Relationships between locomotor forces, hoof position, and joint motion during the support phase of the stride in galloping horses. Acta Anat 1993; 146:200.

63. Barrey E: Investigation of the vertical hoof force distribution in the equine forelimb with an instrumented horseboot. Equine Vet J 1990; 22(suppl 9):35.

64. Auer JA, Butler KD: An introduction to the Kaegi equine gait analysis system in the horse. Proceedings of the Annual Convention of the American Association of Equine Practitioners, 1986; 31:209.

65. Huskamp B, Tietje S, Novak M, et al: Fussungs- und Bewegungsmuster gesunder und strahlbeinkranker Pferde—gemessen mit dem Equine Gait Analysis System (EGA System). Pferdeheilk 1990; 5:231.

66. Adrian M, Grant B, Ratzlaff M, et al: Electrogoniometric analysis of equine metacarpophalangeal joint lameness. Am J Vet Res 1977; 38:431.

67. Ratzlaff MH, Grant BD, Adrian M: Quantitative evaluation of equine carpal lameness. J Equine Vet Sci 1982; 2:78.

68. Taylor BM, Tipton CM, Adrian M, et al: Action of certain joints in the legs of horses recorded electrogoniometrically. Am J Vet Res 1966; 27:85.

69. Ratzlaff MH, Grant BD, Adrian M, et al: Evaluation of equine locomotion using electrogoniometry and cinematography: Research and clinical application. Proceedings of the 25th Annual Convention of the American Association of Equine Practitioners 1979; 381.

70. Fredricson I, Drevmo S, Dalin G, et al: The application of high-speed cinematography for quantitative analysis of equine locomotion. Equine Vet J 1980; 12:54.

71. Drevmo S, Roepstorff L, Kallings P, et al: Application of TrackEye in equine locomotion research. Acta Anat 1993; 146:137.

72. Martine-del Campo LJ, Kobluk CN, Greer N, et al: The use of high-speed videography to generate angle-time and angle-angle diagrams for the study of equine locomotion. Vet Comp Orthop Trauma 1991; 4:120.

73. Knezevic PF, Floss FN: Klinische Ergebniss der rechnergestutzten Bewegungsanalyse beim Pferd. *In* Knezevic PF (ed), Orthopadie bei Huf- und Klauentieren. Hannover, Germany, Schlutersche, 1983, p 140.

74. Floss FN: Grenzen des Einsatzes automatischer Bewegungsanalysesysteme. *In* Knezevic PF (ed), Orthopadie bei Huf- und Klauentieren. Hannover, Germany, Schlutersche, 1983, p 149.

75. Buchner F, Kastner J, Girtler D, et al: Die Hüftbewegung des Pferdes: Vergleichende kinematische Untersuchung bei lahmheitsfreien und spatlahmen Pferden. Pferdeheilk 1992; 8:23.

76. Turner TA: Thermography as an aid to the clinical lameness evaluation. Vet Clin North Am: Equine Pract 1991; 7:311.

77. Purohit RC, McCoy MD: Thermography in the diagnosis of inflammatory processes in the horse. Am J Vet Res 1980; 41:1167.

78. Stromberg B: The use of thermography in equine orthopedics. J Vet Radiol 1974; 15:94.

79. Turner TA, Purohit RC, Fessler JF: Thermography: A review in equine medicine. Compend Contin Educ Pract Vet 1986; 8:855.

80. Turner TA, Fessler JF, Lamp M, et al: Thermographic evaluation of podotrochlosis in horses. Am J Vet Res 1983; 44:535.

81. Vaden MF, Purohit RC, McCoy MD, et al: Thermography: A technique for subclinical diagnosis of osteoarthritis. Am J Vet Res 1980; 41:1175.

82. Stromberg B: Morphologic, thermographic and ^{133}Xe clearance studies on normal and diseased superficial digital flexor tendons in race horses. Equine Vet J 1973; 5:156.

83. Turner TA: Hindlimb muscle strain as a cause of lameness in horses. Proceedings of the Annual Convention of the American Association of Equine Practitioners 1989; 34: 281.

84. Stromberg B: The use of thermography in equine orthopedics. J Vet Radiol 1974; 15:94.

85. Misheff MM, Stover SM, Pool RR: Corticocancellous bone biopsy from the 12th rib of standing horses. Vet Surg 1992; 21:133.

86. Savage CJ, Jeffcott LB, Melsen F, et al: Bone biopsy in the horse. 1. Method using the wing of the ilium. J Vet Med 1991; A38:776.

87. Savage CJ, Tidd LC, Melsen F, et al: Bone biopsy in the horse. 2. Evaluation of histomorphometric examination. J Vet Med 1991; A38:784.

88. Savage CJ, Tidd LC, Østblom LC, et al: Bone biopsy in the horse. 3. Normal histomorphometric data according to age and sex. J Vet Med 1991; A38:793.

89. O'Callaghan MW: Future diagnostic methods. A brief look at new technologies and their potential application to equine diagnosis. Vet Clin North Am: Equine Pract 1991; 7:467.

The Cardiovascular System

COMPONENTS

For the purposes of this section the cardiovascular system will include the heart, the pericardium, and the system of vessels that carry blood to and from the heart through the general systemic and pulmonary systems.

MANIFESTATIONS OF DISEASE

The heart acts as a pump to force blood through the vascular system. Successful transport through the systemic and pulmonary arterial, capillary, and venous systems depends not only on the anatomical integrity of the system, but also on a delicate functional balance between cardiac output, venous return, and vascular tone. The system can be affected by loss of cardiac pumping ability (septal defects, valvular insufficiency, arrhythmias, pericardial effusion or restrictive disease, myocarditis), sepsis (endocarditis, thrombophlebitis, arteritis), reduced venous return (shock in its different forms), or loss of vessel integrity (arteritis, immune-mediated disease, clotting abnormality). The manifestations depend on the extent of compromise and the site involved. Minor loss of pumping ability will produce a slight loss of exercise tolerance, whereas a major reduction creates significant exercise intolerance as well as peripheral edema with right-sided failure and pulmonary edema with left-sided failure. Significant exercise intolerance can be so severe as to result in weakness and collapse. Loss of vessel integrity allows increased movement of fluid into the extravascular compartment with production of edema, and, in certain diseases, there may also be extravasation of blood, seen as petechiation, ecchymoses, and even hematomata. Localized sepsis may involve veins (thrombophlebitis) and heart valves (endocarditis) producing, in addition to mechanical dysfunction, signs ranging from an almost silent syndrome to one of severe toxemia with depression and fever. Such lesions often result in spread of septic emboli to other organs. Diffuse arterial inflammation, such as seen in equine viral arteritis, produces a widespread arterial inflammation with extensive involvement of many organs. Less common anatomic abnormalities such as arteriovenous fistulae with bypass of the capillary circulation can result in pain and lameness. Verminous arteritis, which typically involves the cranial mesenteric artery, is often responsible for intestinal malfunction and injury. When there is incomplete oxygenation of blood because of abnormal circulation, mucosae are blueish (cyanosis) as a result of the increased concentration of reduced hemoglobin.

GENERAL PHYSICAL EXAMINATION

Attitude

It is important to determine whether the disease is affecting the horse to the extent that it is depressed and has lost interest in its environment. This is evident if the horse does not acknowledge the presence of people, does not respond to stimuli such as noise or movement of personnel and other animals, and has a reduced or absent appetite.

Stance

Horses that have difficulty breathing move around very little, and, when they have extreme difficulty breathing, they stand with elbows abducted, head and neck extended, and mouth open.

Physical Condition

Animals with chronic cardiac disease (e.g., cardiac insufficiency, septic endocarditis) often have poor body condition.

Respiration

Cardiac lesions have considerable potential for affecting respiration. Breathing rates are often elevated in response to inadequate oxygenation of the blood that can result from some septal defects or pulmonary edema.

Edema

The increase in intravascular hydrostatic pressure associated with left-sided heart failure causes an increase in net outflow of water from the capillaries in the systemic circulation and, subsequently, edema. The edema is seen first at the sternum and, as it develops, it extends to the ventral thorax and abdomen and eventually to the limbs.

Jugular Pulse

It is normal to see a pulse in the distal one half to one third of the jugular veins just adjacent to the thoracic inlet (Fig. 6-1A). The true jugular pulse is caused by retrograde transmission of pressure waves from the heart and can be an important indication of cardiac abnormality. Both jugular veins should be examined carefully with the horse's head in a normal erect position. The normal pulse consists of a series of pressure fluctuations resulting from atrial contraction, bulging of the atrioventricular (AV) valve, systolic suction during ventricular systole, atrial filling, and atrial emptying. Increased pressures associ-

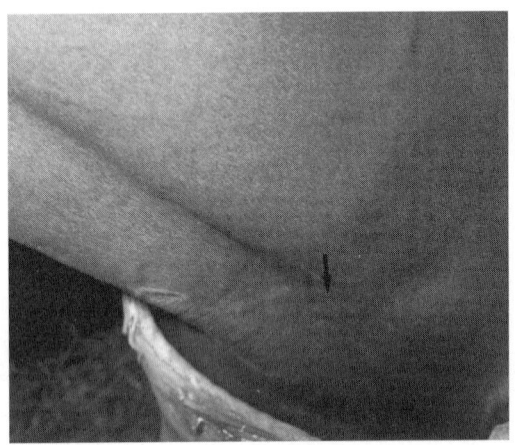

A

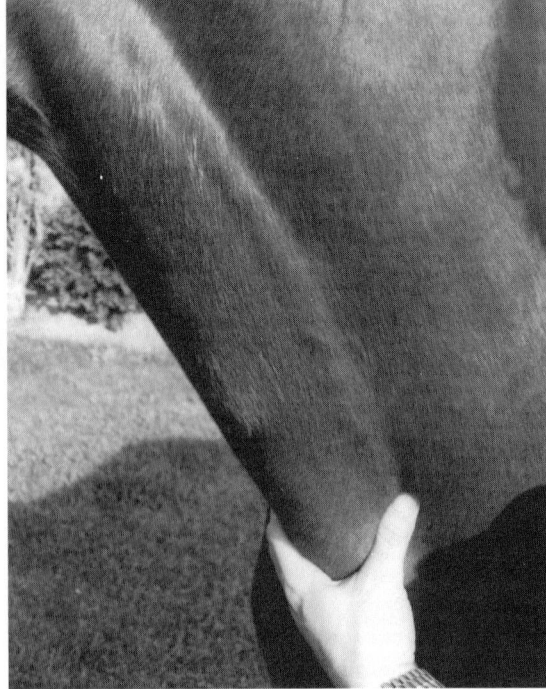

B

▶ **FIGURE 6-1**

Jugular vein. **A.** With the head in a neutral position the jugular vein is usually visible in the ventral third of the cervical region. **B.** Occlusion of the jugular at the base of the neck will abolish a jugular pulse.

ated with any of these events will produce an accentuation of the jugular pulse. Resistance to ventricular filling, atrial contraction against a closed AV valve, and regurgitation of blood through the tricuspid valve all produce retrograde transmission of an exaggerated pressure wave. Careful simultaneous auscultation will often help to determine the cause.

Transmission of the carotid artery pulse is easily confused with a true jugular pulse. However, it is a simple matter to differentiate between the two. Occlusion of the jugular vein at the thoracic inlet will abolish a jugular pulse by preventing retrograde transmission of the pressure wave, but will have no effect on a carotid pulse (Fig. 6-1B).

Pulseless distension of the jugular veins can result from an increase in central venous pressure resulting from congestive heart failure and pericardial disease. Pulseless distention of the vein is also associated with occlusion or reduced flow associated with disease of the vessel itself, such as thrombophlebitis. Thrombophlebitis is characterized by thickening of the vein and by pain on palpation.

Cardiac Impulse

In thin or fit horses the cardiac impulse can be seen on the left side of the thorax immediately caudal and dorsal to the point of the elbow. It should not normally be visible on the right side. Similarly, it is also easily palpable on the left side but not so easily on the right side. The left side is palpated with the left hand and the right side with the right hand. In either case the hand is placed with the palm against the thoracic wall and the fingers are directed cranioventrally beneath the triceps muscles, as far forward as possible (Fig. 6-2). The impulse can be detected between the third and fifth intercostal spaces, being strongest in the fifth left intercostal space.

Arterial Pulse

The arterial pulse is the result of the difference between the systolic and diastolic pressure waves, and it is affected by vessel size, distance from the heart, and the difference between the systolic and diastolic pressures. The ability to detect a pulse is determined mainly by a vessel's proximity to the body surface. Which sites are used is a matter for personal preference. However, the clinician should be familiar with a number of locations because, under certain circumstances, such as

recumbency, excitement, and intractability, the preferred site(s) may be inaccessible or inappropriate. Sites where an arterial pulse can be palpated include the facial, transverse facial, carotid, common digital, saphenous, and coccygeal arteries (Fig. 6-3). For simple examination the most usual site is probably the facial artery, and, when simultaneous cardiac auscultation is required, the radial artery is usually used.

A pulse is characterized by rate, rhythm, intensity, amplitude, and duration. Under normal conditions, the pulse rate and heart rate are identical.

The rhythm should be regular, and, if it is not, one should note whether the irregularity is cyclic or not. If it is cyclic, the variation is likely to result from a corresponding variation in heart rate (e.g., sinus arrythmia), and, if noncyclic, it is probably the result of variation in ventricular filling, whereby there is insufficient blood being pumped into the arterial system for every pulse to be equally palpable (e.g., premature contractions, atrial fibrillation). The extreme of this latter situation is when there is no pulse following the heart beat, and a pulse deficit is said to exist. This

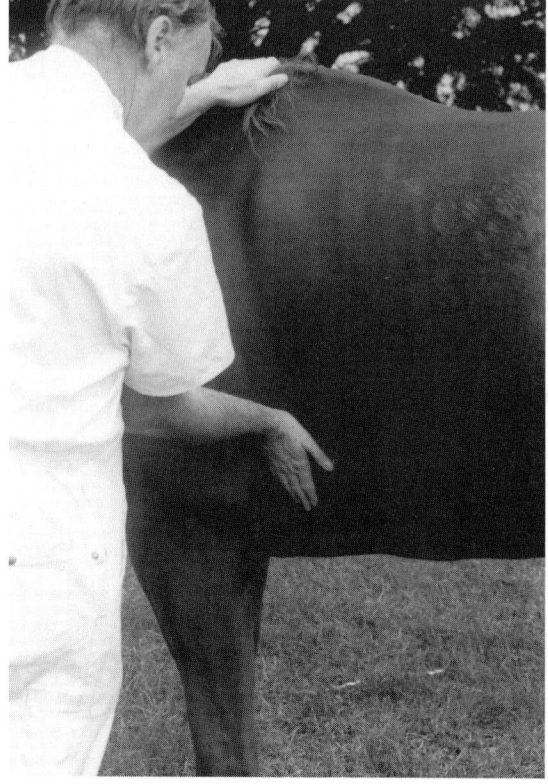

▶ FIGURE 6-2

Palpation of the cardiac impulse.

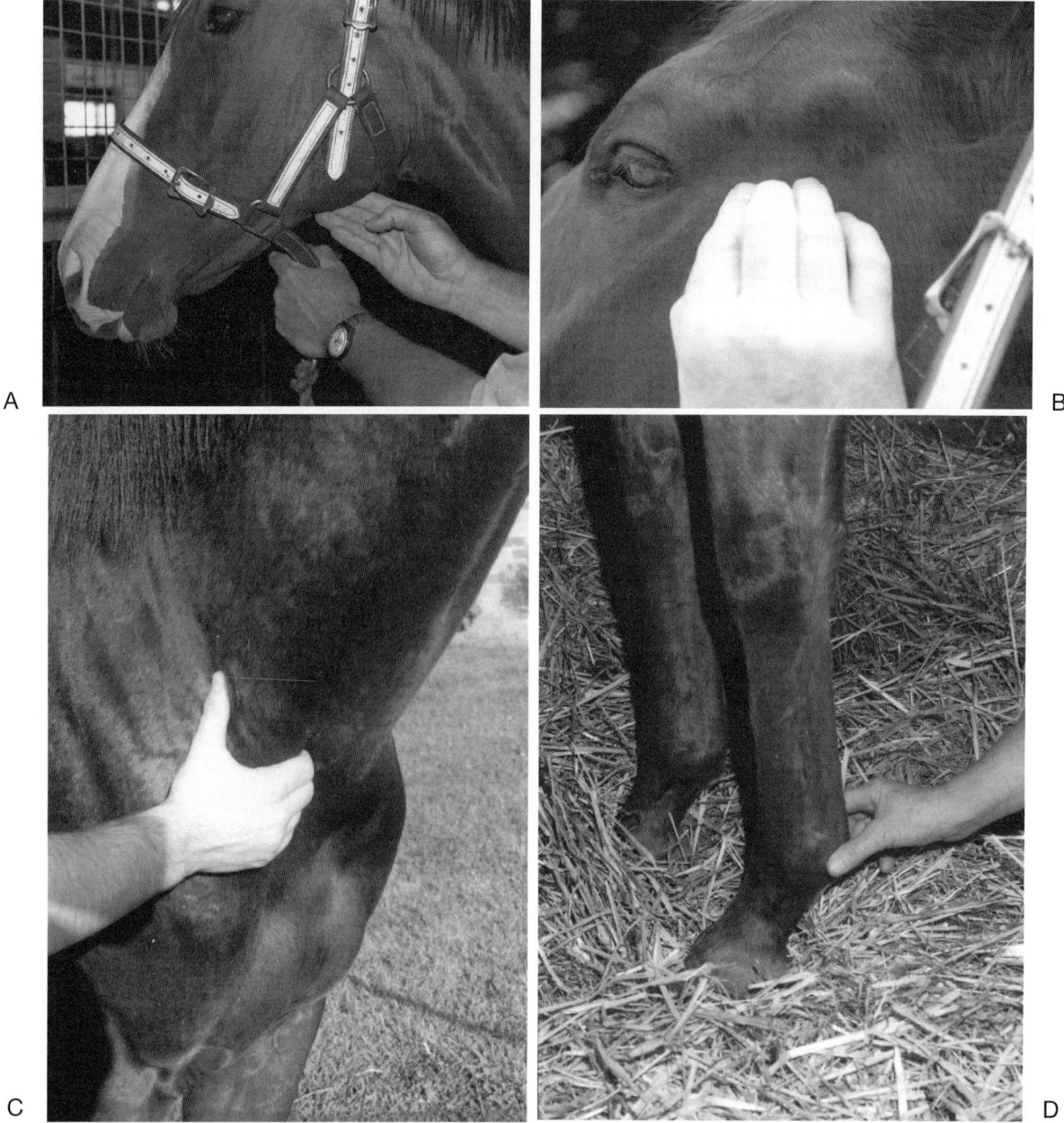

▶ FIGURE 6-3

Sites for palpation of an arterial pulse. **A.** Facial artery. **B.** Transverse facial artery. **C.** Carotid artery. **D.** Digital artery.

should be differentiated from a "dropped beat," where the absence of pulse is the result of the absence of ventricular contraction.

The normal pulse is full and bounding with a distinct rise and fall. Pulses can be defined as weak, normal, or strong. The pulse is weak when the pulse pressure is low, when arterial pressure is low, and when its rise and fall are slower than normal, due to conditions such as reduced cardiac output and arrhythmias. The so-called water

hammer pulse, which rises strongly and then falls very quickly, is associated with large stroke volumes and rapid diastolic runoffs, and it is seen particularly with a patent ductus arteriosus.

Mucous Membranes

Color

Normal mucosae are pink, the color being imparted by a normal content of oxyhemoglobin

---

PULSE RATE

• Horses: 30 to 40 beats per minute (bpm)
• Foals and ponies: Up to 80 bpm

---

in the erythrocytes, and have a capillary refill time of 1 to 2 s. The pink color remains as long as there is sufficient oxygenated hemoglobin within the erythrocytes in the capillary circulation. When the circulating blood volume is low, such as after hemorrhage, the mucosae may be pale because of absence of blood. When the number of erythrocytes is normal but there is an excess of reduced hemoglobin because of an abnormality in erythrocyte oxygenation or stagnation of capillary flow, the mucosae will be blueish in color (cyanotic). For the blue coloration to occur there must be a normal or near-normal hemoglobin concentration. Therefore, in the presence of anemia there may be insufficient reduced hemoglobin to provide discoloration. The mucosae may also be colored brown by methemoglobinemia due to nitrite poisoning and bright red because of cyanide poisoning.

Capillary Refill Time

Digital compression of the gingival mucosa expresses blood from the capillary circulation, causing the mucosa to become pale (Fig. 6-4). When compression is discontinued, the blood returns, and the mucosa becomes pink again. The time taken for the return of color is known as the capillary refill time (CRT) and is used as an approximate, but useful, index of capillary perfusion. The normal CRT is 1 to 2 seconds. The CRT is prolonged when capillary perfusion is low (e.g., hypovolemic and endotoxic shock).

Auscultation

Auscultation is a very important component of the cardiovascular examination. It should be carried out in a quiet environment with the horse relaxed and restrained in the standing position. For optimal results, it is advisable to use both the bell and the diaphragm parts of the stethoscope, designed for lower and higher frequencies, respectively. The shape of the bell section precludes it from being pushed beneath the triceps muscles. A thorough examination involves a systematic evaluation of both sides of the thorax and of all valve areas. Artefacts are introduced by background environmental noise, patient movement, respiration, friction sounds generated by movement of the phonendoscope on hair, and gastrointestinal sounds. As for all evaluations, a systematic examination is necessary, although the precise order of the procedure is at the discretion of the clinician.

Normal Heart Sounds

To ensure access to the appropriate sites for auscultation, the horse should be positioned with the front legs level with one another or, preferably, with the left slightly forward of the right.

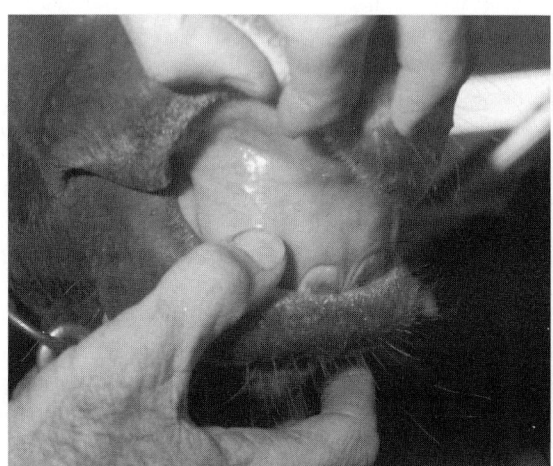 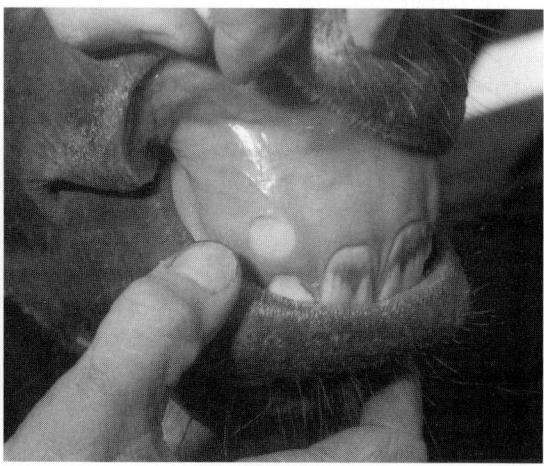

A   B

▶ **FIGURE 6-4**

Testing the capillary refill time (CRT). **A.** Applying digital pressure to blanch the mucosa. **B.** Release of digital pressure reveals the blanched mucosa, which should return to a normal pink color. The time taken to do this is defined as the CRT.

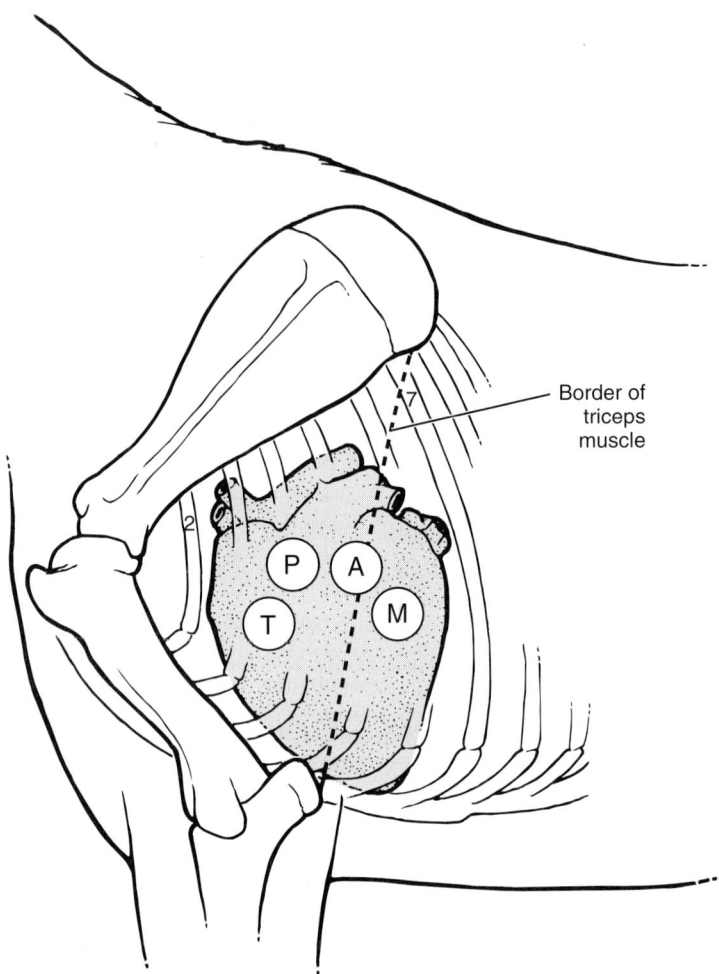

Border of
triceps
muscle

▶ **FIGURE 6-5**

Sites for auscultation of specific valve sounds. (M = mitral, A = aortic,
P = pulmonic, T = trisucspid)

Normal heart sounds are audible tissue vibrations produced by the disruption of laminar flow as blood in the heart and major vessels is accelerated or decelerated. In order to interpret normal and abnormal sounds, the clinician requires a thorough knowledge of the events of the cardiac cycle and of the generation of the sounds that are of clinical relevance. Briefly, the cardiac contraction is initiated in the sinoatrial node in the wall of the right atrium and then extends distally as the impulse is transmitted to the ventricles through the atrioventricular node and the specialized neural pathways present in the interventricular septum. The sequence of events contributing to normal heart sounds are contraction of the atria and filling of the ventricles, ventricular contraction and closure of the atrioventricular valves, closure of the semilunar valves, and rapid filling of the ventricles. The sites where specific valve sounds can best be heard are shown in Figure 6-5.

Four heart sounds can often be heard in normal horses, although, frequently, only two or three are audible. Which sounds are heard depends on the particular horse, heart rate, excitement, the quality and state of repair of the stethoscope, background environmental noise, and the skill and aural acuity of the clinician. The sounds are designated S_1, S_2, S_3, and S_4. However, it is unfortunate that the sound designated as S_4 is actually the first to occur in the cardiac cycle. Therefore, a normal sequence of sounds when all four are audible is S_4, S_1, S_2, S_3, which is confusing for someone just learning the technique. It is useful to remember that the two loudest and most obvious sounds are S_1 and S_2.

- *The fourth heart sound (S$_4$)* is composed of two components. The first, barely audible, is associated with the contraction of the atria and blood flow from the atria to the ventricles and occurs after the P wave of the electrocardiogram (ECG). The second component is associated with closure of the AV valves and is more audible if the (PR) interval is long. Isolated S$_4$ sounds are heard when the interval between atrial and ventricular contractions is long (first-degree AV block) or when there is no ventricular contraction (second-degree AV block). This helps to distinguish a heart block originating from the sinoatrial node (sinoatrial block), when no atrial sound is present, from one where a problem in conduction between the atria and ventricles exists, when an atrial sound will be present (second-degree AV block).

- *The first heart sound (S$_1$)* is related to ventricular contraction, closure of the AV valves, opening of the semilunar valves, and initial ejection of blood. It follows the QRS (ventricular depolarization) complex of the ECG, and is, in turn, followed by the arterial pulse. Splitting of the sound may be detected as a normal finding or an abnormal one associated with lesions that produce asymmetric ventricular contraction. The split sound must be differentiated from the late component of S$_4$. S$_1$ is best heard over and just below the region of the AV valves.

- *The second heart sound (S$_2$)* is associated with closure of the semilunar valves and the rapid reversal of blood flow. Splitting of the sounds can be observed in normal horses, especially during inspiration, when closure of the semilunar valves is not simultaneous. Very obvious splitting is seen in chronic obstructive respiratory disease.

- *The third heart sound (S$_3$)* is associated with the end of rapid ventricular filling. This sound is present in approximately 50% of normal horses and may occur (rarely) as a split sound as a result of asynchronous ventricular filling.

Rhythm

Evaluation of cardiac rhythm is an important component of the overall assessment of cardiac function. To complicate matters, horses exhibit a variety of normal rhythms. In order to detect and help identify abnormal rhythms (arrhythmias or dysrhythmias), the clinician should note the heart rate, the basic rhythm, intensity, and any tendency for splitting of the loudest sounds (S$_1$ and S$_2$), the presence of extra sounds, and the absence of normal sounds (dropped beats). The term *dysrhythmia* means a disturbance of rhythm, and *arrhythmia* means an absence of rhythm.

The normal rate varies greatly with body size and cardiovascular fitness, but it is in general likely to fall in the range of 25 to 50 bpm. Variation in autonomic nervous system activity is responsible for considerable variation in rate, and increased vagal nerve activity is the primary mechanism responsible for arrhythmias regarded as normal in horses.

Variation in rhythm can have many causes. Dysrhythmias associated with increased rates result from increased activity of the normal pacemaker in the sinoatrial node or from subsidiary sites in the atria or ventricles. *Tachycardia* is the term used to describe rates greater than 50 bpm. Those dysrhythmias associated with decreased rates result from depressed pacemaker activity or from frequent failure of impulses to be transmitted along the conducting pathways. The term *bradycardia* is used to describe rates below 26 bpm. Dysrythmias without a significant effect on rate also occur when there are isolated instances of early (premature) or missing ("dropped") beats, although rate is affected if the incidence of such events is high.

As stated, increased vagal tone is a common cause of dysrythmias in horses. However, under normal circumstances, the effects of this hyperactivity are abolished by exercise, excitement, or vagolytic (parasympatholytic) drugs. Sinus dysrhythmia is a waxing and waning of heart rate that may or may not be synchronized with respiration. When it is associated with respiration, an increase in rate is seen upon inspiration.

Although many dysrhythmias can be diagnosed using palpation and auscultation, a definitive diagnosis often requires an ECG examination.

Murmurs

Murmurs are audible vibrations produced as a result of turbulent flow during a normally quiet period of the cardiac cycle. Flow in tubes becomes turbulent when the Reynolds critical number (Re) exceeds a value of about 2,000. According to the following formula:

$$Re = RVD/v \times 2,000,$$
where

v = fluid viscosity
D = fluid density
V = velocity of flow
R = radius of vessel or orifice

In the cardiovascular system, increased velocity (high cardiac output, stenosis of orifices, regurgitation of blood through an incompetent valve) and decreased density (hypoproteinemia, anemia) are frequent causes of murmurs. The precise cause(s) of the murmur are poorly understood, and much of the generated sound is downstream of the structure that is responsible for it. Murmurs are classified as functional or pathological and are described according to their timing and duration, intensity, radiation, and quality.[1-3]

TIMING. Murmurs are first described according to when they occur in the cardiac cycle (systolic, diastolic, or continuous), when they occur within the systolic or diastolic phases, and, last, according to their duration, as shown in the box.

CHARACTER. The character of the murmur can be described according to its acoustic properties. The sound of a murmur can be continuous (plateau), or it can wax (crescendo) and wane (decre-

---

INTENSITY OF MURMURS

- *Grade 1:* Softest audible murmur heard only after careful auscultation.
- *Grade 2:* Faint murmur clearly audible when the stethoscope is placed over its point of maximum intensity (PMI).
- *Grade 3:* Moderately loud murmur.
- *Grade 4:* Loud murmur audible over a wide area but without a palpable thrill.
- *Grade 5:* Loud murmur associated with a thrill.
- *Grade 6:* Loud murmur that remains audible after the phonendoscope is lifted just off the surface of the thorax. Always associated with a thrill.

---

scendo). Murmurs are often described, therefore, as being crescendo, crescendo-decrescendo, decrescendo, or plateau in character.[2,4-6]

INTENSITY. The intensity can be graded at the point of maximum intensity (PMI) with a six-unit system, as shown in the box.[5,7]

RADIATION. The murmur usually radiates in the direction of the turbulent flow, and, although a murmur can radiate almost anywhere, its PMI is a useful clue to its anatomical location.

FUNCTIONAL AND PATHOLOGIC MURMURS. Functional murmurs are those that do not appear to be associated with organic disease. They can occur in any section of the cardiac cycle and are subdivided into systolic and diastolic murmurs. Functional systolic murmurs are audible in over 50% of normal horses and are frequently associated with hypoproteinemia, anemia, and hyperkinetic states such as fever. They appear to be related to the normally rapid flow during the early stages of ventricular ejection and are usually of low intensity, decrescendo or crescendo-decrescendo, extend from early to late systole, and have a PMI over the heart base. Such murmurs are often described as being of the ejection type. Functional diastolic murmurs usually occur in presystole or early diastole. The presystolic murmurs occur between S_4 and S_1 and are related to atrial movements. Those occurring in early diastole shortly after S_2 are probably related to rapid ventricular filling.

TIMING OF MURMURS

- Systolic murmurs
  Pansystolic: Begins with S_1 and extends into S_2.
  Holosystolic: Extends between S_1 and S_2 but does not encroach on either.
  Proto- (early), meso -(mid-), and telo -(late) systolic.
  Presystolic: Heard between S_4 and S_1.
- Diastolic murmurs
  Holodiastolic: Heard between S_2 and S_1.
  Protodiastolic: Heard between S_2 and S_3.
  Mesodiastolic: Heard between S_3 and S_4.
- Continuous murmurs
  Span systole and diastole.

Pathological murmurs are due to turbulent flow related to stenotic or relatively stenotic valves, outflow tracts or great vessels, valvular insufficiency, or abnormal communication between vessels or different cardiac chambers. Causes of some pathological murmurs are mitral regurgitation (holosystolic and pansystolic plateau, and mid-late systolic plateau or crescendo murmurs, with PMI over the mitral valve area), tricuspid regurgitation (holosystolic or pansystolic plateau murmurs with PMI over the tricuspid valve area), and aortic regurgitation (holodiastolic decrescendo murmurs with PMI over the heart base).

The significance of a murmur is often difficult to establish. However, pansystolic mitral and tricuspid murmurs, holodiastolic murmurs and all murmurs with a palpable thrill are usually regarded as being pathological.[5,8] The use of Doppler echocardiography can improve the detection of valvular regurgitation and thus improve understanding of the origins of auscultatory sounds. The prevalence of murmurs, both functional and pathological has been described and is presented in Table 6-1.

Clicks

Systolic clicks are heard in normal horses and are of unknown significance or cause.

▶ TABLE 6–1

PREVALENCE OF AUSCULTATORY FINDINGS IN HORSES OF DIFFERENT BREEDS AND USE (NATIONAL HUNT, FLAT RACERS, AND COMPETITON AND PLEASURE HORSES, $N = 545$)

Auscultatory Findings	Proportion (%)
No murmur	31.7
Early systolic murmur, left side	49.5
Early systolic murmur, right side	8.4
Early diastolic murmur, left side	15.0
Early diastolic murmur, right side	13.4
Pan- or (holo-) systolic murmur	
Compatible with mitral valve regurgitation	3.5
Compatible with tricuspid valve regurgitation	9.0
Holodiastolic murmur (compatible with aortic regurgitation)	2.2
Presystolic murmur	2.2
Second-degree atrioventricular block	19.6
Atrial fibrillation	0.6

Source: Data from Patteson MW, Cripps PJ: A survey of cardiac auscultatory findings in horses. Equine Vet J 1993; 25:409.

Pericardial Friction Sounds or Rubs

Pericardial friction sounds are produced by friction between an inflamed pericardium and the epicardium. They occur during movement of the heart and are therefore heard during systole and diastole. The sounds can be described as "scratchy," but may be "splashy" if gas produced by microorganisms is present as well as fluid. The sounds are present in the early stages of pericardial disease, but disappear at a later stage as fluid accumulates and keeps the layers of pericardium separated. Care should be taken to differentiate these sounds from those associated with the respiratory system, which can be difficult if the respiratory and heart rates are similar or identical.

Lung Sounds

Pulmonary auscultation (see Chapter 3, Auscultation of the Thorax and Upper Airways) is an integral part of the cardiovascular examination because cardiac disease is sometimes manifested by signs related to pulmonary lesions (e.g., cough caused by pulmonary edema). Conversely, pulmonary disease may produce cardiac abnormality (e.g., pulmonary hypertension and cardiac hypertrophy related to chronic respiratory disease).

Thrills

A thrill is the palpable equivalent of a murmur, both resulting from vibrations produced by turbulent blood flow. The thrill becomes palpable when the underlying lesion causes sufficient vibration of tissue for it to be transmitted to the external thoracic wall. A thrill is palpated by placing the palm of the open hand on the thorax overlying the heart. Thrills are associated with the more severe grades of murmur.

Percussion

Gross cardiac enlargement can be demonstrated by employing percussion to outline the area of thoracic dullness overlying the heart. Use of a plexor and pleximeter is described in Chapter 3 (see Percussion of the Thorax). The presence of the triceps muscles makes it necessary to pull the fore limb forward. The normal area of cardiac dullness is demonstrated in Figure 3-4.

Cardiac Evaluation during Exercise

Evaluation during and after exercise is useful when subtle lesions are present, particularly in performance horses.[10] Simple field testing, where heart rate is measured before and after exercise, is the simplest form of testing. Provided that the abnormal rate or rhythm remains after the horse has finished the test, simple auscultation, or even palpation of the pulse, will often allow a diagnosis to be made or, at least, indicate that heart function may be abnormal. For abnormalities that are present only during exercise or that require a standardized test to be detected, other methods must be employed. Heart rate monitors (cardio-tachometer) and electrocardiographic electrodes can be attached to the horse ("on board"), allowing rate and an electrocardiogram to be recorded for later replay or transmitted telemetrically for examination while the exercise test is under way. The most advanced form of testing is with the horse running on a high-speed treadmill under standardized test conditions.

Evaluation of Heart Rate in The Field

The effect of exercise on heart rate can be evaluated by examining postexercise recovery of heart rate and heart rate response to exercise of specified intensity.

PROCEDURE. The procedure varies according to the complexity of the test. The simplest method, which is usually the only one available to most clinicians, is measurement of rate with a stethoscope after exercise. The rate should be recorded immediately after the exercise is finished, and then at 5-minute intervals for up to approximately 20 minutes or longer if recovery is abnormal.

If an on-board cardiotachometer is used, heart rate can also be utilized in other ways,[11] by first recording the velocity required to generate a target heart rate, and, second, the velocity associated with maximum heart rate. A target rate such as 200 bpm is commonly used, and the associated velocity is designated as V_{200}. The velocity at maximum heart rate is termed V_{HRmax}. The velocity is estimated by recording the time taken to cover a known distance.

Use of a treadmill allows close monitoring of heart rate and precise adherence to a standardized test procedure. The treadmill is usually run at an incline of 6°, which imposes maximum workload at less than maximum velocity.

RESULTS. After a strenuous exercise session, heart rate in a fit horse falls very quickly in the first minute or so, and should reach about 100 bpm or

less after about 5 minutes.[12] Maximum rates are in the order of 200 to 240 bpm. Normal variation can be related to factors such as lack of fitness, illness, high environmental temperatures and humidity, and excitement. A reduction in the efficiency of cardiac function will prolong recovery time and be associated with reduced velocity at target heart rates.

Telemetric Electrocardiography

Exercise electrocardiograms can also be recorded with the horse running on or off a treadmill. The data can be stored for playback or viewed during the test. This form of test has special application for the detection and evaluation of dysrhythmias contributing to reduced exercise tolerance.

PROCEDURE. The ECG can be transmitted by radiotelemetry for examination during exercise or can be examined after exercise by being recorded with an on-board recorder or stored on magnetic tape.

RESULTS. The QRS complex is not greatly affected by exercise. Normal responses to exercise include shortening of the PR and QT intervals and superimposition of P waves on preceding T waves,[13] possibly some variation in T waves,[14] and abolition of second-degree AV block.[13] The evaluation of abnormalities such as ventricular ectopic beats[15,16] and atrial fibrillation[15] is facilitated by exercise. Postexercise, dysrhythmias, such as sinus dysrhythmia, are present in some normal horses,[15] and atrial and ventricular ectopic beats not present at rest may be identified.[15-17]

Special Diagnostic Techniques

Pericardiocentesis

Although pericardial disease is rare in horses, it is occasionally necessary to collect and evaluate pericardial fluid that has accumulated secondary to infection, neoplasia, congestive heart failure, or trauma. The process of collection is known as *pericardiocentesis*. The presence of fluid may be deduced from a clinical examination, and signs such as bilateral muffling of heart sounds and jugular distension with increased central venous pressure are strongly suggestive of an increase in the volume of pericardial fluid. Other diagnostic techniques, such as ultrasonography, are very useful for confirming the presence of fluid and, in particular, to help differentiate between pleural and pericardial fluid, increased volumes of which are often present concurrently. It is easier to obtain the pericardial fluid if any coexisting pleural fluid is removed first.

PROCEDURE. To avoid any unexpected movement, which can result in serious damage to the heart, the horse should be adequately restrained. The procedure can be carried out from the right or left side of the thorax. However, the choice may depend on other factors such as coexisting pleural or lung disease and radiographic or echocardiographic findings. An area approximately 10×10 cm, overlying the 5th, 6th, and 7th intercostal spaces and centered over the costochondral junctions, is clipped and prepared for sampling under sterile conditions. The local anesthetic fluid is infiltrated subcutaneously and into the intercostal muscle region in the appropriate intercostal space. A small stab incision is made with the scalpel blade, and the cannula with the syringe attached is then carefully advanced into the thorax, ensuring that it is inserted on the cranial border of the rib so as to avoid the intercostal vessels and nerves. Although the cannula can be inserted directly through the skin, it is better first to make a small stab incision so that it can be inserted without friction from the skin. The absence of "drag" caused by skin friction improves the clinician's ability to detect when contact is made with the heart. During insertion, gentle negative pressure is applied. If the pericardium is thick, as a result of disease, it may be a little more difficult to penetrate. When the heart or a thickened pericardium is touched, it is usually possible to appreciate the movements of the heart associated with each contraction. If an electrocardiogram is being recorded, stimulation of the epicardium will usually produce a premature ventricular

contraction. When this occurs, the needle should be withdrawn a little and the fluid aspirated. Aspiration will not be possible if the fluid is too viscous or if there is chronic fibrosis. The fluid collected should be analyzed in the same manner as fluid from the other body cavities (pleural and abdominal), with the objective of establishing its nature.

RESULTS. Pericardial fluid has the same properties as fluid from the other body cavities (see Appendix D). Although there is considerable overlap of the cytological findings associated with different conditions, the presence of neoplasia may be indicated by characteristic tumor cells, sepsis by increased protein concentration, leucocytosis, and presence of bacteria, and hemorrhage by large numbers of erythrocytes. After acute hemorrhage the fluid will clot quickly.

COMPLICATIONS. Irritation of the epicardium can produce premature ventricular contractions and other dysrhythmias, and, therefore, it is wise to have drugs on hand to manage them. Lidocaine 2% is usually used, and can be injected intravenously or directly into the pericardial sac (initial intravenous dose, 0.5 mg/kg, repeated as necessary every 5 minutes for a total dose of 2.0 to 4.0 mg/kg).

Pericardiocentesis can result in hemorrhage, and the examination should be stopped if there is evidence of sudden bleeding. If the bleeding is sufficient to distend the pericardial sac and compromise cardiac filling and output (tamponade), it will be necessary to attempt removing some of the blood and possibly place an indwelling drain (e.g., Argyle Trocar Catheter, Sherwood Medical Industries, Inc., St Louis, MO).

Electrocardiography

The events associated with cardiac depolarization and repolarization produce varying electrical fields over the body surface where the resulting potential differences between any two points can be measured by means of an electrocardiograph. At any one instant, the activity of the heart comprises a single dipole vector with polarity, direction, and magnitude. The electrocardiograph is a galvanometer, which, after appropriate adjustment for sensitivity and frequency, can record continually the potential difference between different points with a recording device such as a heated stylus on heat-sensitive paper or an ink pen or jet. When a potential difference

---

Materials for Pericardiocentesis

- Intravenous cannula (e.g., Intracath; 12–14 gauge)
- 60-mL syringe
- Scalpel blade (#15)
- Local anesthetic- 2% Lidocaine, 2% mepivacaine
- Sample tubes

exists, a current flows through the electrocardiograph, producing a deflection of the pen with an upward deflection being regarded, by convention, as positive. Flow away from the electrode is negative. The resultant record is the electrocardiogram. The apparatus therefore indicates the polarity of the electrical vectors and also, after calibration and careful placement of electrodes, their magnitude and direction. The recording apparatus is connected to the horse through a number of conducting wires, with a circuit between points known as a lead.

The lead systems used in large animals have been based on Einthoven's triangle. In the simplest system a bipolar lead is used, in which two leads, a negative and a positive, are connected to the horse. The standard bipolar leads (leads 1, 11, and 111) and the augmented unipolar limb leads (aVR, aVL, and aVF) are usually used with an exploring chest lead.

Because of certain anatomical and physiological differences between the human and equine heart, the use of multiple-lead systems in horses is restricted, and it is unlikely that the ECG will prove to be as useful in evaluating the shape and size of the heart as it is in man. As a result, the equine electrocardiograph is used mainly to evaluate disturbances of rhythm and myocardial function in certain systemic states. The fetal ECG can also be recorded (see later).

PROCEDURE. Because the electrocardiogram is a measure of electrical activity, it is important that the horse stand quietly in order to minimize

Requirements for Electrocardiography

▶ Electrocardiograph machine
    Capable of recording leads I, II, III, aVR, aVL, aVF, CV.LA, CR.LA, CF.LA, and CL.LA
    Frequency response of 0.05–80 Hz
    High-input impedance of at least 10 MΩ
    High common mode rejection ratio of at least 60–90 dB
    Patient cable should be at least 20 feet long
    Chest and limb leads should be about 5 feet long

▶ Electrodes (electrode plates or alligator clips with points filed down)

▶ Electrode paste, gel, or solution (obstetrical lubricant with added salt, and methylated spirts saturated with common salt are effective and cheap alternatives to commercial products)[10]

muscle activity.[18] The resting heart rate should be less than 40 bpm. The horse should be positioned so that it is standing squarely with the forelegs opposite one another or, preferably, with the left foreleg slightly in advance of the right (Fig. 6-6A). The ECG machine should be grounded to minimize the chances of electrical shock and mains

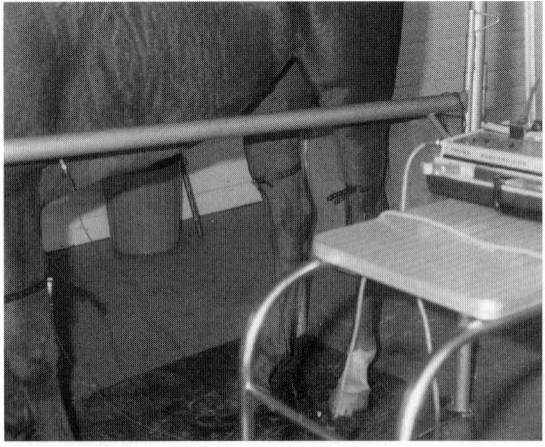

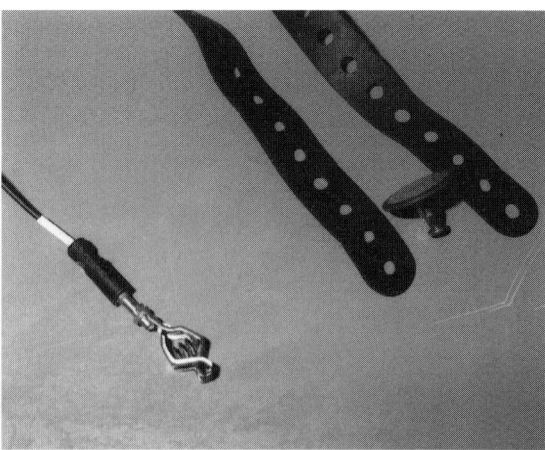

A

B

▶ **FIGURE 6–6**

Electrocardiography. **A.** An electrocardiographic recording session in progress. Note the manner in which the horse is confined and the rubber mat on which it is standing. **B.** Two electrode systems used to attach leads to the horse: alligator clips and rubber strips with flat metal discs.

interference (50–60 cycles per second). The horse is often made to stand on a dry rubber mat to avoid leakage to ground of any mains' current, although this is unnecessary when there is no major source of electrical interference. To maximize conduction, electrical paste is applied to each electrode site. The leads are attached with the alligator clips. Some horses object to alligator clips, in which case flat metal electrodes that are attached with rubber straps are used (Fig. 6-6B). The lead system that is used depends on the clinician as well as the purpose for which the recording is being made. The sites for attachment of the electrodes are described in the following paragraphs. Whatever lead system is used, it is wise to record at paper speeds of 25 and 50 mm/s in order to allow interpretation of complex waveforms. The sensitivity should be adjusted so that a deflection of 1 cm is equivalent to 1 mV and should be recorded on the tracing by activating the STD or CAL button. During recording, electrodes should not be moved or allowed to come into contact with each other. Leads should be identified on the electrocardiograph as they are recorded, calibrations should be made and registered at the beginning and end of recording, and leads 1, 11, and 111 should be recorded again at the end of the procedure. The record should include at least 24 artefact-free complexes of leads 1, 11, and 111 and at least six complexes of the other leads and will, therefore, extend over several minutes. A time marker is placed automatically on the tracing every 3 seconds during recording.

Bipolar Lead System

To assess arrhythmias and myocardial integrity in systemic states and to monitor during anesthesia a simple bipolar lead system is used. The base-apex and Y leads are two examples of such a system. This simple system produces large waveforms and reduces the interference associated with movement of the patient, which has a considerable effect on the quality of the recording when using other, more complicated, lead systems. The base-apex lead is recorded with the right-arm electrode (negative) attached to the skin in the right jugular furrow, approximately one third of the way up the neck (or just cranial to the withers at the base of the neck), and the left-arm electrode (positive) attached to the skin of the thoracic wall, immediately behind the point of the left elbow in the region of the apex beat (note that

the nomenclature on the leads applies to people, and for left and right arm, one should read left and right foreleg). For the Y lead the right-arm electrode is attached over the manubrium and the left-arm electrode is attached to the ventral midline overlying the xiphisternum. The ground (right hind) electrode is attached at any site remote from the heart. Lead 1 is selected.

Other Lead Systems

For more extensive evaluation there is a choice of some other lead systems. One such commonly used system uses the standard bipolar limb leads, the augmented unipolar limb leads, and an exploring chest lead. The electrodes are attached on the caudal aspects of the forelimbs, approximately 10 cm distal to the olecranon, on the cranial aspects of the hind limbs about 5 cm proximal to the tarsus, and on the chest, level with and caudal to the point of the olecranon. The leads are designated as follows:

- *Standard bipolar leads*
  Lead 1. Right and left forelegs
  Lead 11. Right foreleg and left hind leg
  Lead 111. Left foreleg and left hind leg
- *Augmented unipolar limb leads.* These leads pair two of the three limbs used in the standard bipolar leads against the third. As the lead selections are made, the machine automatically changes the combinations, and the specified limb (exploring electrode) gets connected to one pole of the galvanometer and the other two limbs to the other pole (neutral electrode). These leads are designated as follows:
  aVR. Right foreleg
  aVL. Left foreleg
  aVF. Left hind leg
- *Chest leads.* The unipolar chest leads, using Wilson's central terminal as the indifferent electrode, are located over the surface of the thorax in the following manner:
  CV6LL. Sixth left intercostal space at the costochondral junction
  CV6LU. Sixth left intercostal space level with the point of the shoulder
  V10. Over the dorsal spinous process of the sixth thoracic vertebrae
  CV6RL. Sixth right intercostal space at the costochondral junction
  CV6RU. Sixth right intercostal space level with the point of the shoulder

Evaluation of the Electrocardiogram

The electrocardiogram should be examined systematically. Lead 11 is frequently used to calculate heart rate, determine rhythm, and measure the durations of each of the waveforms. Any thorough procedure is satisfactory, and the following can be used as a guide.[18]

- Examine the whole tracing to ensure it is of appropriate quality for evaluation and to detect the presence of arrhythmias. The existence of an arrhythmia may not be apparent until a considerable number of complexes have been examined.
- Calculate the heart rate. This can be done in a number of ways, including:

    Count the number of complexes, using the QRS waves as reference points, that occur during a specified interval (e.g., 30 s), and then multiply the result by an appropriate factor (e.g., 2).

    Multiply paper speed (mm/s) by 60, and divide by the distance (mm) between complexes.

    A very rapid way to calculate the rate is to count the number of large squares between two successive S or R waves and to divide the figure into 300 or 600, for paper speeds of 25 or 50 mm/s, respectively.

- Check the tracing to see whether each cycle contains a normal sequence of P, QRS, and T waves. If not, identify the abnormality and decide whether it is a single event or one that is repeated.
- Identify the origin of any dysrhythmias. Dysrhythmias can be classified according to whether they originate above (supraventricular) or below the ventricle (ventricular).

    Supraventricular dysrhythmias include:
    Sinus tachycardia
    Sinus bradycardia
    Sinus dysrythmia
    Supraventricular premature systoles
    Supraventricular tachycardia
    Atrial fibrillation
    Sinoatrial block
    Atrioventricular block (first, second, or third degree)

    Ventricular dysrhythmias include:
    Ventricular premature systoles
    Ventricular tachycardia

Some dysrhythmias are associated with high vagal tone and are abolished by excitement, exercise, or vagolytic drugs. Examples of these are first- and second-degree heart block, wandering atrial pacemaker, sinus dysrhythmia, sinoatrial block, and sinus arrest. Pathological dysrhythmias are generally characterized by erratic rhythms, premature depolarization, or tachycardia and bradycardia (excluding the physiological forms just described).

- Carefully examine the tracing to identify any pattern that might exist in association with an abnormality of the waveform.
- Measure the intervals of the various components of the complex, using an ×8 to ×10 magnification.
- Vector analysis using a greater selection of leads can be undertaken. However, at present, the usefulness of this form of evaluation in horses has not been established.

RESULTS. The standard waveform and the accepted intervals and segments are depicted in Figure 6-7. It should be remembered that the actual wave will vary considerably depending on the individual, the status of the heart, and the lead that is under examination. The use of standard test conditions will help reduce the variation and familiarize the clinician with the normal tracing.

The durations of the waveforms constituting a depolarization and repolarization cycle from lead 11 of the frontal lead system described are as follows:[19]

P-wave duration	<0.17 s
P-wave peak interval	<0.08s
PR interval	<0.44 s
QRS complex duration	<0.17 s
ST interval	<0.06 s

The magnitudes of the PR and QT intervals are rate dependent and decrease as rate increases. More complete information for the different waveforms and the other lead systems is available elsewhere.[20]

The shapes of the waves vary considerably, even within the same lead. The clinician should become familiar with such variation in order to be able to diagnose any abnormalities with confidence. The shape of the P wave is partly rate dependent, and, as the rate increases, the trough

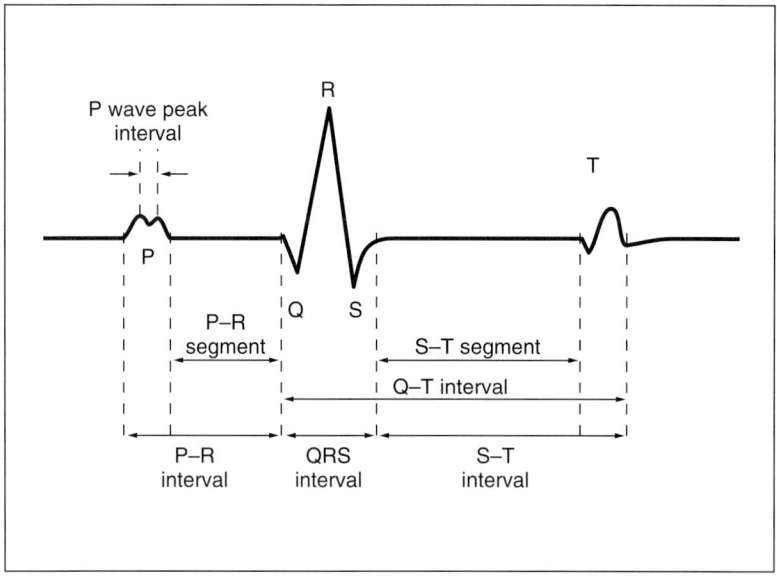

▶ **FIGURE 6-7**
Standard electrocardiogram demonstrating the nomenclature for the various waves, intervals, and segments.

between the two peaks tends to become smaller, or even to disappear, and the first part of the wave may be lost as the second section enlarges. Changes in shape, independent of rate, indicate that the origin of the atrial contraction is changing. The QRS complex is not so affected by an increase in rate until rates more associated with exercise (e.g., greater than 140 bpm) are achieved. The significance of variations in the T wave and the S-T segment has been a point of conjecture for some time. Recent data indicate that variation is physiological and is related to training. The reader is directed to the specific literature for further information.[21]

Fetal Electrocardiography

Fetal electrocardiography[22] is useful to monitor fetal distress during prolonged foaling, to confirm fetal viability, to diagnose twins, and in certain cases, such as in small mares, to diagnose pregnancy.

PROCEDURE. A bipolar lead system is used. The site for attachment of the electrodes is prepared as described for conventional electrocardiography. Self-adhesive or hand-held electrodes can be used, depending on the circumstances and the time over which monitoring is to be conducted. If monitoring is done when the mare is sweating profusely, special care is necessary to ensure that the self-adhesive electrodes do

not fall off. Human antiperspirant, sprayed onto the area of contact is, reportedly, useful in controlling this problem. The left-arm electrode is placed on the dorsal midline in the midlumbar region, and the left-leg electrode about 20 cm cranial to the udder in the ventral midline or to the left of the midline. A ground lead is not usually necessary. Lead 111, paper speed of 25 mm/s, and sensitivity of 1 cm per 1 mV are selected.

RESULTS. Fetal and maternal ECGs are superimposed. The fetal component usually consists only of a QRS complex, with occasional T waves appearing late in pregnancy. The complex can be positive, negative, or bipolar, varying mainly with fetal position. The amplitude of the fetal ECG is quite variable. The amplitude of the maternal ECG can be changed by moving the electrodes, and it is the lowest when the electrodes are on opposite

---

Requirements for Fetal Electrocardiography

- ▶ Electrocardiograph machine
- ▶ Bipolar lead system
- ▶ Electrodes (adhesive or hand-held electrode plates)
- ▶ Electrode gel

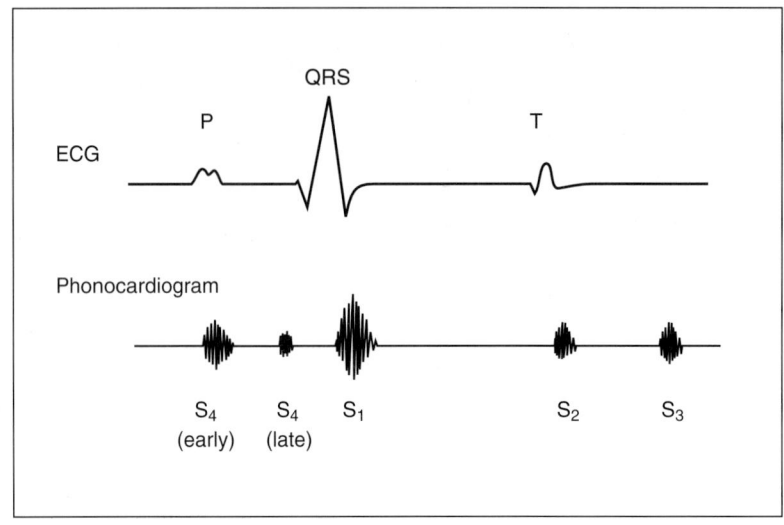

▶ FIGURE 6-8

Relationship between the electrocardiogram and the phonocardiogram.

sides of the abdomen. During gestation fetal heart rate decreases from about 120 to 90 bpm, and the maternal rate increases to about 60 bpm. Diagnosis of pregnancy is best delayed until approximately 150 days of gestation, in order to avoid false-positive diagnoses. When twin fetuses are present, two fetal QRS complexes are present. Moving the electrodes and having the mare walk around a little to stimulate a change in fetal positions will often help in improving identification of twin ECGs.

Fetal tachycardia and bradycardia are defined, respectively, as rates greater or lesser than two standard deviations from the mean. Intermittent tachycardia is normal and occurs especially during parturition. Prolonged tachycardia or excessively high values are indicative of fetal distress, as is bradycardia during parturition.

Phonocardiography

Phonocardiography is the graphical recording of the sounds generated during the cardiac cycle and requires a chest surface microphone and recording device.[23] It is usually carried out simultaneously with electrocardiography and is of considerable assistance in helping to identify sounds that are heard during auscultation. It is of particular value in the investigation of murmurs. Because most equine heart sounds have frequencies below 100 cycles per second (cps) and the normal human ear is capable of detecting frequencies in the range of 20 to 16,000 cps, the phonocardiogram clearly has the potential to improve the evaluation of low-frequency sounds.

A phonocardiogram and electrocardiogram demonstrating the relationship between the electrical and acoustic events occurring during a cardiac cycle are shown in Figure 6-8. The frequency and duration of each sound is relatively characteristic. However, the actual amplitude varies with the site at which the recording is made. The mean frequency and duration for S_1 are 35 to 39 cps and 0.15 to 0.20 secs, and for S_2 they are 57 to 59 and 0.09 to 0.11, respectively. The third sound, S_3, has lower amplitude and duration than S_1 and S_2 (duration of 0.04–0.08 s).

Echocardiography

The application of diagnostic ultrasound to the evaluation of cardiac disease has opened up a whole new world for the clinician. The various forms of the technology have made it possible to examine the form and function of the heart in a manner not possible with the traditional techniques such as palpation, auscultation, radiology, and cardiac catheterization. Unfortunately, much of the equipment is sophisticated and available only in specialized clinics and requires considerable practice and training to produce valid results and to interpret them. Above all else it requires a thorough knowledge of the three-dimensional structure of the heart, so that the clinician can quickly form a mental picture of any proposed section of the heart. The following comments are drawn mainly from a recent review.[24]

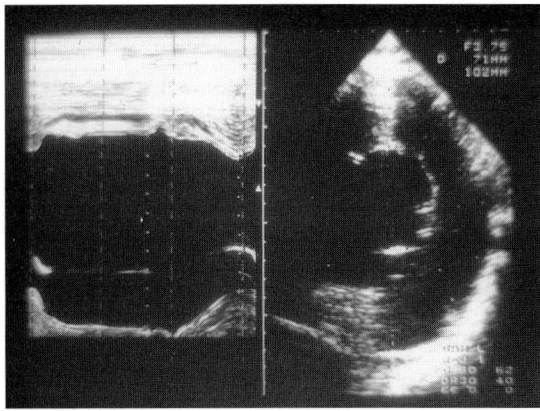

▶ **FIGURE 6-9**

M-mode (left) and two-dimensional (right) ultrasonograms. (Courtesy S. Church.)

M-Mode Echocardiography

M-mode (motion mode) echocardiography provides a one-dimensional representation of the heart and its component parts (Y axis) displayed against time (X axis). It is often called an "ice pick" image because it is composed of a series of closely related points representing repeated signals derived from a particular site at a tissue interface. An ECG is simultaneously displayed so that the cardiac events can be related to the changes in dimension and shape seen in the sonogram. An example of an M-mode sonogram is shown in Figure 6-9. It should be remembered that each series of points in a vertical reference frame represent reflections of ultrasound from different tissue interfaces at one particular time and that the distance between them is related to the actual thickness of the tissues or how far apart they are. As each set of new data is added, the record moves to the right, and by monitoring vertical displacement of the points the clinician can detect changes in the position and thickness of each structure during the cardiac cycle. This form of imaging is now usually performed in conjunction with two-dimensional echocardiography (see later), using the latter technique to guide the placement of the M-mode cursor across the desired structures. Measurements obtained in this way are superior to those using "blind" M-mode echocardiography. Because this methodology has a high sampling rate, it is particularly valuable for measuring subtle variations in movement and thickness of valves and heart wall. The M-mode echocardiogram is routinely used to record the timing of the various events in the cardiac cycle and to measure the size of the cardiac chambers and the thickness of their walls. Measurements are usually made at the end of diastole and systole using the ECG as a guide to these events. End-diastolic measurements are made at the beginning of the QRS complex and systolic measurements during maximum excursion of the ventricular septum.

Data on normal values for cardiac parameters in foals[25,26] and horses[27,28] are available, and experience with diseased hearts is accumulating.

Two-Dimensional Echocardiography

Two-dimensional echocardiography produces a two-dimensional slice of the heart. The image has depth (Y axis) and width but no thickness, and it must be constantly updated to evaluate motion, which is indicated by the changes in shape and position of cardiac structures. Motion is therefore constructed in a fashion similar to the frame-by-frame construction of a movie film. Although more complicated than M-mode echocardiography, the two-dimensional echocardiogram is initially easier to interpret because the image is easier to relate to the three-dimensional form of the heart.

The direction and the plane of the scan must be precisely known to maximize interpretation and reproducibility. The heart can be imaged from either the left or right windows (left or right thoracic views), utilizing long and short axis views. The long-axis plane sections the heart parallel to its long axis (saggital plane), and the short-axis plane is perpendicular to this (coronal plane). Two-dimensional echocardiography is useful for detecting septal defects, valvular lesions, and cardiac dilation.

Although some standardization can be achieved by specifying the location of the transducer on the horse, the considerable anatomical variations between horses and the almost infinite number of possible image planes are serious disadvantages. This problem can be overcome by devising a system of standardizing the image planes, based first on the position of the transducer on the body wall and then on specified intracardiac landmarks.[29] Appropriate imaging of specific structures also requires consideration of the sector rotation of the transducer as well as its angulation.

Doppler Echocardiography

Doppler echocardiography provides a noninvasive means of evaluating blood flow and therefore a way of assessing the significance of heart murmurs.[30] Previously, evaluation was done indirectly by assessing parameters such as chamber enlargement, valve motion, wall abnormalities, and the size of a defect. The technique is based on the Doppler shift, whereby a frequency change occurs when there is relative motion between the source of sound and the receiver. In this case the moving component is the blood, and the receiver is the transducer. With flow of blood toward the transducer, the sound wave is reflected back with an increase in frequency and vice versa. The angle between the ultrasound beam and the vector of blood flow is important in the derivation of Doppler echocardiographic images, but optimal results require that the angle of incidence be as close to zero as possible and certainly less than 20°. As the angle increases from 20° to 60°, the underestimation of velocity increases from 6% to 50%. With some modern equipment it is possible to correct for angle. However, under certain conditions, this may overestimate velocity. The velocity is displayed with spectral analysis with normal flow, in which blood cells are moving at a uniform velocity in the same direction, producing a narrow line on the spectral tracing. The tracing broadens when flow is disturbed by variation in direction and velocity.

PULSED-WAVE DOPPLER ECHOCARDIOGRAPHY. This form of Doppler echocardiography involves the transmission of a pulse of ultrasound to a preselected depth in the tissue and the recording of the reflected wave. The cycle is then repeated, with the pulse repetition frequency being limited by the distance to the target. The maximum velocity that can be measured is a function of the transducer and the distance to the target. The low-frequency transducers used are in the order of 2.25 MHz, and the maximum depth of investigation is approximately 18 cm. This can place some regions beyond the range of the equipment. Superimposition of the Doppler echocardiogram on a two-dimensional echocardiogram can be used to evaluate the extent of regurgitation through a valve or flow through a shunt, a process called *flow mapping.* The principle is based on the fact that such disordered flow produces a broadening of the spectral tracing that, when superimposed on the two-dimensional image, provides an index of the area of affected flow and therefore an estimate of the severity of the defect.

CONTINUOUS-WAVE DOPPLER ECHOCARDIOGRAPHY. Continuous-wave Doppler echocardiography uses two ultrasonic crystals that function simultaneously, one continuously emitting an ultrasonic signal and the other continuously receiving it. The advantage of this system over the pulsed-wave system is that there is no limitation on the maximum velocity that can be measured. However, because there is no range resolution, flow is detected along the entire axis of the ultrasound beam. This technique is usually performed without guidance from two-dimensional echocardiography, although some equipment has the ability to combine the two methods.

If the peak velocity is known, it can be used to obtain noninvasively pressure differences between chambers as well as cardiac output. However, it is often impossible to obtain this information because the ability to measure accurately peak velocities is compromised by the equine anatomy, which frequently makes it difficult or impossible to keep the angle between the ultrasound beam and the direction of flow to less than 20°.

COLOR FLOW DOPPLER ECHOCARDIOGRAPHY. Color flow Doppler echocardiography involves the superimposition of a two-dimensional color image of blood flow on a two-dimensional echocardiographic image. The ultrasound is emitted in bursts, and the pulse repetition frequency depends on the time between each burst. The image is a composite of the spatial distribution of mean velocities rather than peak velocities. The mean frequency shift information is color-coded for direction and velocity, with three types of Doppler maps commonly used: red and blue, enhanced, and velocity variance. Flow toward the transducer is usually red, and flow away is blue. The enhancement maps are used to demonstrate higher velocities, and the variance, using an overlay of green, records different velocities and flow directions. Color flow Doppler echocardiography therefore provides information about the direction, velocity, and turbulence of flow. Data concerning location are supplied by two-dimensional echocardiography. The restrictions imposed by depth and angle are similar to the ones found in other forms of Doppler echocardiography. The method can be used to refine continuous-wave Doppler echocardiography by ensuring that the sensor is located in the area of highest velocity.

Procedures for Standardized Imaging for Guided Two-Dimensional, M-Mode, and Doppler Echocardiography

The examination is carried out on the awake, standing, and, when possible, unsedated horse.[29] It is important that there is no motion during the examination. To obtain optimum images, the hair should be clipped from an area in the region of the fourth to fifth intercostal spaces on the right and left sides of the thorax centered just above the olecranon. This corresponds to a strip overlying the caudal border of, and just caudal to, the triceps muscles. Acoustic coupling gel is placed on the skin as well as on the transducer. Correct positioning of the transducer requires the foreleg to be slightly advanced and abducted. To image from the right hemithorax, the transducer is placed at the fourth or fifth intercostal space just dorsal to the olecranon process, and from the left hemithorax caudal to the olecranon process and dorsal to the left apical pulse. Although orientation can be achieved by using standardized intercostal locations, the technique can be refined by using a combination of the transducer locations just described and certain intracardiac landmarks. From the right side the reference image is a long-axis view of the ventricular inlets, and from the left it is a long-axis view of the left atrium and ventricle, from which the other standardized views can be obtained by varying the location, rotation, and angulation of the transducer.[29] The two-dimensional images obtained in this way are then used to guide the placement of the cursor for accurate M-mode measurements, the placement of Doppler sampling gates, and the overlay of Doppler color flow maps. A simultaneous ECG is used to define the events within the cardiac cycle. End-diastolic measurements are taken at the beginning of the QRS complex, and systolic measurements are taken during maximum excursion of the ventricular septum. When tissue interfaces are parallel to the beam measurements are made using the "leading edge trailing edge method," and, when they are perpendicular, the "leading edge method" is used. Specific details of the techniques can be found in the references.[29,30]

Radiography and Nuclear Cardiology

Radiography

Although radiographic examination of the human and small animal heart is extremely valuable and commonly carried out, similar, comprehensive evaluation of the equine heart is not possible.[31] In small ponies and foals it is sometimes possible to achieve the necessary radiographic projections. However, the results are seldom adequate, even in smaller equines. The sheer size and well-developed shoulder musculature of the larger horses are the main barriers. Penetrating the dorsal and caudal regions of the thorax is usually possible, and useful images of the dorsal and caudal cardiac borders can be produced. Extension of the forelimb can improve the chances of seeing the cranial thorax in small horses and foals. In plain radiographs the manifestations of cardiac disease include cardiac enlargement (cardiomegaly), alteration in lung density reflecting changes in lung perfusion and pulmonary edema, and pleural effusion.

Cardiomegaly is the result of cardiac dilation, muscular hypertrophy, or both. In other species indices of cardiomegaly include tracheal elevation, increased sternal and diaphragmatic contact, and variation in cardiac outline. Although high-quality radiographs are difficult to obtain in large horses, similar criteria apply whenever diagnostic radiographs can be taken. Increased lung density may be associated with overperfusion (left-to-right shunts) and venous congestion (left heart failure). Overperfusion can result in enlargement of vessels and an increase in the number of visible vessels, and underperfusion (right-to-left shunts) is manifested as decreased density. The gradual development of left heart insufficiency produces venous congestion, interstitial edema, and, finally, alveolar edema. Edema is manifested as a patchy or granular increase in density seen best in the dorsocaudal regions. Pleural effusion will cause a loss of visualization of the heart and lungs in the ventral thorax. These signs can also accompany noncardiac disease such as pneumonia and neoplasia, and the exact pattern of radiological abnormality will vary with the disease and its severity.

Angiocardiography

Angiocardiography is a contrast radiographic technique whereby a radiograph is used to detect the presence of intravascularly administered contrast material as it passes through the heart or through the region of specific interest. By outlining vessels, cardiac chambers and valve orifices, and by demonstrating abnormal communication between chambers and vessels, the technique is useful for investigating some aspects of cardiac anatomy and function. Unfortunately, the size of the animal places severe limitations on its application to horses. Consequently it is really useful only in very small animals such as small ponies and foals.

The contrast material can be deposited into a peripheral vessel by direct injection or into a specific vessel or the heart through a catheter positioned with its tip located in the region of interest, for nonselective or selective studies, respectively. Both methods usually require rapid injection of material and then a series of rapid radiographic exposures, both of which are extremely difficult in large animals. As a result of this, the technique has been used mainly to investigate congenital abnormalities in neonates.

Angiography

Contrast radiography to evaluate peripheral vessels (angiography) has an application in horses of all sizes. Conditions in which this technique is useful include mycosis of the guttural pouch, shunts, and AV fistulae. The most common indication has been to investigate arterial lesions related to guttural pouch mycosis.[32]

Scintigraphy or Nuclear Angiocardiography

Nuclear angiocardiography is an imaging technique that does not face the same size limitations as traditional radiography. It involves intravenous injection of a radioactive tracer and then monitoring of its subsequent passage through the heart lungs and great vessels with a gamma camera. The images are recorded on film or as digital files if appropriate conversion and computer facilities are available. Following digital conversion of the analog signal, the data can be analyzed with special software to allow quantitative cardiac studies.

The first of these computerized studies is known as first-pass nuclear cardioangiography (FPNC) and the second as gated-equilibrium nuclear cardioangiography (GENA). FPNC follows the passage of the tracer through the right heart, lungs, and left heart, and a 30-s acquisition is usually adequate to image the full sequence. Abnormal findings include prolonged transit time (congestive heart failure), enlargement of cardiac chambers (valvular malfunction, myocardial failure), simultaneous visualization of the left and right ventricles (intracardiac shunts), and slower-than-normal clearance ("washout") of the tracer from vessels or cardiac chambers (valvular malfunction, myocardial failure).

In another method, GENA, data acquisition is triggered by a signal from a simultaneously recorded ECG, which allows the collection of a series of images from an identical time in the cardiac cycle. Such studies require a stable blood pool of tracer and minimal patient movement (recumbent anesthetized horses).

Blood Pressure Recording

Blood pressure measurement is a routine procedure in human medicine, where it is regularly carried out as part of the clinical examination. It is rarely used for this purpose in equine medicine, but, instead, it finds its major role in monitoring the anesthetized patient and in certain circumstances, when information concerning blood pressure is specifically indicated, such as shock, cardiac disease, and in research investigations of the cardiovascular system. Blood pressure can be recorded in the heart, arteries, and peripheral and central veins. With specialized equipment capillary pressures can also be measured. Measurement of arterial pressure can be indirect, with a pressure cuff, or direct, with a needle or catheter inserted into the vessel.

Arterial Pressure

DIRECT ARTERIAL PRESSURE. To obtain direct arterial blood pressure a catheter or needle is placed in the artery and connected to a measuring device, usually a pressure transducer.[33] The most common application of this form of measurement is patient monitoring during anesthesia, where accuracy and the ability to record rapid pressure fluctuations are required.

Procedure. There is considerable variation in personal preference for equipment and procedure. An important difference between the measuring devices is that the aneroid barometer yields only mean arterial pressure, whereas a pressure transducer can measure systolic and diastolic pressures. The following method is just one of the many that could be described. The artery of choice, usually the facial or transverse facial artery, is clipped and prepared for sterile puncture. The extension tubing and stopcock are connected and flushed with heparinized saline. The artery is localized using the pulse as a guide. When using a cannula, as opposed to a "Butterfly" needle, it is preferable to make a small incision in the skin to facilitate insertion.

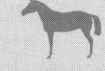

Materials for Measuring Direct Arterial Pressure

‣ Vascular cannula (cannula-over-the needle [e.g., Travenol Quick-Cath], "Butterfly" needle [Abbot], 3–5 cm, 18–20 gauge for adults; 3 cm, 20–22 gauge for foals)

‣ Three-way stopcock

‣ Plastic tubing to connect system to measuring device

‣ Material to attach cannula to skin (suture, superglue, or adhesive tape)

‣ Short extension tube

‣ Heparinized saline (2 units/mL)

‣ Continuous infusion valve (optional)

‣ Pressure-measuring device (aneroid barometer, transducer [e.g., Statham] and recorder)

The device is slowly inserted until blood flows. The cannula is then inserted fully while holding the needle, the needle is removed, the extension tubing and stopcock attached, and the whole system is then connected to the transducer and flushed with heparinized saline as necessary to establish and maintain patency. The cannula should be attached to the skin with a suture, superglue, or adhesive tape. To maintain patency during recording the system can be flushed intermittently through the three-way stopcock or with a continuous-infusion device. Pressure measurements vary with the difference in height between the transducer and the heart, which is important if accurate values are necessary but not if only approximate values or identification of variation in pressures are required. In any case the position of the transducer relative to the heart should be recorded. After removing the cannula, maintain digital pressure over the site for a few minutes to prevent the formation of hematomata.

Arteries that are readily accessible for direct pressure recording include:[34]

• Dorsal metatarsal a
• Transverse facial a
• Facial a
• Digital aa

The aneroid barometer records mean arterial pressure, and the strain-gauge transducer with a recorder displays systolic and diastolic pressures.

Complications. Hematoma formation is the most common complication. Hematomata form quickly when blood is able to leave the vessel through a needle puncture, which can occur during insertion if the vessel is penetrated more than once or, usually, when the procedure is completed and the catheter is removed. People often experience pain and a stinging sensation when a hematoma is present, and it is likely that horses also do. Hematomata formation is minimized first by careful placement of the catheter and then by maintaining firm digital pressure over the artery after the catheter is removed. If possible, a pressure bandage is also useful, especially if the horse is to recover from anesthesia and elevation in blood pressure is expected.

INDIRECT ARTERIAL PRESSURE. There are a number of different methods for deriving indirect blood pressure measurements that are acceptable estimates of direct arterial pressure. In people, blood pressure is routinely measured indirectly by placing an inflatable cuff around the upper arm, and similar techniques have been developed for horses, with the cuff being placed around the base of the tail as well as the lower leg. The method consists of occluding the artery by inflating the cuff to a pressure greater than systolic pressure and then allowing it to deflate while monitoring the return of a pulse distal to the cuff. The pressure in the cuff can be measured with an aneroid manometer, mercury column, or a transducer, but the main component is the device used to record the return of the distal pulse.

Methods to detect pulse return include systems based on auscultation (stethoscopic detection of Korotkoff sounds with or without amplification by microphone), palpation (manual detection of pulse), identification of pressure fluctuations with an oscillometer or xylol pulse detector, and Doppler ultrasonic techniques to detect blood flow or motion of the arterial wall. Not all systems are efficient or suitable for use in horses. The methods used most commonly are those based on ultrasonic technology, from which systolic and diastolic pressures are derived, and the oscillometric evaluation of pressure fluctuations in the cuff, from which systolic, diastolic and mean arterial pressures are derived. The accuracy and reproducibility of the methods depend on numerous factors, a very important one being the width of the cuff relative to the structure it is placed around. The middle coccygeal artery has become the standard site for indirect blood pressure measurement in horses. The optimum cuff-width-to-tail-circumference ratio varies depending on whether systolic or diastolic pressures are being measured. However, as the use of different cuffs is impractical, a compromise between the two is reached. Using a Doppler ultrasound method to detect flow, a ratio for cuff width to tail circumference of approximately 0.5 will provide systolic pressures about 9% lower and diastolic pressures about 9% higher than the actual pressures in the middle coccygeal artery.[35] With the oscillometric method, a ratio of 0.20 to 0.25 is recommended.

Procedure. The procedure can be carried out on conscious or anesthetized horses. If conscious, the horse should be relaxed, but not tranquilized, and the head should be in a normal position (blood pressure is reduced by tranquilization and lowering the head and increased by raising the head). The cuff is wrapped firmly around the base of the tail, with the bladder centered over the middle coccygeal artery. If the oscillometric method is being used, no further steps are necessary. For the Doppler methods care should be taken to position the probes over the artery and to use an ultrasonographic coupling gel to maximize acoustic contact.

The oscillometric method records systolic pressure as the point when bladder pressure fluctuations begin to increase in amplitude; mean arterial pressure when maximum bladder pressure fluctuations occur; and diastolic pressure when fluctuations stop decreasing. To use the Doppler methods, the cuff is inflated to a pressure about 20 mmHg higher than the expected systolic pressure and then deflated at about 2 to 3 mm Hg per heart beat. Systolic pressure is taken as the first audible sound occurs (using blood flow or wall-motion detectors), and diastolic pressure when a distinct second sound occurs (using flow detector), when there is a change in pitch, volume, or both, when two distinct sounds disappear, or when a constant rumble is heard (using wall-motion detectors).

The values obtained can be corrected to heart level or left unchanged as coccygeal uncorrected values (CUCV). Correction to heart level is done by adding or subtracting 0.77 mmHg for each 1 cm the site of measurement is above or below the heart. Correction to heart level in the standing horse is done using the notch on the lateral tuberosity of the humerus (shoulder level), and

---

NORMAL ARTERIAL BLOOD PRESSURE (Mean ± SD, measured indirectly)[36]

- Systolic pressure 111.8 ± 13.3 mmHg
- Diastolic pressure 67.7 ± 13.8 mmHg

---

in the recumbent horse the olecranon (elbow level) is used as the reference point. If correction is made, results are expressed as coccygeal, shoulder-corrected values (CCVsh), or coccygeal elbow-corrected values (CCVe).

Results. Some normal values for resting arterial blood pressure in horses are presented in the box. The values at which a reading can be regarded as hyper- or hypotensive is at present not well established. There is apparently no effect of age or sex on pressure. Although the class of horse does have an influence, the basis for this is not known but may simply be a consequence of temperament.

Intracardiac and Outflow Tract Pressures

Pressures in the heart and its outflow tracts are usually measured for research purposes and investigation of cardiac anomalies. To measure right-heart and pulmonary artery pressures, a catheter must be inserted into a large vein and then passed into the right atrium, right ventricle, and then out into the pulmonary artery. To measure aortic and left-heart pressures, the catheter must be passed retrograde up an artery.

Some values for intracardiac and outflow tract pressures are presented in the box.

INTRACARDIAC AND OUTFLOW TRACT PRESSURES[37] (systolic/diastolic mmHg)

- Right atrium   12–28/–2 – +5
- Right ventricle   30–59/–4 – +14
- Pulmonary artery   34–48/14–22
- Pulmonary artery wedge   13/3
- Left ventricle   140–148/15–17
- Aorta   131–144/86–100
- Carotid artery   142–157/98–119

Central Venous Pressure

Central venous blood pressure is a measure of venous return to the heart, vasomotor tone, and of the heart's efficiency as a pump. Most forms of shock are characterized by reduced venous return and venous pressure. Loss of vasomotor tone will also reduce venous pressure. Failure of the heart to pump because of weakness, valvular stenosis, or insufficiency, or abnormal flow as a result of communication between chambers or vessels will cause venous pressures to rise. Venous pressure can be recorded from any of the large veins. However, it is usual to measure central venous pressure from a site close to the right atrium where it is not affected by venous valves. It is therefore, a measure of blood returning from the head and neck as well as the limbs and trunk.

PROCEDURE.   Central venous pressure is usually measured in anesthetized horses, although it is quite a simple matter to record it in cooperative, conscious animals. The site of insertion of the catheter, usually the jugular vein, is clipped and then prepared for aseptic venepuncture. The trochar is inserted into the vein and directed toward the heart. The catheter is then inserted through the trochar and into the central venous system far enough to reach the anterior vena cava or right atrium. To avoid accidentally severing the catheter, it is most important that it is not withdrawn through the trochar while the trochar is still in the vein. The trochar should be withdrawn as soon as the catheter is in position. The catheter is then attached to the fluid-filled tubing and the measuring device, which is posi-

---

> ### CENTRAL VENOUS PRESSURE: Normal Values
> ....
> - Anesthetized horses
>   Dorsal recumbency: 5–10 cm water
>   Lateral recumbency: 20–30 cm water
> - Standing horses: <10 cm water

---

tioned at heart level. Heart level is taken as the point of the shoulder. Whether a pressure transducer or a calibrated tube is used, it should have the facility of flushing the system between measurements with heparinized saline. Measurement is made by opening the stopcock to establish communication between the intravenous catheter and the measuring device.

RESULTS.   Venous pressure does not fluctuate like arterial pressure and is instead represented by a steady recording with minor fluctuations representing cardiac or respiratory movements. Because they are so low and because of the way in which they are usually measured, venous pressures are usually reported in centimeters of water (cm H_2O). The value obtained is greatly dependent on where the zero point is positioned.

COMPLICATIONS.   Although the method is relatively safe, complications can occur:

- *Loss of the catheter.* This occurs when the catheter is severed by withdrawing it through the trochar while the trochar is still within the vein. The severed piece of catheter will usually be transported to or through the heart, depending on how stiff it is. Embolus of a catheter is a serious matter as cardiac and pulmonary trauma and thrombosis with secondary embolism, maybe septic, can occur. Retrieval of a catheter can be achieved, especially if it is radio-opaque. However, it is preferable to avoid the complication by never pulling the catheter back through the trochar while it is within the vein.
- *Cardiac arrhythmias.* These may occur if the catheter enters the heart, but are rare unless the catheter is very stiff. Use of appropriate catheters will usually avoid this problem.
- *Abnormal placement of the catheter.* The catheter can be passed inadvertently into

---

Materials for Measuring Central Venous Pressure

- Intravascular silastic catheter of sufficient length to reach the central venous circulation
- Venous trochar
- Measuring devices (pressure transducer or calibrated plastic manometer attached to a vertical support)
- Connecting tubing and three-way stopcock
- Heparinized saline (2 units/mL)

vessels other than the central venous system. Extreme fluctuations of pressure associated with thoracic movements are an indication of improper placement. Correct positioning can be ensured by passing the catheter into the heart and then withdrawing it into the atrium or vena cava. Entry of the catheter into the heart is confirmed by using a pressure transducer and recording device to identify cardiac pressures and the characteristic waveforms. Relevant pressures (systolic/diastolic) are:[37]

- Right atrium: 12–28/–2 to +5 mmHg
- Right ventricle: 30–59/–4 to +14 mmHg
- Pulmonary artery: 34–48/14–22 mmHg

R E F E R E N C E S

1. Leatham A: A classification of systolic murmurs. Br Heart J 1955; 17:574.
2. Leatham A: Auscultation of the heart: Heart murmurs. Lancet 1958; 2:757.
3. McKusik VA: Cardiovascular sounds. Circulation 1957; 16:270–290 and 414–436.
4. Detweiler DK, Patterson DF: The cardiovascular system. In Catcott EJ, Smithcors JF (eds), Equine Medicine and Surgery. Santa Barbara, American Veterinary Publications, 1972, pp 277–347.
5. Littlewort MCG: The clinical auscultation of the equine heart. Vet Rec 1962; 74:1247.
6. Smith CR, Smetzer DL, Hamlin RL, et al: Normal heart sounds and murmurs in the horse. In Proceedings of the 8th Annual Convention of American Association of Equine Practitioners, 1962, p 46.
7. Long KJ: The clinical assessment of heart murmurs in the horse. NZ Vet Ass Equine Newsletter June 1990; p 4–8.
8. Glendinning SA: Significance of clinical abnormalities of the heart in soundness. Equine Vet J 1972; 4:21.
9. Patteson MW, Cripps PJ: A survey of cardiac auscultatory findings in horses. Equine Vet J 1993; 25:409.
10. Evans DL: The cardiovascular system: Anatomy, physiology, and adaptations to exercise and training. In Hodgson DR, Rose RJ (eds), The Athletic Horse. Philadelphia, Saunders, 1994, ch 7, p 129.
11. Evans DL, Rose RJ: A method of investigation of the accuracy of four digitally displaying heart rate meters suitable for use in the exercising horse. Equine Vet J 1986; 18:129.
12. Ecker G: Using the heart rate monitor. Equine Vet Ed 1991; 3:232.
13. Senta T, Smetzer DL, Smith CR: Effects of exercise on certain electrocardiographic parameters and cardiac arrhythmias in the horse: A radiotelemetric study. Cornell Vet 1970; 60:552.
14. Steel JD, Hall MC, Stewart GA: Cardiac monitoring during exercise tests in the horse: 3. Changes in the electrocardiogram during and after exercise. Aust Vet J 1976; 52:6.
15. Holmes JR: An investigation of cardiac rhythm using an on-line radiotelemetry/computor link. J S Afr Vet Assoc 1974; 45:251.
16. Holmes JR, Alps BJ: The effect of exercise on rhythm irregularities in the horse. Vet Rec 1966; 78:672.
17. Holmes JR: Cardiac arrhythmias on the racecourse. In Gillespie JR, Robinson NE (eds), Equine Exercise Physiology, ed 2, Davis, CA, ICEEP Publications, 1987, p 781.
18. Australian Equine Veterinary Association: Guidelines for Equine Electrocardiography. Sydney 1981.
19. Rose RJ, Hodgson DR (eds): Cardiovascular System. In Manual of Equine Practice. Philadelphia, Saunders, 1993, ch 5, p 175.
20. Fregin GF: Electrocardiology. In Cardiology. Vet Clin Nth Am: Equine Pract 1985; 1:419.
21. Evans DL: T waves in the equine electrocardiogram: effects of training and implications for race performance. In Persson SGB, Lindholm A, Jeffcott LB (eds): Equine Exercise Physiology, 3rd ed, Davis CA, ICEEP Publications, 1991, p 475.
22. Coles CM: Fetal electrocardiography. In Robinson NE (ed), Current Therapy In Equine Medicine, Philadelphia, Saunders, 1987, p 152.
23. Reef VB: Evaluation of the equine cardiovascular system. Vet Clin North Am: Equine Prac 1985; 1:275.
24. Reef RB: Advances in echocardiography. Vet Clin North Am: Equine Pract 1991; 7:435.
25. Stewart JH, Rose RJ, Barko AM: Echocardiography in foals from birth to three months old. Equine Vet J 1984; 16:332.
26. Lombard CW, Evans M, Martin L, et al: Blood pressure, electrocardiogram and echocardiogram measurements in the growing pony foal. Equine Vet J 1984; 16:342.
27. Lescure F, Tamzali Y: Valeurs de référence en échocardiographie T M chez le cheval de sport. Revue Med Vet 1984; 135:405.
28. Paull KS, Wingfield WE, Bertone JJ, Boon JA: Echocardiographic changes with endurance training. In Gillespie JR, Rose RJ (eds), Equine Exercise Physiology, ed 2, Davis, CA, ICEEP Publications, 1987, p 34.
29. Long KJ, Bonagura JD, Darke PGG: Standardized imaging technique for guided M-mode and Doppler echocardiography in the horse. Equine Vet J 1992; 24:226.
30. Long KJ: Doppler echocardiography—clinical applications. Equine Vet J 1993; 5:161.
31. Koblik PD, Hornof WJ: Diagnostic radiology and nuclear cardiography. Their use in assessment of equine cardiovascular disease. Vet Clin North Am: Equine Pract 1985; 1:289.
32. Colles CM, Cook WR: Carotid and cerebral angiography in the horse. Vet Rec 1983; 113:483.
33. Taylor PM: Techniques and clinical application of arterial blood pressure measurement in the horse. Equine Vet J 1981; 13:271.
34. Rose RJ, Rossdale PD: Techniques and clinical application of arterial blood collection in the horse. Equine Vet J 1981; 13:70.
35. Parry BW, McCarthy MA, Anderson GA, Gay CC: Correct occlusive bladder width for indirect blood pressure measurement in horses. Am J Vet Res 1982; 43:50.
36. Johnson JH, Garner HE, Hutcheson DP: Ultrasonic measurement of arterial blood pressure in conditioned Thoroughbreds. Equine Vet J 1976; 8:55.
37. Fregin GF: The cardiovascular system. In Mansmann RA, McAllister ES (eds), Equine Medicine and Surgery, vol 1, ed 3, Santa Barbara, CA, American Veterinary Publishing, Inc. 1982, p 645.

Examination of the Female Reproductive System

COMPONENTS

The female reproductive tract has internal and external components. These include the vulva; tubular components consisting of vestibule, vagina, cervix, uterus, and fallopian tubes; and ovaries. Only the vulva is visible to unassisted examination.

In addition to a knowledge of basic anatomy, the clinician examining the female reproductive tract requires detailed knowledge of certain specific regions because of their relevance to disease. This concerns mainly the conformation of the vulva, vestibule, vagina, and cervix in relation to predisposition to infection and the structure and morphological changes of the uterus and ovaries during the various stages of the reproductive cycle. The most frequent examinations of the tract are carried out to diagnose the presence and duration of pregnancy.

The normal vulva has firmly sealed lips, is almost vertically positioned and lies so that approximately two thirds lie below the level of the ischial arch. A specific variation of this normal structure, seen in older mares and also as a conformational abnormality, is where the anus and vulva are displaced cranially into the pelvis so that the vulval lips are sloping dorsocranially and lie in an exposed position beneath the anus where the chances of fecal contamination are increased.

The vestibule and vagina are tubular structures that are normally collapsed. An obvious constriction, the vulvovaginal constriction, is present just cranial to the urethral opening.

MANIFESTATIONS OF DISEASE

Because the reproductive tract is mainly an internal system, the manifestations of disease are often not visible to an external examination. The obvious exceptions, are lesions of the vulva where evidence of inflammation (reddening, exudation, erosion, ulceration, vesicles, swelling), neoplasia (swelling, erosion, ulceration, bleeding), and trauma are easily seen. Similar processes that occur internally, within the tubular system, produce external signs only when the volume of exudate or blood is sufficient for it to flow to the exterior. Detecting internal lesions requires the use of a variety of examination techniques and equipment. Systemic signs often associated with internal lesions include pyrexia, depression, weight loss, inappetance associated with infection; abdominal enlargement associated with accumulation of intrauterine fluids; pain associated with ovarian lesions; and hemorrhagic shock associated with arterial rupture.

RESTRAINT

Restraint is particularly important because the examiner has to stand behind the mare, in a potentially dangerous position. The degree of restraint and the actual method used depend on the examiner, the available facilities, and the temperament of the mare. The objectives are, of course, to prevent the mare from kicking the examiner or injuring herself, while allowing a thorough examination.

Most examinations are carried out in a crush, with or without a twitch. When a crush is not available, the examiner can be protected by placing bales of hay or straw behind the mare, by working with the mare positioned in or beside a doorway, and by preventing the mare from kicking with careful use of sidelines or hind leg hobbles. Kicking can often be prevented simply by lifting a foreleg on the same side as the one on which the examiner is standing. Whatever meth-

ods are used, the mare should be handled gently and carefully.

GENERAL PHYSICAL EXAMINATION

The general physical examination consists of the following components carried out in a sequence that may vary between clinicians.

Examination of the Tail, Vulva, and Perineum

The vulva is examined to check conformation and for evidence of injury. The normal vulva is oriented almost vertically, about two thirds of it lie below the ischial arch (Fig. 7–1A). It should have no scars, and no exudate should be present. Old or emaciated mares or those with specific conformational abnormalities may have a sunken anus with an associated craniodorsal displacement of the vulva (Fig. 7–1B). The vulva should be checked for wounds or scars from previous parturition trauma or Caslick's surgery.

The variation in vulval conformation has been characterized by the Caslick Index (CI), which is

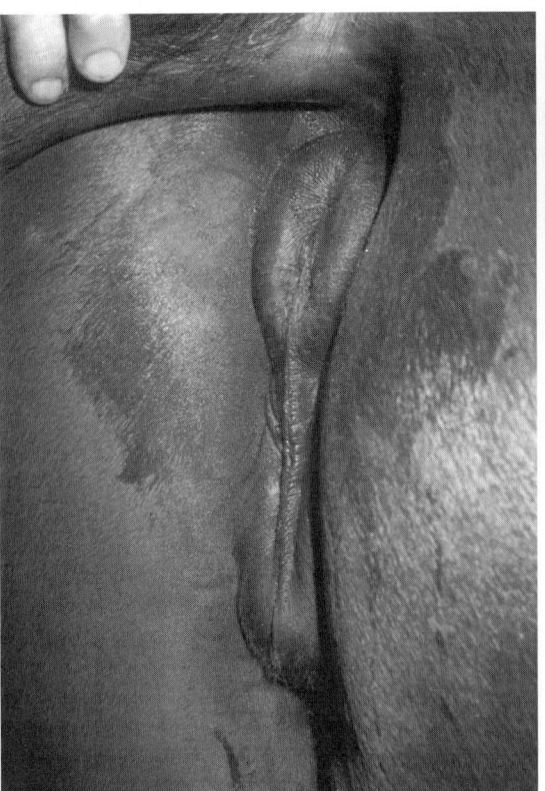

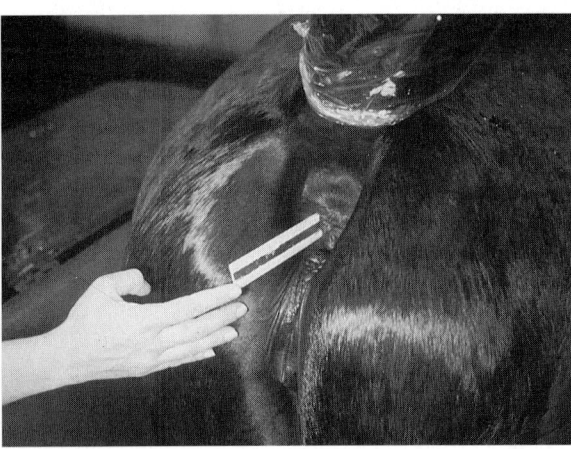

B

▶ **FIGURE 7–1**

Vulval and anal conformation. **A.** Normal. Note the vertical orientation of the vulva as it lies directly below the anus. **B.** Abnormal. Displacement of the anus and malalignment of the vulva in an old mare. Note the cranial displacement of the anus and the oblique alignment of the dorsal part of the vulva as it has become displaced up and over the pelvic brim. (Courtesy A. O. McKinnon.)

A

used as an index of predisposition to infection.[1] The index equals the effective length (cm) of the vulva (distance between the dorsal vulval commissure and the pelvic floor) multiplied by the angle of declination. Vulvoperineal conformation can also be classified as follows:

- *Type I.* <2–3 cm of vulva dorsal to pelvic floor, CI < 100
- *Type II.* 6–7 cm of vulva dorsal to pelvic floor, CI > 50
- *Type III.* 5–9 cm dorsal to pelvic floor, CI 50– > 100

As the conformation becomes increasingly abnormal, there is greater predisposition to pneumovagina, which in turn predisposes to bacterial contamination of the vagina and uterus and ultimately to infection. Urovagina, which is characterized by displacement of the urethral orifice cranial to the ischium, also occurs and also contributes to infection.

Speculum Examination of the Vagina and Cervix

This form of examination requires good restraint because, in order to see properly, the examiner must stand behind the horse and bend over a little. To avoid contamination of the vagina, the perineum and vulva should be cleansed with warm water and a suitable antiseptic. The speculum should be lubricated and, after separating the vulval lips with the fingers, is inserted in a dorsocranial direction to clear the pelvic brim. Resistance is often met at the vestibulovaginal junction. As the speculum is fully inserted air rushes into and dilates the vagina. There are many different types of specula, which can be made from metal, plastic, or cardboard. The usual metal speculum is the familiar duck-billed instrument that, although effective, requires a separate light source and is difficult to clean, particularly for multiple examinations. The plastic instrument commonly used has the advantage that the plastic insertion barrel can be easily cleaned and sterilized and, because they are cheap and separate from the light source, a number of preprepared barrels can be carried (Figure 7-2). The cardboard instrument has a silvered interior wall that allows light from a separate light source to be reflected.

The conformation of the vagina is important in brood mares. The normal vagina slopes dorsally, but as tissues lose support and become lax,

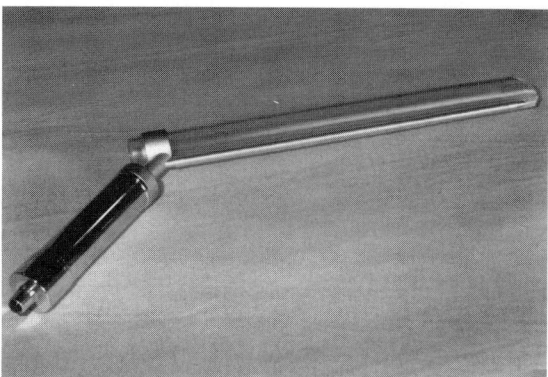

▶ **FIGURE 7–2**
Vaginal speculum.

the vagina and vestibule are displaced cranially. This may lead to urovagina (urine pooling, or vesicovaginal reflux), a condition in which the vagina slopes downward in a cranial direction, allowing urine to pool caudal to the cervix, contributing to chronic infection. The urine can be seen lying in a pool immediately cranial to the cervix (Fig. 7-3).

Palpation of the Vagina and Cervix per Vaginam

Manual examination of the vagina is easily performed by inserting the lubricated, gloved hand through a previously prepared vulva. The fingers can be used to examine the urethral opening, the hymen, vagina, and cervix. The cervix can be penetrated at all stages of the reproductive cycle.

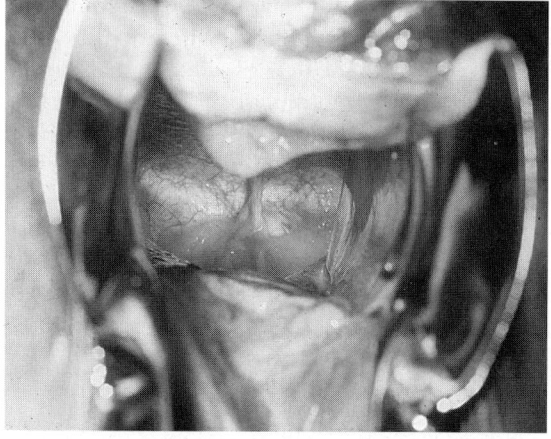

▶ **FIGURE 7–3**
Urovagina. Note the presence of urine that has pooled in the cranial part of the vagina and is covering the cervix. (Courtesy A. O. McKinnon.)

Palpation of the Cervix, Uterus, and Ovaries per Rectum

The principles of a safe rectal examination are described in Chapter 11 (see per Rectum Palpation of the Abdomen). It is very important that care be taken to ensure that the mare is relaxed and that the examination is carried out carefully. This is sometimes difficult in stud practice where a large number of mares, many of them young, must be examined quickly.

Optimal examination of both ovaries is easiest when the clinician uses the left hand to palpate the right ovary and vice versa. This is not absolutely necessary, but, if the time is taken to become familiar with two-handed palpation, it can be useful.

As when palpating any structure per rectum, it is important that the hand always pass beyond the structure being examined and then be brought back to it, to ensure that there is minimal tension in the rectal wall during the examination. It is most important that the hand not be pushed forward or laterally against a taut rectum.

The ovaries often lie lateral to the broad ligament and must be brought around the cranial edge of the ligament so that they can be palpated.

Examination of the uterus per rectum is usually done to check for pregnancy but also for pyometra, neoplasia, and torsion. The uterus consists of a body and two horns, with the body lying on the floor of the pelvis and the horns extending laterally and dorsally toward the ovaries. The horns and body are supported laterally by the two broad ligaments that extend cranially to cover the ovaries. The thickness and muscular tone of the uterus vary with the stage of the reproductive cycle, the age of the mare, and whether or not she has had any foals. The ovaries are bean shaped and also vary considerably in shape, depending on follicle and corpus luteum development. They are also bigger in older and larger mares. The ovary is covered by the broad ligament except where the ovulation fossa is located on the cranio-medial surface.

Uterine Changes Associated with Pregnancy

After ovulation, the tone in the uterine wall begins to increase, so that at about 2 to 3 weeks it is turgid and feels pipelike.[2] A swelling, the site of the developing conceptus, is palpable at the base of one of the horns, and this gradually enlarges in the subsequent days. As the conceptus enlarges, the ability to identify its age precisely decreases. Some significant factors that help with age identification are as follows:

- 60 days: Conceptus is about 12 cm in diameter and tone is maintained in the adjacent body and nonpregnant horn.
- 60–90 days: The swelling enlarges and extends into the body and other horn, gradually becoming less tense as fluid accumulates.
- 90 days: The swelling occupies the complete uterus and the ability to differentiate between body and horns is beginning to be lost.
- 90 days and later: As the structures continue to enlarge the uterus extends over the cranial brim of the pelvis.

Cervical and Vaginal Changes Associated with Pregnancy

The characteristic change with pregnancy is the gradual accumulation of very sticky mucus over the surface of the cervix, which may form a cervical plug, and the cranial vaginal walls. The contours of the cervix disappear, and although it can always be penetrated by a finger it should be remembered that this can introduce contaminants as well as cause abortion. The anestrus cervix is also dry and pale but is relaxed. During estrus the mucosa is red-pink in color, its secretions are fluid, and the cervix is relaxed and edematous. After ovulation the cervix begins to lose its reddish color and it becomes paler, smaller, and less edematous. In diestrous it is moist and pale, and has tone that causes it to project into the vagina.

Ovarian Changes Associated with Pregnancy

- 120–150 days: The corpus luteum of pregnancy persists
- 18–40 days: Numerous follicles (up to 3–4 cm diameter) that rarely ovulate can be palpated.
- 40–120 days: There is much follicular activity with ovulation as well as luteinization of follicles that have not ovulated.
- 120 days–term: Follicular activity regresses and the ovaries become smaller and harder.
- As the weight and size of the uterus increase, its cranial displacement automati-

cally involves the ovaries being pulled cranially and medially. After about 5 months they usually cannot be palpated.

Diagnosis of Twins

It is important to diagnose the presence of twins because twinning rarely leads to a normal healthy foal. Manual palpation is inferior to ultrasonography in its ability to detect twins, especially when it is realized that in approximately 30% of pregnancies the twin conceptuses occupy the same horn. When the conceptuses are in different horns, the accuracy is improved but diagnosis is still not easy and requires considerable expertise.

SPECIAL EXAMINATION PROCEDURES

Ultrasonography of the Ovaries and Uterus per Rectum

Ultrasonography has become a routine and important component of the reproductive examination. Its value lies in the ability to present a two-dimensional picture of structures from which a mental three-dimensional image can be constructed. In particular, the recognition of fluid is enhanced, which is important to differentiate ovarian structures and intrauterine fluid.

The objectives of the ultrasound examination are to:

- Establish whether the mare is pregnant or not.
- Diagnose multiple pregnancies.
- Locate site of development of conceptus.
- Identify any uterine or ovarian abnormalities.

PROCEDURE. The mare is restrained in stocks for optimum safety of the clinician, mare, and

---

Materials Required for Ultrasonography of the Ovaries and Uterus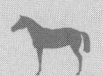

- Ultrasound Machine (5- or 7.5-MHz sector or linear array transducer)
- Ultrasonographic coupling gel
- Rectal examination sleeve

---

equipment, and the rectum is emptied of feces. It is best to carry out a preliminary rectal palpation to establish orientation and to gain an impression of uterine tone, position, and any obvious problems. The surface of the transducer is coated with ultrasonic coupling gel and then placed in a rectal examination sleeve and carefully inserted into the rectum, orientated so that the ultrasound waves are directed ventrally. Some clinicians do not bother to place the transducer in a rectal sleeve. However, with this practice, greater effort is required to keep it clean.

Ultrasonography of the Uterus

After locating an image of the uterus, the probe is moved systematically along a uterine horn, examining a continually changing set of cross sections.[3] The procedure is continued laterally past the tip of the horn, confirmed by visualization of the ovary. The probe is then brought back along the horn, across the bifurcation, and the examination repeated on the opposite horn. The uterine body and cervix are examined next by moving the probe caudally. The mobility of the conceptus in early pregnancy diagnosis dictates that a systematic and thorough examination be made.

If a fetal sac is located, it should be examined in detail to differentiate it from cysts, fluid, or a second conceptus. This part of the examination is best done by locating the sac and then rotating the probe from side to side to enable the precise outline of the sac to be seen a number of times.

Some factors that are important regards interpretation are as follows:

- *Days 1–16 postovulation.* The conceptus is mobile during this time, and examination carries the risk that pregnancy or twins may not be identified.
- *Days 17–21 postovulation.* The conceptus lodges in one horn during this time and, because it is no longer mobile, accuracy of diagnosis is improved. In cases of bicornuate twins one conceptus can be more easily crushed at this time.
- *Days 21–25 postovulation.* A heart beat and an embryo become evident, allowing differentiation between cysts and a conceptus.
- *Day 35 postovulation.* Endometrial cups begin to develop around this time. Therefore the examination just prior is the last chance to confirm a single pregnancy, and to re-

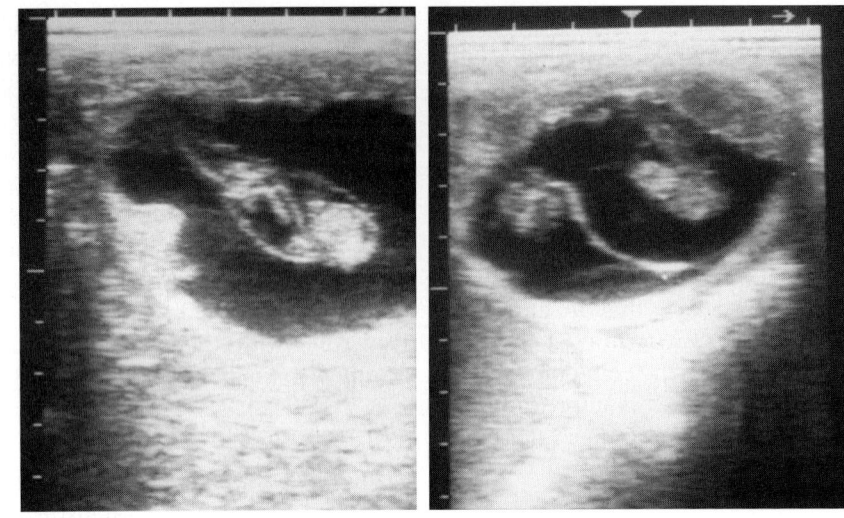

A   B

▶ **FIGURE 7-4**

Ultrasonogram of a pregnant uterus. **A.** A single embryonic vesicle is present. The vesicle consists of an anechoic, approximately circular structure, that contains the echogenic fetus attached to its umbilical cord. In this case it is 47 days postovulation. (Courtesy A. O. McKinnon.) **B.** A case of twins, showing two fetuses. (Courtesy A. O. McKinnon.)

move a conceptus before endometrial cups begin to secrete chorionic gonadotrophins. Removal of a conceptus after this time is unlikely to be followed by a fertile heat.

- *Day 40 postovulation.* Certification around this time is preferred by insurance companies because the chances of missing a twin are virtually nil and subsequent loss of a conceptus is greatly reduced.

Specific information concerning fetal identification and evaluation of fetal age have been described.[3] Some examples of pregnancy are shown in Figure 7-4. In addition to fetal identification, the ultrasonographer must be familiar with the normal ultrasonographic anatomy during the various stages of the estrus cycle as well as pathological changes such as fluid accumulation, cysts, air, adhesions, tumors, hematomata, and fetal remnants (Fig. 7-5). The reader is referred to the published literature for a description of how to evaluate these variations.[4]

Ultrasonography of the Ovary

The ovary can also be examined in great detail by ultrasonography.[5] As mentioned, the ovary may lie lateral to the broad ligament and should be repositioned as described. Fat and intestine can also sometimes hinder examination, necessitating manipulation of the probe, ovary, or offending structure. Imaging is directed mainly toward the

follicles and corpora lutea, although the evaluation of pathological processes such as hematomata, abscesses, neoplasia, and cysts is greatly enhanced by ultrasonography.

Follicles. Follicles appear as black (anechoic), approximately circular structures. Variation in shape is usually caused by pressure from an adjacent structure, such as another follicle, luteal tissue, or ovarian stroma. Sometimes the apposing walls are not visible, thus giving an irregular outline to the image. Follicles usually have a smooth, well-defined outline, and measurement is usually made from one internal surface to the other, excluding the wall that is often hard to define accurately. Measurements are made on a frozen image using the plane of maximum diameter. Nonspherical follicles can be measured by averaging measurements made in two directions.

In general, follicles begin as round bodies and gradually increase in size, change shape from a spherical to a conical or pear form, and increase their wall thickness (Fig. 7-6A). Selection of which follicle is to undergo ovulation occurs on average six days before ovulation, at which time the other follicles start regressing. Relatively large follicles appear necessary for ovulation. Diameters of the order of 45 ± 6 mm are typical and are somewhat smaller if double preovulatory follicles are present. Ovulation is characterized by loss of fluid and collapse of the follicle over a period of about 5 to 7 minutes. During this time the

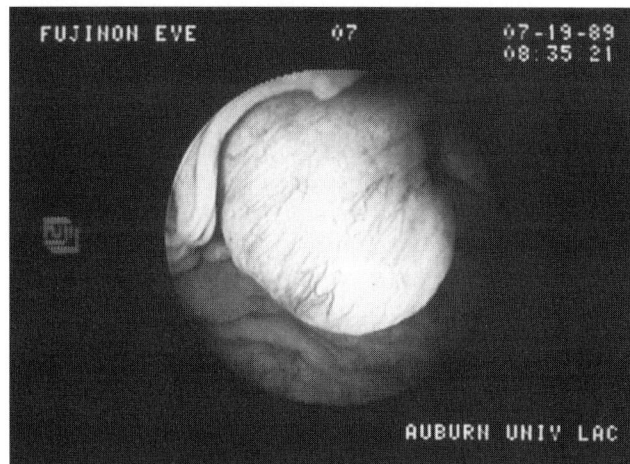

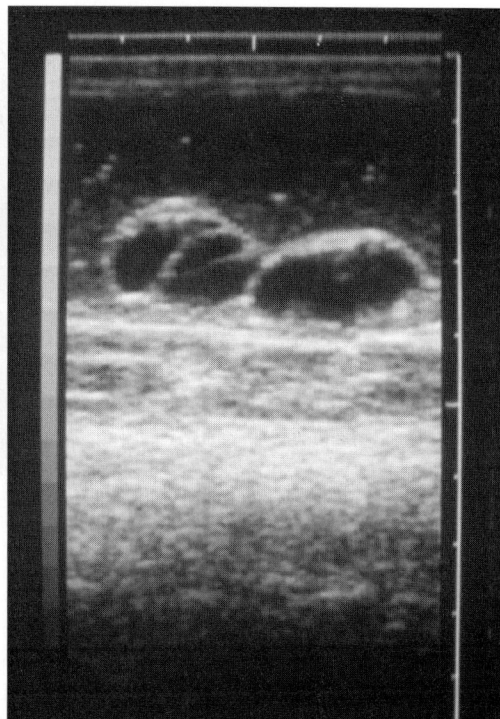

▶ **FIGURE 7-5**

Endometrial cysts. **A.** Endoscopic photograph showing a single cyst. **B.** Ultrasonogram of a uterus containing some endometrial cysts. Note the locular structures consisting of an anechoic interior retained within hyperechoic boundaries. (Courtesy A. O. McKinnon.)

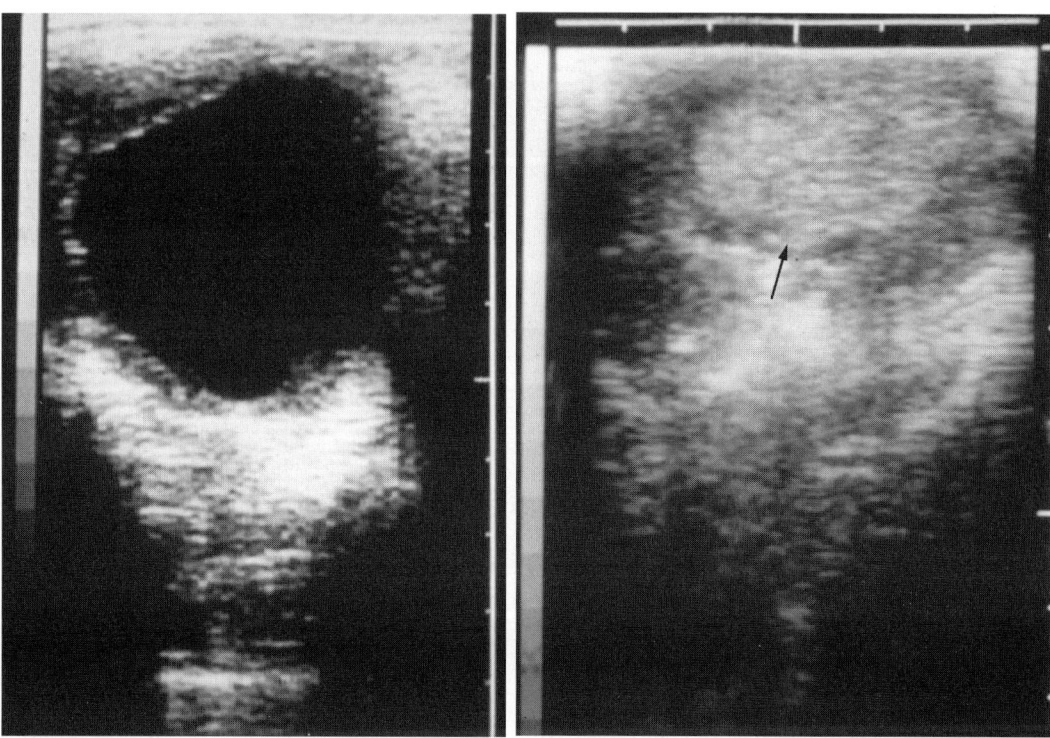

▶ **FIGURE 7-6**

Ovarian ultrasonography. **A.** Follicle. The follicle is represented by the circular structure with the fluid-filled, anechoic interior. (Courtesy A. O. McKinnon.) **B.** Corpus luteum. (Courtesy A. O. McKinnon.)

contents of the follicle remain anechoic. Ovulation may therefore by observed or can be inferred by loss of a follicle previously present, appearance of an ovulation fossa, and later by appearance of a corpus luteum.

The Corpus Luteum. The corpus luteum can be detected throughout its functional life during diestrus and pregnancy. It is visible in most mares from the day of ovulation until well into the second half of the interovulatory interval. The structure of the gland varies from being uniformly echogenic to having a large anechoic central region occupying about 50% of the total area in about 50% of cases (Fig. 7–6B). The central region is gradually organized and as a result becomes more echogenic with a variety of focal spots and bands.

Examination of the Placenta

Although an examination of the placenta is often necessary to detect disease, the most frequent reason for placental examination by a clinician is to ascertain if the complete placenta has been expelled during parturition.[6] Normally, the foal is born through a tear in the allantochorion, at its cervical pole, and the intact placenta is expelled

soon afterward, usually within 1 hour. The foal may be born enclosed in the amnion. The umbilical cord ruptures at a predetermined location close to the foal's abdomen.

The equine has diffuse epitheliochoriol placentation, and the fetal membranes consist of the allanto-chorion, amnion, and hippomanes (Fig. 7-7). The outer surface of the allanto-chorion is the surface that was in contact with the uterus and has the appearance of red velvet, while the inner surface is smooth and glistening. The white amnion is separate from the allanto-chorion and is that part of the placenta that is in immediate contact with the foal. The hippomanes are soft structures, $5 \times 10 \times 15$ cm, that form in the allantoic cavity. The amnion should be translucent but may contain scars as evidence of previous infection. The amnion is attached to the umbilical cord. The intra-amniotic section of the umbilical cord is longer than the intra-allantoic part.

The umbilical cord contains the two umbilical arteries and one vein, and varies between approximately 30 and 100 cm in length. A remnant of the yolk sac is usually located somewhere along the cord in the intra-allantoic section, varying from a minor structure to one of about 5 cm in size. The placenta can be divided according to

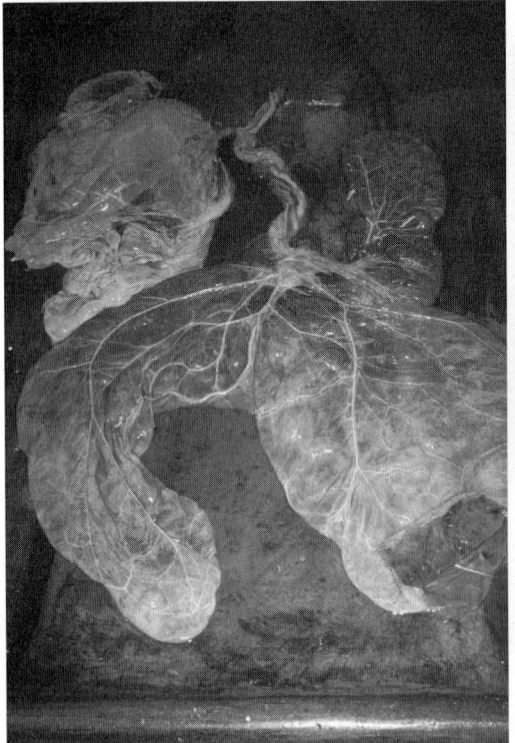

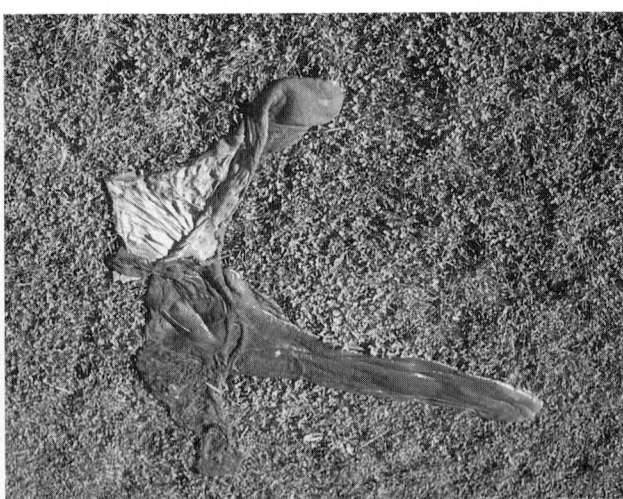

B

▶ **FIGURE 7–7**

Placenta. **A.** Note the umbilical cord extending from the amnion to the larger organ, the allanto-chorion, which is displayed with its inner surface outermost. **B.** The allanto-chorion is arranged with its chorial (outer) surface on show. (Courtesy J. H. Hyland.)

A

whether it was located in the body or the pregnant or the nonpregnant horn of the uterus. The body is the largest and thinnest part, and close examination of its junction with the pregnant horn will reveal small smooth avillous areas ($5 \times 3 \times 2$ cm) previously occupied by the endometrial cups. The cervical end of the placenta is also white and avillous with a stellate appearance.

Visible abnormalities of the placenta include avillous areas (inadequate nutrition), black, bruised or scarred regions (infarction), edema and inflammation (infection). Diagnostic procedures used to evaluate the placenta include:

- Clinical examination and measurement
- Microbiological examination
- Submission of full-thickness sample in formalin for histological examination

Collection of Samples for Microbiological Evaluation

Collection of samples from the female reproductive tract is a very common procedure, generally carried out to identify the cause of uterine infection or to ensure that the stallion is not bred to a mare carrying an infection.[7]

PROCEDURE. The mare should be restrained in a crush or placed beside a doorway so that the clinician cannot be kicked. A twitch or sedation should be used if necessary. The tail should be bandaged and then held aside while the region is prepared and then sampled. The perineal region should be cleansed of gross contamination and then dried with a paper towel. Antiseptic agents should not be used.

Materials for Collection of Samples for Microbiological Examination

---

- Standard hospital swabs (small swab for clitoral sinus, standard swab for clitoral fossa)
- Antiseptic-free, sterile lubricant (e.g., K-Y jelly)
- Transport medium (e.g., Amies charcoal transport medium [Medical Wire and Equipment Co. Ltd., Corsham, Wiltshire, UK])

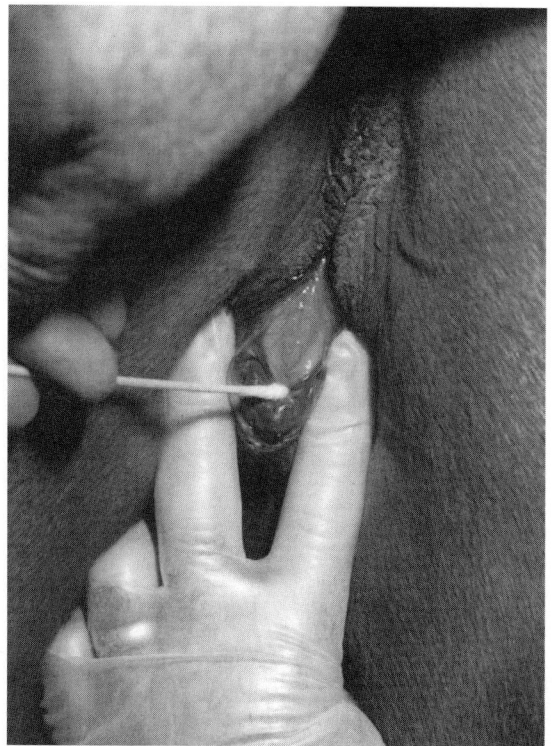

▶ **FIGURE 7–8**

Clitoral swabbing. The clitoris has been everted and a swab is positioned in the central clitoral sinus.

Clitoral Swabbing

The clitoral region is sampled to identify potential venereal disease organisms, in particular the organism responsible for contagious equine endometritis (CEM). Using a gloved hand, the vulva is manually opened with the thumb and first finger while holding the second finger at the base of the commissure. The clitoral fossa is swabbed by rubbing the larger swab around the full extent of the fossa, and the smaller swab is then used to swab the central clitoral sinus (Fig. 7–8). If a delay in processing is expected, the swabs are placed in transport medium and processed as described in Appendix C.

Cervicouterine Swabbing

Cervicouterine swabbing is carried out during estrus when the chances of obtaining a reliable swab are maximized. Because the uterus is located at the end of a long tubular structure, there is considerable chance that any sample will be contaminated. To avoid this, swabbing can be done with the assistance of a speculum or by a guarded manual method. A commonly used spec-

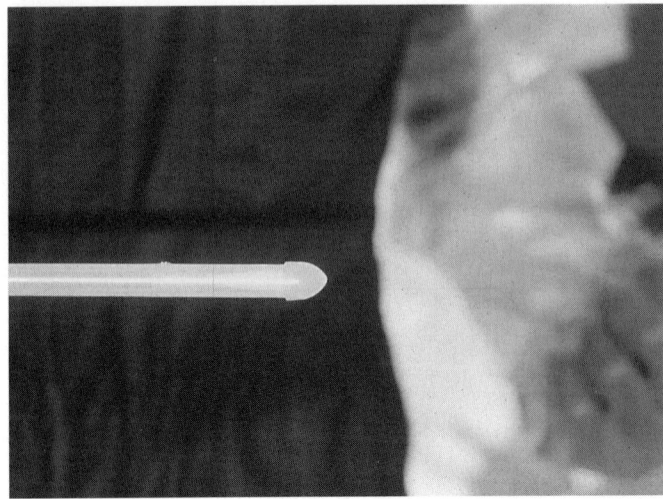

▶ FIGURE 7-9

Guarded swab for endometrial swabbing. Note the cap, which is displaced once the swab is positioned within the uterus. (Courtesy A. O. McKinnon.)

ulum has been described earlier. The disadvantage of the metal speculum is that it must be resterilized between each horse, but the thinner disposable ones are so narrow that visualization is difficult.

The vulva should be cleaned with warm water and dried with a paper towel. The speculum is first lubricated, passed through the vulval lips, and then directed into the cranial vagina. There is usually some resistance at the vestibulovaginal junction. The guarded swab (Fig. 7-9) is then directed through the speculum, into the cervical canal that is recognized as the site from which the edematous folds radiate, and then into the lumen of the uterus. The cap guarding the end of the swab is displaced by advancing the swab stick within the outer guard. The swab is then rotated a few times against the endometrium, withdrawn into the outer guard, and removed. To use the guarded, protected technique, the swab, contained in its outer protective guard, is inserted into a sterile sleeve (Fig. 7-10A). The end of the swab, contained in the sleeve, is held in the palm of the hand, which is inserted through the vulval lips and advanced into the cranial vagina. The index finger is inserted into the cervical orifice. The guarded tube is advanced along the side of the index finger and is then pushed sharply through the end of the sleeve and then on into the lumen of the uterus (Fig. 7-10B). After ensuring that the unit is within the uterus, the swab is extended, rotated against the endometrium, and withdrawn into its guard. The complete unit is withdrawn into the sleeve, and the sleeve and swab unit are removed from the vagina. If a delay in processing is expected, the sample should be placed in a transport medium and processed as described in Appendix C.

Although bacteria are generally responsible for uterine infections, yeasts and fungi are also often present, especially as complicating factors in mares that have received antimicrobial agents. Isolation of an organism does not always mean that it is responsible for an infection, as numerous organisms are present as contaminants. The following list contains some of the organisms known to be causes of infection and also some generally regarded as likely to be contaminants:

- Organisms frequently associated with uterine infections:
  Bacteria: Beta-hemolytic *Streptococci*, *Escherichia coli*, *Pseudomonas aeruginosa*, *Klebsiella pneumoniae*
  Fungi and yeasts: *Candida albicans*, *Aspergillus* spp.
- Organisms often regarded as contaminants: *Staphylococcus* spp., Alpha-hemolytic *Streptococci*, *Enterobacter* spp., *Proteus* spp., *Pasteurella* spp.

Collection of Samples for Endometrial Cytology with Lavage

Uterine cytology involves collecting and evaluating cells from the lumen and endometrial surface of the uterus.[8] By enabling material representing a large surface area to be examined, the method has some advantages over the more specific endometrial biopsy. Its value lies in allowing a better assessment of the significance of bacteria in the uterus.

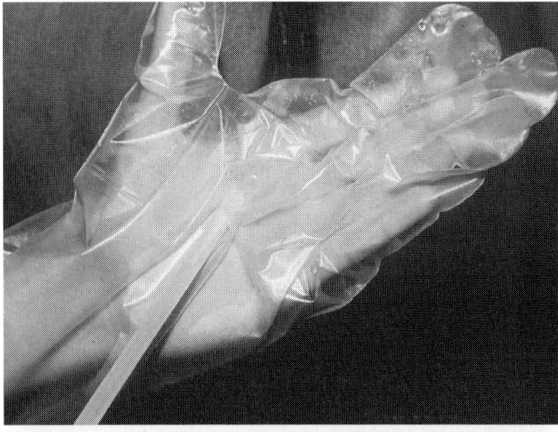

A

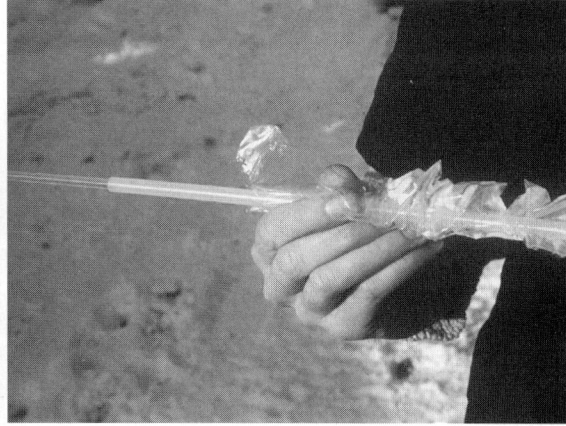

B

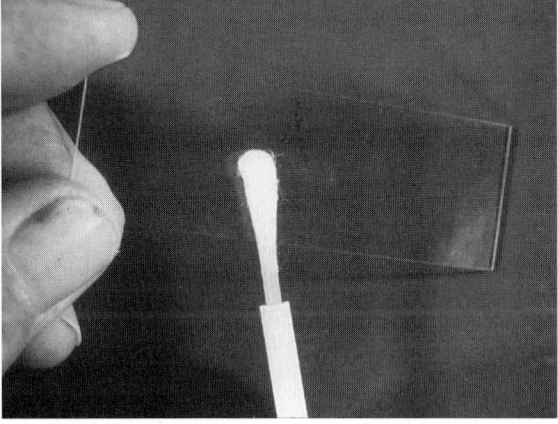

C

▶ **FIGURE 7-10**

Protected swab technique. **A.** The end of the swab is inserted through the palm of a rectal sleeve, prior to inserting the arm into the vagina. (Courtesy A. O. McKinnon.) **B.** The picture shows the outer casing of the swab protruding from the end of the glove and the swab stick protruding from the casing after the protective cap has been dislodged. Penetration of the glove and dislodgement of the cap are done once the apparatus has been positioned in the cervical canal. **C.** Swab is rolled on to a dry sterile microscopic slide immediately after collection of the sample for cytological examination (the same or a second swab can then be used for bacteriology). (Courtesy A. O. McKinnon.)

PROCEDURE.   The mare is restrained and prepared as described. After putting on the obstetrical sleeve, the tip of the pipette is protected in the palm of the hand and guided into the vagina and then to the entrance to the cervix. The pipette is inserted carefully through the cervix and passed into the uterus. The saline is injected, and negative pressure is applied immediately and maintained for a minute or so while the pipette is moved around in the uterus to ensure a reasonable collection of fluid from as wide a region as possible. The volume of fluid obtained varies considerably but is adequate for cytological purposes. The fluid is submitted for evaluation or placed in a tube containing about 10 mL of 40% ethanol to preserve cellular morphology for a few days. Cytology is conducted after staining with Diff Quik (American Scientific Products, McGaw Park, IL) or, for better cell definition Sano's modification of Pollack's trichrome method.

RESULTS.   The findings vary with the time of the reproductive cycle as well as with the type and extent of pathological change. The advan-

tage of the technique is that the cells are sampled from a large surface area, which improves the chances of detecting abnormality. The endometrium has a significant seasonal fluctuation characterized by an inactive winter period (winter anestrus), followed by a transitional spring period, an active spring period, which is the active breeding season, and a transitional fall period.

Materials for Collecting Samples for Uterine Cytology

▶ Sterile pipette with attached rubber or plastic tubing, or guarded balloon-tipped catheter

▶ Sterile 0.9% saline

▶ 60-ml syringe

▶ Obstetrical sleeve

▶ 40% ethanol

Variation associated with infection and pregnancy are superimposed over the basic cycle. The main characteristics of each of the groups are described in the box. It should be remembered that each period blends with the next, rather than undergoing an immediate and distinct change.

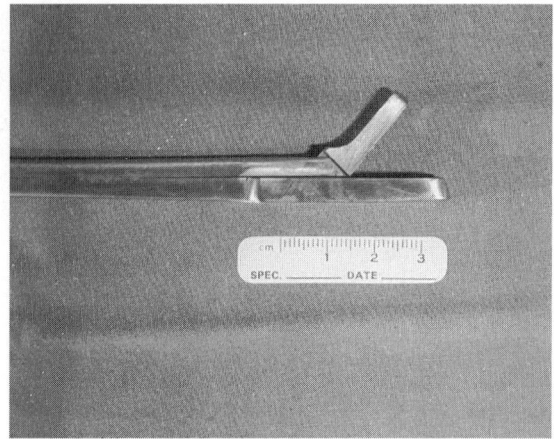

▶ **FIGURE 7-11**
Basket-jawed uterine biopsy instrument. (Courtesy A. O. McKinnon.)

Endometrial Biopsy

An endometrial biopsy is useful for allowing an histological evaluation of the endometrium.[9] The usual biopsy instrument has large jaws that enable a large sample to be safely collected (Fig. 7–11). The sample can be taken at any time of the reproductive cycle, usually during mid-diestrus when glandular activity is under progesterone influence comparable with that found in pregnancy. Biopsy during estrus has the advantages that the cervix is more easily penetrated, resistance to accidentally introduced bacteria is increased, and endometrial swabbing and culture can be carried out at the same time.

PROCEDURE. The mare should be restrained and the perineal and vulval region prepared as described. The obstetrical sleeve is placed on the clinician's preferred arm, and a little lubricant applied. The end of the biopsy instrument is held in the palm of the gloved hand that is inserted into the vagina and then guided to the cervix. The handles of the instrument are controlled with the other hand. The index finger is inserted into the cervix, and the forceps is then passed along the ventral surface of the finger and on into the uterus. The gloved hand is removed from the vagina, inserted in the rectum, and cupped so as to hold the jaws of the forceps in the palm, although separated from it by the ventral wall of the rectum and the dorsal wall of the uterus. Gentle forward pressure on the forceps and downward pressure by the hand in the rectum then forces a portion of the dorsal wall of the uterus into the jaws of the biopsy forceps. The

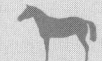

▶ Biopsy forceps (60-cm Pillings biopsy
   punch [Pilling Surgical Instrument Co.
   Fort Washington, PA])

▶ Obstetrical sleeve

▶ Obstetrical lubricant

▶ Bouin's fixative

▶ 70% alcohol or 10% buffered neutral
   formalin

specimen is then collected by closing the jaws and pulling the instrument caudally. The biopsy site(s) is at the junction between the uterine body and horn, plus any other site dictated by rectal findings. The biopsy can also be collected without the assistance of a hand in the rectum. Although one biopsy is thought to be adequate in mares without identifiable abnormalities,[10] there is some indication that it may not always be sufficient.[11]

The sample(s) is processed as follows, however the laboratory requirements may vary:

- Bouin's fixative for 2 to 4 hours.
- 70% alcohol or 10% buffered neutral formalin.

RESULTS. The procedure is relatively safe and free of pain except, perhaps, for some discomfort when the instrument is inserted through the cervix.[12] The biopsy should be interpreted after the other factors related to fertility have been considered. There are several systems in use for classifying the histological findings with respect to prognosis for fertility. These systems have been summarized and are based on consideration of evidence of inflammation and fibrosis.[8] It is important that the normal endometrium and its variations during the reproductive cycle be understood. Normal physiological changes include tall ciliated columnar cells and active glands in estrus, cuboidal epithelium and inactive glands in diestrus, and inactive epithelium with few glands in anestrus. The normal findings and a system for classification of the uterine biopsy are presented in the box.[13,14]

The classification is closely related to fertility, with rates of 80% to 90% and 10% being typical for

groups I and III, whereas the prognosis for the intervening two groups is spread evenly between these extremes.

Collection of Amniotic Fluid

Amniotic fluid analysis is a regular procedure in man and has recently been investigated in horses with the objectives of perfecting the technique and establishing data for determining fetal health and gestational length.[15,16]

In the preparturient mare the procedure is carried out with the sedated mare restrained in stocks. The abdomen is ultrasonically scanned (5- or 3-MHz sector scanner) until a collection of amniotic fluid is located. Then the region overlying it is prepared for a sterile centesis and injected with local anesthetic. The needle (22-cm, 18-gauge spinal needle) used for aspiration is inserted

---

**ENDOMETRIAL BIOPSY:
NORMAL FINDINGS**

- *Anestrus.* Endometrial glands are inactive and atrophic, although a few nonatrophic glands may be present. Gland branches are narrow, and the epithelium of glandular ducts is often low columnar with paler cytoplasm than the deeper glands. Luminal and glandular epithelial cells are cuboidal or squamous. Epithelial cells have increased cytoplasmic basophilia. Edema of lamina propria is rare.

- *Transitional–winter.* There is a resumption of glandular activity, with luminal and glandular epithelial cells often at different stages of activity. Luminal and upper glandular epithelial cells are first to become active and may be columnar while deep inactive cells are low cuboidal.

- *Estrus.* Luminal and glandular epithelial cells are columnar and pale-staining, with vacuoles in basal portion of the luminal epithelium. Polymorph neutrophils are often present in capillaries beneath the epithelium and lamina propria. Edema of lamina propria may be present.

- *Diestrus.* Epithelium varies from columnar to cuboidal. The glandular branches are often tortuous.

ENDOMETRIAL BIOPSY: CLASSIFICATION

- *Category I.* Normal or very slight abnormality.
- *Category IIA.* Slight to moderate, diffuse cellular infiltration of the stratum compactum; scattered, frequent inflammatory foci in stratum compactum or stratum spongiosum; frequent, scattered fibrotic changes associated with individual gland branches, less than two fibrotic, glandular nests per 5.5 mm linear field in four or more fields; palpable lymphatic lacunae; or partial endometrial atrophy late in physiological breeding season.
- *Category IIB.* Mares with more than one of the changes specified in Category IIA; or widespread, diffuse, and moderately severe foci of inflammation; widespread and uniformly distributed fibrosis of individual gland branches; or average of two to four fibrotic nests per 5.5 mm linear field in four or more fields.
- *Category III.* Mares with more than one of the changes specified in Category IIB; or severe or irreversible changes (widespread periglandular fibrosis, inflammation, palpable lymphatic lacunae, or endometrial hypoplasia).

---

through the biopsy guide of the ultrasound transducer, and then, under ultrasound guidance, it is directed into the amniotic fluid. Amniotic fluid can also be collected by needle aspiration under direct vision during parturition before rupture of the amnion.

At present, the fluid can be analyzed microbiologically and to assess the percentage phosphatidylglycerol, lecithin to sphingomyelin ratio, and cortisol and creatinine concentrations as possible indicators of fetal maturity.

Uterine Endoscopy (Hysteroscopy)

Although not a new technique, the flexible fiber-optic endoscope has made endoscopic examination of the uterus a relatively easy procedure.[17] It is not a routine procedure, but it can be carried out when indicated by the findings of other examinations such as rectal palpation or ultrasonography. The examination requires a suitable endoscope and light source and also the ability to distend the uterus to convert the collapsed, tubelike organ into a hollow cavity that is easy to examine.

PROCEDURE. Hysteroscopy can be carried out during estrus or diestrus.[18] If done during diestrus, distension is more readily achieved because the cervix is closed. If pyometra, metritis, and retained placenta are the indications for examination, the examination is done when dictated by relevant signs.

The mare is restrained in stocks, and sedation and some form of analgesia are usually necessary. Uterine distension is easier if the feces are first manually removed from the rectum. A tail bandage is applied and the perineal region prepared by being washed with warm water and then dried with disposable towels. The obstetrical sleeve is placed on the clinician's arm and some lubricant applied. The pipette, attached to the tubing, is then guided into the vagina and inserted through the cervix into the uterus. Three to four liters of warm sterile water are then infused into the uterus to distend it for examination. The endoscope is guided manually through the cervix, the guiding hand remains in the vagina to assist in later manipulation of the endoscope. The uterine lumen is examined systematically in its distended state to detect obvious abnormalities. Samples for bacteriology can be aspirated through a catheter, and tissue biopsy can be taken with appropriate forceps, both inserted through the instrument channel of the endoscope. The uterine folds cannot be examined when the uterus is distended, but, after aspirating the fluid from each horn, they again become visible and can be examined. The cervix is examined as the endo-

---

Materials for Hysteroscopy

- Fiber-optic endoscope (1 m long)
- Light source
- 3 to 4 liters of warm, sterile water
- Sterile rubber or plastic tubing connected to a plastic pipette
- Obstetrical sleeve

scope is withdrawn. The normal cervical canal is lined with a smooth mucosal membrane. Hysteroscopy can reveal abnormalities such as endometrial cysts, endometrial fibrosis, endometritis, adhesions, and atrophy.

R E F E R E N C E S

1. Pascoe RR: Observations of the length and angle of declination of the vulva and its relation to fertility in the mare. J Reprod Fertil (Suppl) 1979, 27:299.
2. Allen WE: Fertility and Obstetrics in the Horse. Oxford, Blackwell, 1988, ch 7, p 30.
3. McGladery AJ, Rossdale PD: Ultrasound scanning of the mare for the early diagnosis of pregnancy. Equine Vet Educ 1992; 4:198.
4. Curnow EM: Ultrasonography of the mare's uterus. Equine Vet Educ 1991; 3:190.
5. Ginther OJ: Ultrasonic imaging of equine ovarian follicles and corpora lutea. Vet Clin North Amer: Equine Pract 1988; 4:197.
6. Cottrill CM: Placental evaluation in the field. Equine Vet Educ 1991; 3:204.
7. Allen WE: Swabbing techniques and diagnosis of endometritis. In Fertility and Obstetrics in the Horse. Oxford, Blackwell, 1988, p 71.
8. Roszel JF, Freeman KP: Equine endometrial cytology. Vet Clin North Amer: Equine Pract 1988; 4:247.
9. van Camp SD: Endometrial biopsy of the mare. A review and update. Vet Clin North Amer: Equine Pract 1988; 4:229.
10. Bergman RV, Kenney RM: (1975) Representativeness of a uterine biopsy in the mare. Proceedings of the 21st Annual Convention of the Amer Assoc Equine Pract 1975; p 355.
11. Waelchli RO, Winder NC: Distribution of histological lesions in the equine endometrium. Vet Rec 1989; 124:271.
12. Doig PA, McKnight JD, Miller RB: The use of endometrial biopsy in the infertile mare. Can Vet J 1981; 22:72.
13. Doig PA, Waelchli RO: Endometrial biopsy. In Mckinnon AO, Voss JL (eds), Equine Reproduction. Malvern, PA, Lea & Febiger, 1993, ch 26, p 225.
14. Kenny RM, Doig PA: Equine endometrial biopsy. In Morrow DA (ed), Current Therapy in Theriogenology, 2nd ed. Philadelphia, Saunders, 1986, p 117.
15. Schmidt AR, Williams MA, Carleton CL, et al: Evaluation of transabdominal ultrasound-guided amniocentesis in the late gestational mare. Equine Vet J 1991; 23:261.
16. Williams MA, Schmidt AR, Carleton CL, et al: Amniotic fluid analysis for ante-partum foetal assessment in the horse. Equine Vet J 1992; 24:236.
17. Leidl W, Schallenberger-Pottiez U: Hysteroscopy in the mare. Vet Med Rev 1976; 2:203.
18. Wilson GL: (1988) The use of fiberoptics in the visual assessment and clinical diagnosis of the endometrium. Equine Vet Pract 1988; 8:395.

A D D I T I O N A L   R E A D I N G S

Ginther OJ: Ultrasonic Imaging and Reproductive Events in the Mare. Cross Plains, WI, Equiservices, 1986.
Mckinnon AO, Voss JL (eds): Equine Reproduction. Malvern, PA, Lea & Febiger, 1993.

Male Reproductive System

COMPONENTS

The male reproductive system extends from the testicles through the tubular epididymis, ductus deferens, and urethra to the penis and prepuce. Along the way it constitutes part of the spermatic cord, passes through the inguinal canal, receives contributions from the intrapelvic organs or accessory sex glands, and shares part of the conduit with the urinary system. The system is under endocrine control.

MANIFESTATIONS OF DISEASE

By virtue of its location, much of the system is internal and is not accessible to visual examination. Fortunately, examination of the internal components by rectal palpation and ultrasonography, examination of the semen, and evaluation of endocrine function allow a comprehensive assessment to be made. The major focus is on reproduction, where malfunction varies from reduced to complete infertility. In addition to lesions of the reproductive system, reproductive malfunction can be related to serving difficulty caused by disease in the musculoskeletal system or to behavioral abnormalities associated with management, environment, and temperament. Lesions in the system that reduce fertility include infection (urethritis, seminal vesiculitis, ampullitis, epididymitis, orchitis) and contamination of semen with blood (hemospermia) or urine (urospermia). Infection can be venereal in nature. Trauma to the testes, penis, and prepuce produces swelling and, depending on the type of trauma, bleeding. Paralysis of the penis (rabies, tranquilizers) is seen as loss of ability to retract the penis, often associated with erection (priapism). Penile and preputial neoplasia (squamous cell carcinoma, melanoma) produce lesions that include swelling and ulceration. Pain and swelling in the scrotum can be caused by torsion of the testicle, inguinal herniation of the intestine, and orchitis and periorchitis. The signs of partial or complete failure of testicular descent (cryptorchidism) vary with the extent of the abnormality and whether it is bilateral or unilateral. Cryptorchid testes may be intraabdominal or located in or just outside of the inguinal canal. Cryptorchid testicles have an increased susceptibility to neoplasia and are associated with abnormal blood hormone levels. Many problems, such as seminal vesiculitis, can be detected only by rectal palpation, ultrasonography, and examination of semen and glandular secretions.

RESTRAINT

During examination of the reproductive tract of the male horse restraint is required for rectal palpation, while the penis, prepuce, and testicles are examined, and during catheterization or endoscopic examination of the urethra. In most horses restraint is easily achieved. However, in others, especially breeding stallions, it can be more difficult and even quite dangerous. The procedures for safe rectal examination are described in Chapter 11 (see Palpation of the Abdomen per Rectum). Examination of the penis, prepuce, and testicles may require stocks that contain a side doorway that can be opened to provide access. Examination of the penis will also require tranquilization to ensure that it is extended. Regardless of the method of restraint used the safest position for the clinician is beside the horse adjacent to the thorax. This does not mean that a horse cannot kick someone standing in this position, but the chances of being kicked are greatly diminished. It is vastly more dangerous to stand adjacent to or behind the hind limbs.

GENERAL PHYSICAL EXAMINATION

Examination of the Prepuce and Penis

For examination, the penis must be partly or completely extended from the prepuce. There are a number of ways to stimulate penile extension:

- Stallions can be stimulated to protrude the penis by exposure to a mare in estrus. This also allows an evaluation of the erection mechanism.
- Penile protrusion also occurs when the horse urinates, which can be stimulated in many horses by placing them in a stall with hay. This procedure is very successful in competition horses familiar with the process of regular urine collection for drug surveillance.
- Urination and penile protrusion are also produced 15 to 20 minutes after administration of a diuretic (furosemide, 0.5–1.0 mg/kg IV).
- Manual exteriorization is possible in some horses, but it is usually resented. This is done by inserting a gloved hand into the prepuce, grasping the penis gently, and by applying steady traction to overcome slowly the tension in the retractor muscles.
- Tranquilization is the usual method of causing good penile relaxation and protrusion, allowing a thorough examination to be made.

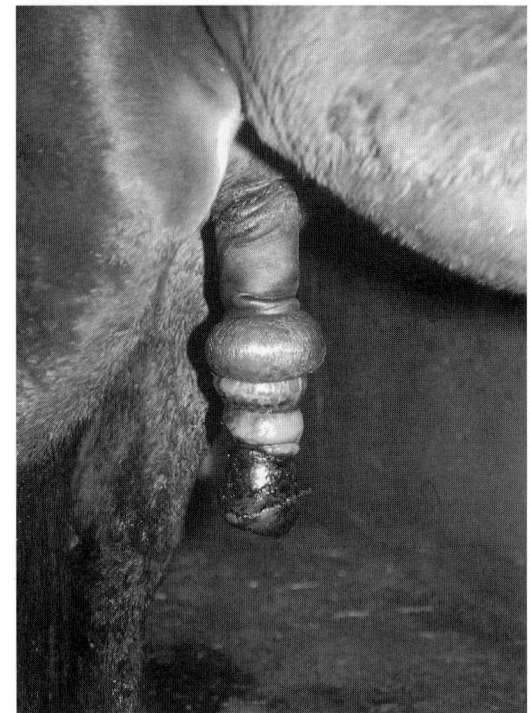

▶ FIGURE 8–1

Paraphimosis. The penis has been injured through the incorrect application of a stallion ring (a device used to discourage masturbation), resulting in swelling and loss of ability to retract the penis.

Drugs most often used include xylazine (0.5 mg/kg IV) or acetylpromazine (0.04–0.06 mg/kg IV). Complications such as penile paralysis and priapism can occur, although the mechanisms are not well understood. To minimize the chances of injury to the penis after drug-induced relaxation, every care should be taken to ensure that the horse is not allowed to go free in the paddock until the penis has been retracted. Persistent prolapse is initially handled by manually repositioning the penis in the prepuce and ensuring that it stays there by closing the prepuce with towel clamps or by using a support bandage. Under no circumstances should the penis be allowed to remain in the prolapsed position for longer than 2 hours before these measures are taken. The development of penile edema is a very serious indication of pending complications, which can result in chronic paraphimosis (Fig. 8–1).

The penis is usually examined for lesions such as neoplasia or viral infection (Fig. 8–2). The structure of the prepuce and the manner in which

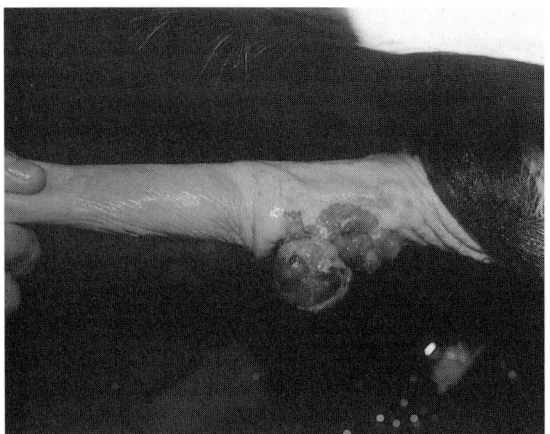

▶ **FIGURE 8–2**

Squamous cell carcinoma of the penis.

it is folded when the penis is retracted should be understood. The end of the urethra extends from the penis as the urethral process and is a site of disease processes such as habronemiasis (Fig. 8–3). The prepuce contains a thick material, known as smegma, that accumulates at the base of the penis. The urethral fossa surrounds the urethral process and communicates dorsally with the urethral diverticulum, which also accumulates smegma.

Examination of the Testicles and Spermatic Cords

The position of the testicle can be visually assessed. Both testicles are usually of similar size, each lying with its long axis parallel to the long axis of the horse, with one slightly cranial to the other. The normal testicle is firm, smooth, and resilient. Palpation is carried out by gently squeezing the testicle, simultaneously stabilizing it in the scrotum with the other hand placed dorsally (Fig. 8–4). The head of the epididymis lies on the craniodorsal pole, the body on the lateral aspect, and the tail on the caudal pole, all of which can be palpated. Identification of the tail is facilitated by identifying the caudal ligament of the epididymis, palpated as a small firm nodule attached to the tail. Occasionally a testicle is rotated so that the cranial pole faces caudally, which appears to be asymptomatic, although more extensive rotation produces pain and vascular obstruction. Testicular dimensions can be measured with calipers. Normal dimensions for length, width, and height are 9 to 10 cm, 5 to 6 cm, and 5 to 5.5 cm, respectively, and total scrotal width should be at least 10 cm (average of three measurements) in mature stallions.[1]

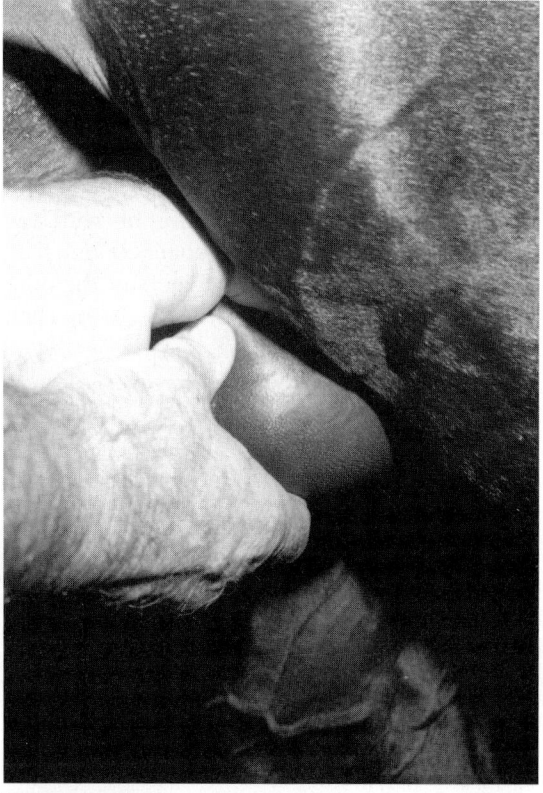

▶ **FIGURE 8–4**

Palpation of a testicle. The testicle is held in the scrotum with one hand while the other hand is used to conduct an examination by palpation.

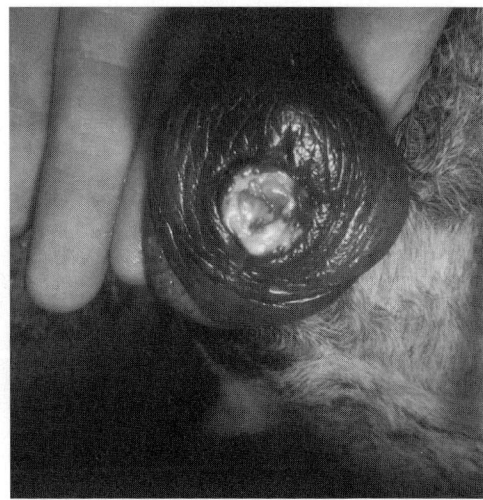

▶ **FIGURE 8–3**

Habronemiasis *(H. muscae),* an inflammatory process involving the urethral process and the urethral fossa.

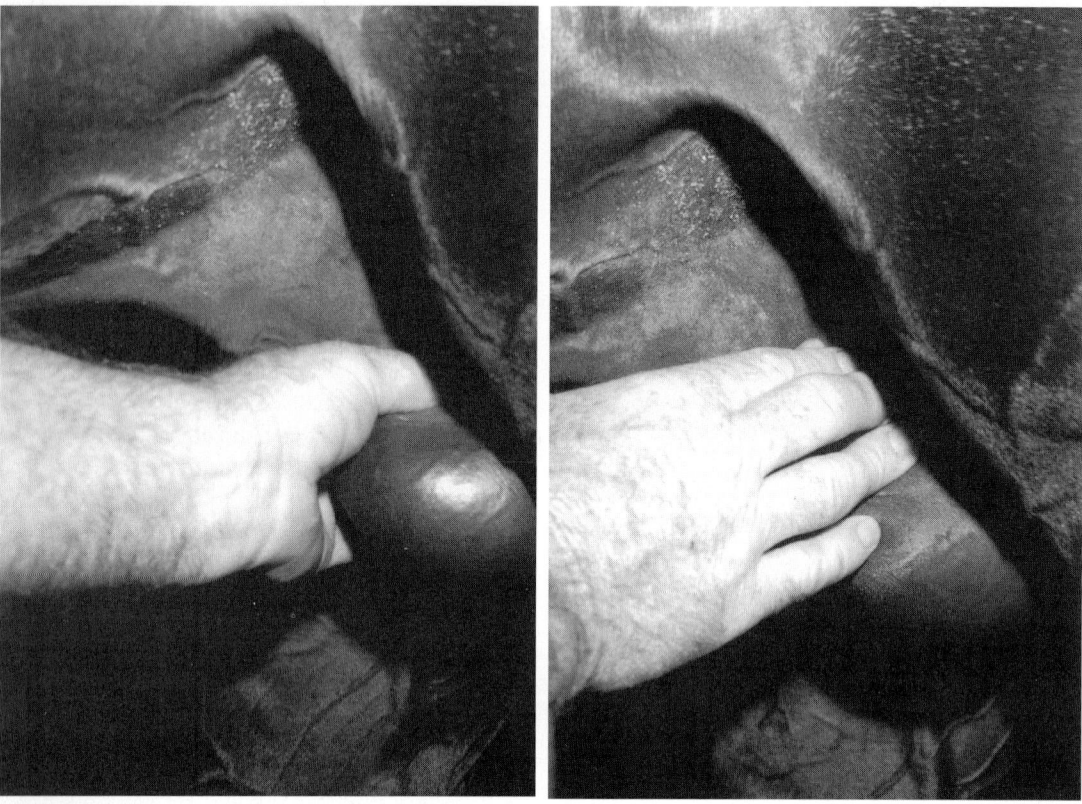

A   B

▶ **FIGURE 8-5**

Palpation of the spermatic cord. **A.** One-handed. **B.** Two-handed.

The spermatic cord is examined by gentle palpation through the neck of the scrotum. This can be done with one hand by squeezing the cord between fingers and the thumb, or with two hands by using the tips of the fingers of one hand to press the cord against the fingers of the other hand placed medial to the cord (Fig. 8-5). There should be no pain or swelling, as such abnormal findings can indicate an abscess, hematoma, hernia, or torsion (Fig. 8-6). The cord contains the spermatic artery, the spermatic vein in the form of a meshwork of vessels termed the pampiniform plexus, and ductus deferens, all contained in the vaginal tunics, plus the cremaster

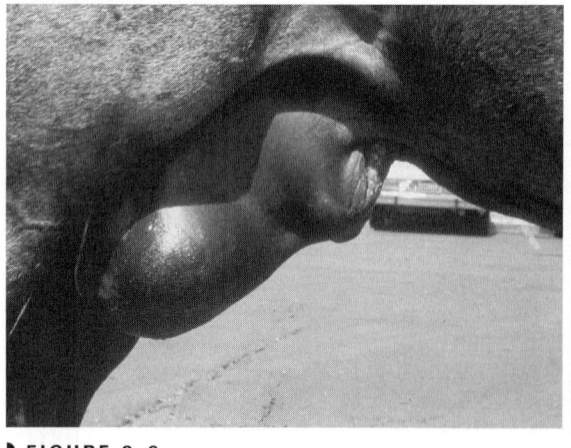
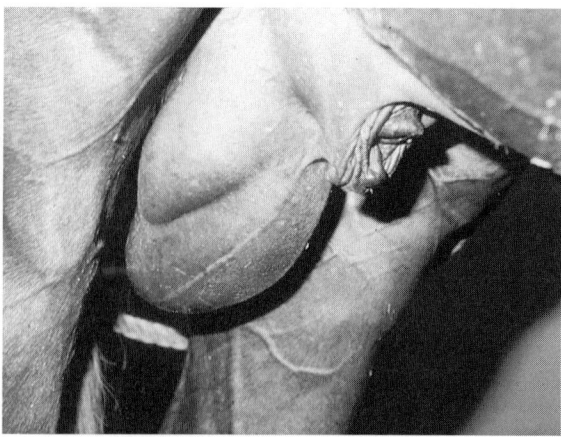

A   B

▶ **FIGURE 8-6**

Testicular and scrotal lesions. **A.** Acute traumatic hematoma with scrotal and preputial edema. **B.** Direct inguinal hernia on the left side.

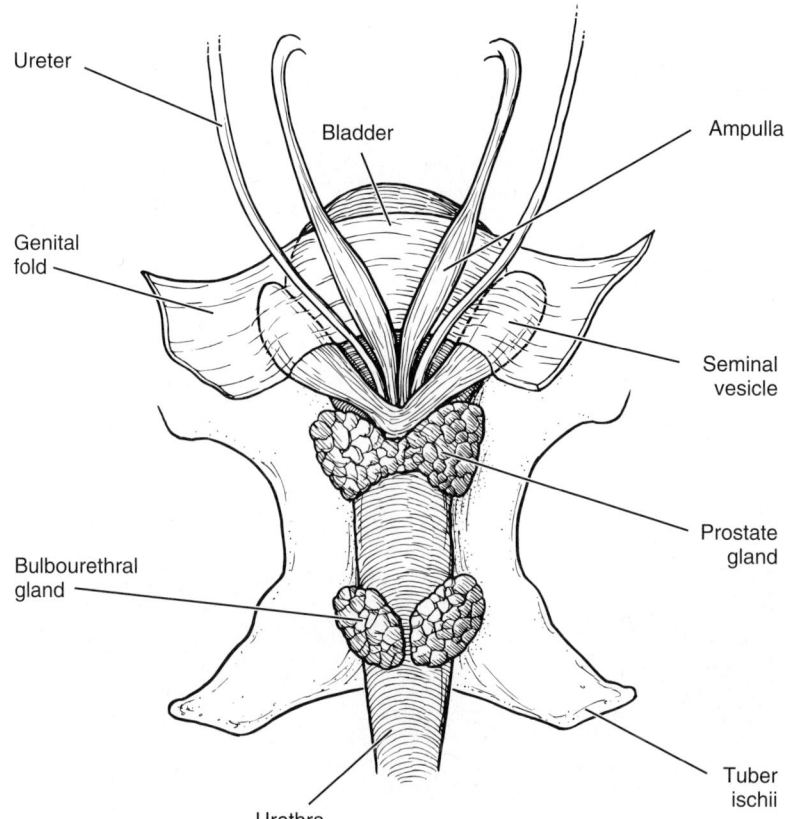

Ureter

Bladder

Ampulla

Genital
fold

Seminal
vesicle

Prostate
gland

Bulbourethral
gland

Tuber
ischii

Urethra

▶ **FIGURE 8–7**

Accessory sex glands of the male.

muscle, which is attached to the outer surface of the tunics. These structures are not all identifiable and identification varies to a large extent with tissue thickness.

Examination of the External Inguinal Ring

The external inguinal ring is traversed by the spermatic cord and can be palpated by passing the fingers dorsally and laterally to the scrotum. The ring is a fenestration in the fascia of the insertion of the external abdominal oblique muscle. The usual reasons for examining the ring are to diagnose cryptorchidism and inguinal herniation. Cryptorchid testicles can often be located adjacent to the ring.

Palpation of the Accessory Sex Glands and Internal Inguinal Ring per Rectum

The accessory sex glands can be palpated per rectum, although their small size and flaccidity make it a rather unreliable procedure. In the stallion, the prostate, vesicular glands (seminal vesicles) bulbourethral glands, and ampullae of

the ductus deferens can be palpated. Teasing results in enlargement of these glands, noted especially with the large vesicular glands. The location of the organs is demonstrated in Figure 8-7. The prostate is firm and painless on palpation and is about 2×4 cm in size. It is located when the examiner's arm is inserted to about the level of the wrist. The vesicular glands are immediately cranial to the prostate and situated laterally. The bulbourethral glands are located caudally and are difficult to palpate because of the overlying bulbourethral muscle. The ampullae are further cranial and are much softer. The internal inguinal rings can be palpated cranial and ventral to the pelvic brim on either side of the midline. They are slitlike structures and should be free of intestine and adhesions. Within each inguinal ring is the vaginal ring, 2 to 3 cm in diameter, where the spermatic artery and vas deferens can often be palpated.

Collection of Samples for Microbiological Evaluation

Bacterial examination is usually done in breeding stallions to detect carriers and therefore avoid

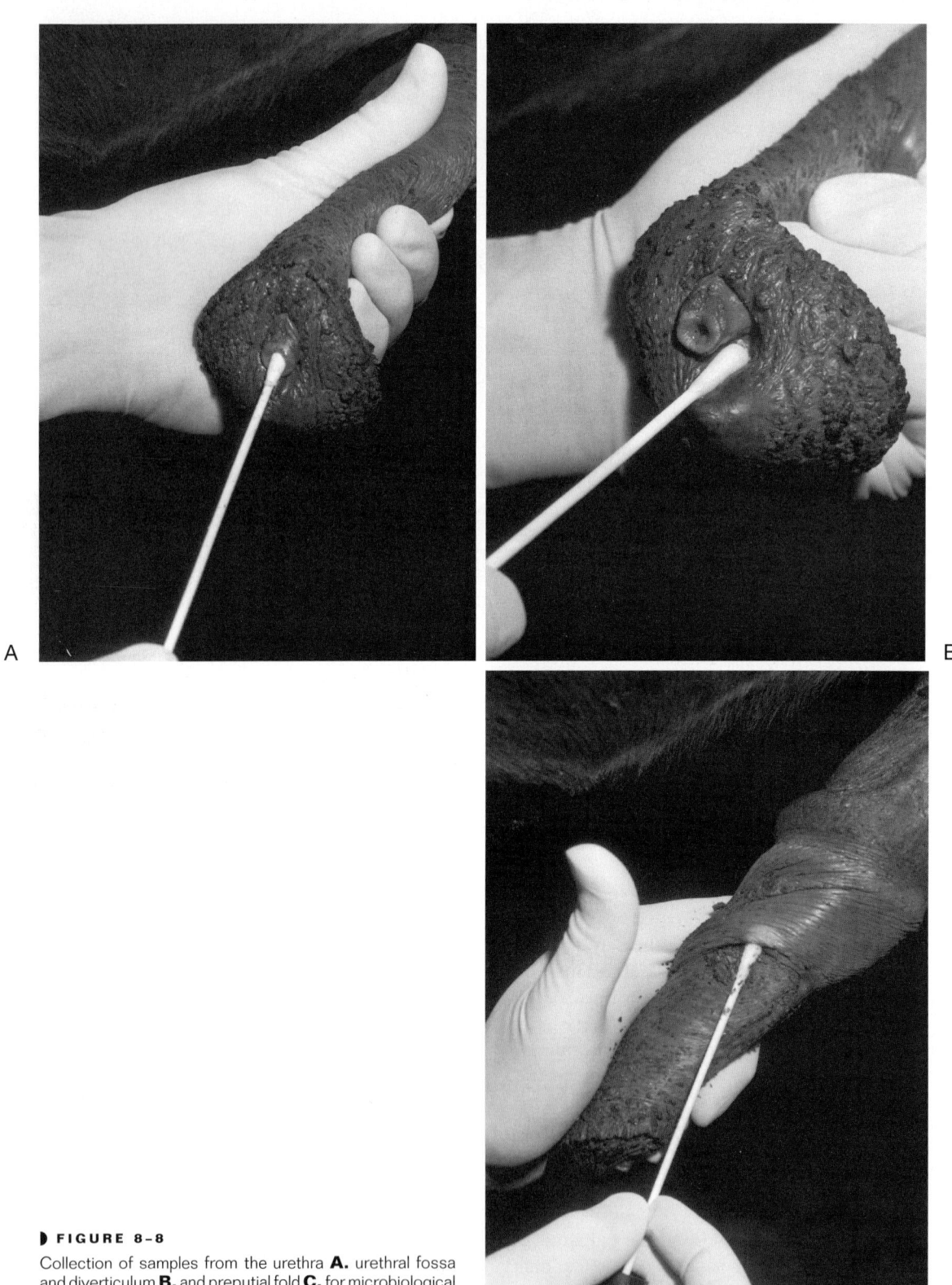

▶ **FIGURE 8–8**

Collection of samples from the urethra **A.** urethral fossa
and diverticulum **B.** and preputial fold **C.** for microbiological
examination. (Courtesy H. Meier.)

Materials for Swabbing the Penis and Prepuce

▶ Gloves

▶ Tranquilizers (e.g., xylazine, 0.5 mg/ kg IV)

▶ Swabs

▶ Transport medium

transmission of infection to the mares.[2] The procedures for collection vary between countries, but the international significance of contagious equine metritis has produced a relatively standard set of procedures. A minimum recommendation is to swab the stallion once per year. More frequent swabbing is indicated if infection or infertility are present. The urethra, urethral fossa, urethral diverticulum, and preputial fold should be swabbed.

PROCEDURE. The penis should be exteriorized (see Examination of the Prepuce and Penis), although this precludes a preejaculate sample. The penis is held in the gloved left hand while the other hand is used to manipulate the swab sticks, which can be handled either separately or simultaneously by inserting each swab between a different finger space (Fig. 8–8). The urethra, urethral fossa, urethral diverticulum, and preputial fold are swabbed in order, with the latter being most likely to be resented by the stallion. Swabs dampened with sterile water or transport medium can be used.

RESULTS. Active infection of the genital tract is not common. The main problem is the carrier state that facilitates the spread of organisms between mares via the stallion. Organisms often associated with reduced fertility include *Taylorella equigenitalis,* beta-hemolytic streptococci, *Escherichia coli, Pseudomonas aeruginosa,* and *Klebsiella pneumoniae* (capsule types 1, 2, and 5). In addition to the presence of microorganisms, an active infection in the stallion is likely to be associated with inflammatory cells and the other signs of inflammation, such as redness, blood, and swelling.

SPECIAL EXAMINATION

Ultrasonography of the Testes, Penis, and Accessory Sex Glands

Ultrasonography is used to measure testes, to identify intratesticular masses and accumulation of fluid in the vaginal tunics, lesions of the cavernous spaces of the penis, and undescended testicles in crytorchid horses, and to examine the internal genital organs. The techniques are relatively simple.

PROCEDURE. The penis must be exteriorized, as described, and held firmly in one hand while the probe, which is coated with coupling gel, is held against the penis with the other hand. The probe is then moved along the penis as dictated by the requirements of the examination.

Examination of the testicle is also easily accomplished. The testicle is stabilized for examination by grasping the scrotum proximally with one hand and using the other to manipulate the probe. By moving the probe around, the testicle and epididymis can be imaged. Ultrasonography can also be used to localize cryptorchid testicles with a high degree of accuracy.[3] A 5.0 MHz transducer is used to carry out an examination from outside the abdomen and then transrectally. The probe is placed over the external ring and then moved to image the canal and external inguinal ring region as thoroughly as possible. The examination is then continued transrectally by inserting the probe and then, beginning at the pelvic brim, it is swept from side to side while gradually moving cranially.

The internal organs are examined in the same manner as those of the female tract.[4,5] The rectum is emptied of feces, and the probe (7.5 MHz), coated with coupling gel and enclosed in an ob-

Materials for Ultrasonography of the Testes, Penis, and Internal Genital Organs

▶ Ultrasound machine with 5.0 or 7.5-MHz linear or sector transducer

▶ Ultrasound coupling gel

▶ Obstetrical sleeve

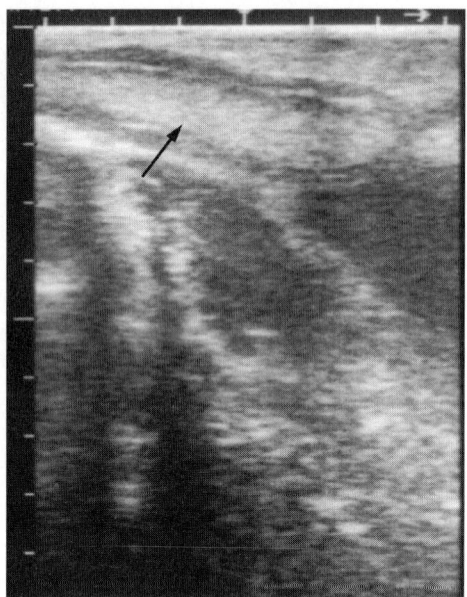

▶ FIGURE 8-9

An ultrasonogram of an impacted ("plugged") ampulla. (Courtesy A. O. McKinnon.)

stetrical sleeve, is inserted into the rectum and held against the ventral wall of the rectum with the beam directed ventrally. The bulbourethral glands, pelvic urethra, prostate gland, seminal vesicles, ampullae of the vas deferens, the masculine uterus, and the excretory ducts can be imaged and measured. Each gland is scanned over its length to evaluate size, shape, and fluid content.

The *vesicular glands* are located dorsolateral to the bladder and are difficult to image unless they are distended. If the glands contribute gel to the ejaculate, postejaculation imaging will show that the lumen has decreased in size or has become invisible, depending on the state of emptying. The *ampullae* lie medial to the vesicular glands, and dorsolateral to the bladder. The lumen increases in size after teasing and decreases after ejaculation. An ultrasonogram of an impacted ampulla is shown in Figure 8-9. The *prostate gland* lies immediately caudal to the attachments of the above glands to the urethra. The image of each gland is characterized by hypoechoic bands that radiate from the region of urethra. The gland increases in size and fluid content after teasing and decreases after ejaculation. The *bulbourethral glands* are located caudal to the other glands. In longitudinal section the image consists of a mottled isoechoic central glandular region, surrounded by a hypoechoic border, corresponding to the bulboglandularis muscle. These glands

respectively increase and decrease in size after teasing and ejaculation. The *pelvic urethra* is seen as a hypoechoic circular region, corresponding to the urethralis muscle, surrounding a mottled central region.

Radiology of the Genital System

There is little indication for a radiological examination of the genitalia. Plain and contrast radiography can be used to image the urethra to detect strictures and obstructions such as urethral calculi.

Semen Collection

Semen is collected to establish the morphological and functional status of sperm, thereby establishing the fertility of the stallion and allowing an evaluation of certain disease states. The usual methods of obtaining a semen sample are as follows:[6]

- *Collection of the ejaculate from the vagina after service.* This is easy to do but suffers the disadvantages that it indicates only if sperm are present, may be contaminated, and is not representative of the total ejaculate.
- *Condom.* Collection with a condom also is convenient. However, the stallion may resent its application, and the condom may be dislodged and the ejaculate lost. When used successfully, it provides a good sample.
- *Artificial vagina (AV).* The AV is the usual method and most often provides a good sample that is easily examined. This is the method that will be described.

Semen Collection with an Artificial Vagina

There are a number of different AVs available, the basic components being an outer casing that is used for transport and support, an inner rubber liner(s), and a collection bottle. In-line gel filters are available for most models. An example of AV is shown in Figure 8-10.

PROCEDURE

Preparation of the AV. The apparatus must be washed before use with a mild antiseptic, flushed at least three times with clean water, rinsed with 70% alcohol, and then air-dried. The internal temperature of the AV should be at 45°C (113°F) at the time of service, so it is usual to fill

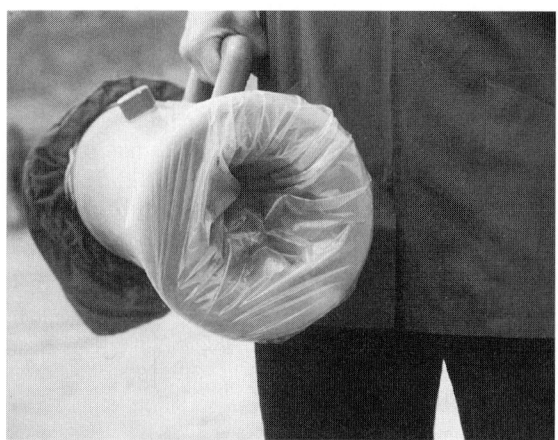

Artificial vagina (AV) of the Colorado type prepared for use. Note the handle, water filler cap, inner plastic liner, and protective cover for the collection bottle. (Courtesy A. O. McKinnon.)

Materials for Semen Collection with an Artificial Vagina

▶ Mare in estrus

▶ Hobbles for the mare

▶ Artificial vagina

▶ In-line gel filter

▶ Dial thermometer

▶ Tail bandage

▶ Sterile lubricant (nonspermicidal, such as K-Y jelly)

the liner with water at a higher temperature (e.g., 50°C; 122°F) to compensate for some prior heat loss. Before use, some sterile nonspermicidal lubricant should be placed in the palm of the gloved hand and then applied to the cranial two thirds of the liner. The pressure in the liner must be adjusted to provide the correct pressure on the penis. The pressure in the Missouri AV can be manually increased during service, but other makes require adjustment by adding air.

Preparation of the Stallion. The stallion's penis should be washed with water at a temperature of 42°C (108°F). Plastic disposable gloves should be used. A mare in estrus is used to stimulate protrusion of the penis. The water is placed in a bucket lined with a plastic liner.

Preparation of the Mare. To collect semen while the stallion serves, a mare in estrus, the "jump" mare, is usually used to stimulate the stallion so that sexual behavior can be better evaluated. Occasionally a dummy mare, or phantom, is used. The mare used should be tractable and her perineal region should be washed with an antiseptic detergent, rinsed, dried with disposable towels, and her tail covered with a sock, obstetrical sleeve, or completely bandaged (a shorter length is acceptable if the tail can be held aside during collection). The tail bandage should be changed and the mare rewashed between stallions. To avoid accidents and to protect the stallion, the mare is usually hobbled and twitched.

Semen Collection. The person holding the AV is in a potentially dangerous position, and in many institutions and on many studs will wear a

protective helmet and strong, hard footwear. The stallion is led up to the left side of the mare and allowed to tease her while moving toward her rear end. The collector stands on the near side just behind the stallion handler. When the penis is erect, the stallion may be allowed to mount and then, while the stallion handler controls him and ensures that the collector is not injured by the stallion's foreleg, the collector quickly but gently guides the penis onto the AV. Sometimes, by accident the stallion will serve the mare, and it is therefore important that such service cannot cause infection or unwanted pregnancy. The AV is held firmly in the right hand with the left hand on the bottom, and supported by pushing against the mare's thigh during the ejaculation (Fig. 8-11). Ejaculation is confirmed by placing the fingers of

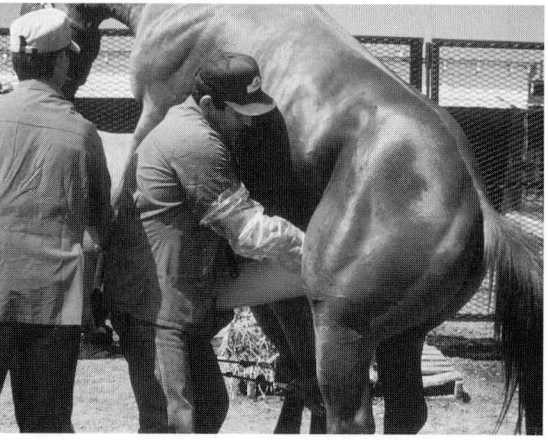

▶ **FIGURE 8-11**

Collection of semen using a mare and artificial vagina (AV). Note the position of the collector and the stallion holder, and how the AV is supported against the mare (Courtesy A.O. McKinnon).

the right hand around the penis and noting the pulsations that normally occur. The ejaculate is collected by directing the AV slightly ventrally and then gently lowering it while supporting the penis, so that the semen flows into the collection tube. At the completion of service the right hand can be used to strip residual semen from the urethra into the AV. The pressure in the liner can also be reduced to allow any trapped semen to flow to the collection tube. The presence of white frothy semen in the urethral orifice indicates that ejaculation has occurred. The semen sample is then transferred quickly to the laboratory, either in the AV or in a separate collection tube, during which time it must be protected from ultraviolet light and temperature changes. To avoid accidents, the mare and stallion are immediately separated from one another.

Semen Processing. The semen sample must be kept warm by placing it immediately in a water bath or incubator kept at 37°C, to await processing:

- *Density and mass activity.* A drop of gel-free semen is placed on a warm slide and examined under ×100 magnification. Density is an estimate of sperm concentration and mass activity is a measure of activity and depends on density and motility.
- *Motility.* To evaluate motility, a drop of semen is pipetted onto a warm slide, covered with a cover slip, and examined under phase-contrast (×200). Although percentage motility, percentage progressive motility, spermatozoal velocity (scale 0–4), and longevity can be assessed, percentage progressive motility is the most important. Progressive motility is motility resulting in forward progression of sperm. Motility is assessed, subjectively, as the mean of values obtained from 3 to 5 fields per coverslip while moving in a straight line across the specimen. To avoid clumping of sperm, which hinders evaluation, the sample can be diluted 1:20 with warmed semen extendor or 5% glucose. Estimates should be made on both raw and extended semen so that any effect of extendor can be assessed.
- *Percentage live sperm.* This parameter is assessed on a sample stained with nigrosin-eosin. A drop of semen is added to a warmed vial containing eight drops of the stain and allowed to stand for 3 minutes be-

fore a drop is transferred to a warm slide and smear made. After air-drying the unmounted smear is examined under oil immersion (×1,000 magnification). The dead spermatozoa take up the eosin and stain pink against the dark background of the nigrosin.
- *Volume.* Volume is measured in the collector or in a special warmed receptacle. Alternately, it can be measured after all other tests have been made.
- *Color.* Color is checked grossly for discoloration indicative of blood, debris, or urine.
- *pH.* The pH of the gel-free portion is measured with a pH meter.
- *Concentration.* Concentration can be measured automatically with an electronic counter or manually in a hemocytometer chamber.[2] For manual measurement the following steps are carried out. (1) Dilute the semen 1:200 using a red cell hemocytometer pipette. (2) Place a drop on the grid of the chamber, and cover with a cover slip. (3) Use a ×40 objective to focus, and count the number of sperm in five of the large squares. Count in squares that lie diagonally across the grid, and, to avoid counting twice those sperm that lie across a border, count those that touch the bottom and the left sides of each square. Repeat the count using another diagonal, and calculate the mean value for five squares (not each individual square) and multiply this by 10,000 to arrive at sperm/mm.[3] Dilution can also be carried out with a system used for measuring platelets and white blood cells, which requires different dilution and multiplication factors. Use of a spectrophotometer (Spectronic 20, Bausch & Lomb, Rochester, NY) requires precalibration with construction of a standard curve based on comparisons between hemocytometric and spectrophotometric data. A precalibrated instrument (Equine Sperm cell Counter, Animal Reproduction Systems, Chino, CA) is available.
- *Total number of sperm.* The total number of sperm is calculated by multiplying sperm concentration (10^6-mL) by the volume (mL) of the gel-free portion of the ejaculate.
- *Morphology.* Although morphology can be assessed on unstained, buffered formalin-fixed samples with phase-contrast microscopy, the simpler option is to use a nigrosin-eosin stained sample and oil immersion mi-

croscopy. The sample is processed as follows: Six drops of stain are added to a test tube held in the water bath and left for 2 minutes to equilibrate before adding one drop of semen and shaking gently. One drop of the mixture is transferred to a slide and a smear made. After air-drying, the sample is examined at ×1,000 magnification and results recorded for at least 200 cells. With the nigrosin-eosin stain, dead cells stain pink (eosin), and the nigrosin provides the background stain. The results can be broadly grouped as normal sperm (including those with abaxial tails), abnormal heads, detached heads, proximal droplets, distal droplets, abnormal midpieces, and abnormal tails. Further subdivision is based on shape, size spatial arrangement, malformation, and injury to the head, acrosome, midpiece, and tail. The number of normal sperm is obtained by adding the number of normal live sperm and sperm with distal cytoplasmic droplets.

EVALUATION OF THE STALLION. Important aspects include the ability to produce and maintain an erection and to insert the penis in the vagina and ejaculate and lack of sexual vices. A discussion of sexual behavior dysfunction in the stallion is not pertinent for this text. However information is readily available in the published literature.[7]

Semen Evaluation. The ejaculate is produced by six to nine urethral contractions and consists of spermatozoa (80% in first three jets of semen), seminal plasma from the accessory glands, and gel (in the latter portion of the ejaculate) from the seminal vesicles. Some normal values are presented in the box.

No parameter is 100% accurate as a criterion of fertility, although the percentage of progressively motile sperm (those able to swim foreward) is thought to be the best indicator. In addition, although a stallion may be capable of fertilizing one mare, the need to fertilize a number of mares for a commercial stud must also be considered. In such cases, some measure of both semen output and quality is required. Collection of two samples, 1 hour apart in a sexually rested stallion and measurement of daily sperm output are useful in this context. In general, the second sample can be expected to be similar to the first, although the total number of sperm will be about half that of the first. Daily outputs of sperm in young and

---

NORMAL VALUES FOR SEMEN (MEAN; RANGE IN PARENTHESIS)[8]

	Mean	Range
Appearance: Whitish, opaque, liquid (resembling skimmed milk)		
Gel-free volume (mL)	45	(20–150)
Sperm concentration (10^6/mL)	175	(60–350)
Total sperm/ejaculate (10^9)	9	(2–25)
pH	7.4	(7.2–7.6)
Motile sperm (%)	75	(60–90)
Progressively motile sperm (%)	50	(40–90)
Morphologically normal sperm (%)	50	(40–85)

---

mature stallions should be 4×10^9 and 6×10^9, respectively. Daily sperm output is closely related to testicular size. Some causes of reduced sperm production include testicular degeneration, overuse, small testes, and incomplete ejaculation.

Endoscopy of the Genital System

Flexible endoscopes allow easy examination of the urethra and the urethral openings of the intrapelvic genital organs.[9]

PROCEDURE. The horse is sedated and the penis exteriorized (see Examination of the Prepuce and Penis). A tail bandage is useful, as it will prevent the horse from switching its tail into the face of the clinician or contaminating the equipment. The horse should be restrained in a crush so that it cannot move around and damage the

---

Materials for Endoscopy of the Urethra and Intrapelvic Genitalia

▸ Flexible endoscope (maximum diameter, 1.0 cm, minimum length, 100 cm) that has been sterilized or properly cleaned
▸ Sterile lubricating jelly containing xylocaine
▸ Gloves

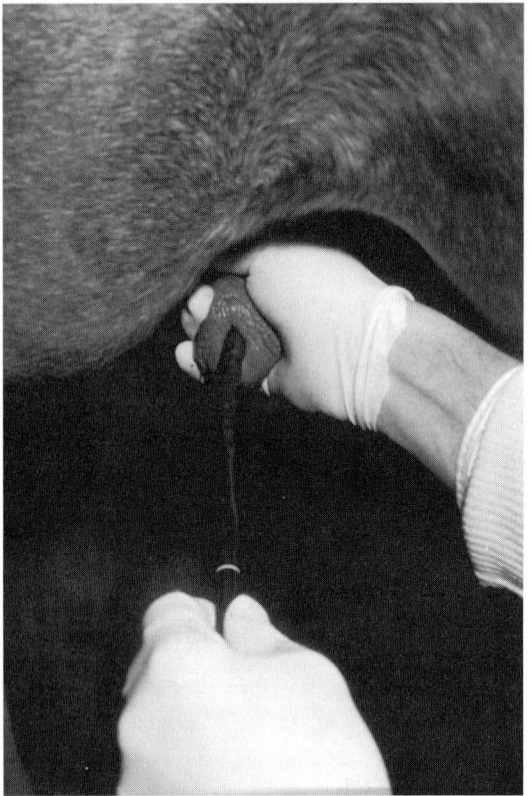

▶ **FIGURE 8-12**

Urethral endoscopy. Insertion of the lubricated flexible endoscope into the urethra.

equipment or kick the operator. The person holding the penis should stand beside the horse's flank facing toward the rear. The penis should be grasped proximal to the glans and traction applied slowly to extend it fully. The urethral process and surrounding fossae and glans should be carefully washed with an antiseptic and then flushed clean with water.

A small amount of sterile lubricant is applied to the endoscope and the urethral process. The assistant holds the penis above the glans with one hand and guides the endoscope into the urethra with the gloved other hand (Fig. 8-12). As the endoscope is advanced, the urethra should be inflated with air to improve visualization of the mucosa. This is done by covering the air outlet of the endoscope and squeezing the penis gently to prevent air from passing back around the endoscope. Care is necessary to avoid overinflating the system, which will cause discomfort. If the presence of the endoscope or the air stimulates a desire to urinate, the hold on the penis should be relaxed and the penis should be directed ventrally to allow urine to flow easily around the endoscope.

The normal urethra is pink, and the mucosa is arranged in longitudinal folds that change to a reddish color and become smooth if inflated. Overinflation allows the vessels of the underlying corpus spongiosum to be seen. As the trauma from the endoscope readily produces hyperemia, it is important that the evaluation be completed during insertion, rather than during the withdrawal of the endoscope. As the endoscope is inserted, some resistance is appreciated as it passes around the ischial arch and enters the pelvic inlet, bringing the lumen of the intrapelvic urethra into view (Fig. 8-13). Immediately, the papillae of the ducts of the bulbourethral glands

A 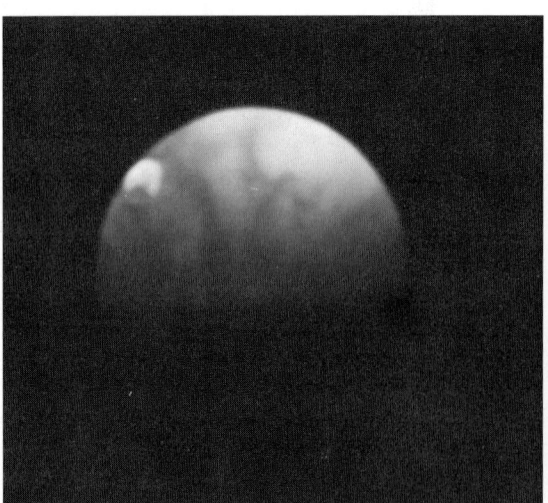 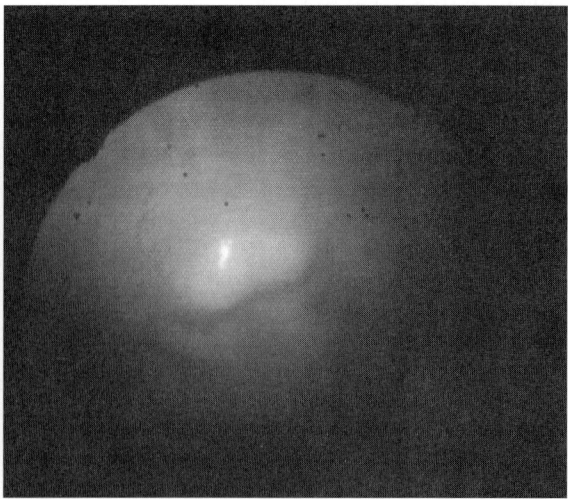 B

▶ **FIGURE 8-13**

Urethral endoscopy in the male horse—intrapelvic openings of the accessory sex glands. **A.** Openings to bulbourethral glands with colliculus seminalis in the background. **B.** Colliculus seminalis with left and right ejaculatory duct-openings in sight.

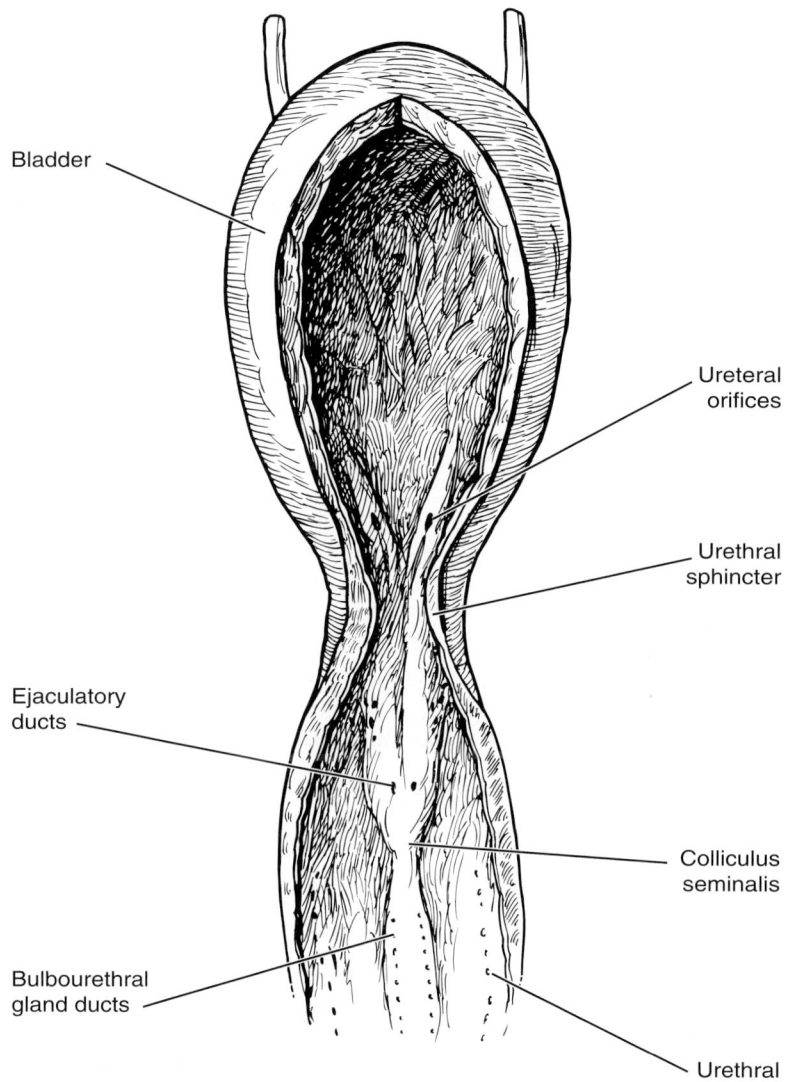

Bladder

Ureteral
orifices

Urethral
sphincter

Ejaculatory
ducts

Colliculus
seminalis

Bulbourethral
gland ducts

Urethral
gland ducts

▶ **FIGURE 8-14**

Diagram showing the urethral openings
of the accessory sex glands.

are seen arranged in two parallel rows just off the
dorsal midline of the urethra. At the same level the
openings of the urethral glands are seen as similar
structures on the lateral walls.

Advancing the endoscope 2 to 3 cm brings the
colliculus seminalis into view, seen as a prominent
papilla on the dorsal midline. On each side of this
structure are the openings of the left and right
common ducts of the ductus deferens and the
vesicular glands, which are usually difficult to
find. Lateral and proximal are the prostatic ducts,
which are small and also difficult to see. The
bladder sphincter is located 2 to 3 cm cranial to
the colliculus seminalis. These anatomical features are shown in Figure 8-14.

Lesions associated with hemospermia are often
located in the intrapelvic region of the urethra. An
example of urethritis is shown in Figure 8-15. The

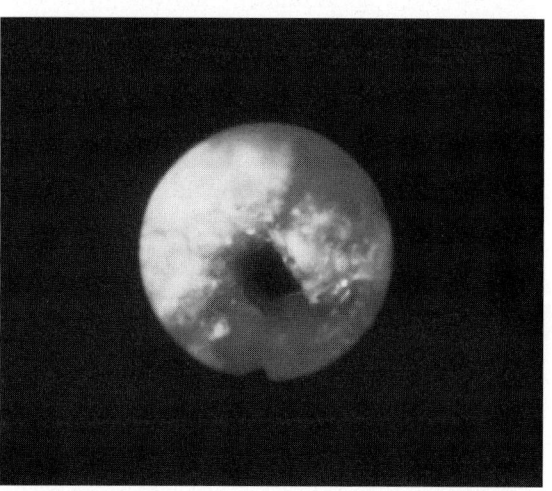

▶ **FIGURE 8-15**

Urethral endoscopy. Urethritis—Note the swollen and irregular
mucosa.

> ## Materials Required for Open Biopsy of the Testicle
>
> ▶ #11 scalpel blade
> ▶ Surgical instrument kit
> ▶ Suture material (3/0 absorbable of choice)

> ## Materials for Aspiration Biopsy of the Testicle
>
> ▶ Sterile syringe (10 mL)
> ▶ 23-gauge needle
> ▶ Local anesthetic (Lidocaine or mepivacaine)

bladder and ureteral openings of both sexes are not important in the context of reproduction and will be described in the section dealing with the urinary tract.

Biopsy of the Testicle

Biopsy of the testicle is not a routine procedure and is rarely done because of the fear of complications such as sperm granuloma or intratesticular bleeding. Available methods include open, needle, and aspiration biopsy. Because of minimal invasiveness, the latter two techniques are preferred.

Open Biopsy

PROCEDURE. The procedure is best done as a sterile procedure under general anesthesia with a standard skin preparation. The testicle is manipulated and stabilized in the scrotum by squeezing it manually from above. This tenses the scrotal skin in which a 2-cm ventral incision is made midway between the cranial and caudal poles. An incision of similar size is made in the underlying parietal layer of the vaginal tunic, followed by a stab incision through a nonvascular region of the visceral tunic. The stab incision is about 1 cm deep. An elliptical piece of tissue about 2 mm wide is excised. The visceral and parietal tunics are closed separately with absorbable suture material. The skin is apposed with a subcuticular suture pattern, which bypasses the need to remove sutures.

COMPLICATIONS. Open biopsy has the potential for serious sequelae such as bleeding, excessive inflammatory response, and testicular degeneration. However, when carried out carefully, in particular taking care to avoid visible blood vessels, the procedure is relatively benign.[10] Notwithstanding this, one of the less invasive methods is preferred, especially in valuable stallions.

Aspiration Biopsy

PROCEDURE. The biopsy is carried out using appropriate restraint with the horse standing. A few milliliters of local anesthetic solution can be injected into the scrotal tissues, but this is usually unnecessary. The needle is inserted into the testicular tissue and connected to the syringe, and suction is applied while the needle is redirected in a few different directions to ensure collection of material. The plunger of the syringe is then released and the needle and syringe withdrawn.

Needle Biopsy

PROCEDURE. This is a more invasive procedure than aspiration biopsy, and therefore restraint is more critical and local anesthesia is necessary. The testicle is held by an assistant and a few milliliters of anesthetic solution are injected into the scrotal skin. A small stab incision is made through the skin but not into the testicle. The biopsy instrument is inserted through the incision and into the testicle. The sample is collected as described in Appendix F.

COMPLICATIONS. Possible complications with both methods are sperm granuloma, intratesticular bleeding, and infection. With the aspi-

> ## Materials for Needle Biopsy of the Testicle
>
> ▶ Tru-cut biopsy needle
> ▶ Local anesthetic, (Lidocaine or mepivacinae)
> ▶ #11 Scalpel blade
> ▶ 5-mL syringe and 23-gauge needle

ration method, complications are rare, but it is advised that biopsy be used only when definitely indicated and after other diagnostic possibilities have been considered. This is even more important when it is realized that the biopsy is most likely to be necessary in a breeding stallion in which complications are most likely to be of significance.

R E F E R E N C E S

1. Thompson DL, Pickett BW, Squires EL: Testicular measurements and reproductive characteristics in stallions. J Reprod Fertil Suppl 1979; 27:13.
2. Allen WE: Examination of the stallion for breeding soundness. *In* Fertility and Obstetrics in the Horse. Oxford, Blackwell, 1988, p 136.
3. Jann HW, Rains JR: Diagnostic ultrasonography for evaluation of cryptorchidism in horses. J Am Vet Med Assoc 1990; 196:297.
4. Little TV, Woods GL: Ultrasonography of accessory sex glands in the stallion. J Reprod Fertil Suppl 1987; 35:87.
5. Weber JA, Geary RT, Woods GL: Changes in accessory sex glands of stallions after sexual preparation and ejaculation. J Am Vet Med Assoc 1990; 196:1084.
6. Pickett BW: Collection and Evaluation of Stallion for Artificial Insemination. *In* Mckinnon AO, Voss JL (eds), Equine Reproduction. Malvern, PA, Lea & Febiger, 1993, ch 79, p 705.
7. McDonnell SM: Sexual behaviour dysfunction in stallions. *In* Robinson NE (ed): Current Therapy in Equine Medicine, 3rd ed. Philadelphia, Saunders, 1993, p 668.
8. Jasko DJ: Stallion seminal characteristics and fertility. *In* Robinson NE (ed): Current Therapy in Equine Medicine, 3rd ed. Philadelphia, Saunders, 1992, p 671.
9. Sullins KE: Urinary tract. *In* Traub-Dargatz JL, Brown CM (eds): Equine Endoscopy. St Louis, Mosby, 1990, ch 12, p 145.
10. Delvento VR, Amann RP, Trotter GW, et al: Ultrasonographic and quantitative histologic assessment of sequelae to testicular biopsy in stallions. Am J Vet Res 1992; 53: 2094.

Urinary Tract

9

COMPONENTS

The urinary tract extends from the urethral opening to the kidneys. With appropriate methods, all of the tract can be examined, although the anatomical differences between the sexes means that examination of the male and female urethra is conducted differently.

MANIFESTATIONS OF DISEASE

The prime function of the urinary tract is to excrete some of the end products of metabolism and to participate in the maintenance of fluid and electrolyte homeostasis. Interference with this group of functions results in a variety of abnormal fluid and electrolyte values that at first are detectable only by measuring appropriate blood and urine parameters. As disease progresses and exhibits increasingly greater disruption of homeostasis, the main systemic sign of reduced function is depression. The tubular nature of the tract renders it susceptible to obstruction, which can occur with neoplasia, urolithiasis, and infection. Local signs of disease include exaggerated efforts to pass urine, associated with obstruction; abnormal frequency of urination; variation in total urine output; dribbling of urine; and presence of abnormal urine constituents such as blood, crystals, pigments, and inflammatory cells. Microscopic examination of urine sediment is important in determining the disease process, where abnormal findings include blood, crystals, cellular casts,

leucocytes and bacteria, and neoplastic cells. Crystals, calcium carbonate in alkaline urine, and triple phosphate in neutral and acid urine, are commonly found, and their presence does not necessarily indicate disease. Bacteremia and toxemia accompany severe infection, such as cystitis and pyelonephritis, and contribute to depression and fever.

RESTRAINT

Examination of the urinary tract involves procedures that place the clinician in danger of being kicked. Injury can be avoided by observing the procedures described in the sections dealing with the male and female genital tracts.

GENERAL PHYSICAL EXAMINATION

Visual Inspection

Unassisted visual inspection of the urinary tract is limited to the penis and external urethral orifice in the male, and the vulva and urethral opening in the female, to observing the physical act of micturition (urination) and to the appearance of the urine.

Posture Adopted during Micturition

The male horse extends the penis from the prepuce and adopts a wide-based stance, with the

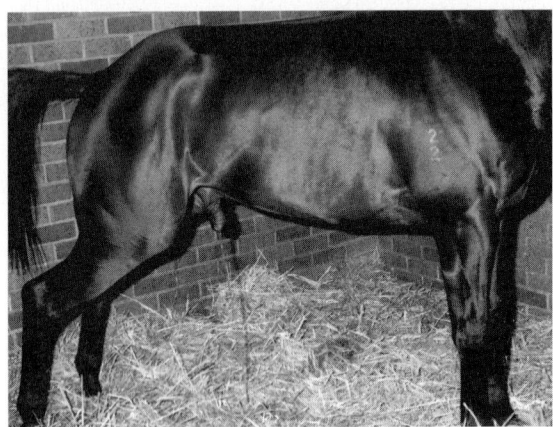

▶ **FIGURE 9–1**

Stance for urination in the male horse.

front legs forward of a normal position and the hind legs placed caudally (Fig. 9–1). The horse often takes quite a few seconds to get himself into position. The urine is at first expelled forcibly in a steady stream and then finally in a series of spurts. Male horses, especially stallions, can often be stimulated to urinate by being placed in a stall with hay on the floor or by rustling the hay with a fork. The female stands with her hind legs spread apart and adopts the position with less preliminary activity than shown by the male (Fig. 9–2). She also urinates by expelling the urine forcibly in a stream and then in spurts.

Some abnormal clinical findings regarding posture and expulsion of urine include:

- Inability to adopt the normal posture due to back or limb pain.
- Failure to produce a strong stream of urine due to obstruction from calculi, bladder atony, or neurological deficits.

Appearance of Urine

Equine urine often has a heavy content of mucus and calcium carbonate crystals, giving it a thick, yellow appearance that is often a matter of concern for an owner. This material is mainly expressed with the last of the urine at the end of micturition. The urine should be assessed for color and presence of abnormal constituents.

Volume of Urine and Frequency of Micturition

The volume of urine varies with water intake, physical activity, and environmental temperature. Increased or decreased output can occur in association with disease. Frequent passage of small volumes of urine, due to irritation or simply overflow from a full but paralyzed bladder, may give the impression that larger than normal volumes are being produced. Collection and measurement over 24 hours is a more accurate method of establishing urine output.

Collection of Urine

Urine can be collected in a container during spontaneous urination ("free catch"), by catheter, or in some cases in foals by cystocentesis. As stated, male horses can often be stimulated to urinate by being placed in a stall that has a liberal layer of straw bedding and then by rustling the straw. Urination can also be stimulated by admin-

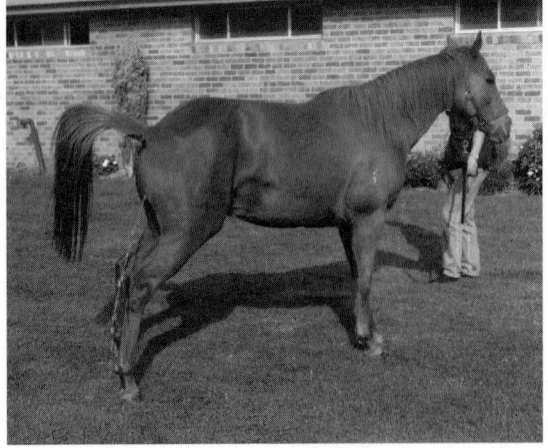

▶ **FIGURE 9–2**

Stance for urination in the female horse.

istering a diuretic (furosemide, 0.5–1.0 mg/kg IV), although samples are not suitable for quantitative studies. Urine is collected usually for chemical analysis and cytological evaluation. However, when infection is suspected, culture and antibiotic sensitivity are required. An uncontaminated sample, collected by catheter or cystocentesis is necessary if culture for organisms is required. A midstream, voided sample may be suitable if the penis and prepuce or the vulva have been cleaned and dried beforehand.

"Free-Catch" Collection of Urine during Spontaneous or Stimulated Urination

This requires a small receptacle, such as plastic beaker, which can be attached to a long handle. The long handle allows the receptacle to be placed quickly in a position to catch the urine without disturbing the horse (Fig. 9–3).

Bladder Catheterization in the Female

The female bladder is easily catheterized, either blindly, under direct vision, or with digital assistance. Catheterization is most easily achieved with a curved metal catheter, although a plastic pipette is satisfactory. For blind catheterization the curved catheter is best, as its curvature and

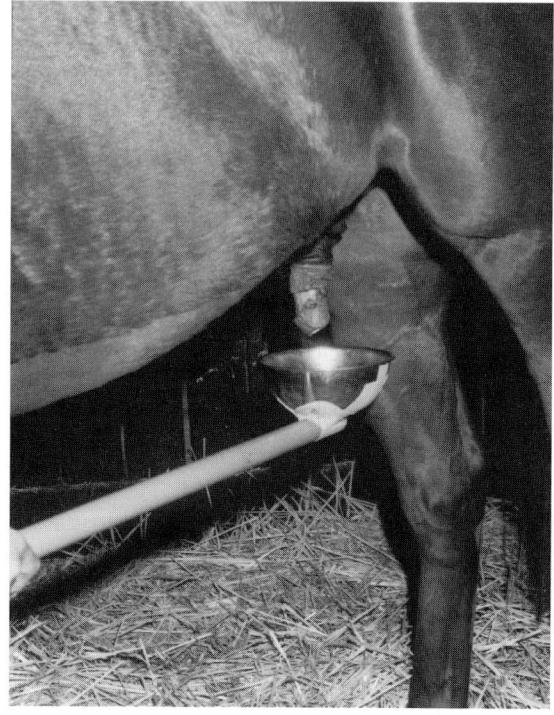

> **FIGURE 9-3**

Collection of urine by "free-catch."

> ### Materials for Catheterization of the Male Bladder

> ▶ Male urinary catheter
> ▶ Sterile lubricant (such as K-Y jelly)
> ▶ Sterile gloves
> ▶ Detergent antiseptic (e.g., Povidone iodine or chlorhexidine)

rigidity ensure it will slide easily into the urethral orifice.

The mare should be restrained in stocks and the tail held to one side. For blind catheterization the curved metal catheter is inserted through the ventral aspect of the vulva and pushed cranially, ensuring that the curvature is directed ventrally and that the tip is in contact with the floor of the vagina. The urethral orifice is located immediately caudal to the hymen remnant, and on most occasions the catheter passes easily through it and into the bladder without the mare showing resentment. For catheterization with digital assistance the gloved and lightly lubricated hand is passed into the vagina, and the urethral orifice is located and dilated with the first or second finger. The orifice is usually closed but dilates easily when pressure is exerted with the exploring finger. The catheter is then inserted beside the finger. If a speculum is used the catheter is passed toward the region of the orifice that cannot usually be seen because it lies beneath the remnant of the hymen. The catheter should be directed beneath the hymen, and it will usually pass easily into the urethra.

Bladder Catheterization in the Male

The male bladder is usually catheterized to collect urine for evaluation of infection or to check the patency of the urethra in cases of urolithiasis.

PROCEDURE. The patient is tranquilized (see Chemical Restraint in Chapter 1) and restrained in stocks that have a side access to the penis. Tranquilization is necessary to cause relaxation and protrusion of the penis, as well as to quieten the horse. Care must be taken to avoid penile complications associated with sedation and tranquilization (see Chemical Restraint of the Adult Horse in Chapter 1). The clinician should stand beside the horse's left flank, facing backward, and take the extended penis just behind the glans in the left hand. If necessary, gentle traction is applied until the penis is extended far enough to allow the catheter to be inserted without its becoming contaminated. The penis is then directed laterally so that the urethral orifice and urethral diverticulum can be cleansed with a detergent antiseptic such as povidone iodine or chlorhexidine. A small amount of lubricant is placed on the urethral opening and the catheter, which is then slowly inserted with the gloved right hand. The catheter is demonstrated in Figure 9-4.

There is usually some resistance and maybe a response from the horse (downward movement of tail) as the catheter passes around the ischial arch and then into the pelvic urethra and bladder. Once in the bladder there is usually a flow of urine. However, on occasions, negative pressure applied by syringe is necessary.

Laboratory Evaluation of Urine

A full evaluation of urine is not required for all situations, but when it is, the sample should be divided and submitted for urinalysis, consisting

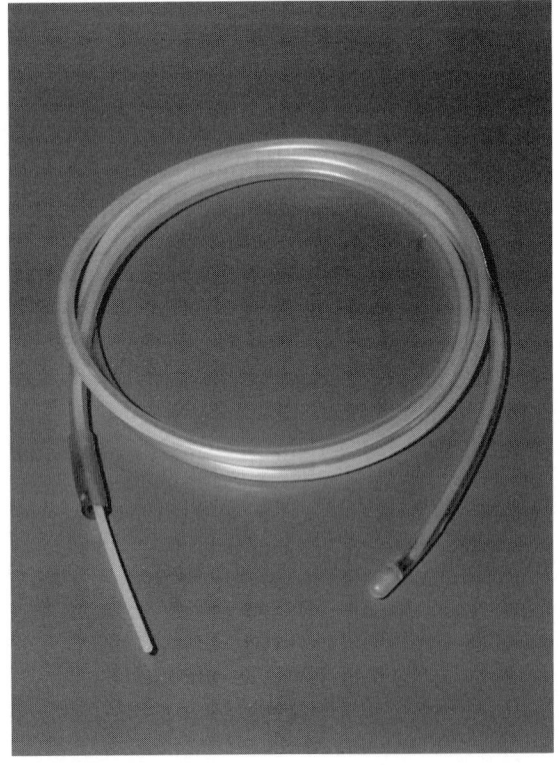

▶ FIGURE 9-4

Catheter for collection of urine from the male horse.

(depending on circumstances) of: microscopy for cytology, casts, and crystals; measurement of specific gravity; stick tests; chemical tests; and bacterial culture and sensitivity testing. As deterioration of leukocytes and bacterial viability begins rapidly, urine must be processed within 20 minutes or stored at 5°C, when these entities are significant in the context of the case. A smear is usually made immediately to allow a Gram stain and examination for cells and bacteria to be made.

SPECIFIC GRAVITY. Specific gravity is measured with a refractometer, normal values being 1.008 to 1.040 for adults, and 1.001 to 1.025 for foals.[1]

STRIP OR DIPSTICK TESTING. Stick tests are used to estimate pH, glucose, protein, blood, ketones, and bilirubin.[1] Normal values for pH are 7.5 to 8.5 for adults, and 5.5 to 8.0 for foals. Normal urine contains no protein (none to trace), glucose, or bilirubin. Care is required when interpreting the stick tests because of the tendency for false-positive results for protein when urine is concentrated, in which case protein should be estimated with the sulfosalicylic acid procedure. Stick tests are often positive for blood and the pigments hemoglobin and myoglobin, differentiation of which requires more detailed laboratory analysis.

CHEMICAL AND BIOCHEMICAL ANALYSIS. Chemical and biochemical analysis includes calcium, chloride, phosphorus, potassium, sodium, creatinine (Cr), and gammaglutamyl-transpeptidase (GGT). Some of these values can be combined with the plasma values to calculate urine plasma ratios, renal clearances of creatinine and electrolytes, fractional excretion of electrolytes, and the ratio of urine GGT (UrGGT) to urine creatinine (UrCr). The relevant formulae and normal values are:[2]

- Urine/plasma ratios (normal)
  U/P osmolality ratio = 2–6
  U/P urea nitrogen ratio = 20–124
  U/P creatinine ratio = 2–344
- Ratio of urine GGT to urine creatinine (normal <25)
  UrGGT/UrCr
    = UrGGT (IU/mL)/UrCr(mg/dL) × 0.01
- Fractional excretion of substance x relative to creatinine (FEx)
  FEx = Urx/Px × PCr/UrCr × 100 (where P = serum)

FE Na = 0.032–0.52%
FE PO$_4$ = 0%–>20%
FE K = 23.3%–48.1%
FE Cl = 0.59%–1.86%
FE Ca = 0%–6.73% >2.5% when fed adequate calcium

- Renal clearance of substance x (Cx) (pooled or timed urine samples) [mL/min/kg]

Cx = Urx/Px × VUr/time/kg BW (where V = volume, BW = body weight)

Normal:
C$_{creatinine}$ {horses} = 0.96–2.80
C$_{Na}$ = 0.003–0.009
C$_K$ = 0.538–1.05
C$_{Cl}$ = 0.013–0.031

CYTOLOGY. Cytology is conducted after centrifugation. Casts are tubular structures formed in the renal tubules from protein, cells, and debris, and, when present, they indicate tubular disease. Crystals are very common, especially calcium carbonate. Under light microscopy a concentration of more than five red cells or leukocytes per high-power field is abnormal, with red cells indicating hemorrhage and leukocytes indicating septic or nonseptic inflammation. The presence of bacteria increases the probability of infection. Tumor cells may also be present.

MICROBIOLOGY. Instructions pertinent to clinical bacteriology can be found in Appendix C. As stated, a smear and Gram stain are often carried out immediately after collection to allow rapid identification of bacteria and to help determine whether further microbiological investigation will be necessary.

Palpation of the Bladder, Kidneys, and Ureters per Rectum

The principles of rectal palpation are described in Chapter 11 (see Palpation of the Abdomen per Rectum). The normal *bladder* is not palpable when it is empty and relaxed. When distended with urine, it is easily palpated, lying in the region of the pelvic brim as a relatively firm and circumscribed structure. Chronic cystitis often produces a thickened bladder wall, and calculi can be palpated as hard structures within the bladder. Distension because of obstruction (e.g., calculus) places the bladder wall under considerable pressure, which can lead to rupture. The *intrapelvic urethra* in the male is palpable as a thick muscular tube lying on the pelvic floor between the anus and the bladder neck. In females, the urethral opening is located in the ventral midline of the vagina, immediately caudal to the remnant of the hymen. The *ureters* are not palpable unless thickened or enlarged by obstruction (calculus) or disease (infection). Normally, only the left *kidney* is palpable, and then only the caudal pole. Enlargement, because of disease (e.g., cyst) makes palpation easier and can, on occasions, bring the right kidney within range. A pain response is sometimes associated with kidney disease.

SPECIAL EXAMINATION PROCEDURES

Radiography

Radiography of the urinary tract is limited mainly to ponies and foals because of the restriction imposed by size. In foals, intravenous pyelography is useful to investigate the kidneys, ureters, and bladder. Cystography is useful in bladder studies, and contrast cystography can demonstrate bladder rupture, patent urachus, and cystitis.[3]

Plain radiographs should be carried out before contrast studies. Positive contrast studies use a mixture of equal volumes of sterile saline and a water-soluble contrast material placed in the bladder by catheter. If carried out in the conscious foal, a few milliliters of a local anesthetic will control bladder discomfort. The bladder should be gently distended to its full volume, which often requires a preliminary radiograph(s). Lateral and ventrodorsal exposures are made. After removal of the contrast material, air can be injected to allow a negative-contrast study. Double-contrast studies, which use a combination of positive and negative techniques, is also possible. In the case of a patent urachus, the contrast material can also be delivered through the urachal remnant.

Intravenous pyelography requires general anesthesia and ventrodorsal exposures. The bladder is prepared by removing all urine by catheter. After injection of 100 mL of a water-soluble contrast material (e.g., Urografin, Schering Corp., Kenilworth, NJ) intravenously, exposures are made at 5-minute intervals. The angle of the exposures may require changing in order to improve the definition of structures, in particular the ureters. The material eventually accumulates in the bladder, allowing a positive-contrast study after about 20 minutes.

Measurement of Bladder and Urethral Pressures

Urinary continence ultimately depends on co-ordination between the detrusor muscle and urethral function, which can be disrupted by neurogenic (e.g., cauda equina syndrome) and nonneurogenic causes (e.g., calculi). Measurement of pressures within the bladder and urethra can help to evaluate problems associated with urination. Cystometrography, urethral pressure profilometry, and simultaneous cystometry and uroflowmetry have been used to investigate urodynamics. The latter technique has not been reported in horses.

Cystometrography consists of the measurement of bladder pressures and volumes when the bladder is filled with fluid or gas, producing data for tone, capacity, and compliance of the bladder, as well as the threshold volume and pressure required to trigger micturition. This technique has been used in mares, and differences were found between normal mares and incontinent ones.[4] Urethral and bladder pressures have been reported in male horses, using intravesicular pressure (IVP), maximal urethral closing pressure (MUCP), and the ratio between MUCP and IVP.[5] The bladder and urethral pressures were measured by recording the pressure within the cuff of a cuffed catheter inserted into the bladder and then withdrawn through the urethra.[5] The IVP was calculated by subtracting the cuff pressure

---

Materials for Endoscopy of the Male Urinary Tract: Urethra and Bladder

- Flexible endoscope (minimum length, 100 cm, maximum diameter, 1 cm)
- Sterile lubricant (e.g., K-Y jelly)
- Gloves
- Detergent antiseptic (Povidone iodine, chlorhexidine)

---

outside the urinary tract from the pressure inside the bladder, and the MUCP by subtracting the IVP from the maximal urethral pressure. Similar bladder and urethral pressure profiles have been carried out in mares.[6]

Catheterization of the male bladder requires sedation. However, the effects of adrenergic drugs on bladder function preclude their use. Xylazine is recommended as it had no significant effect on pressures in mares at a dose of 1.1 mg/kg IV.[6]

RESULTS. Normal pressure levels for horses, mares, and ponies are found in the box.

Endoscopy of the Male Urinary Tract: Urethra and Bladder

Endoscopy is indicated to facilitate a diagnosis when clinical signs or laboratory data indicate that lesions of the urinary tract could be present.[7]

PROCEDURE. For a flexible endoscope 100 cm and 1 cm are the minimum acceptable length and diameter, and a slightly longer instrument is necessary if the horse is very large or the penis becomes partially erect. With this length the endoscope must be fully inserted and, accordingly, the clinician's head must be placed low down and close to the penis, which can be dangerous with some horses. Using a videoendoscope, thus allowing the image to be seen on a monitor, is a much safer procedure. The endoscope, including the biopsy channel, should be prepared as described in Appendix A.

The procedure for insertion is virtually identical with that just described for catheterization, except that an assistant usually holds the penis and inserts the endoscope while the clinician controls the endoscope and conducts the examination. With the horse tranquilized and restrained in

---

Urethral and Bladder Pressures

- Male horses and geldings (mean ± SD cm H_2O)[5]
    - IVP = 10.3 ± 1.7
    - MUCP = 129.8 ± 19.6
    - MUCP: IVP = 13.2 ± 2.5
- Mares[6]
    - Stimulation pressure for micturition = 91.4 ± 16.5 cm H_2O
    - MUCP = 49.1 ± 19.4 cm H_2O
- Ponies[6]
    - Stimulation pressure for micturition: 86.0 ± 14.4
    - MUCP = 37.7 ± 14.4

stocks, the assistant, standing beside the horse and facing backward, takes the extended penis just behind the glans in the left hand. If necessary, gentle traction is applied until the penis is extended far enough to allow insertion of the endoscope without its becoming contaminated. The penis is then directed laterally so that the urethral orifice and urethral diverticulum can be cleansed with a detergent antiseptic such as povidone iodine or chlorhexidine. A small amount of lubricant is placed on the urethral opening and the endoscope, and the instrument is then slowly inserted by the assistant, using the gloved right hand. The clinician should begin examination of the urethra as soon as the endoscope is being inserted.

The urethra is normally collapsed, and it is necessary to insufflate it to obtain a better view of the mucosa. This is done by gently squeezing the penis to prevent retrograde escape of the air around endoscope. Sometimes too much air is injected and the horse is stimulated to urinate. If this occurs the assistant should relax the hold on the penis and direct it ventrally and away from the operators, allowing urine and air to pass around the endoscope. The normal urethral mucosa is pale pink in color and arranged in longitudinal folds. As the urethra is distended, the folds disappear and the mucosa becomes darker in color as the underlying background vasculature of the corpus spongiosa becomes visible. Examination of the mucosa should be carried out during insertion because contact with the endoscope produces hyperemia, which may be misconstrued as inflammation if the examination is conducted while the endoscope is being removed. Conditions such as urethritis or urolithiasis are readily identified (Fig. 9-5).

As with a catheter there is usually some resistance and maybe a response from the horse (downward movement of tail) as the endoscope passes around the ischial arch and then into the pelvic urethra and bladder. The openings of the accessory sex glands can be seen as the pelvic urethra comes into view (see Endoscopy of the Genital System in Chapter 8).

The urethral sphincter is usually closed, but injecting some air and gentle forward movement of the endoscope quickly overcome sphincter tone. There is usually some urine in the bladder, which will aid orientation. Excess urine should be evacuated with a separate catheter or through the suction channel of the endoscope. The bladder

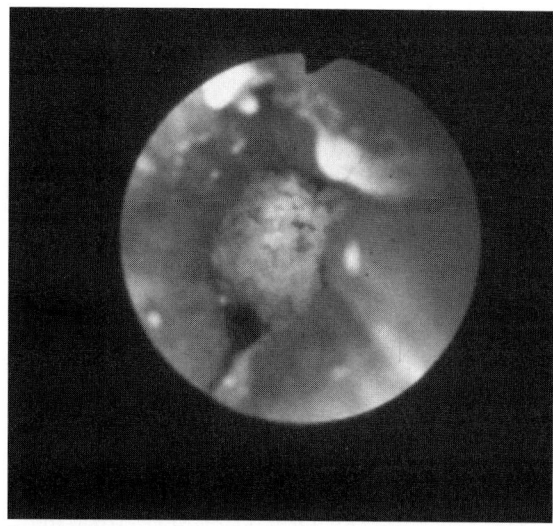

▶ **FIGURE 9-5**
Endoscopic view of a urethral calculus.

mucosa is also pink-red in color but is usually darker than that of the urethra. Some horses have a diverticulum in the region of the urachus.

The slitlike urethral openings lie dorsally in the neck of the bladder and can be seen if the endoscope is slightly withdrawn. Intermittent jets of urine can be seen entering the bladder from the ureters. The ureters can be catheterized relatively easily by inserting a catheter through the endoscope and then directing it into a ureteral orifice (Fig. 9-6). Ureteral catheterization requires coordination between the endoscope and the catheter.

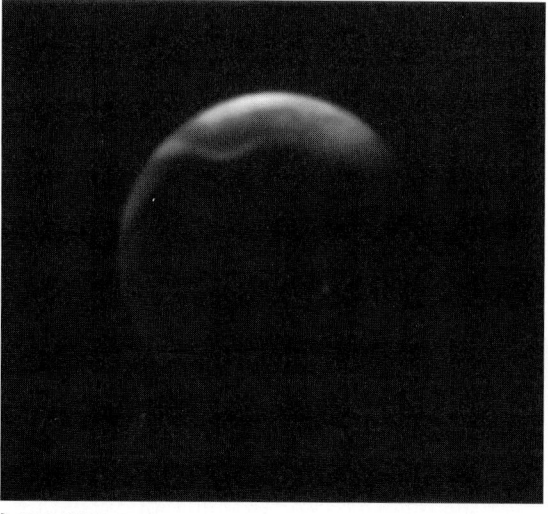

▶ **FIGURE 9-6**
Bladder endoscopy. Ureteral orifices in the dorsal aspect of the bladder.

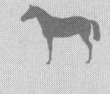
Endoscopy of the Female Urinary Tract: Urethra and Bladder

The indications for catheterization of the female urinary tract are similar to those for the male tract.

PROCEDURE. The technique is simpler than in the male horse because the urethra is much shorter, has a greater diameter, and is more distensible. However, despite the different urethral dimensions, the ready availability of longer endoscopes used more regularly in the other anatomical regions means that an endoscope much longer than necessary is often used. The mare should be restrained in stocks and tranquilized if necessary. The tail should be bandaged or held aside by an assistant, and the vulva should be washed with a detergent antiseptic and dried. The endoscope, including the biopsy channel, should be prepared as described in Appendix A. Some lubricant is placed on the tip of the endoscope and the gloved hand of an assistant, who guides the endoscope to the urethral opening. The endoscope is then inserted into the opening and on into the bladder. Sometimes the assistant's finger must be used to dilate the urethral opening while insertion is carried out. The clinician begins the examination while insertion is taking place. Once the endoscope is in the bladder, the appearance and procedure for urethral catheterization are as described for the male tract.

Ultrasonography of the Bladder, Kidneys, and Ureters

Bladder

Ultrasonography of the bladder is useful to identify calculi, perforations, and tissue masses involving the wall.[8] The examination would usually follow a rectal examination that had indicated bladder pathology.

PROCEDURE This is a transrectal procedure, and therefore it involves inserting the probe into the rectum. The rectum is first emptied of feces, and a liberal coating of coupling gel is then applied to the probe, which is placed in an obstetrical sleeve and guided into the rectum. Some clinicians push the probe into the rectum and then insert their hand and arm, others prefer to carry the probe loosely in the palm of the hand. The probe is positioned over the bladder and moved around so as explore the neck of the bladder and the bladder itself. Choice of probe is related to the depth of the lesion and the thickness of the bladder (7.5 MHz is suitable on most occasions and 5.0 MHz when there is significant tissue thickness).

Kidneys

The kidneys are usually scanned percutaneously, although a transrectal approach is also sometimes useful.[8] Because of the anatomical differences between the kidneys, better images are obtained by using a 3- or 3.5-MHz probe with a 20-cm field of view for the left kidney, and a 3- or 3.5-MHz probe with a 15-cm field of view for the right kidney. For ponies or foals, a 5-MHz probe can be used.

PROCEDURE. The imaging is usually done with the horse under suitable restraint and standing in stocks. This allows the operator to concentrate on the procedure and minimizes the chances of damage to the equipment. The hair should be clipped from the examination site and the coupling gel applied to the skin. If a suitable image cannot be obtained, the skin should be shaved to produce the best possible acoustic coupling. Obesity and dehydration are factors that can reduce the quality of the image. Occasionally the presence of gas-filled loops of intestine and also a large spleen will hinder imaging of the left kidney, necessitating transrectal examination.

The locations of the kidneys vary slightly between horses, which means that the first step is to locate them. As a general rule the right kidney will be found deep to the last two or three intercostal spaces and ventral to the lumbar processes. The right kidney has the shape of a blunt-pointed equilateral triangle, with the cranial portion lying in the renal fossa of the caudate process of the liver. Adjacent structures include the base of the cecum with its gas cap, lying ventromedial, and the caudal vena cava, lying deep to it. The bean-shaped left kidney is imaged best through the left paralumbar fossa, where it lies medial to the spleen. The left kidney may also be located cranially beneath the last few ribs.

After each kidney is located, the following aspects should be evaluated:

- External dimensions
- External contours
- Size of the pelvis and its recesses
- Distance between surface and corticomedullary junction

The cortex is seen as an homogenous rim that is usually more echoic than the medulla. The me-

dulla is characterized by a series of hyperechoic columns, contrasting with the relatively hypoechoic background. The renal parenchyma is visible as a patchy, but uniformly, echoic structure, and the pelvis is outlined by a rim of echogenic tissue. Some abnormal findings include:

- Enlargement (acute nephrosis, neoplasia)
- Opacities in the pelvis or its recesses associated with acoustic shadows (calculi)
- Loss of differentiation between the cortex and medulla and decreased size (chronic disease)

Examples of normal and abnormal kidneys are demonstrated in Figures 9–7 and 9–8.

Ureters

Imaging of the ureters is usually carried out transrectally, because of their small size and location.[8] Occasionally, when they are greatly enlarged, they will be seen during transabdominal imaging of the kidney. Ureters are not routinely imaged unless there is specific indication to do so, such as rectally located enlargements or hydronephrosis.

PROCEDURE. The procedure is similar to that for bladder imaging, although the probe must be directed dorsally to image the proximal ureter. Once located, it can be followed along its course

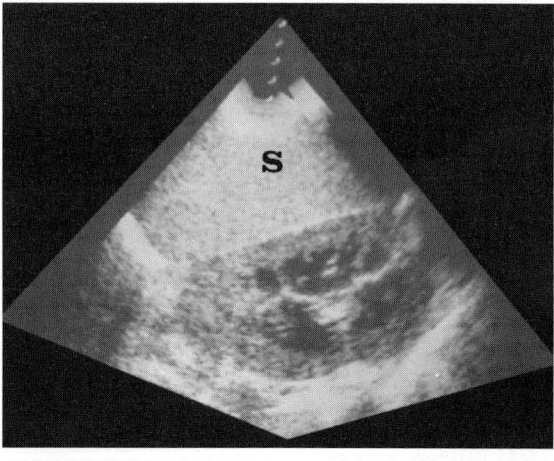
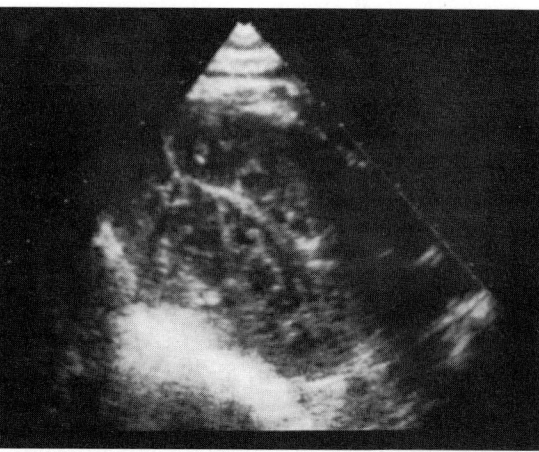

A   B

▶ **FIGURE 9–7**

Ultrasonograms of the normal left and right kidneys. **A.** Ultrasonogram of the left kidney obtained with a 3-MHz sector transducer placed in the dorsal left flank, just caudal to the 18th rib. The more superficial spleen (S) acts as an acoustic window to the kidney. The normal renal cortex is less echogenic than the spleen. The hyperechoic pelvis is surrounded by hypoechoic medulla. Deep to the kidney, hyperechoic echos arise from the adjacent bowel. (Courtesy R. H. Wrigley.) **B.** Ultrasonogram of the right kidney obtained with a 3-MHz sector transducer placed in the dorsal aspect of the right 17th intercostal space. The centrally located hyperechoic line results from echoes generated by the walls of the pelvis and is surrounded by the hypoechoic medulla. The outer border of the kidney represents the cortex. Deep to the kidney high-intensity echoes arise from the gas and contents of the underlying colon. (Courtesy R. H. Wrigley.)

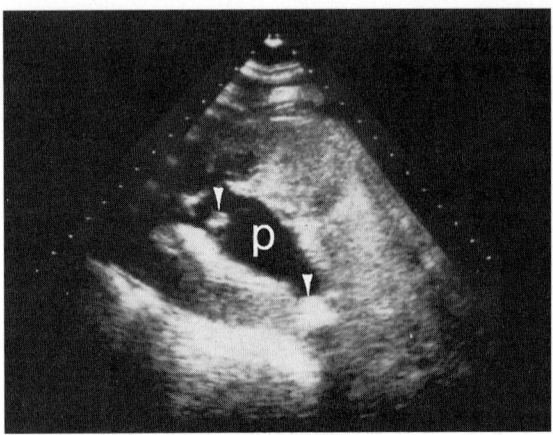
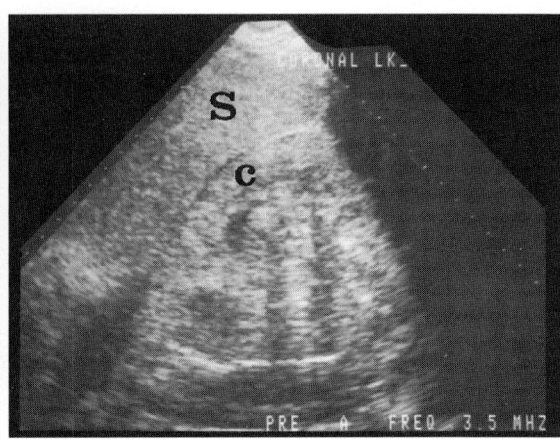

A
B

▶ **FIGURE 9-8**

Some examples of abnormal kidney ultrasonograms. **A.** Calculi and hydronephrosis. Dorsal ultrasonogram of the right kidney made with a 5-MHz sector transducer demonstrating a dilated pelvis (P) and calculi *(arrows)* with characteristic far-field shadowing in the renal pelvis. (Courtesy R. H. Wrigley.) **B.** Chronic degeneration. Dorsal ultrasonogram of the left kidney made with a 3-MHz sector transducer. The echogenicity of the renal cortex (C) and the overlying spleen (S) are similar. There is reduced corticomedullary/pelvic echo differentiation. The diagnosis was membranoproliferative glomerulonephritis. (Courtesy R. H. Wrigley.)

toward the bladder provided it is sufficiently enlarged.

Renal Biopsy

Percutaneous renal biopsy is occasionally used to obtain samples of renal tissue however, the technique is associated with risk of injury to the kidney, and a decision to carry out such a biopsy should only be made after the risks have been weighed against the benefits of the extra information so gained. Although biopsy can be carried out blindly, the chances of penetrating a large vessel, the spleen, or intestine are reduced by utilizing ultrasonic guidance. Defects in the clotting mechanism, which predispose to bleeding, should be ruled out by appropriate laboratory tests, before carrying out this procedure.

Ultrasonically Guided Percutaneous Renal Biopsy

The accuracy of inserting a biopsy needle into the kidney can be improved by using ultrasonography.[9]

PROCEDURE. Use of ultrasound allows both left and right kidneys to be biopsied. Biopsy is usually preceded by a standard ultrasonographic examination so that the clinician will know in advance what the region of interest is and the exact site for skin penetration as well as the angle and depth of penetration. For diffuse disease, the above data may allow biopsy to be carried out

without further use of the transducer. However, biopsy of focal lesions may require that the transducer be in use, either adjacent to the needle or with the needle inserted through it. The site for biopsy is prepared for a sterile procedure, and a local anesthetic solution is injected into the skin and muscles through which the needle will pass. If the transducer is to be used beside the needle, it must first be placed in a sterile sleeve containing a little sterile coupling gel. Then using more gel to ensure a good contact, it is applied to the skin. If the transducer contains a biopsy guide, the needle is inserted through it. The procedure should be carried out under sterile conditions. The biopsy

---

Materials for Ultrasonically Guided Renal Biopsy

▶ Biopsy needle (Tru-cut biopsy needle, [Travenol Laboratories, Inc., Deerfield, IL] Temno biopsy needle [Products Group International, Inc., Boulder, CO])

▶ Ultrasound machine

▶ Sector Transducer (3–3.5 MHz)

▶ Sterile coupling gel

▶ Local anesthetic solution (e.g., 2% Lidocaine or 2% Mepivacaine)

needle is imaged as a linear object and is directed into the region of interest under guidance from the sonogram.

Blind Percutaneous Renal Biopsy

Blind biopsy is usually suitable only for the left kidney because of its caudal location. Blind biopsy is carried out with the kidney stabilized by a hand inserted in the rectum. The kidney is localized by rectal exam, and the best site for skin penetration is decided on with the assistance of a second person, who observes the movement in the flank as the kidney is pushed against the abdominal wall. After preparing the biopsy site, the kidney is again manipulated and stabilized against the internal wall of the abdomen, and the needle is carefully and slowly inserted. The needle may enter the abdominal cavity and pass directly into the kidney, or, if the direction is not precise, it may pass beside the kidney. Penetration of the kidney is perceived by detecting movement of the kidney, or the needle itself is felt if it misses the kidney. In the latter case it must be redirected carefully. Care should be taken to avoid puncturing the rectum, as well as making the kidney move during the procedure. It is important that the needle be in-serted in the caudal pole away from the pelvis and renal vessels and that it not pass right through the kidney.

R E F E R E N C E S

1. Rose RJ, Hodgson DR (eds): The urinary system. *In* Manual of Equine Practice. Philadelphia, Saunders, 1993, ch 9, p 295.
2. Brobst DF, Parry BW: Normal clinical pathology data. *In* Robinson NE (ed), Current Therapy in Equine Medicine, 2nd ed. Philadelphia, Saunders, 1987, p 725.
3. Butler JA, Colles CM, Dyson SJ, et al (eds): The alimentary and urinary systems, and miscellaneous techniques. *In* Clinical Radiology of the Horse. Oxford, Blackwell, 1993, pp 500, 519.
4. Kay AD, Lavoie JP: Urethral pressure profilometry in horses. J Amer Vet Med Assoc 1987; 191:212.
5. Ronen N: Measurements of urethral pressure profiles in the male horse. Equine Vet J 1994; 26:55.
6. Clark ES, Semrad SD, Oliver JE, et al: Cystometrography and urethral pressure profiles in healthy horses and pony mares. Amer J Vet Res 1987; 48:552.
7. Sullins KE: Urinary Tract. *In* Traub-Dargatz JL, Brown CM (eds): Equine endoscopy. St Louis, Mosby, 1990, ch 12, p 145.
8. Rantanen NW: Diseases of the abdomen. Vet Clin North Am (Equine Pract) 1986; 2:67.
9. Modransky PD: Ultrasound-guided renal and kidney biopsy technique. Vet Clin North Am (Equine Pract). 1986; 2:115.

The Eye and Adnexa

The eye is a very delicate and specialized structure, and more than any other organ it requires examination by a specialist. Despite this, a clinician with an understanding of ocular anatomy and function can carry out a surprisingly thorough examination.

COMPONENTS

The eye and adnexa include the eyelids, including the third eyelid (nictitating membrane, nictitans); the conjunctiva; and the bulb consisting of the cornea, sclera, uveal tract, anterior and posterior chambers, optic nerve, nasolacrimal ducts and punctae, and muscles.

MANIFESTATIONS OF DISEASE

The manifestations of disease vary depending on which ocular components are involved and what type of process is present. In general, systemic diseases that affect the eye and adnexa cause bilateral signs, whereas unilateral signs are more likely to result from local disease. There is an extensive nomenclature describing ocular abnormalities, including:

- Exophthalmos: Prominent globe
- Prolapse: Dislocation of the globe from the orbit and beyond the eyelids
- Buphthalmos: Enlargement of the globe
- Enophthalmos: Globe positioned caudally in the orbit
- Anophthalmia: Complete absence of the globe
- Microphthalmia: Partial absence of the globe
- Strabismus: Deviation of the eye from its normal axis
- Ptosis: Drooping of the upper eyelid
- Blindness: Lack of central perception
- Blepharospasm: Persistent contraction of the orbicularis muscle as a result of irritation to the conjunctiva, cornea, and eyelids
- Photophobia: Increased sensitivity to light
- Conjunctivitis: Inflammation of the conjunctiva
- Superficial and deep perilimbal hyperemia: Superficial vessels usually larger and less numerous than the deeper vessels and indicate superficial inflammation rather than deep inflammation in the uveal tract
- Staphyloma: Protruberance of the corneoscleral region lined with uveal tissue
- Keratoconus: Thinning and protrusion of the cornea
- Anisocoria: Difference in pupil size
- Mydriasis: Dilation of the pupil
- Miosis: Constriction of the pupil
- Chemosis: Conjunctival edema
- Epiphora: Overflow of tears from the eye
- Hyphema: Blood in the anterior chamber
- Acqueous flare: Increased protein and turbidity of anterior chamber
- Hypopyon: Presence of leucocytes in the anterior chamber

RESTRAINT, SEDATION, AND ANESTHESIA

Because of the difficulty in controlling movement of the horse's head as well as the eye itself, and because there is often a considerable chance that the ocular examination will produce further injury (e.g., rupture of the globe when a corneal ulcer is present), restraint, analgesia, and sedation are extremely important.

Restraint and Sedation

With quiet horses it is sufficient to have the head restrained with head gear such as a bridle, headstall, or halter. If the horse is agitated or continually moves its head, a nose twitch and sedation are often required. Horses usually resent repeated interference with an eye, and manipulation, drug administration, and sample collection become more difficult as the number of interferences increases. Methods of physical restraint and sedation are listed in the box.

Anesthesia for Ocular Examination

In addition to sedation and physical restraint, topical and conduction block anesthesia are often necessary, especially when there is a painful lesion present and also to facilitate opening of the eyelids.

Topical Anesthesia

Although the globe, conjunctiva, and much of the adjacent eyelids and skin can be anesthetized by blocking the ophthalmic nerve, topical anesthesia is the preferred method for anesthesia of the cornea and conjunctiva. Various solutions are available for topical ophthalmic use.

PROCEDURE. Instilling an anesthetic solution into the eye is simple and can be done in many

---

> ### PREFERRED TOPICAL OPHTHALMIC ANESTHETIC SOLUTIONS
>
> - 0.5% proparacaine hydrochloride
> - 0.5% tetracaine hydrochloride

---

ways, but each requires that the eye be partially open. A simple method that is well tolerated by the patient and does not waste solution is to evert the lower lid with the thumb or finger and then place a few drops of solution into the conjunctival sac. Alternatively, solution can be squirted into the eye from a tuberculin syringe minus needle or from a normal hypodermic syringe and 25-gauge needle hub (Fig 10-1). Several applications over a few minutes are necessary for optimal effect.

Conduction Block Anesthesia

Conduction block anesthesia requires a perineural deposition of anesthetic solution.[1]

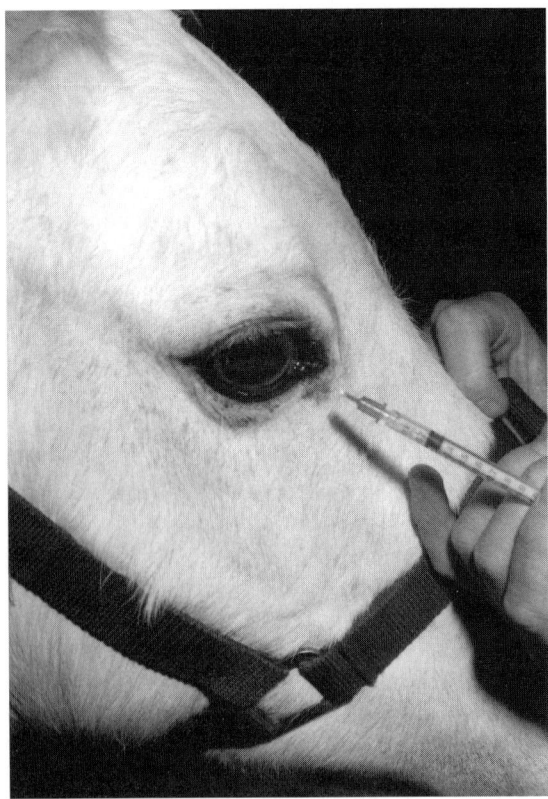

▶ **FIGURE 10-1**

Using a tuberculin syringe and needle hub to squirt anesthetic solution into the eye.

> ### RESTRAINT AND SEDATION DURING OCULAR EXAMINATION
>
> - Restraint: Twitch, stocks (depending on temperament)
> - Sedation (e.g., xylazine 0.5–1.0 mg/kg IV or xylazine, 0.5 mg/kg plus butorphanol 0.02 mg/kg IV)

Materials for Conduction Block Anesthesia

▸ Local anesthetic solution
   2% Lidocaine hydrochloride
   2% Mepivacaine hydrochloride
▸ Syringe (10 mL)
▸ Needle (25 gauge, ⅝")

PROCEDURE

Auriculopalpebral Nerve Block to Achieve Eyelid Akinesia. Because of its extremely strong orbicularis oculi muscle, the equine eye is often difficult to open, which can make examination difficult or impossible—and sometimes dangerous when there is a possibility that the globe may rupture. If this muscle is paralyzed by conduction block of the auriculopalpebral nerve at a site along its course adjacent to the zygomatic arch, the eyelid can be opened easily, although sensory function is retained. Although there are three sites where the anesthetic agent can be injected, the writer prefers the site where the palpebral branch can be palpated as it lies on the zygomatic arch (Fig. 10-2). It is a simple matter to inject 3 to 5 ml of anesthetic solution subcutaneously over the nerve.

Sensory Conduction Block. Ocular examination does not routinely require special sensory anesthesia. However, for a biopsy, it may be necessary. The sensory innervation of eyelids and surrounds is supplied by the frontal, infratrochlear,

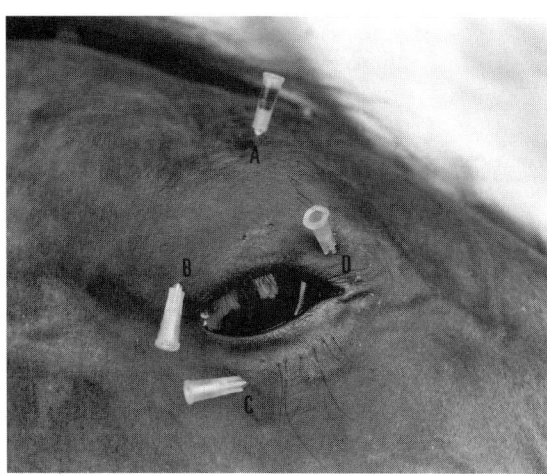

▸ **FIGURE 10-3**

Needles in place to produce sensory anesthesia of the conjunctiva and cornea. Frontal nerve **(A)**, lacrimal nerve **(B)**, zygomatic nerve **(C)**, and infratrochlear nerve **(D)**.

zygomatic, and lacrimal nerves, all branches of the trigeminal nerve. The sites for injection are shown in Figure 10-3. The *frontal nerve* is the sensory nerve most commonly anesthetized, where it emerges from the supraorbital foramen (at this site it should be remembered that the medial portion of the auriculopalpebral nerve described, which is a motor nerve, will also be blocked). It can be anesthetized within or as it emerges from the foramen to desensitize the middle two thirds of the upper eyelid. The foramen can be palpated beneath the first finger if the thumb and second finger are placed on either side of the zygomatic arch where it begins to widen toward its junction with the temporal bone (Fig. 10-4). A 25-gauge,

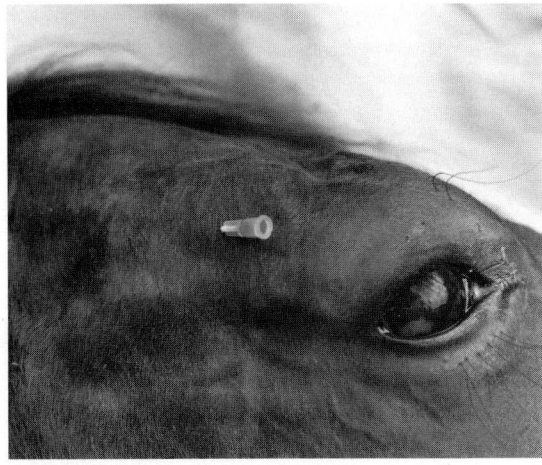

▸ **FIGURE 10-2**

Auriculopalpebral nerve block. The palpebral branch of the auriculopalpebral nerve can be palpated as it courses over the zygomatic arch.

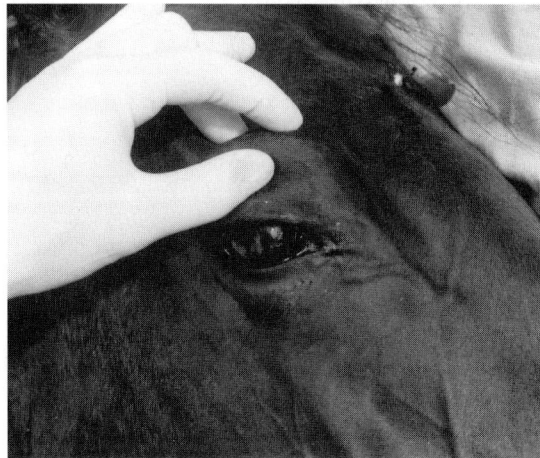

▸ **FIGURE 10-4**

Location of the supraorbital foramen. The foramen lies below the first finger when the thumb and second finger are placed across the zygomatic arch where it begins to widen toward the temporal bone.

⅝″ needle can be inserted into the foramen and 1 to 2 ml of solution injected, taking care not to inject it into the accompanying artery and vein. To anesthetize the *lacrimal nerve* a 25-gauge ⅝″ needle is inserted medial to the lateral canthus just beneath the dorsal rim of the orbit, and 2 to 3 ml of solution is injected. The *zygomatic nerve* is anesthetized by inserting a 25-gauge ⅝″ needle

beneath the lower lid about 2 cm medial to the lateral canthus. The needle is directed medially just inside the ventral rim of the orbit, and 2 ml of solution is deposited. The *infratrochlear nerve* is anesthetized by inserting a 25-gauge ⅝″ needle in the skin of the upper lid just lateral to the medial canthus and injecting 2 ml of solution adjacent to the notch in the upper rim of the orbit.

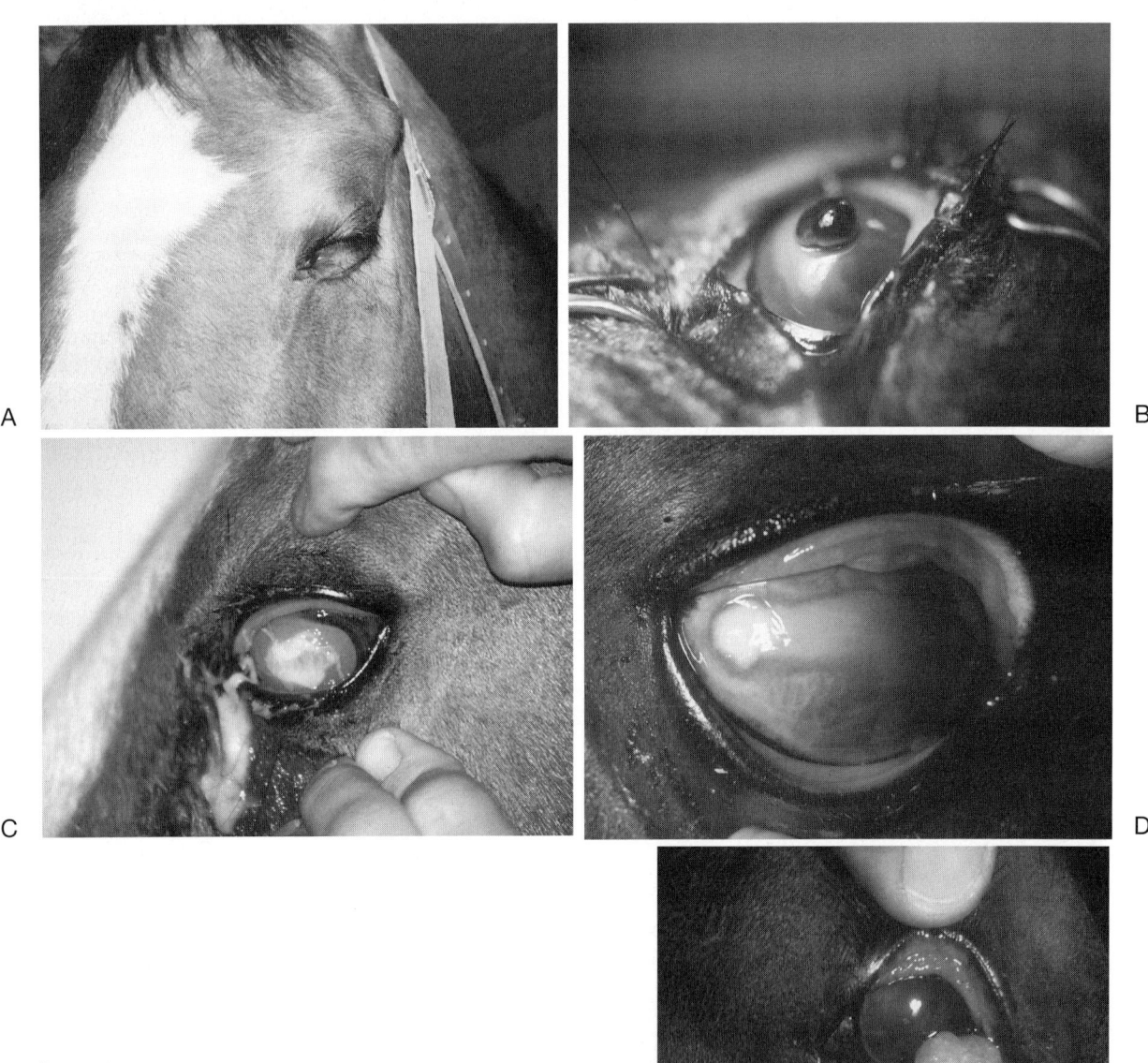

▶ **FIGURE 10-5**

Some examples of ocular conditions. **A.** Blepharospasm. Eyelids are closed as a result of hypersensitivity to light. **B.** Iris prolapse. The prolapsing iris is seen as a circumscribed dark-colored mass emerging through a defect in the center of the cornea. **C.** Corneal perforation with drainage of exudate and aqueous humor. **D.** Chronic glaucoma with secondary stromal abscess. Note the enlarged globe, the extensive superficial neovascularization, and the stromal abscess located adjacent to the lateral canthus. **E.** Squamous cell carcinoma of the nictitans. Note the mass in the region of the medial canthus involving the nictitans and conjunctiva of the lower eyelid.

GENERAL EXTERNAL EXAMINATION

The first part of the examination should be conducted outside or in a well-lit area where a good visual examination can be carried out.

Visual Examination

The first part of the exam is to evaluate the eyes and adjacent regions for symmetry, eyelid function, abnormal discharges, signs of trauma, and swelling. Although this is mainly visual, palpation is also very important in assessing the integrity of the osseous orbital rim and zygomatic arch, the supraorbital fossa, and intraocular tension. Signs of ocular pain (e.g., photophobia, blepharospasm), conjunctivitis (e.g., exudate and edema), protrusion (exophthalmos), enlargement (buphthalmos) or collapse (enophthalmos) of the globe, obvious corneal lesions such as edema and laceration should be searched for, and the size of the pupil should be examined. This can usually be done virtually without restraint, but, in many horses, especially those with ocular pain, more extensive examination will require some form of restraint or sedation, as described. Some ocular abnormalities are shown in Figure 10–5.

Palpation

The orbital rim can be palpated for evidence of fractures or foreign bodies. Examination can often be facilitated by inserting a gloved and lubricated finger between the globe and the orbital rim. The

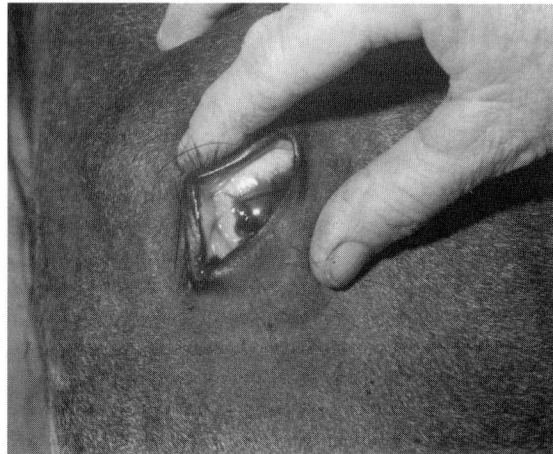

▶ **FIGURE 10–6**

Manual prolapse of the nictitans. The first finger is being used to depress the globe, thus allowing the nictitans to extend ("prolapse") across the cornea to where it can be examined.

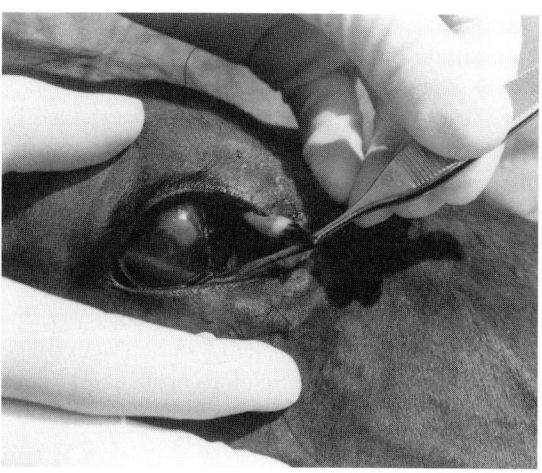

▶ **FIGURE 10–7**

Examination of the bulbar surface of the nictitans. After the application of topical anesthetic solution, fine forceps are used to lift the membrane away from the globe, thus allowing its inner surface to be examined.

nictitating membrane (NM) is not normally visible unless its function is disturbed by conditions such as tetanus or if it contains a lesion. It can be brought into view ("prolapsed") by depressing the globe through the upper eyelid with the finger, although this apparently simple procedure does require practice (Fig. 10–6). Once the technique has been mastered, there is little or no resentment from the horse, and the NM comes easily into view. The bulbar surface of the NM can be examined by grasping it with hemostats or thumb forceps (requires anesthesia) and then lifting it away from the globe (Fig. 10–7). The lids should be carefully examined for continuity, extra cilia (distichiasis or ectopic), edema, and foreign bodies.

Ocular Reflexes

Pupillary Light Reflexes (Direct and Indirect)

Pupillary light reflexes (PLRs) are tested with a focal light (Fig. 10–8) and are best carried out as part of a dark-room examination (see later). Light is shone into each eye separately, the direct PLR is present when the ipsilateral pupil constricts in response to light, and the indirect (consensual) PLR is present when constriction occurs in the other eye. The neurological pathways involved in this important reflex are shown in Figure 10–9. Briefly, the stimulus of increased light is detected by the retina and transmitted through the optic nerve to the contralateral pretectal area of the brain stem, where bilateral stimulation of parasympathetic nuclei of the oculomotor nerves occurs with subsequent stimulation and contraction of the sphincter pupillae muscle of the iris in both eyes.[2] The pathways involved in pupillary dilation as a result of decreasing light intensity are also demonstrated.

Eyelid Ocular Reflexes

MENACE REFLEX. This test is made by threatening the eye with the hand or a finger (Fig. 10-10). Care should be taken to ensure that wind currents are not generated in so doing and that the eyelids or cilia are not touched, as these will produce a similar response based on appreciation of touch rather than sight.

CORNEAL AND PALPEBRAL REFLEXES. These tests are carried out by gently touching the cornea or the upper or lower eyelids, respectively. The response is the same in each case, although slightly different pathways are tested.

It is important to realize that these reflexes do not necessarily indicate that the horse has vision.

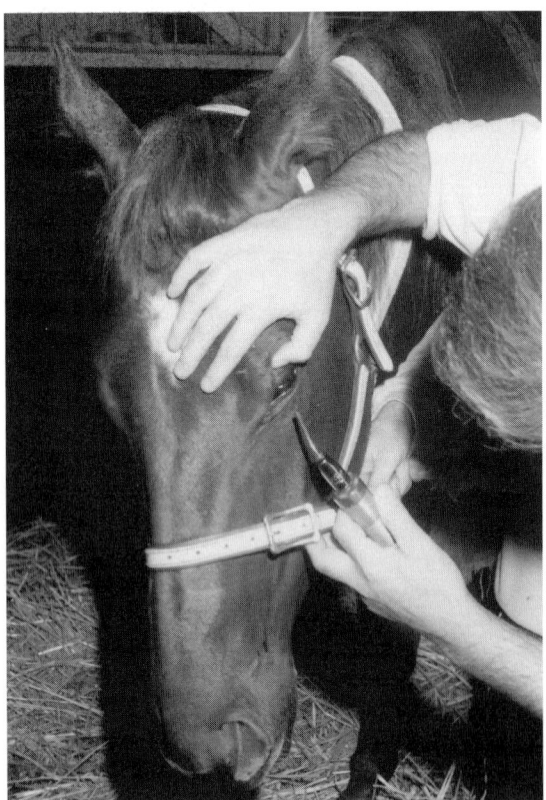

▶ **FIGURE 10-8**

Testing pupillary light reflexes with a focal light source. This test is carried out in a darkened room.

They are primarily protective reflexes designed to produce rapid eyelid closure and head movement in order to prevent injury. The detail of these reflexes is summarized in Table 10-1.

TESTING FOR VISION. Making the horse negotiate an unfamiliar obstacle course is also useful in detecting vision deficits. Each eye can be tested separately by blindfolding the other eye. Eyes can be masked by taping an opaque material over the orbit or by using a towel or drape tucked into the headstall. The test can be carried out in reduced light to test dark adaptation. Naturally, care should be taken to avoid accidents by selecting appropriate obstacles and speed and by maintaining control over the horse with a long lead.

DARK-ROOM EXAMINATION

A thorough examination of the eye and adnexa is best done in a darkened room with the horse adequately restrained.[3,4] Most stalls are suitable for this purpose, although, when this is not possible, a cloth sheet that will not transmit light can be placed over the head of the horse and the examiner (Fig. 10-11). This procedure is accepted by most horses, as are most of the various examination procedures.

The anterior segment is usually examined with a focal light source, focused or unfocused. Because it is deeper in the eye and behind the lens, the posterior segment is best examined by direct ophthalmoscopy (direct ophthalmoscope), indirect ophthalmoscopy (monocular or binocular indirect ophthalmoscope or hand-held +20-diopter lens plus focal light) or by focal light.

Focal Light Examination

Focal light examination is the easiest, most frequently used, and most important method for examining the eye in veterinary practice (Fig. 10-12). The term *focal light* refers to a light that uses a condensing lens to focus the light beam, which, by virtue of its focus, is able to penetrate deeper into the eye than a nonfocused beam. Magnification glasses are useful as they leave the other hand free to control the horse.

The Cornea

Examination is best carried out with a focal light directed onto the cornea from different angles.

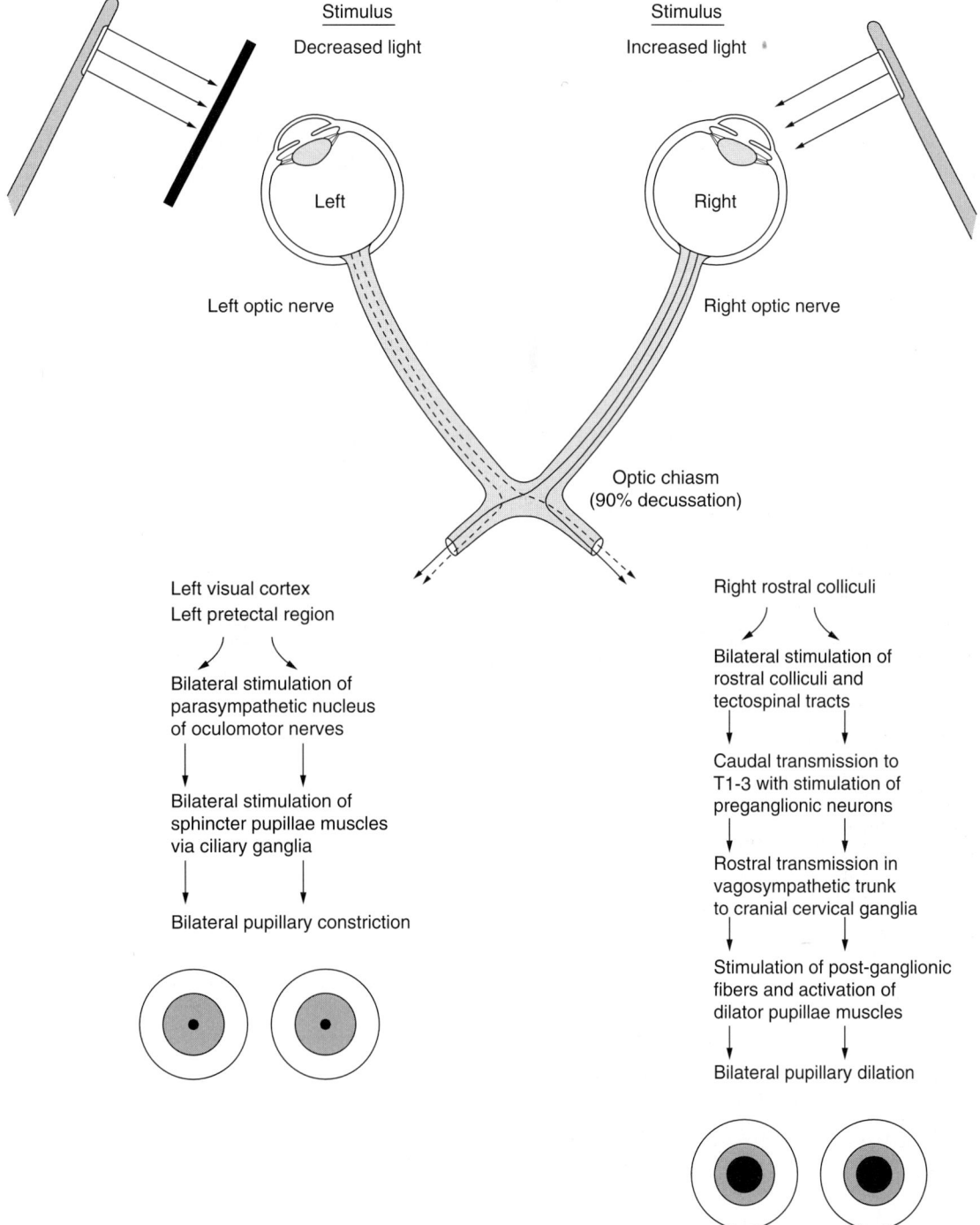

FIGURE 10–9

Neurological pathways involved in the pupillary light reflexes. The pathways involved in the constrictor response to increased light and the dilator response to decreased light are demonstrated.

The normal cornea is transparent, and its surface is smooth, glistening, and evenly curved. It should be examined carefully for ulcers, wounds, foreign bodies, focal infections, defects, and deep or superficial vascularization. The peripheral pale band adjacent to the limbus is normal and represents the site of the insertions of the pectinate ligament.

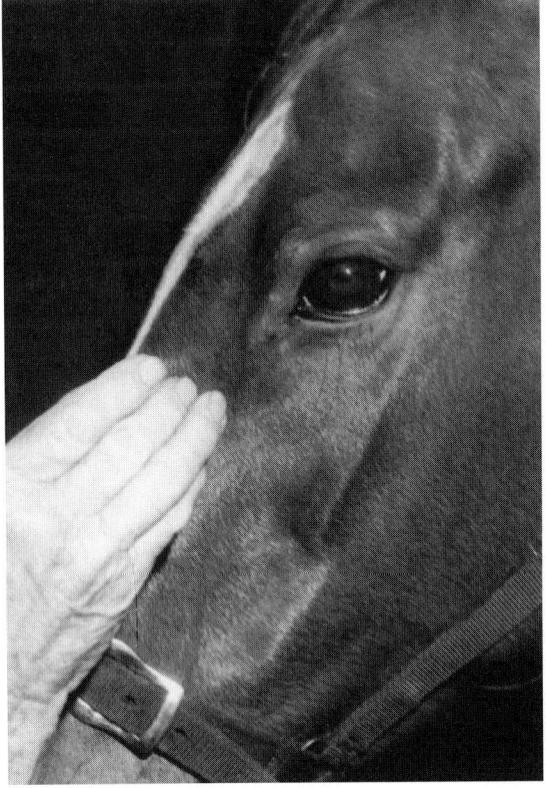

▶ **FIGURE 10–10**
Menace reflex. The eye is threatened with the fingers, taking care to avoid any contact or to produce any air currents.

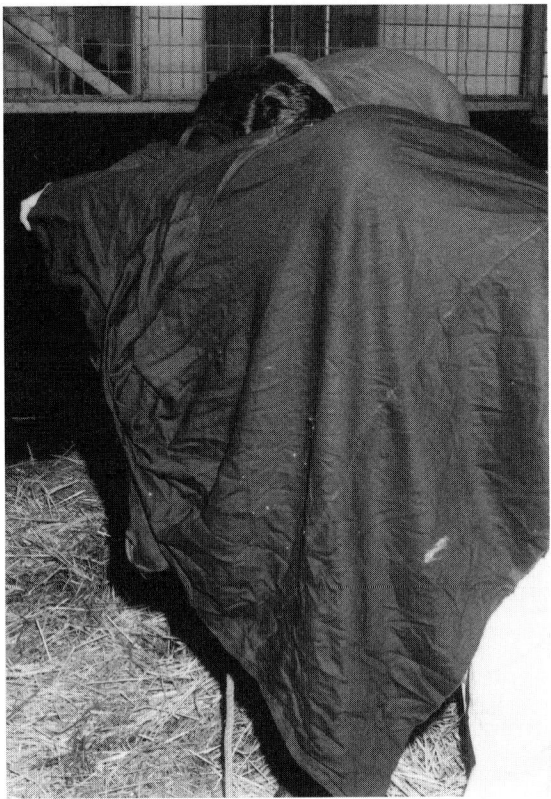

▶ **FIGURE 10–11**
Using an opaque cloth to allow examination of the eye in darkness.

The Iris

The iris is normally dark brown but is often lighter in light-colored horses. The iris is evaluated for changes in color, position, shape, texture, and presence of cysts, adhesions, and corpora nigra. The latter, usually rounded structures attached to the iris, vary greatly in size and number and are ocasionally free in the anterior chamber. The pupil should be evaluated for size.

The Lens

Complete examination of the lens requires that the pupil be dilated (mydriasis), necessitating use

▶ **TABLE 10–1**
SUMMARY OF EYELID OCULAR RESPONSES

	REFLEX		
	PALPEBRAL	MENACE	CORNEAL
Stimulus	Touch eyelid	Threaten	Touch cornea
Afferent	Opthlamic nerve (upper lid) Maxillary nerve (lower lid)	Optic nerve	Ophthalmic nerve
Efferent	Facial nerve	Facial nerve	Facial nerve
Effectors	Eyelid muscles	Eyelid muscles	Eyelid muscles
Effect	Blink	Blink	Blink

Requirements for Dark-Room Examination

▶ Darkened room or head sheet
▶ Magnification (16- to 20-diopter hand lens [×5–6], magnifying glasses [e.g., Neitz, ×4])
▶ Focal light source (penlight, Finoff transilluminator, Heine Accumat illuminator)
▶ Direct ophthalmoscope
▶ Indirect ophthalmoscope
▶ Short-acting mydriatic (1% tropicamide)

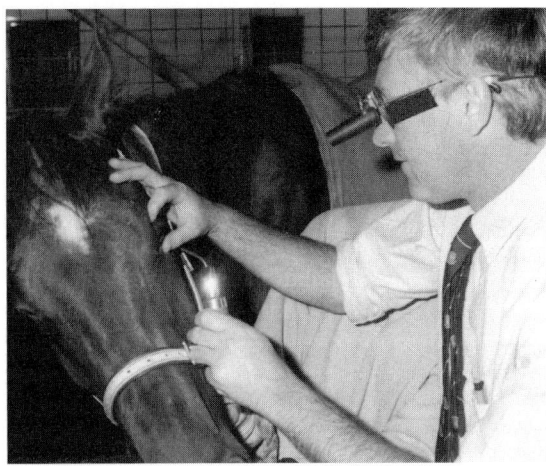

▶ **FIGURE 10-12**

Focal light examination with the assistance of magnifying spectacles.

of a short-acting mydriatic such as 1% tropicamide. Atropine should not be used because its duration of action is too long. The lens is examined for cataracts, suture lines, and position. The normal lens is transparent and difficult to see.

INDIRECT OPHTHALMOSCOPY. Indirect ophthalmoscopy can be performed with either a monocular or a binocular instrument, as well by simply using a hand-held lens and a focal light source.[5] The hand-held lens and focal light do not involve expensive equipment, are extremely useful as screening devices, and are appropriate for most examinations. Although the indirect binocular instrument has the advantages of stereopsis, a greater field of view, better view of the peripheral regions of the fundus, and better depth perception, it has the disadvantages of being expensive and of requiring more practice.

Both the monocular instrument, which is hand-held, and the binocular instrument, which is hand-held or mounted on the examiner's head, have a built-in light source (Fig. 10-13). The instrument is merely aimed into the eye. For monocular indirect ophthalmoscopy with hand-held focal light and lens, the light source is held adjacent to the examiner's eye and aimed into the pupil from a distance of about 60 cm until a reflection of the tapetum is seen. The lens, held at arm's length in the other hand is then placed in the line of sight and moved toward or away from the eye so as to give a sharp, but inverted, tapetal image (Fig. 10-14).

Direct Ophthalmoscopy

Direct ophthalmoscopy requires the direct ophthalmoscope and is particularly useful for examining the fine details of the disc.[5,6,7] The instrument should have a series of lens to facilitate an examination of the various regions of the eye; a small aperture for examining an undilated pupil, a large aperture for dilated pupils, a fixation aperture to allow measurement of lesions, a red-free (green) aperture to improve the identification of arteries (black) and veins (blue), and a slit aperture to improve the detection of variation in retinal surface contour and enhance examination of the anterior segment (Fig. 10-15A).[4] Routine examinations can be carried out in the undilated eye but, for detailed examination and for examination of the peripheral fields, mydriasis is required.

With direct ophthalmoscopy first the lens selector is set at zero and the instrument held vertically against the examiner's eyebrow and the bridge of the nose (or against the examiner's glasses if these are worn) and about 40 to 50 cm from the patient's eye (Fig. 10-15B). The examiner can use the same eye to examine the patient's left and right eyes or the left eye to examine the left eye and vice versa. The horse's head is supported by the examiner's free hand, placed so that the upper lid is controlled by the index finger and the lower lid by the thumb. The light beam is directed into the eye and a reflection of the tapetum obtained that will be used as a background for viewing the other structures. Opacities between the tapetum

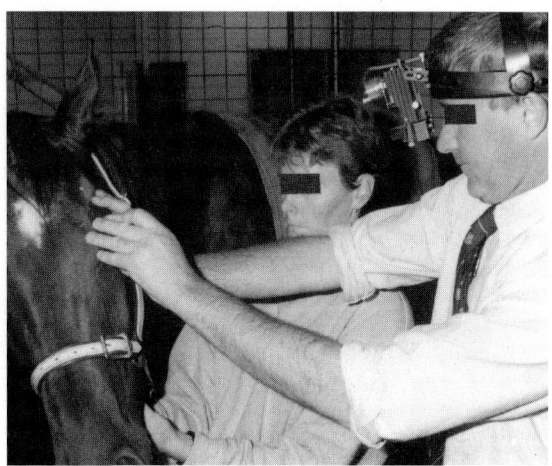

▶ **FIGURE 10-13**

Binocular indirect ophthalmoscopy with a Mentor indirect ophthalmoscope.

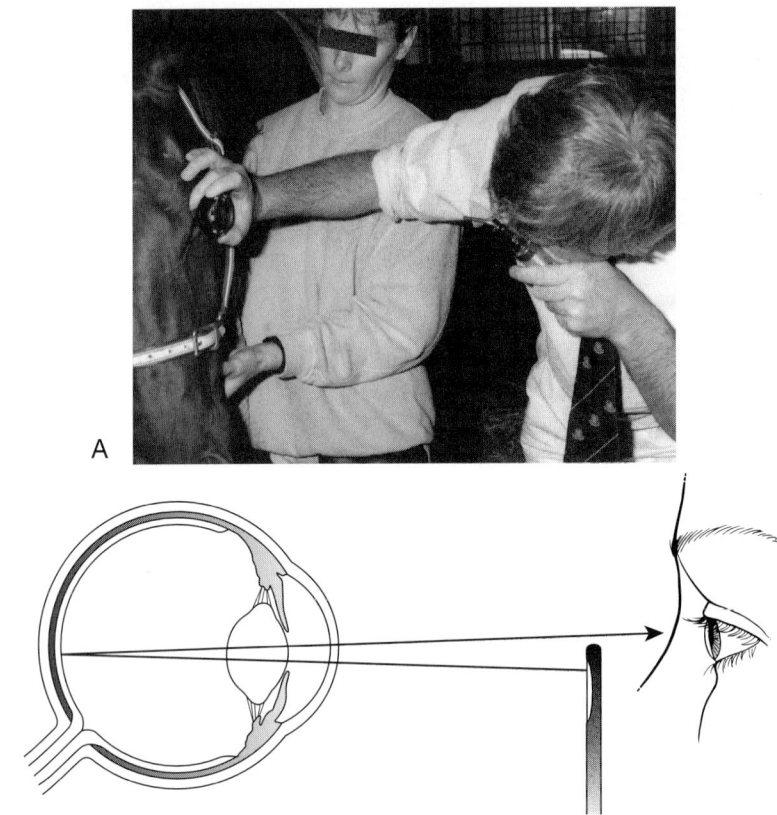

▶ FIGURE 10–14

Monocular indirect ophthalmoscopy. **A.** Monocular indirect ophthalmoscopy with hand-held lens and focal light source. **B.** Demonstration of the principle of light reflection from the tapetum.

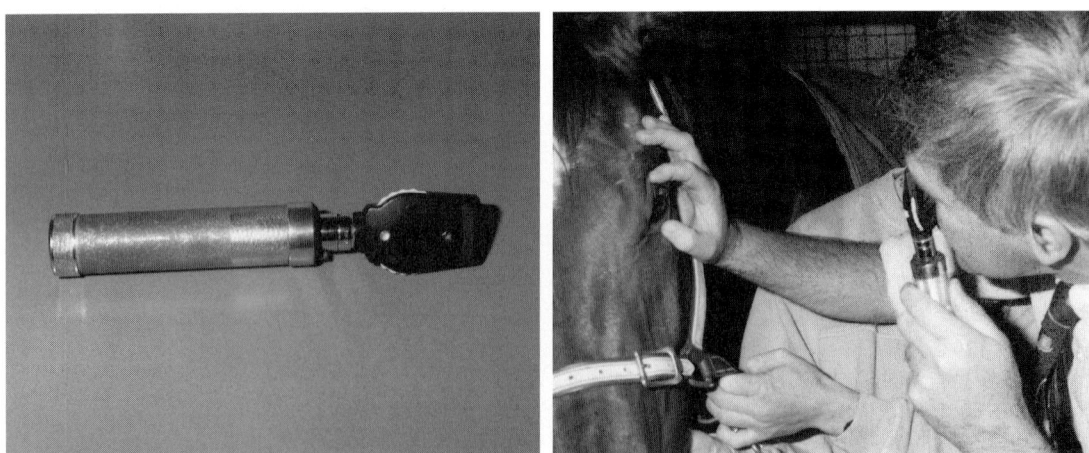

▶ FIGURE 10–15

Direct ophthalmoscopy. **A.** Direct ophthalmoscope with fittings. **B.** Direct ophthalmoscopy. The free hand is placed on the horse's head for support and protection, and the clinician's left eye is being used to examine the horse's left eye.

OPTHALMOSCOPIC SETTINGS FOR THE NORMAL EQUINE EYE	
Structure	Diopters
• Cornea	+15 to +20 diopters
• Iris	+12 to +15
• Lens (anterior capsule)	+12 to +15
• Lens (posterior capsule)	+8 to +12
• Vitreous	+2 to +8
• Fundus and optic disc	+2 to −2

and the viewer (i.e., in the cornea, anterior chamber, lens, and vitreous) block the tapetal reflection and appear as black spots. Their location can be ascertained by noting how the position of the lesion changes as the angle of view changes as the horse's or the examiner's eye moves: Opacities cranial to the optical axis of rotation (posterior lens capsule) appear to move in the same direction as the horse's eye, and vice versa. The opposite applies for movement of the examiner's eye. At this distance structures deep to the lens are usually not visible. As the instrument moves progressively closer to the eye, the deeper structures come into view, the lens at about 30 cm and finally the fundus, first at about 15 cm and then clearly at a distance of a few centimeters. The sharpness of the fundus may be improved by varying the diopter settings between −2 and +2, although the exact settings vary with the visual acuity of the examiner. The fundus and disc are then examined, noting the lens settings. The normal disc setting is within 1 diopter of the fundus setting. A more negative disc setting indicates depression (e.g., glaucoma, atrophy), and a more positive setting indicates elevation (e.g., neoplasia). By using higher positive lens settings, the vitreous, lens, anterior chamber, and cornea can be carefully examined with the instrument held within a few inches of the eye.

The vitreous body is also transparent but may contain fibrils and floating bodies, as well as remnants of the hyaloid artery adjacent to the posterior lens capsule in neonates.

The equine fundus is shown in Figure 10–16. It is characterized by the dorsal, bright-colored, reflective tapetum and the ventral, brown, nonreflective nontapetal region, the optic disc, and blood vessels. The optic disc lies in the nontapetal region ventral (inferior) and lateral (temporal) to the central axis. It is round in young animals and becomes more oval with age. It contains a peripheral pale zone, an intermediate pinkish zone, and a central yellowish zone. Approximately 50 to 70 small blood vessels are located radially around the periphery of the disc and extend onto the retinal surface for a distance of about one disc diameter. Choroidal vessels, which are darker in color and are broader, are especially seen when the tapetum is underdeveloped. Although the tapetum is usually yellow or green, its color varies considerably with coat color, as well as within a tapetum and between the left and right eyes. It contains a number of small blue, brown, or red spots known as the "stars of Winslow," which are choroidal vessels seen in cross-section. Abnormal findings include congenital developmental defects (colobomas) of retina and choroid, retinal hemorrhages, detachment, scars, and depigmentation, and disc atrophy with loss of vessels and color.

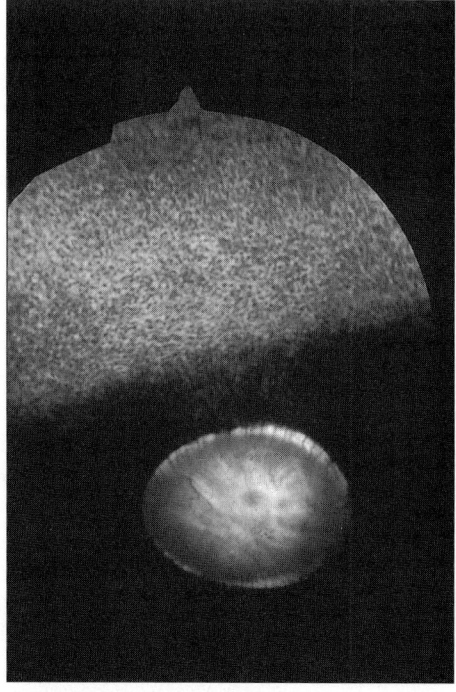

▶ **FIGURE 10–16**

Photograph of the equine fundus. Note the dorsal tapetal region and the ventral nontapetal region that contains the optic disc and its associated peripheral vessels. (Courtesy R. Blogg.)

COLLECTION OF SAMPLES FOR IDENTIFICATION OF MICROORGANISMS AND CYTOLOGICAL EXAMINATION

Material can be obtained as a swab, scraping, or impression smear.[8] Samples for bacteriological and or fungal culture should be obtained before any substances have been applied topically.

Ocular Swabbing

Ocular swabbing can be done without anesthesia and therefore provides a suitable sample to culture microorganisms.

Procedure

The procedure is facilitated by anesthesia of the auriculopalpebral nerve to produce akinesia of the upper eyelid (see Anesthesia for Ocular Examination). A commercial culture swab is moistened with transport medium or sterile saline and then applied to or wiped across the region of interest (Fig. 10-17). When appropriate, it is also useful to rotate the swab to improve the collection of material, particularly with ulcers, where rotation elevates the undermined edge of the lesion to expose microorganisms that may have been shielded from lacrimal lavage and topical agents. Samples are often collected from the conjunctiva in the ventral fornix adjacent to the nasal canthus. Care should be taken to ensure that only the region of interest is swabbed so as to avoid contaminating the sample. Samples should be collected from the center as well as the periphery of the lesion. If blood and Sabouraud's agar plates are available the sample can be innoculated directly onto them.

Scraping

A scraping is usually carried out to collect material suitable for microscopic examination. As it requires anesthesia it should be done after samples for culture and sensitivity were collected.

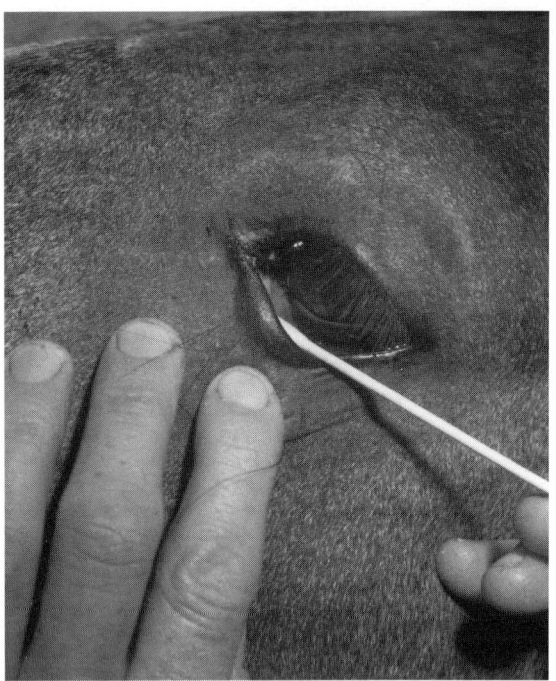

FIGURE 10-17
Swabbing the conjunctival sac with a cotton-tipped swab.

If general anesthesia is used, this does not apply, as there is no need for topical anesthesia then.

PROCEDURE. The procedure is carried out under topical anesthesia and, if necessary, upper eyelid akinesia (anesthesia of the auriculopalpebral nerve). A twitch or heavy sedation may be required in fractious horses. It is a simple procedure, but it requires adequate restraint to ensure that further ocular injury is not produced by sudden movement of the horse's head. The ventral conjunctival fornix, or specific lesion, is scraped with the selected instrument, and the

---

Materials for Ocular Swabbing

- Commercial culturette (Becton Dickinson and Co., Cockeysville, MD)
- Transport medium or sterile saline

Materials for Ocular Scaping

- Glass microscope slides
- Instrument to scrape material off tissue (Kimura iris spatula, blunt end of scalpel blade)
- Topical anesthetic (0.5% proparacaine)
- Fixative (spray or immersion)
- Cellular stain (Giemsa or Gram for bacteria, new methlyene blue for fungi)

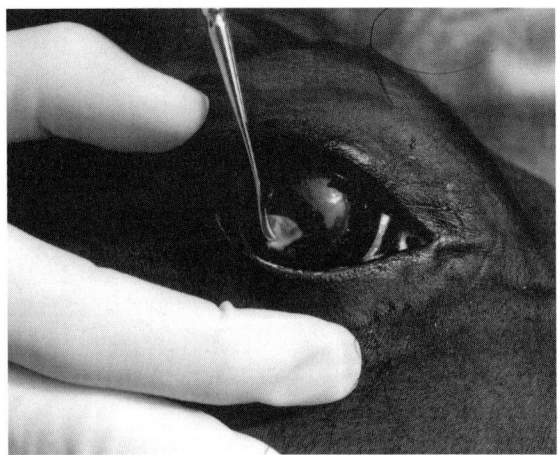

▶ **FIGURE 10–18**
Corneal scraping carried out under anesthesia.

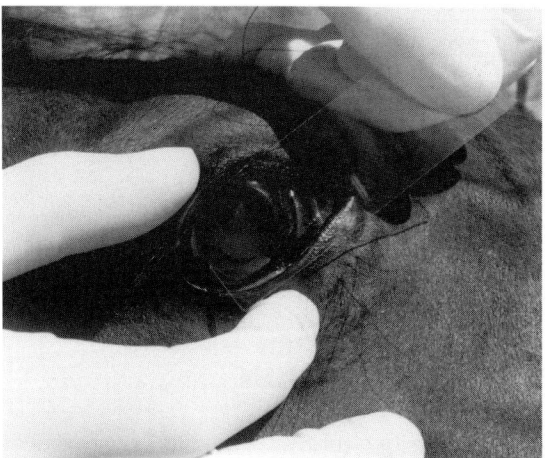

▶ **FIGURE 10–19**
Corneal impression smear using a microscopic slide.

material it collects is spread onto the slides in preparation for staining and examination (Fig. 10–18).

Impression Smear

Impression smears are not made on a routine basis but are useful for rapid identification of mycosis and neoplasia.

PROCEDURE. A smear is made by applying a glass microscopic slide directly to the region of interest, which may be the cornea, conjunctiva, or a tumor (Fig. 10–19). When deep fungal lesions are present in the cornea, it may be necessary to scrape away the superficial tissue and debris before making the smear.

Normal Ocular Flora

Microorganisms can be found in most normal eyes, specifically Gram-positive, aerobic, non-pathogenic bacteria, although gram-negative rods, *Neisseria,* and environmental fungae are also identified. The flora isolated vary with disease status, season, and environment. Bacteria commonly found in normal eyes include *Staphylococcus, Corynebacterium,* and *Bacillus* species and fungi including *Aspergillus, Penicillium, Alterna-*

ria, and *Cladosporium* species.[9,10] In diseased eyes gram-negative bacteria such as *Pseudomonas* and *Escherichia* are common, as well as fungi, which tend to be opportunistic in the presence of trauma and prolonged antibiotic therapy.[11]

Conjunctival Biopsy

A conjunctival biopsy is useful for identifying tumors and isolating *Onchocerca microfilaria.*[12]

PROCEDURE. After the conjunctiva have been desensitized with topical anesthetic solution, Adson tissue forceps (or similar) are used to elevate a piece of conjunctiva, that is then snipped off with strabismus scissors. If necessary, bleeding can be controlled by topical application of 10% phenylephrine. For histological examination the tissue sample is pinned to a piece of cardboard and fixed. To identify *microfilaria* the tissue is sliced, incubated at 37°C in saline, and the supernatant examined.

Materials for Conjunctival Biopsy

- ▶ Forceps (e.g., Adson's)
- ▶ Scissors (e.g., strabismus)
- ▶ Topical anesthetic solution (0.5% proparacaine)
- ▶ 10% phenylephrine

Materials for Collection of a Smear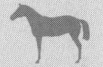

- ▶ Microscope slide

MEASUREMENT OF TEAR PRODUCTION

It is possible to test the efficiency of tear production (lacrimation) by measuring the extent to which tear fluid is absorbed by a strip of absorbent paper. Schirmer tear strips are commercially available as absorbent strips 40 × 5 mm in size with a notch 5 mm from the end. To accommodate greater tear production, filter paper cut to a larger size can also be used.

PROCEDURE. The test is usually made without topical anesthesia. A strip is folded over at the notch and the tip is placed inside the temporal third of the lower lid between it and the cornea, as demonstrated in Figure 10–20. The strip is removed, usually after 60 seconds, and the

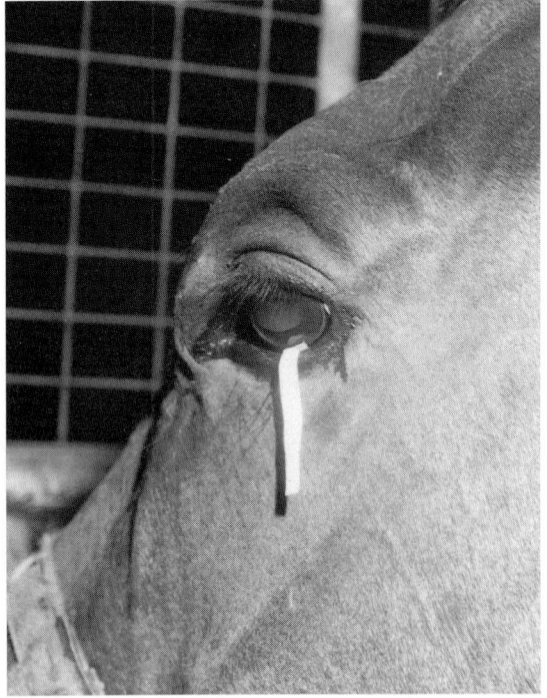

▶ **FIGURE 10–20**
Measurement of tear production with absorptive paper.

distance the fluid has moved along the strip from the notch is measured.

Fluorescein Staining of Corneal Lesions

Fluorescein is water soluble and will not penetrate intact cornea or conjunctiva. The basis of the test is that corneal defects will retain topically applied stain after the remainder has been washed away by eyelid action or by saline lavage. This enhances ability to identify corneal lesions. The test is simple to carry out and a vital part of ocular examination.[1]

PROCEDURE. The test is carried out by wetting the strip with the eyewash solution or saline and then applying it to the eye. Dry strips should not be used, and even wet strips may be irritating to a painful eye. To avoid pain and trauma the eyewash solution can be stained with the fluorescein and then squirted onto the eye with a syringe. This can be done by placing a little of the solution and a fluorescein strip in a beaker and then aspirating the stained fluid into a syringe that is then used to squirt it into the eye.

Evaluation of Nasolacrimal Duct Patency

The nasolacrimal system allows fluid to pass from the eye to the nasal cavity. On each side the system consists of two puncta, each opening into a canaliculus that joins to form a lacrimal sac that then continues as the nasolacrimal duct to enter the nasal cavity through a punctum lying near the mucocutaneous junction. The existence

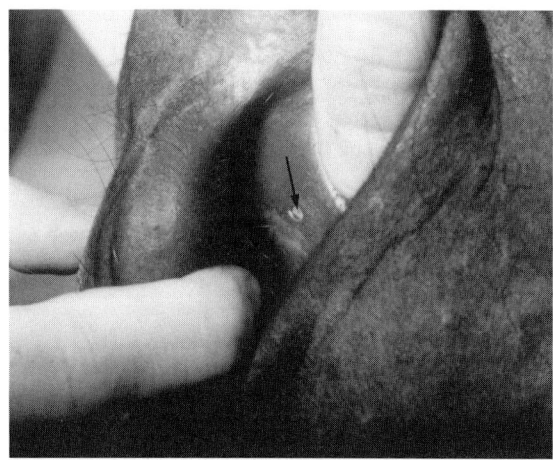

▶ **FIGURE 10-21**
Nasal punctum of the nasolacrimal duct.

of the puncta is easily ascertained by examining the eyelids and nasal passage.[15]

TESTING PATENCY BY PASSAGE OF FLUID. The patency of the system can be assessed by placing fluorescein in the eye, as described above, and waiting for it to appear at the nostril after 5 to 15 minutes or by flushing. The disadvantage of the dye method is the time required for the dye to appear and the fact that dye passage can be hindered by mucus. The most common method of assessing patency is by flushing the duct from the nasal punctum, and less often from the lacrimal punctum. The nasal punctum lies ventrally just inside the nasal passage at the mucocutaneous junction, usually in the pigmented cutaneous portion (Fig. 10–21). The opening is usually easy to find because the nonpigmented lining of the duct contrasts with the pigmented surrounds. Catheterization is also possible from the proximal end, but this is more difficult and is most easily done under general anesthesia. The lower punctum is slightly larger and is therefore easier to catheterize.

Materials for Nasolacrimal Duct Catheterization

▶ Syringe (30 ml)
▶ Catheter (1–2 mm, such as flexible tomcat urinary catheter, polyethylene tubing [PE 90])
▶ Lacrimal cannula (20–22 gauge)

PROCEDURE. To insert the catheter the horse's head is restrained and the nostril is held open. When the orifice of the duct has been located, the catheter can be easily inserted for a few centimeters, but extra assistance is often necessary to ensure that it can pass further up the duct. It is important to remember that the duct curves around the lateral wall of the nasal passage and that this curvature sometimes hinders passage of the catheter. On no account should the catheter be forced, because the duct is easily torn. To ensure that the catheter follows the duct, a finger can be placed over the catheter to hold it against the lateral nasal wall and so guide it around the curvature. After insertion it is a simple matter to inject fluid under pressure to assess ductal patency. The sudden emergence of fluid from the proximal puncta will frighten many horses, so flushing should be done carefully and with adequate restraint.

To flush the duct from the proximal end, a catheter or lacrimal cannula is inserted through a lacrimal punctum, which is relatively difficult in the standing horse (Fig. 10–22). Because the lower punctum is larger it is easier to catheterize.

DACROCYSTORHINOGRAPHY. The system can also be demonstrated radiographically by injecting contrast material from the proximal or distal openings (Fig. 10–23).[16] The distal approach is easier, as described above for flushing, although this may fail to identify any accessory blind endings to the duct that sometimes occur. The procedure is identical to that described for flushing the duct. Although 60% barium sulfate

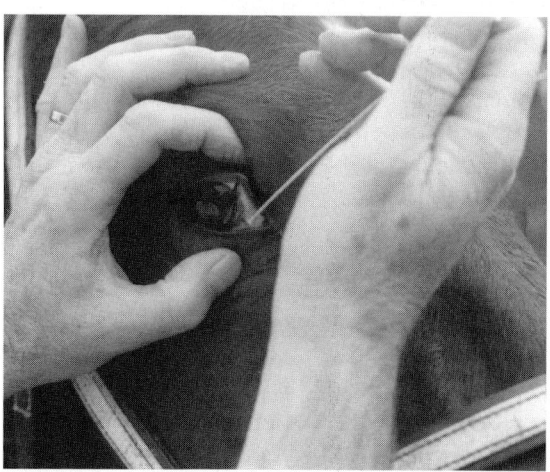

▶ **FIGURE 10-22**
Cannulation of the lower lacrimal punctum with a tomcat urinary catheter.

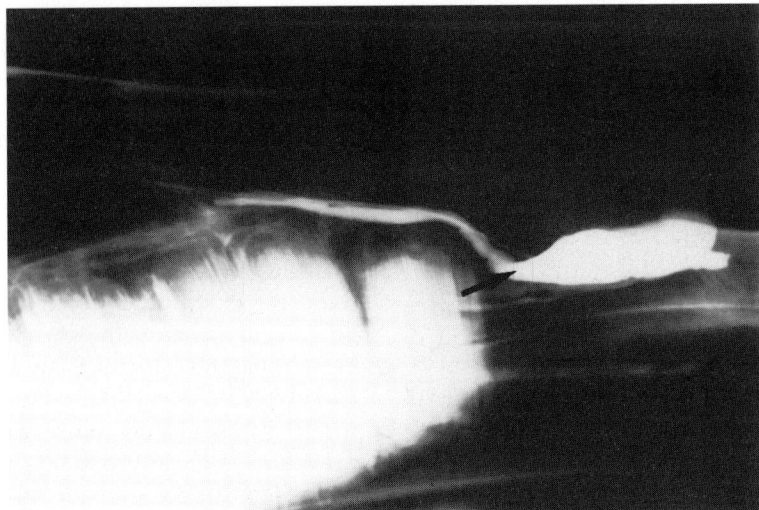

▶ **FIGURE 10-23**
Nasolacrimal duct containing positive contrast material. It is dilated because of distal atresia.

(Hypaque) is a suitable contrast agent, the agents used for intravenous contrast studies (diatrizoate meglumine or sodium renograffin) are preferred.

SPECIAL EXAMINATION PROCEDURES

Intraocular Tonometry

Intraocular pressure is often measured in man and to a lesser extent in small animals. However, it is not a common practice in equine medicine, probably because of the low incidence of glaucoma. *Direct tonometry* involves direct measurement of intraocular pressure with a manometer or transducer, but this is not clinically feasible. *Indirect tonometry* involves measurement of intraocular tension by measuring the tension in the cornea. Digital palpation (digital tonometry) is useful, easily performed, but inaccurate, especially when regular monitoring is required. Digital tonometry is carried out by placing the first finger on the upper lid and then gently applying pressure so as to depress the eyeball (Fig. 10-24). This can also be done by placing the finger directly on the cornea, which requires topical anesthesia. Obvious variation in intraocular pressure is easily detected with digital tonometry.

Indirect tonometry is more accurate and measures the force necessary to indent (Schiotz tonometer) or flatten (applanation tonometer) a small section of the cornea. The Schiotz tonometer is not well suited to the horse and the applanation method is recommended.

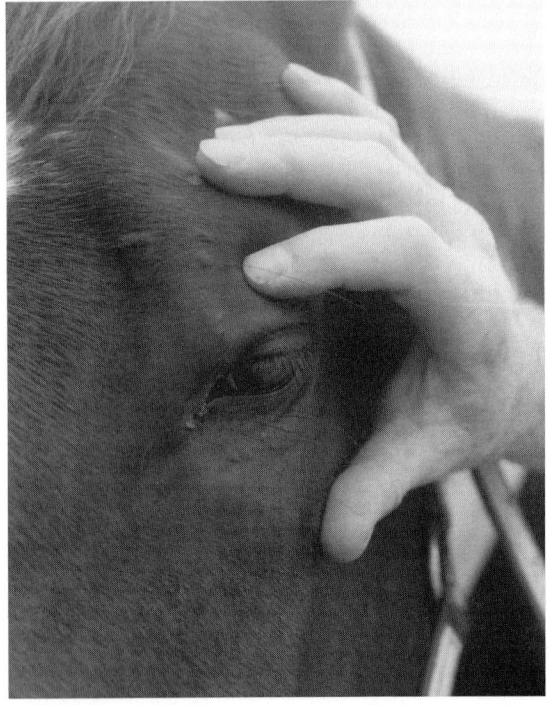

▶ **FIGURE 10-24**
Digital tonometry. The intraocular pressure is estimated by pushing the first finger against the globe.

Materials for Indirect Tonometry

▶ Topical anesthetic solution
▶ Applanation tonometer (Ton-O-Pen, MacKay-Marg)

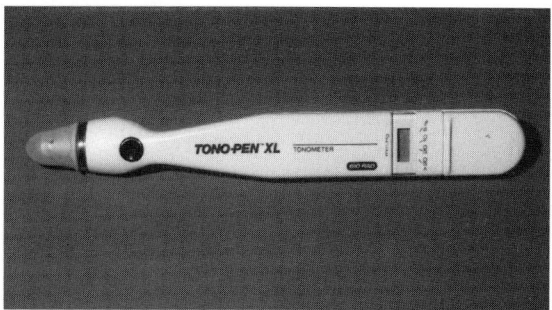

▶ **FIGURE 10-25**

A Ton-O-Pen applanometer, used for measuring intraocular pressure.

PROCEDURE. The horse should be sedated, appropriately restrained, and the cornea anesthetized with topical anesthetic solution. An auriculopalpebral nerve block can also be used to paralyze the upper eyelid, if required, without affecting intraocular pressure.[17] General anesthesia with xylazine-ketamine is also reported to have no effect on intraocular pressure.[18] Measurements are made by applying the tip of the probe at right angles to the cornea and recording the results (Fig. 10-25). The Ton-O-Pen is probably the most appropriate instrument to use because it is easier to handle and transport and because the MacKay-Marg tonometer is no longer available. Results from the Ton-O-Pen are given as an averaged digital readout, and those from the other instrument are produced as a calibrated graphic output. Both instruments slightly underestimate intraocular pressure.

Although the pressure can fluctuate rapidly up to 10 mm Hg in excited horses, significant differences are not usually seen between the normal left and right eyes.

Electroretinography

Electroretinography records the retinal response to light. It is a measure of the integrity of the outer part of the retina and the pigmented

---

Materials for Electroretinography

▶ Electroretinography apparatus (active, reference, and ground electrodes, chart recorder, AC amplifier, photostimulator, and filters as necessary, oscilloscope, flash generator, flash tube)

---

epithelial layer, but it is not a test of vision. It is best regarded as a general response of the retina as a whole rather than a technique to diagnose focal lesions. In the clinical sphere it is useful for evaluating retinal function when opacity in the lens or cornea precludes the usual methods of examination, trauma, and certain inherited retinal diseases such as night blindness (congenital stationary night blindness) in Appaloosa horses.

PROCEDURE. Electroretinograhy is carried out under general anesthesia.[19] Placement of the electrodes is variable, but the location of the reference electrode at the medial canthus and of the ground electrode on the tip of the ipsilateral ear is acceptable. The active electrode is either a contact lens or saline-soaked agar wick.

The retina is stimulated to light of varying intensity, wavelength, and flash duration, and the response is detected by electrodes amplified and then displayed on an oscilloscope or paper recorder. The normal electroretinogram is demonstrated in Figure 10-26, and consists of A-, B-, and sometimes C-waves. The first two are rapid, and the third is slow.

Biomicroscopy

The slit lamp, or biomicroscope, allows the transparent structures of the eye to be examined in optical section. It is useful for evaluating the structures as deep as the cranial vitreous and provides good illumination and magnification.[20] The major limitations are the expense and the restriction of view. Table, or fixed, models are of little value for horses where a portable instrument is required; an example is the portable hand-held Kowa model (Fig. 10-27). The major components are illumination and binocular microscopic observational systems.

Fluorescein Angiography

The ability of fluorescein to fluoresce with maximal emission at 520 to 530 nm after illumi-

---

NORMAL VALUES FOR INTRAOCULAR PRESSURE

• *Horses* (conscious)[17]
   23.5 ± 6.1 mm Hg (MacKay-Marg)
   23.3 ± 6.9 mm Hg (Ton-O-Pen)
• *Ponies* (xylazine-ketamine anesthesia)[18]
   23.5 ± 4.5 mm Hg (MacKay-Marg)

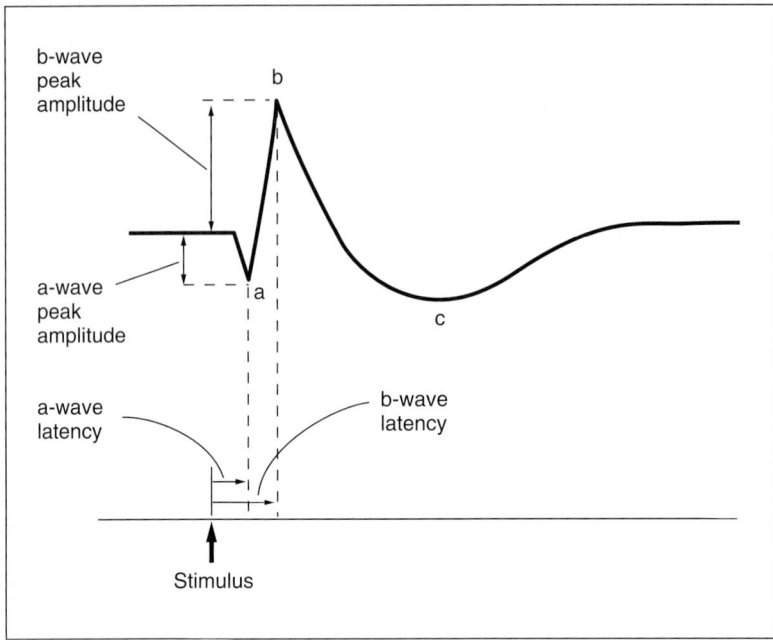

▶ FIGURE 10-26

Electroretinogram. Diagram of the response of the retina to light.

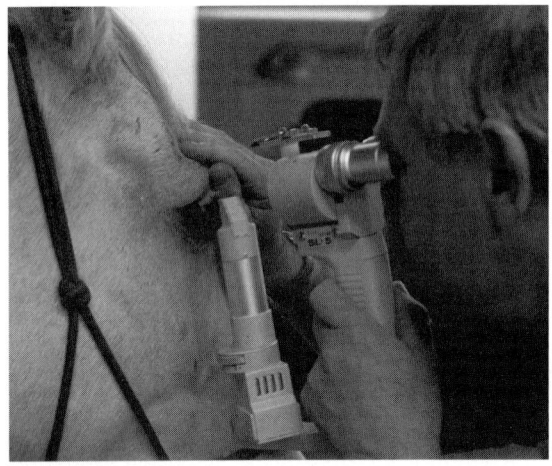

▶ FIGURE 10-27

Slit lamp biomicroscopy using a hand-held Kowa slit lamp biomicroscope.

nation by light with wavelength of 485 to 500 nm allows certain aspects of the ocular vasculature to be studied, including the pulsation of retinal and choroidal vessels, permeability of the vasculature in association with inflammation and neovascularization, and pigmentary abnormalities.[20] The procedure involves the intravenous injection of fluorescein followed by serial photography over 20 to 30 minutes, with about 30 exposures in the first 30 seconds, allowing the circulation to be monitored and divided into different phases as follows:

- Choroidal phase: Choroidal vessels filled
- Arteriolar phase: Retinal arterioles filled
- AV phase: Arterioles and venules filled
- Venous phase: Arterioles and venules emptying, veins filling
- Late phase: Certain tissues staining (e.g., optic nerve head)

Gonioscopy

Gonioscopy is the examination of the filtration (iridocorneal) angle and requires the application of a contact lens (gonioscopy lens or goniolens) to the cornea to refract the image of the angle, thereby allowing it to be viewed directly.[21] The instrument is used to determine whether the angle is open or closed, obstructed, and to check for neoplasia, foreign bodies, and inflammatory exudate. It has limited application in horses because of the low incidence of glaucoma. Under normal circumstances, light rays reflected from the drainage angle enter the cornea from its posterior surface and then undergo total internal reflection. This is countered by placing a lens on the external surface of the cornea, thus allowing rays from the drainage angle to be viewed directly through the lens.

Materials for Gonioscopy

▶ Goniolens (e.g., Koeppe, Franklin, Barkan)

▶ Magnification (magnifying glasses,[e.g., Neitz loupe, Storz optivisor], otoscope)

▶ Light source (transilluminator [e.g., Finoff], focal light [e.g., auriscope, Heine, Accumat])

▶ Artificial tears (e.g., Adsorbotear; [Alcon Labs, Fort Worth, TX])

▶ Topical anesthetic (0.5% proparacaine hydrochloride)

PROCEDURE. The procedure usually requires general anesthesia, although in tractable animals, sedation and topical anesthesia will suffice. A few drops of the artificial tears (or normal saline) are placed in the concavity of the goniolens that is then gently placed on the cornea. When using the Barkan lens, which has tubing and a syringe attached, more fluid is injected after the lens is in place, to ensure the removal of all air bubbles. The iridocorneal angle is examined with illumination and extra magnification as required.

Ultrasonography of the Globe and Orbit

Ultrasonography of the globe and orbit can be useful for detecting intraocular masses, foreign bodies, and retrobulbar lesions; assessing the size of the globe; detecting retinal detachment behind a catatact; and evaluating the osseous integrity of the orbit. The ultrasound can be directed through the cornea or through the eyelids, depending on which region is being imaged.

R E F E R E N C E S

1. Hakanson NE, Merideth RE: Ocular examination and diagnostic techniques in the horse part 1: Examination of the adnexa and extraocular structures. Equine Pract 1987; 9(5):7.
2. Blythe LL: Neurologic examination of the horse. Vet Clin North Amer: Equine Pract 1987; 3:255.
3. Hakanson NE, Merideth RE: Ocular examination and diagnostic techniques in the horse part 2: Assessment of vision and examination of intraocular structures. Equine Pract 1987; 9(10):6.
4. Miller WW, Crenshaw KL: The basics of in-clinic ophthalmic examinations. Vet Med Nov. 1988:1154.
5. Crispin SM, Matthews AG, Parker J: The equine fundus 1: Examination, embryology, structure and function. Equine Vet J Supplement 10, Equine Ophthalmology 2, 1990:42.
6. Matthews AG, Crispin SM, Parker J: The equine fundus 11: Normal anatomical variants and colobomata. Equine Vet J Supplement 10, Equine Ophthalmology 2, 1990:50.
7. Matthews AG, Crispin SM, Parker J: The equine fundus 111: Pathological variants. Equine Vet J Supplement 10 Equine Ophthalmology 2, 1990:55.
8. Blogg JR: The Eye in Veterinary Practice. Extraocular Disease. Philadelphia, Saunders, 1980, p 69.
9. Moore CP, Heller N, Majors LJ, et al: Prevalence of ocular micro-organisms in hospitalized and stabled horses. Am J Vet Res 1988, 49:773.
10. Whitley RD, Burgess EC, Moore CP: Microbial isolates of the normal equine eye. Equine Vet J Supplement 2, Equine Ophthalmology, 1983:138.
11. Moore CP, Fales WH, Whittington P, et al: Bacterial and fungal isolates from equidae with ulcerative keratitis. J Am Vet Med Assoc 1983; 182:600.
12. Slatter D: Conjunctiva. In Slatter DE (ed): Textbook of Small Animal Surgery, 2nd ed, Philadelphia, Saunders, 1985, ch 83, p 1183.
13. Marts BS, Bryan GM, Prieur DJ: Schirmer tear test measurement and lysozyme concentration of equine tears. J Equine Med Surg 1977, 1:427.
14. Williams RD, Manning JP, Peiffer RL: The Schirmer tear test in the equine: Normal values and the contribution of the gland of the nictitating membrane. J Equine Med Surg 1979; 3:117.
15. Harling DE: Epiphora and lacrimal system dysfunction in the horse. Equine Pract 1988; 10(5):27.
16. Latimer CA, Wyman M, Diesem CD, et al: Radiographic and gross anatomy of the nasolacrimal duct of the horse. Am J Vet Res 1984; 45:451.
17. Miller PE, Pickett JP, Majors LJ: Evaluation of two applanation tonometers in horses. Am J Vet Res 1990; 51:935.
18. Smith PJ, Gum GG, Whitley RD: Tonometric and tonographic studies in the normal pony eye. Equine Vet J Supplement 10, Equine Ophthalmology 2, 1990:36.
19. Wouters L, de Moor A, Moens Y: Rod and cone components in the electroretinogram of the horse. Zentralblatt für Veterinärmed 1980; 27A:330.
20. Gelatt, KN: Ophthalmic examination and diagnostic procedures. In Gelatt KN (ed), Veterinary ophthalmology, 2nd ed. Philadelphia, Lea & Febiger, 1991, ch 4, p 224.
21. Blogg JR: The Eye in Veterinary Practice. Extraocular Disease. Philadelphia, WB Saunders Company. 1980, p 70.

A D D I T I O N A L   R E A D I N G S

Barnett KC: A Color Atlas of Veterinary Ophthalmology. London, Wolf Publishing, 1990.

Blogg JR: The Eye in Veterinary Practice. Eye Examination of the Performance Horse. Malvern, Australia, Chilcott Publishing, 1985.

Lavach JD: Large Animal Ophthalmology, vol 2. St Louis, Mosby, 1990.

Slatter DH: Fundamentals of Veterinary Ophthalmology. Philadelphia, WB Saunders Company, 1980.

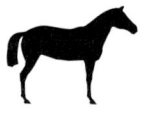

The Alimentary Tract

11

COMPONENTS

The alimentary tract extends from the oral cavity to the anus and includes the teeth, salivary glands, tongue, esophagus, stomach, and small and large intestines.

MANIFESTATIONS OF DISEASE

The alimentary tract is concerned with the intake, processing, and absorption of food and water and the excretion of waste. The manifestations of disease are related to malfunction of these systems and include:

- *Abnormality of prehension.* Inability to take food into the mouth (prehend) is associated with conditions such as poor occlusion of incisor teeth, and paralysis of tongue or jaw.
- *Excessive salivation.* Excess saliva may be associated with excess production or inability to swallow because of pain (foreign body) or obstruction (esophageal foreign body)
- *Vomiting.* Horses do not exhibit projectile vomiting. However, gastric content will flow from the mouth and nares when the stomach is grossly distended.
- *Abnormality of swallowing.* Swallowing malfunction can be the result of physical obstruction (e.g., pharyngeal or esophageal

foreign body, esophageal diverticulum) or nerve deficit (e.g., guttural pouch mycosis with lesion of the glossopharyngeal nerve). Signs include exaggerated efforts to swallow and flow of food, water, and saliva from the nares.
- *Abnormality of mastication.* Chewing can be altered or prevented by the pain of stomatitis or tooth disease.
- *Abdominal distension.* The abdomen becomes distended when there is an accumulation of gas (tympany) or ingesta (obstruction) in the intestines.
- *Poor body condition.* Reduced efficiency of digestion and absorption results in loss of condition.
- *Change in character of feces.* The appearance of feces can be altered by a number of factors, such as infection, change in intestinal flora (dietary change), presence of foreign material (e.g., sand), poor digestion and absorption (malabsorption syndromes), excitement, parasitism, and prolonged transit.
- *Pain.* Pain is caused by distension and obstruction, and signs of pain are common in equine intestinal disease. Pain is manifest by pawing the ground, rolling on the ground, frequent lying down and standing up, and assuming odd recumbent positions.
- *Foul-smelling breath.* Oral disease, especially involving the teeth, often produces a foul odor.

CLASSIFICATION OF BODY CONDITION

0 Very poor

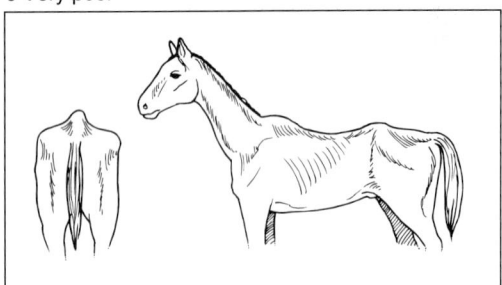

Very sunken rump
Deep cavity under tail
Skin tight over bones
Very prominent spine and pelvis
Marked ewe neck

1 Poor

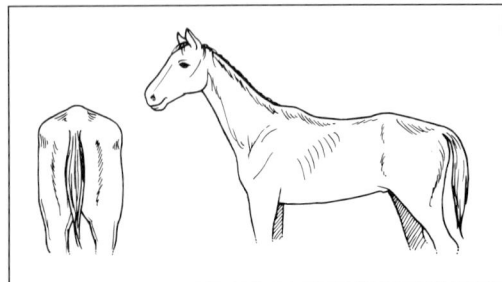

Sunken rump
Cavity under tail
Ribs easily visible
Prominent spine and croup
Ewe neck - narrow and slack

2 Moderate

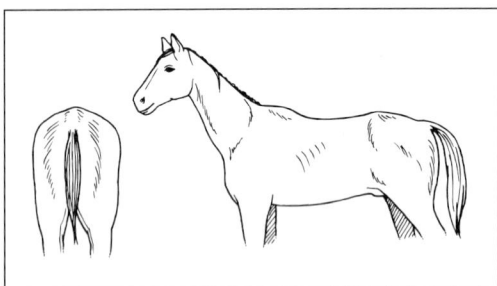

Flat rump either side of spine
Ribs just visible
Narrow but firm neck
Spine well covered

3 Good

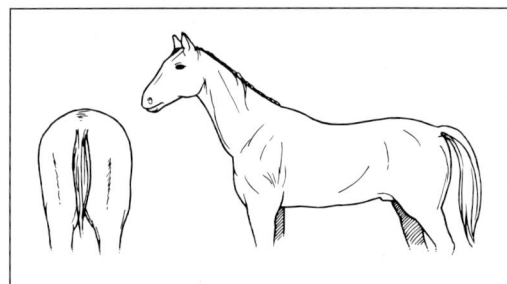

Rounded rump
Ribs just covered but easily felt
No crest, firm neck

4 Fat

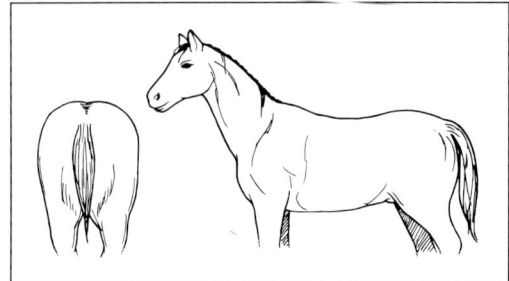

Rump well rounded
Gutter along back
Ribs and pelvis difficult to palpate
Slight crest

5 Very fat

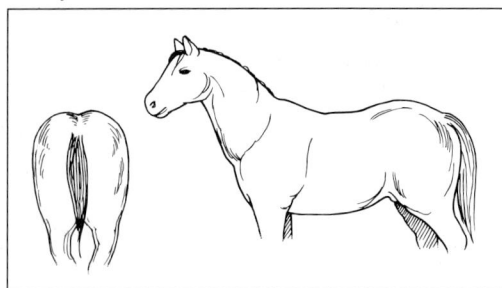

Very bulging rump
Deep gutter along back
Ribs not palpable
Marked crest
Folds and lumps of fat

▶ **FIGURE 11-1**

Body condition classification. (From Huntington PJ: Condition Scoring and Weight Estimation of Horses. Ag Note 2816-85. Melbourne, Department of Natural Resources and Environment, 1985. Reprinted with permission.)

GENERAL PHYSICAL EXAMINATION

Body Condition

The general body condition is easily evaluated by visual examination. Chronic intestinal disease invariably results in loss of condition characterized by a loss of subcutaneous fat and muscle mass, resulting in the skeletal structures' becoming progressively more visible (Fig. 11-1).[1]

Prehension, Mastication, and Swallowing

These functions are evaluated by allowing the horse to drink and graze. If food is given by hand, prehension cannot be properly evaluated. Ability to graze from the ground requires that there are no painful lesions preventing the extension and lowering of the head and neck and opening and closing of the mouth. Incisor teeth must be capable of grasping grass, which is difficult when they are malaligned because of age, disease, or trauma.

The cheek teeth are used to grind food and, with the tongue, participate in mixing it with saliva (mastication). Coordination between the tongue and jaws is required to move food toward the esophagus in preparation for swallowing. Problems that compromize chewing include lingual pain (laceration), dental pain (fracture, periapical abscess), dental malformation, supernumerary teeth, overgrowth of teeth, absence of teeth, and sharp edges of the occlusal surfaces resulting from abnormal wear. When any of these conditions are present, a horse will often cease chewing and drop a portion of partly masticated food from its mouth, a process known as "quidding."

The masticated food eventually passes to the oropharynx from where it passes into the esophagus. The bolus is visible as it passes down the esophagus on the left side of the neck in the region of the jugular furrow. The act of swallowing (deglutition) requires considerable coordination and can be interrupted by painful or obstructive lesions or neurological deficit (e.g., guttural pouch mycosis).

The Teeth and the Oral Cavity

Unassisted Examination of the Teeth and Oral Cavity

The incisor teeth are examined first. To do this, stand to the left side of the horse, support the

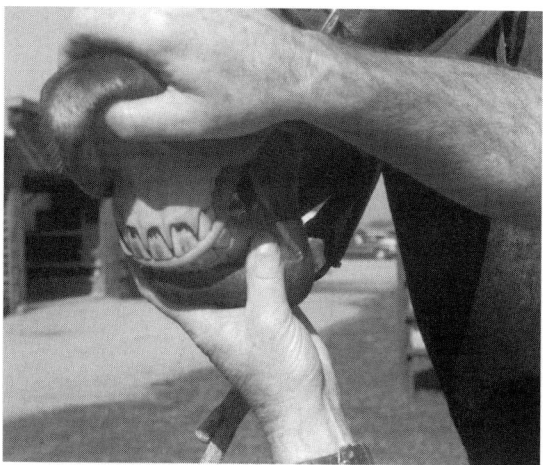

▶ FIGURE 11-2
Examination of the incisor teeth.

head by placing the left hand under the lower jaw, and then use the thumb and first finger of the right hand to separate the lips and bring the incisors into view (Fig. 11-2). The incisors should be checked, noting especially if they occlude normally and if they are normal in number and orientation. The rostral cheek teeth can be cursorilory examined by forcing the horse to open its mouth. Although a full examination of the cheek teeth requires the use of a mouth gag, cursory visual examinations and palpation are possible. The visual examination is made possible by forcing the horse to open its mouth, which is done by placing the thumb in the interdental space and pressing it against the hard palate (Fig. 11-3). Another way of making a horse open its

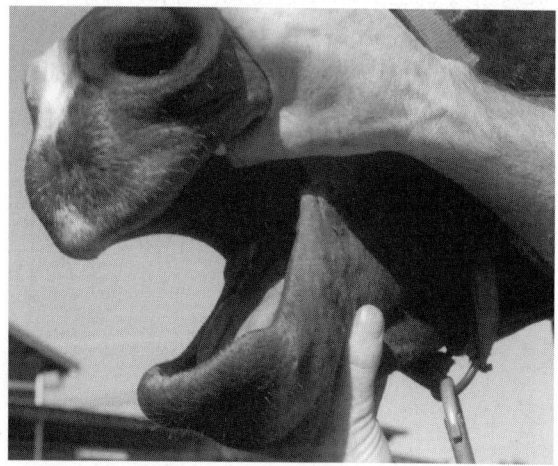

▶ FIGURE 11-3
Method of stimulating a horse to open its mouth by placing the thumb through the interdental space and against the hard palate.

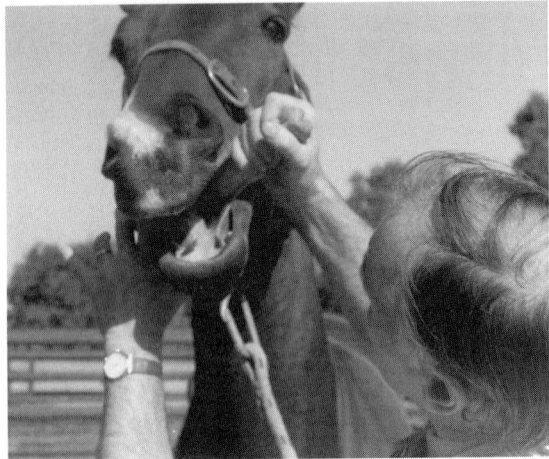

▶ **FIGURE 11-4**

Retraction of the tongue to allow examination of the cheek teeth.

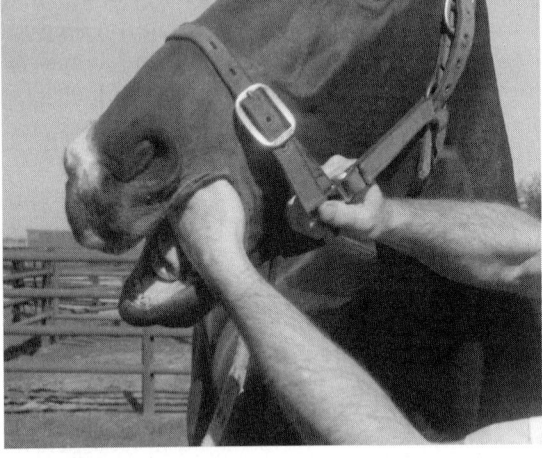

▶ **FIGURE 11-5**

Palpation of the cheek teeth without a mouth gag. In this photograph the left hand is being used to palpate the left upper and lower arcades.

mouth is to grasp its tongue and pull it gently out and to one side, taking care to avoid excessive traction that can tear the frenulum (Fig. 11-4). To palpate the cheek teeth in the left dental arcades without using a gag, the clinician must stand on the left side, hold the head stall with the right hand, and insert the left hand into the mouth through the interdental space (Fig. 11-5). The fingers must be close together, and the hand must be cupped, as demonstrated. As the cupped hand is forced into the mouth, the back of the hand forces the tongue between the opposite (right) arcades, thus preventing the horse from closing its mouth and injuring the clinician. The left arcades are then examined with the fingers. It is important that the hand remain cupped; otherwise, the horse will be able to close its mouth. To examine the right arcades, the clinician stands on the right side and uses the other hand in identical fashion. This procedure is potentially dangerous and must be done only when the horse is tractable and well restrained.

Examination of the Teeth and Oral Cavity with a Gag

A safe and thorough examination of the teeth requires a mouth gag (Fig. 11-6). The Hausmann and Swale gags demonstrated are two of a number in use. The Swale's gag is easier to apply, but there is a tendency for teeth to fracture because of the small area of contact with the teeth and the gag. The Hausmann gag, preferred by the author, opens the mouth by applying pressure to all the incisor teeth, thus distributing the load. The Hausmann gag is applied by placing the strap behind the ears. As the strap is being tightened, the dental plates are forced between the incisor

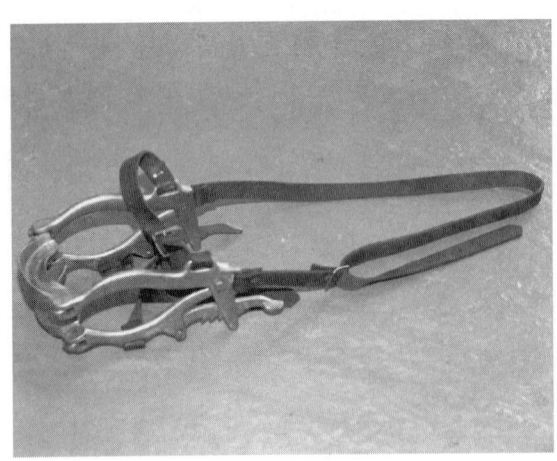

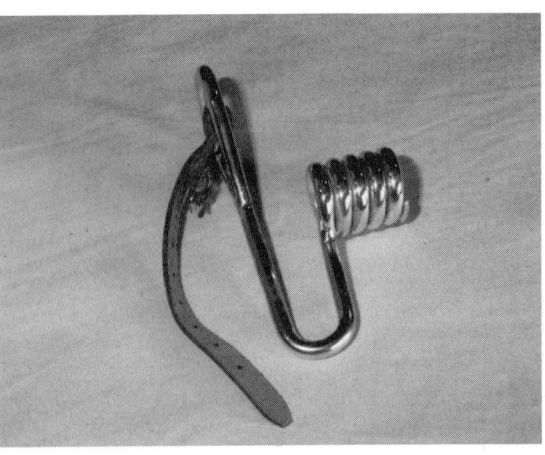

A   B

▶ **FIGURE 11-6**

Opening the mouth by mechanical means. **A.** Hausmann mouth gag. **B.** Swale's mouth gag.

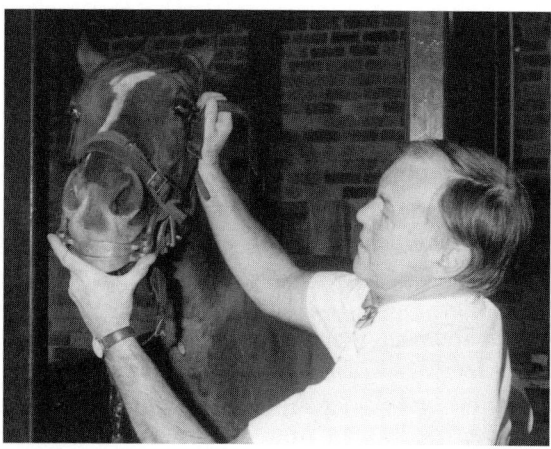
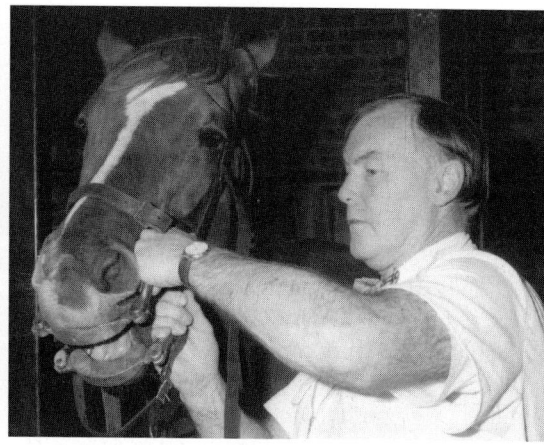

A   B

▶ **FIGURE 11-7**

Hausmann mouth gag. **A.** Placing the gag with the strap behind the ears and the dental plates between the teeth. **B.** Opening the mouth by pulling the arms of the gag apart.

teeth (Fig. 11-7). Most horses tolerate the procedure and readily open their mouths. Once in place, with the plates against the labial surfaces of the incisor teeth, the side handles are pulled apart to open the mouth. A visual examination and palpation of the mouth and teeth can then be carried out quite easily. A pen light is useful to examine the caudal regions. The teeth are examined for fractures, deformity, malocclusion, and sharp edges.

The Salivary Glands

Disease of the salivary glands and their ducts is not common in horses. There are three main, paired, discreet glands; the parotid, mandibular (submaxillary), and sublingual; and several minor less defined glands; the buccal, labial, lingual, and palatine. The diseases of the salivary glands and ducts are reviewed elsewhere.[2]

The largest, and clinically most important, of these glands is the parotid gland, located caudal and medial to the vertical ramus of the mandible and extending dorsally to the base of the ear. The gland secretes a primarily serous fluid, which is transported to the oral cavity through the parotid (Stenson's) duct. The duct traverses the ventromedial aspect of the mandible with the facial artery and vein before passing dorsally to enter the oral cavity on the parotid papilla opposite the third or fourth upper premolars. The most common lesion of this gland is a salivary fistula caused by a laceration of the duct. This duct is involved because its exposed location predisposes it to trauma. The fistula is usually obvious when the horse is feeding, as saliva squirts from

the severed duct. Salivary calculi, composed mainly of calcium carbonate, also occur and cause distension of the duct proximal to the site of obstruction. Duct atresia and heterotopia rarely occur.

The mandibular salivary gland lies medial to the parotid gland. Its duct passes rostrally on the medial side of the mandible to enter the oral cavity on the sublingal caruncle situated ventral to the tongue and just rostrolateral to the frenulum of the tongue. The sublingual salivary gland lies between the tongue and the medial aspect of the mandible, extending from the incisors to the region of the lower molar teeth. There are many small ducts, which open separately onto the sublingual fold. Rupture of a gland or duct produces a fluid-filled swelling known as a sialocele or salivary mucocele. Ranula is the term given to a similar swelling, lying on the floor of the mouth, caused by dilation of a duct.

Other conditions affecting the glands include neoplasia (most frequently melanoma), ptyalism caused by irritation, and slaframine toxicosis caused by ingestion of *Rhizoctonia leguminicola.*

Radiographic visualization of the parotid gland and its duct is possible.[3] Water-soluble radiographic contrast material can be infused into the gland by catheterization of the duct, either from its opening into the mouth, or from a site in the duct caused by a wound or created by surgical incision. In view of the problems with duct healing, the first method is recommended. A volume of 35 mL of contrast medium (0.08 mL/kg body weight) provides good definition of the duct and some glandular filling.[3] Glandular definition can be improved by increasing the volume of contrast. Glandular involution may occur when Renografin-76 is used as the contrast material.[3]

Abdominal Distension

The abdomen can be distended by gas, ingesta, or fluid. Distension is easily seen, but the cause of distension must be ascertained by other means. The presence of gas is inferred from the tympanitic sound ellicited by percussion with the fingers. Gas is usually within the gut but can also be free in the abdomen (e.g., gut rupture, occasional cases of peritonitis). Gas can also be identified by percutaneous needle puncture through the left or right paralumbar fossa. Although needle puncture is usually not necessary as a diagnostic tool, it is often carried out to relieve intra-abdominal pressure to improve respiration or to allow other examinations, such as rectal palpation, to be carried out. When there is a large volume of ingesta (e.g., intestinal impaction) or fluid (e.g., bladder rupture), percussion elicits a dull sound. Fluid can also be intraluminal or free within the abdomen. Fluid can be detected by pushing the fist against the abdominal wall and then listening for fluid sounds after it has been quickly withdrawn (ballottement) or, in foals, by shaking the abdomen (succussion). Free fluid also is detected by tactile percussion, in which percussion is carried out on one side of the abdomen with the fingers of one hand while the palm of the other hand is held against the opposite side of the abdomen to detect transmission of the fluid waves resulting from the percussion. Intraluminal fluid is not easily detected with tactile percussion. Problems of the gastrointestinal tract are the usual cause of abdominal distension, but an oversized fetus(es), ovarian tumor, and fetal hydrops are some other possible causes.

Abdominal Auscultation

Abdominal auscultation is an important part of the clinical examination, especially in horses that are showing signs of abdominal pain. Although there is a general consensus that auscultatory findings have prognostic significance in colic cases, little data correlating the sounds heard during auscultation with specific parts of the gastrointestinal tract exists. A stethoscope is used to auscultate the left and right sides and the ventral aspect of the abdomen. The organs lying beneath the left and right body walls are demonstrated in Figure 11-8. It is usual to begin in the left or right paralumbar fossa and then progress ventrally. It is advisable to listen for a minute or so at each site, although, in many cases, a much longer time is necessary to hear and interpret adequately what is occurring. Auscultation for up to 5 to 10 minutes may be necessary to evaluate appropriately abdominal sounds, especially those originating in the cecum and large colon. Cecal and colonic sounds associated with propulsion are infrequent, loud, and distinctive sounds that wax and wane,[4] occur every few minutes, and last 10 to 20 seconds. In general, small intestinal sounds tend to be more fluid in character and of higher pitch than large intestinal sounds. In the right paralumbar fossa the high-pitched, gurgling sounds like water running down a pipe are, rightly or wrongly, often described as originating from the ileocecal region, and sounds in the left paralumbar region are taken as originating from the small intestine. Because of the absence of appropriate standards and of the inability to identify the source of a sound precisely, clinicians tend to report sounds as being absent, reduced, normal, or increased. It has been shown that experienced clinicians are relatively consistent for intraobserver interpretation, although there is less consistency between observers.[5]

Increased activity is noticed after feeding and drinking and with enteritis and partial obstructions. The fluid sounds are greatly increased with enteritis. Loss of activity (ileus) results in the absence of normal sounds and the appearance of tinkling sounds as gas bubbles rise to the surface of the fluid. The tinkling sounds are most frequently heard when gas bubbles rise to the surface and emerge in the cecal gas cap. Presence of sand in the large intestine can often be detected from the grating noise produced as it is moved along by peristalsis. Auscultation can be combined with percussion to define more accurately the presence of gas in an organ, particularly the cecum.

Passage of a Nasogastric Tube

Passing a nasogastric tube is an important procedure with which all clinicians should be familiar. Some indications for the procedure include: decompression of the stomach, diagnosis of esophageal patency, diagnosis of intestinal function, and administration of medication. The ability to carry it out correctly also is important because of the ease with which the tube can be accidentally passed into the trachea.

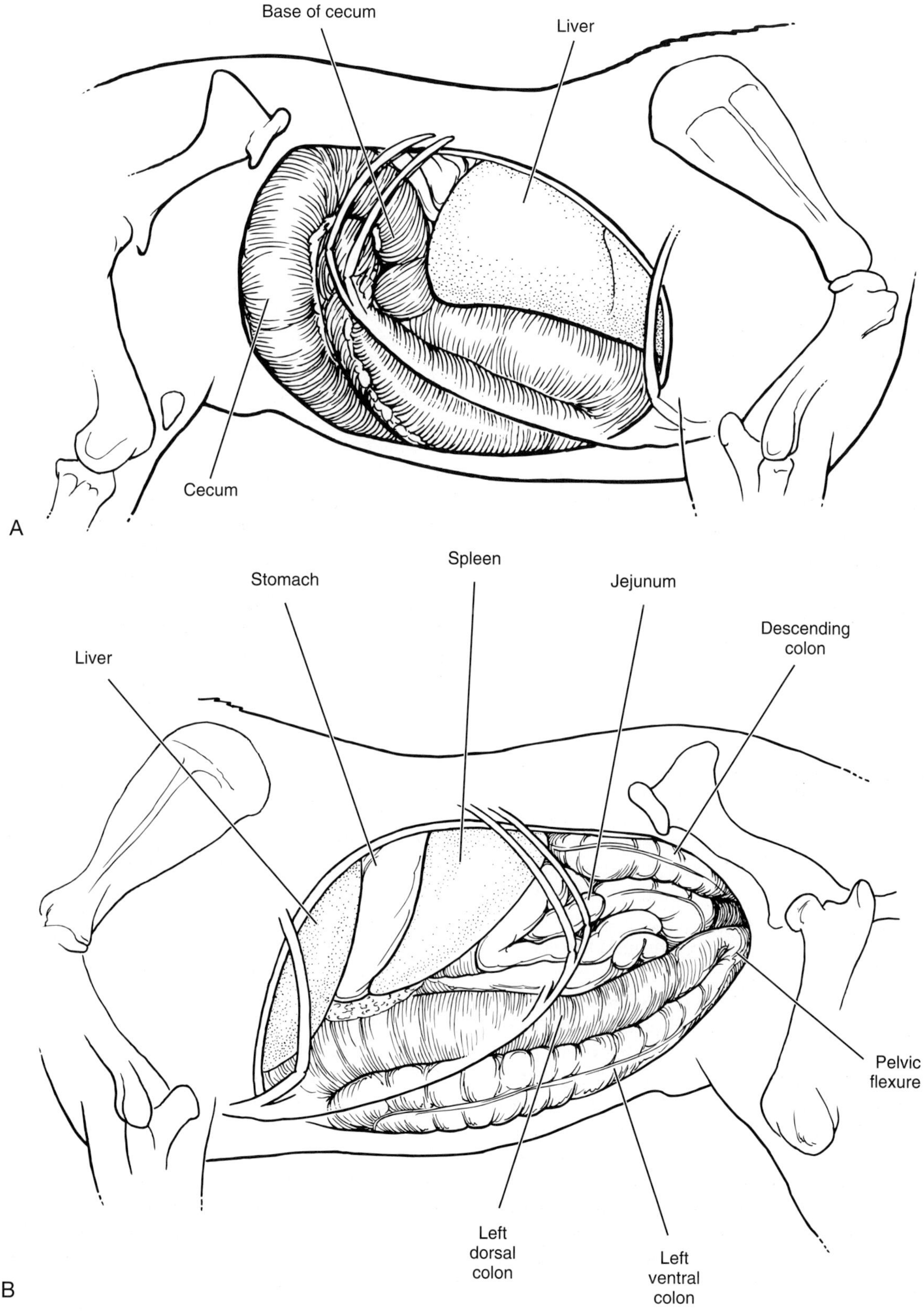

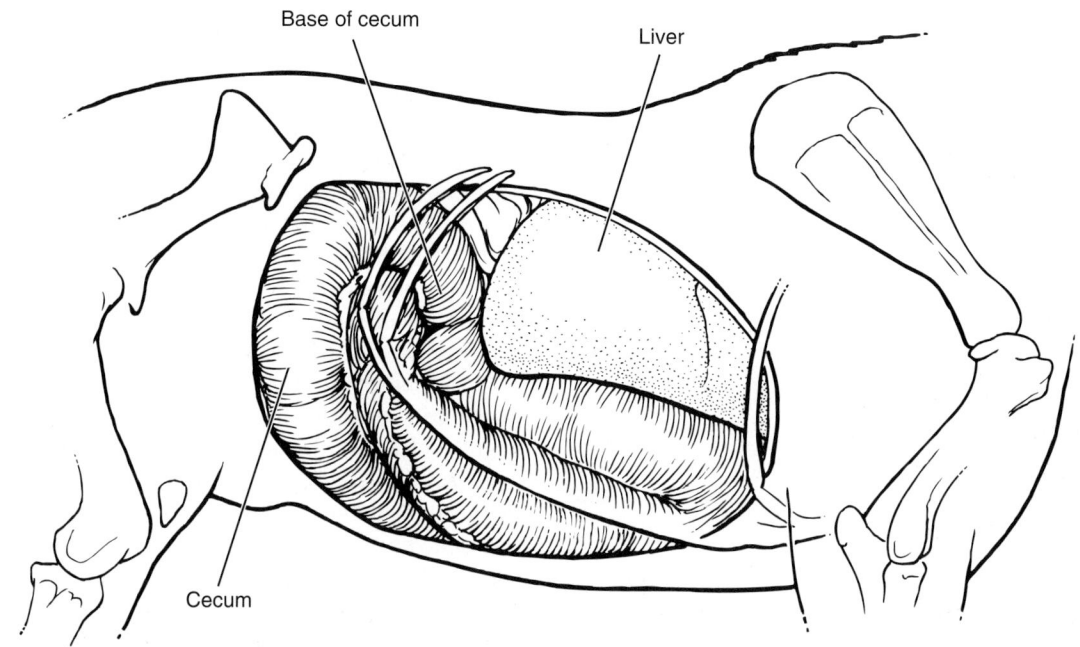

Base of cecum

Liver

Cecum

A

Stomach

Spleen

Jejunum

Descending
colon

Liver

Pelvic
flexure

Left
dorsal
colon

Left
ventral
colon

B

▶ **FIGURE 11-8**

Location of intestinal structures. **A.** Right side. **B.** Left side.

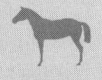

Materials for Passing a Nasogastric Tube

▶ Nose twitch

▶ Nasogastric tube (rubber or plastic, 8 to 10 feet)

    Small foals: ⅜-inch outside diameter (O.D.)

    Older foals and routine use in adults: ⁹⁄₁₆-inch O.D.

    Very large horses: ¾-inch O.D.

▶ Lubricant (obstetrical gel or water if tube is very smooth)

PROCEDURE. A ⁹⁄₁₆-inch tube is suitable for older foals and routine use in most adults. A length of 8 to 10 feet is adequate. When the tube needs to be passed a number of times, a smaller tube can be used to minimize trauma to the tissues of the nasal passage. When the tube is being used to decompress the stomach, it is advisable to use a larger tube to reduce the chance of ingesta blocking the opening at the end. For the beginner, it is useful to place two marks on the tube, one that will be level with the external nares when the end of the tube is about to enter the esophagus, and the other for when the tube is about to enter the stomach. The end of the tube should be beveled and smooth, and there should be a distal and a side opening. Old and rough tubes should not be used. The tube should be coiled up between use so that it will retain a curve during use, thus facilitating insertion through the ventral meatus.

There are many different ways to pass a nasogastric tube, but the important thing is to avoid injury by using a procedure that is safe in all situations. The procedure described here fulfills these requirements. The horse should be adequately restrained, the extent of which depends on the horse's temperament and the skill and experience of the clinician and holder. The usual restraint consists of a nasal twitch, although this is not always necessary. If the horse is dangerous and has a tendency to strike with the forelegs, it can be placed in stocks and perhaps sedated. Other ways of handling the difficult horse include placing it behind a low door or gate, or on the other side of a dividing partition. When stocks are

not used, the horse can be backed into a corner to prevent it from backing away during the procedure. The clinician and holder should stand on the same side of the horse, usually the left, with the holder standing beside the horse's shoulder. The twitch is applied as described (see Aids to Restraint in Chapter 1). The twitch should be positioned toward the right side of the muzzle and rotated in an anticlockwise direction, so as to open the external nare and allow the tube to be passed directly into the nasal passage. Failure to do this means that the tube must be forced obliquely into the nasal passage, which is traumatic and resented by the horse. The clinician stands in front of the holder with the tube draped over the shoulder, to prevent it from dragging on the ground and collecting dirt, which can damage the delicate nasal mucosae (Fig. 11-9A). Tubes should always be lubricated on all surfaces entering the nasal passage, although excessive lubrication makes the tube unmanageable. Very smooth tubes can be lubricated by being dipped in water, but commercial lubricant is required for all other surfaces, especially when the procedure is to be carried out frequently during a short time or when the horse is dehydrated. When a commercial lubricant is used, a suitable volume should be placed on the distal end of the tube so that it will be transferred to the nasal mucosa and so help lubricate the remainder of the tube as it passes.

The palm and fingers of the right hand are placed over the bridge of the nose, and the thumb is inserted into the nasal passage (Fig. 11-9B). The hand over the bridge of the nose prevents the horse from throwing its head into the air. The tube, held in the left hand about 12 inches from the end, is passed through the external nare and *directed along the floor of the nasal passage beneath the thumb.*

The tube must traverse the nasal passage in the ventral meatus. Failure to do this will result in injury to the nasal turbinates, causing profuse bleeding. It is important that this first part of the insertion be carried out smoothly and quickly, as it is the part of the procedure most likely to be resented. After the first part of the insertion is completed, the tube is stabilized by holding it against the floor of the nasal passage with downward pressure from the right thumb (Fig. 11-9C). The left hand is then transferred about 18 inches along the tube, which is then grasped and, after releasing the thumb pressure, pushed further into the nasal passage.

The objective is to stimulate the horse to swallow and take the tube into the esophagus. The stimulus to swallow is the presence of the tube in the dorsal part of the nasopharynx. To ensure that the tube reaches and stimulates the correct region, the horse's head must be held in a neutral to flexed position. The tendency that most horses have of extending the head during insertion must be countered, as it results in passing the tube directly into the larynx. When the tube reaches and contacts the caudal part of the pharynx, the clinician can detect a characteristic resilient sensation. If the tube has passed into the middle or dorsal meatus, it meets firm resistance and

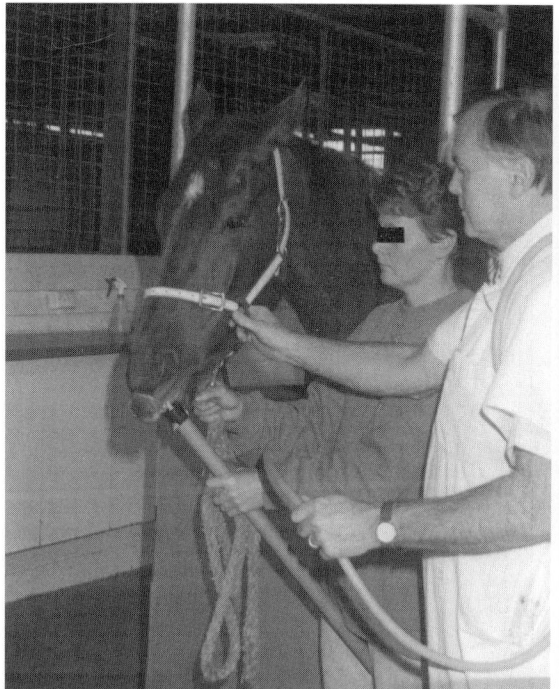

A

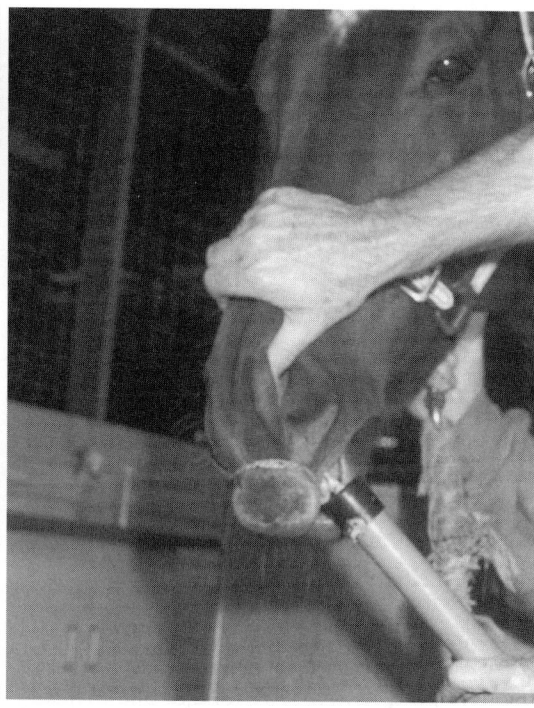

B

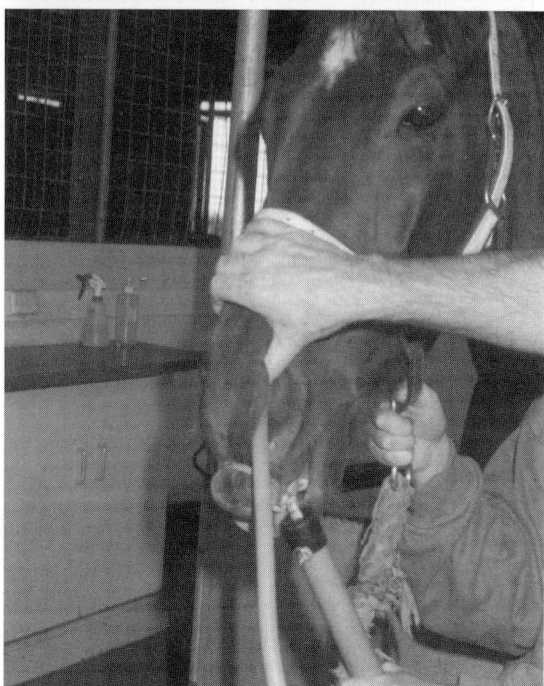

C

▶ **FIGURE 11–9**

Passage of a nasogastric tube. **A.** Preparation. Nose twitch in place with clinician and assistant standing on the same side of the horse. **B.** Right hand positioned over the nose with thumb inserted into the left nasal passage to ensure the nostril is open to receive the tube. **C.** Stabilization, with the thumb, of the partially inserted tube, enabling the left hand to release the tube and grasp it further distally before continuing with insertion.

its onward passage will be prevented by the ethmoidal turbinates. If the tube is forced onto the turbinates, crackling sounds will be heard as the turbinates are deformed or injured. The tube should be withdrawn immediately and redirected into the ventral meatus, if there is any suspicion that it has passed dorsally. After the tube contacts the dorsal pharynx, the clinician should be ready to push the tube onward as swallowing occurs. With experience this is all done in a coordinated series of movements. If swallowing does occur, the tube should be withdrawn a few inches and then advanced to stimulate the wall of the pharynx and esophageal opening again. Other methods are to maintain contact with the pharynx while awaiting swallowing and also to blow into the tube. If all fails, success is often met by passing the tube through the opposite nasal passage.

The presence of the tube in the esophagus is usually apparent to the experienced clinician. However, until experience is gained and occasionally for even experienced clinicians, its exact position is difficult to ascertain. There are a number of ways to check whether the tube is in the esophagus or the trachea. Although only one of these may be routinely used, it is advisable to be familiar with them all because there will be occasions when one's preferred indicator is not effective or cannot be utilized. Such situations can arise when the horse is anesthetized and cannot swallow, when it is recumbent, especially in left lateral recumbency, and when it is resisting intubation. Some guidelines are listed in the box.

After the tube is safely in the esophagus, it is advanced until it passes through the cardia and enters the stomach.

COMPLICATIONS. Complications include epistaxis, administration of fluids into the respiratory tract, rupture of the esophagus, and miscellaneous trauma. The most frequent complication is epistaxis resulting from injury to the ethmoidal turbinates. Fortunately it is self-limiting, but in compromised patients it can be fatal. The potentially serious sequelae of accidental administration of fluids into the respiratory tract dictate that all clinicians be meticulous in ensuring that the tube is in the esophagus before proceeding. Esophageal rupture is likely to occur only if the tube is advanced when an obstruction is present. Despite complications, the technique is safe provided that the clinician is careful and ensures that the tube

---

METHODS OF LOCATING THE SITE OF NASOGASTRIC TUBE

- In the esophagus
  The tube is usually visible on the left side of the neck (except when the esophagus passes dorsal to or to the right of the trachea).
  There is normally a slight resistance to passage of the tube.
  Blowing into the tube is met with slight resistance, distends the esophagus, and often results in reflux of stomach gases.
  Tube can be palpated within the esophagus on the left side of the neck.
  Characteristic gurgling noises are heard when the tube is in the stomach.
- In the trachea
  Horses will sometimes cough (do not rely on this!).
  There is no resistance to passage of the tube.
  The tube can be heard to rattle against the walls of the trachea if it is shaken from side to side.
  There is no resistance to blowing into the tube, and passage of air coordinated with breathing can be detected.

---

traverses the ventral meatus and enters the esophagus.

Abdominocentesis

Abdominocentesis is the collection of a sample of intraabdominal fluid. It is a very valuable and frequently performed procedure. It is especially useful in the routine examination of horses with colic, weight loss, or peritonitis.

PROCEDURE. The preferred site for abdominocentesis is the ventral midline about 6 inches caudal to the xiphoid process. This site corresponds with the lowest part of the abdomen when viewed from the side. In pregnant mares or when there is an accumulation of ingesta or fluid in the intestinal tract, particularly in the cecum and colons, this site often results in inadvertent penetration of the organ. In these cases, judgment is required to select an appropriate alternate site.

To avoid penetrating the spleen, the left paramedian site should be avoided. In adults the puncture can be made with a needle or with a teat cannula after a stab incision has been made. In foals the needle method is recommended because they have very little subperitoneal fat, which makes accidental injury of intestine with the scalpel blade more likely. The principles are shown in Figure 11–10A.

Most horses do not object to the procedure, although care must be taken to prevent the clinician from being kicked in the head. The horse is best restrained in a crush with a side opening, and the clinician should stand beside the horse's thorax, and facing toward the rear.

Use of a Teat Cannula. After preparing the skin, 5 mL of local anesthetic is infiltrated into the subcutaneous tissue overlying the linea alba. The linea alba can be palpated as a firm ridge lying

---

Materials for Abdominocentesis

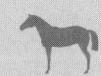

▸ Instrument for abdominal penetration (4″ teat cannula or 18-gauge, 1.5-inch needle)

▸ Sterile surgical gloves

▸ Hair clippers (#40 blade)

▸ Local anesthetic (2% lidocaine hydrochloride, 2% mepivacaine hydrochloride)

▸ Syringe (5 mL, 25-gauge, ⅝-inch needle)

▸ Scalpel blade (#15)

▸ Materials for skin preparation (such as detergent antiseptic [Betadine, Hibiclens], 70% alcohol, iodine tincture)

▸ Sample containers (varies with required tests)

    EDTA tube (purple-top Vacutainer) for cytology, total protein determination

    Plain tube (red-top Vacutainer) for biochemistry and electrolyte measurement

    Sodium fluoride tube (gray top Vacutainer) for lactate measurement

    Bacterial culture media for aerobic and anaerobic culture

---

directly in the midline. Use enough solution to produce a visible skin bleb so that the site of anesthesia can be identified for the centesis. The scalpel blade is held in the gloved hand between the thumb and first finger, with about 1.5 cm exposed. After ensuring that the blade is aligned accurately, using the linea alba, palpated with the second finger as a reference, the exposed length of the blade is then inserted through the skin and partway into the linea alba. Full penetration of the linea alba is not necessary. The teat cannula, with some gauze swabs wrapped around its base to prevent blood from running down its shaft and contaminating the sample, is then inserted into the stab wound, pushed completely through the linea alba, and then advanced slowly until fluid is obtained. It is tempting to carry out the insertion procedures under direct vision, but, as the horse is most likely to kick at this time, the writer recommends retracting one's head during the insertion of the blade and the cannula. There is often resistance as the peritoneum is penetrated. If fluid does not flow immediately, the cannula can be rotated or gently redirected, although it is advisable to be patient, as fluid often takes a few moments to appear. If firm resistance is met, the cannula should not be pushed any further. If fluid cannot be obtained, success is often had if the horse walks a few steps, or an alternate, more caudal site(s), is used. Accidental penetration of an internal organ will stabilize the tip of the cannula and provide resistance to any manipulation. Therefore, if resistance is detected, manipulation should be done very carefully to avoid iatrogenic injury.

Use of a Needle. Abdominocentesis with a needle is easier than with a cannula and is preferred in foals. Otherwise, method selection is largely a matter of personal preference, although using a needle, because of the sharp point, carries an increased chance of laceration or puncture of internal viscera. The length of the needle usually used, 1.5 inch, is often too short for large horses with ample subperitoneal fat. The simplicity of needle puncture makes it easier and faster to carry out a number of punctures when obtaining fluid is difficult. No anesthesia is required, and there is no need for a preliminary scalpel stab incision. Otherwise, the method is similar to that described when using the cannula, although, because the needle can easily penetrate an organ, insertion should be done a little slower and more carefully. Walking a horse to encourage fluid flow is not

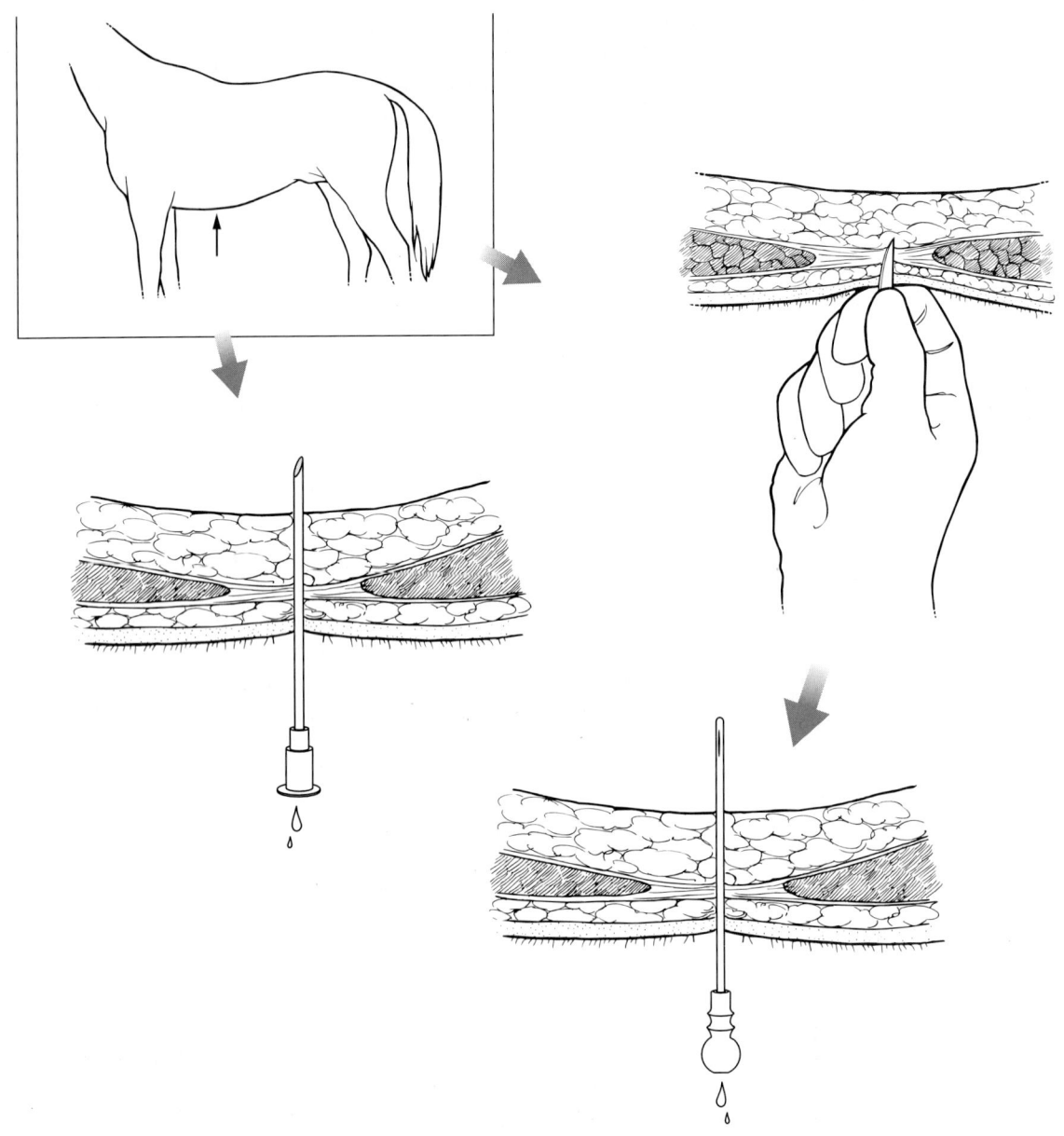

A

▶ **FIGURE 11–10**

Abdominocentesis. **A.** Use of a needle or a teat cannula.

recommended when using a needle because of the increased possibility of iatrogenic injury.

Processing of Samples. The minimum protocol is to collect a sample of fluid into EDTA for gross and cytological examination. Depending on the case, additional samples may be required to allow measurement of electrolytes and biochemical parameters as well as microbiological evaluation. As bacteria are often difficult to isolate, it is useful to add some of the fluid to a bacterial enrichment media, for later plating and more successful identification. The appropriate procedures are described in Appendices C and D.

RESULTS. Peritoneal fluid reflects the status of the peritoneal surfaces of the abdomen and is useful in identifying conditions such as infection, neoplasia, compromisation of intestinal vasculature, rupture or perforation of intestine, hemorrhage, and rupture of bladder. Grossly, normal peritoneal fluid is clear, straw-colored, serous, and does not clot. The characteristics of normal peritoneal fluid for adults and foals are shown in Table 11–1. There is a considerable range in normal values as well as overlap between different pathological conditions. Therefore, evaluation must always be made after considering the

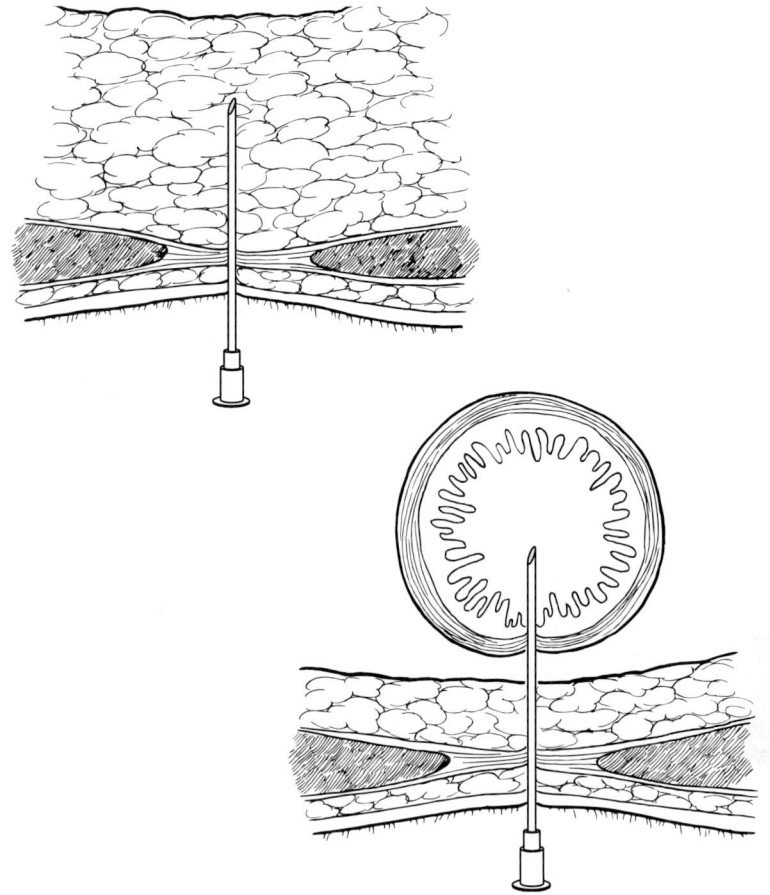

B

▶ **FIGURE 11–10** *Continued*
B. Complications. Accidental puncture of the intestine and failure to penetrate the abdominal cavity because of excessive subperitoneal fat or using a needle or cannula of insufficient length (above).

clinical situation. Although interpretation is not always easy, some basic principles greatly assist evaluation:

- *Inflammation.* Acute inflammation results in elevation of nondegenerate neutrophils and the content of fibrinogen. In chronic inflammation the increase in neutrophils is not usually so marked, and there is also an increase in mononuclear cells and macrophages.
- *Sepsis.* In addition to signs of inflammation, sepsis is characterized by degenerate neutrophils or neutrophils with toxic changes and, often, free or intracellular bacteria.
- *Bowel rupture or perforation.* Although signs of inflammation may not be well developed, the fluid has the odor of intestinal content, and plant material is usually present. There is a mixed population of bacteria, most of which are extracellular.

- *Neoplasia.* Signs of neoplasia are similar to those of chronic inflammation, with the possible addition of exfoliated tumor cells and degenerate neutrophils if tumor necrosis factor is present.
- *Intraabdominal hemorrhage.* With acute bleeding the cell types are similar to peripheral blood, although fewer in number. As the process becomes chronic, there is an increase in macrophages, presence of hypersegmented and pycnotic neutrophils, erythrocytophagia, and very few platelets.
- *Inadvertent splenic puncture.* Presence of blood with a packed cell volume higher than peripheral blood, increased numbers of lymphocytes, and no erythrocytophagia.

Luckily, much information can be obtained by careful visual examination of the sample before any laboratory procedures are conducted. This is useful because samples are often collected

▶ TABLE 11–1

REFERENCE VALUES FOR PERITONEAL FLUID IN ADULTS (MEAN ± 2 SD OR RANGE) AND FOALS (MEAN ± 1 SD)

White Blood Cells (×10⁹/L)	Neutrophils (%)	Mononuclear Cells (%)	Lymphocytes (%)	Eosinophils (%)	Protein (g/L)	Specific Gravity	Reference
Adults							
4.33 (1.50–10.10)	45.2	47	7.8 (1.0–19.0)	0 (0–5)	8* / 14†	1.010 (1.008–1.012)	45
3.25 (1.89–4.61)	43.1 (24.4–61.8)	33.8 (17.3–50.2)	20.4 (4.5–36.3)	2.5 (0.8–5.8)	9 (7–11)‡ / 16.9 (10.2–23.6)‡	1.005 (1.000–1.015)	46
3.31 (±0.7)	63.8 (±8.1)	1.4 (±1.3)	21.3 (±6.2)	0	12.9‡ (±4)	—	47
2.10 (0.5–4.6)	90 (80–98)	7.4 (1–17)	4.4 (1–11)	2.1 (0–7)	10.5* (1–25)	1.013 (1.006–1.030)	48
3.24 (0.20–9.0)	59.5 (36–78)	30.4 (3–50)	10.0 (0–29)	0.1 (0–3)	11‡ (1–34)	1.001 (1.000–1.093)	49
Foals (age 68.2 ± 36.7 days) all values ×10⁹/L							
0.451 (±0.322)	0.230 (±0.318)	0.211 (±0.152)	0.003 (±0.005)	0	12⁺ (±3) / 16* (±2.5)	1.013 (±0.0015)	50

*Refractive index.
†Biuret method.
‡Technique not quoted.

from emergency cases, such as colic, when immediate laboratory evaluation may not be available. Some common findings and diagnoses are as follows:

- *Frank blood.* Acute hemorrhage or accidental splenic puncture.
- *Serosanguinous fluid.* Compromisation of intestinal vasculature, neoplasia.
- *Increased turbidity.* Sepsis.
- *Plant material and an odor of ingesta.* Intestinal perforation, accidental intestinal puncture.
- *Clotting.* Increased fibrinogen associated with inflammation

Interpretation can be complicated further by contamination with blood during collection, as well as by collection after abdominal surgery. As little as one drop of blood in 1 mL of fluid produces significant discoloration, although this is counterbalanced by the fact that the number of white cells, protein values, and the packed cell volume are little altered.[6] Therefore, a reddish color should not be taken as pathognomonic of vascular compromise. After celiotomy, evaluation is compromised by the fact that celiotomy, especially after manipulation of viscera, is associated with an inflammatory response.[7,8] At least for the small colon, the response is not greater when there has also been resection and anastomosis.[9] These changes can persist for at least a week. Therefore, postoperative evaluation of peritoneal fluid depends heavily on the clinical condition of the patient and the presence of bacteria and toxic and degenerate neutrophils.

COMPLICATIONS. The complication rate is very low.[10] Complications include penetration (enterocentsis) or laceration of intestine, penetration or laceration of the spleen, failure to obtain a sample, and subcutaneous abscessation (Fig. 11–10B). Although the potential significance of the complications should not be understated, the main problem is that sample contamination makes diagnosis more difficult. Complications can be almost eliminated by careful attention to technique.

Palpation of the Abdomen per Rectum

Per rectum palpation of the abdomen and its contents is a most important part of the clinical examination of a number of different body systems. Although this section is directed primarily

Materials for Examining the Abdomen and Its Contents per Rectum

- Shoulder-length rectal sleeve
- Obstetrical lubricant
- Stocks or other form of protection for clinician
- Rectal relaxant (Propantheline bromide, 0.014 mg/kg IV)

toward examining the alimentary tract, the principles of the rectal examination of all systems are similar. Regardless of which system is to be examined, the procedure must be carried out competently and with the utmost safety for both horse and clinician.

PROCEDURE. The method of restraint to be used is the first consideration both to protect the clinician and to restrict the horse's movement. There are many ways of doing this, largely related to the temperament of the horse and the available facilities:

- *Stocks.* A set of stocks is the most common means of restraint, although some horses will not tolerate them, and an alternative method must be found. Most stocks have a rear door that can be closed or some form of railing(s) that can be positioned in slots or rings (Fig. 11–11). These do not prevent a horse from

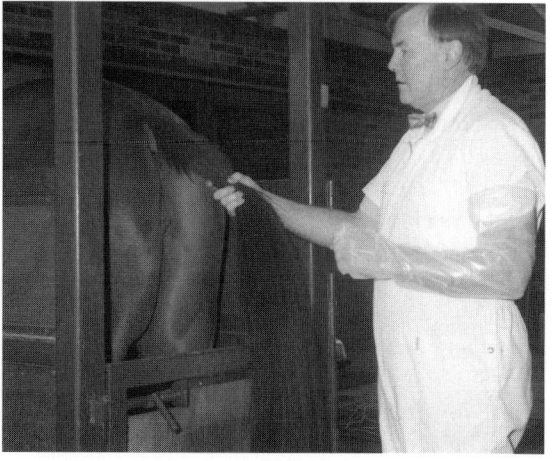

▶ FIGURE 11–11
Rectal examination. Use of stocks.

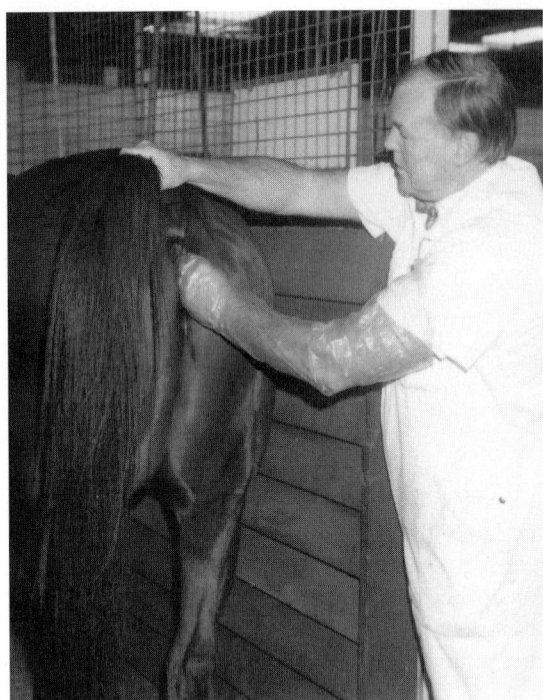

A

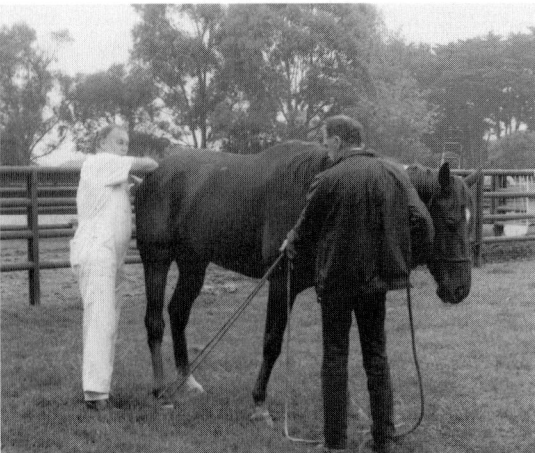

B

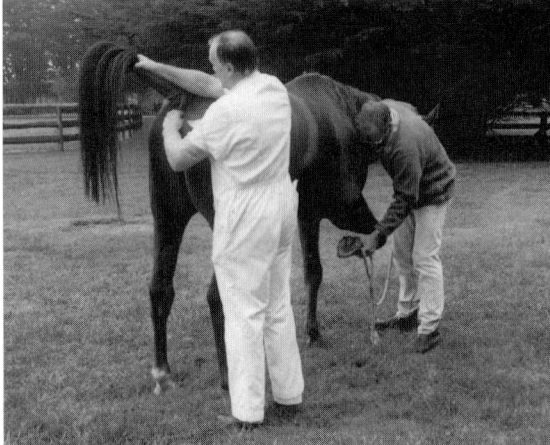

C

▶ **FIGURE 11–12**

Rectal examination. Alternative methods of protecting the clinician. **A.** Standing beside a doorway. **B.** Use of sidelines. **C.** Picking up the ipsilateral forelimb.

kicking, but will protect the clinician. Because horses can still kick, the apparatus should be constructed in a way that minimizes the chances of a horse injuring itself while kicking. In addition to this, some stocks are padded. To place a horse in a set of stocks the front and rear doors are opened and the horse is led in through the rear door. For some horses it is also necessary to open a side door. Once inside, the doors are closed and the horse is held by the headstall or tied up. Many horses will reverse out through the back door if the front door is closed before they have entered the stocks fully. The rear protection, door, or railing must be high enough to prevent the horse from kicking over it and low enough to prevent the clinician from receiving an arm injury if the horse lowers its rear quarters.

- *Standing beside a door.* When stocks are not available or if a horse will not accept the stocks, useful protection is obtained by positioning the horse in a doorway or beside a sturdy partition (Fig. 11–12A). The clinician can then proceed with the examination by standing to one side of the horse and behind the protective barriers.

- *Hobbles and sideline.* When none of the preceding restraints are available, kicking can be controlled to a certain extent by using a sideline or a set of breeding hobbles (Fig. 11–12B). A single sideline applied to the left hind leg is used for a right-handed examiner, and vice versa. The examiner stands adjacent to the leg to which the line is attached. Breeding hobbles are applied to both hind limbs.

- *Elevation of a foreleg.* Some protection from kicking can be obtained by having an assistant pick up and hold one foreleg (the left foreleg for a right-handed examiner and vice versa (Fig. 11–12C).

- *Twitch.* Using a twitch is sometimes necessary, regardless of other restraint.

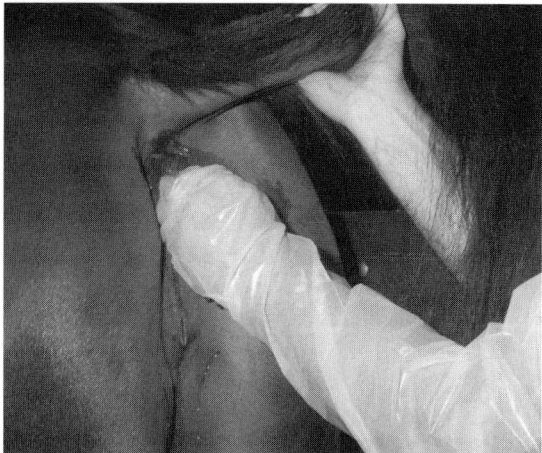

▶ **FIGURE 11-13**

Rectal examination. Insertion of gloved and lubricated hand into the rectum.

With the horse in position and restrained, the examiner dons a rectal sleeve and applies a liberal amount of lubricant to the glove and the arm. The horse's tail can be bandaged or, more commonly, is held to one side by an assistant or the examiner. This is done to allow free access to the anus, important in those horses that hold their tail firmly over the perineal region and also to avoid carrying tail hairs into the rectum, which can produce significant laceration of the mucosae. Some of the lubricant is transferred from the glove to the horse's anus and the fingers of the coned hand are then gently inserted through the anus and into the rectum (Fig. 11-13). As the anus is dilated, the mucosa should be examined for evidence of inflammation, presence of mucus, and evidence of trauma.

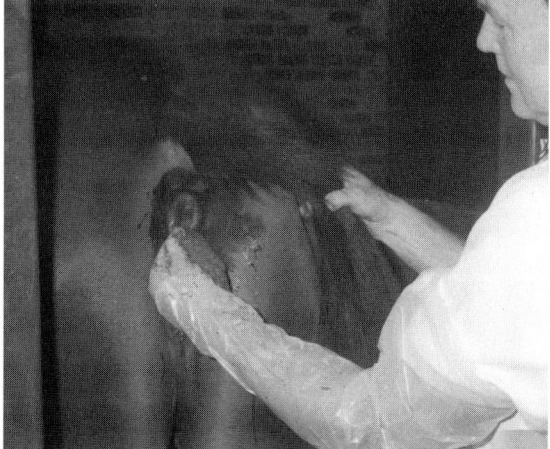

▶ **FIGURE 11-14**

Rectal examination. Evacuating feces from rectum.

Feces, either unformed or in ball form, are usually encountered in the rectum. These are removed by passing the hand cranial to all or some of the fecal mass and then, "scooping" them caudally with the palm of the hand (Fig. 11-14). This can be completed in one procedure, but, more often, a number of efforts are necessary. Even when no feces are present, and the procedure is theoretically unnecessary, it is advisable, before full insertion is made, to withdraw the hand to inspect for the presence of blood because rectal perforation, as a result of manual rectal examination, is relatively common and a careful preliminary search for blood can be proof that a perforation existed prior to the current exam. *Be aware that a lay person, and not only a veterinarian, may have carried out an earlier rectal examination!*

The arm is then inserted as deeply as possible into the flaccid rectum. As a rule, it is advisable to insert the arm beyond the depth of the structures to be examined because examination of organs close to the anus after just partial insertion will usually make the horse strain (tenesmus). After full insertion, the hand can then be brought back toward the organ(s) of interest, which can then be examined through a flaccid (relaxed) rectal wall. However caution should be observed (see box).

If a contraction is detected, the clinician has the options of allowing the arm to be expelled or leaving it in place and allowing the contraction to pass over it. The strength of the contraction and the experience of the clinician determine which of these options is taken, although, as a general rule, strong contractions should never be resisted. In most circumstances when a horse is straining against the arm and resents the examination, gentleness and use of copious amounts of lubricant will allow the examination to be completed, albeit this will take longer. When tenesmus cannot be controlled as described, rectal

> ### WARNING
> ....
> *Attempts to insert an arm or to proceed with the rectal palpation when the horse is actively straining or when the rectal wall is undergoing contraction carries a high risk of producing a perforation and should be avoided at all costs.*

METHODS OF CONTROLLING TENESMUS DURING A RECTAL EXAMINATION

- Propantheline bromide (0.014 mg/kg IV) to abolish rectal motor innervation
- Epidural anesthesia to abolish rectal sensory and motor innervation
- Intrarectal administration of local anesthetic (50 mL xylocaine) to abolish rectal sensory innervation
- Reduce ability to increase intraabdominal pressure (insertion of a nasogastric tube into trachea or of a needle percutaneously into trachea)

relaxation can usually be achieved with one of the methods listed in the box.

When the arm is extracted after the procedure, it should be inspected for the presence of blood. Blood always indicates that trauma has occurred but does not necessarily denote a significant injury.

RESULTS. The successful performance and interpretation of per rectal palpation requires considerable experience. It should be remembered that only a small portion of the abdomen is within reach of a clinician's arm (Fig. 11–15). The following guidelines can be used to assist evaluation (Fig. 11–16):[11]

Normal Findings

- Soft fecal balls are present in the rectum. Feces may be unformed when horses are grazing lush pasture.
- Rectal mucosa is folded and thin.
- The abdomen gives a general impression of "emptiness." Organs are more easily palpated if they are enlarged and made firmer by disease or obstruction.
- Fecal balls are palpable in the caudal abdomen. They lie within the small colon and can be moved freely in all directions.
- The caudal border of the spleen lies against the left abdominal wall.
- The caudal pole of the left kidney is palpable dorsally, lying to left of the midline.
- The nephrosplenic ligament can be palpated as it runs between the spleen and the left kidney.
- The nephrosplenic space can be palpated lying dorsal to the nephrosplenic ligament and between the dorsal part of the spleen and the caudal pole of the left kidney. A few fingers can be inserted into this space.

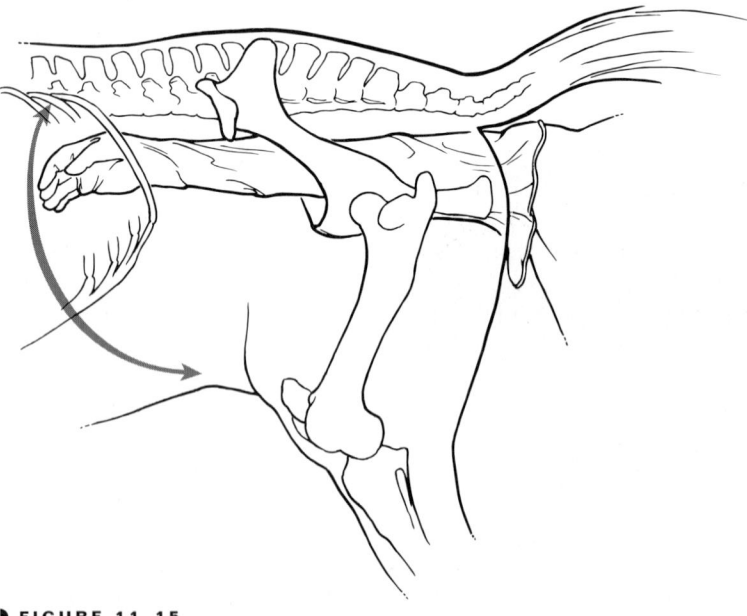

▶ **FIGURE 11–15**

Rectal examination. Approximate extent of abdomen within range of per rectum examination.

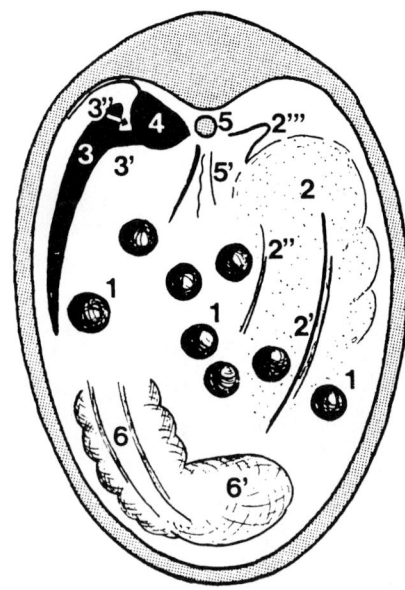

▶ **FIGURE 11–16**

Rectal examination, normal findings. Structures usually palpable include fecal balls within the small colon (1), cecal base (2), ventral (2') and medial (2'') cecal tenia, mesenteric attachment of cecum to roof of the abdomen (2'''), spleen (3), mesenteric attachment between spleen and left kidney (3'), nephrosplenic space (3''), left kidney (4), aorta (5), root of cranial mesenteric artery (5'), left colons with ventral tenia (6), and pelvic flexure (6'). (From Kopf N: Rectal examination of the colic patient. *In* Robinson NE (ed), Current Therapy in Equine Medicine, ed 3. Philadelphia, Saunders, 1992, p 197. (Reprinted with permission.)

- The cecum lies in the right section of the abdomen. Although the cecum itself is sometimes palpable as a soft viscus with a doughlike content and a dorsal gas cap, the ventral taenia is the only part that is always palpable. The taenia is palpated as a band running diagonally from the upper right side of the abdomen toward the ventral midline. Occasionally the medial taenia, as well as the dorsal cecal attachment to the right of the aorta, can be identified.
- The aorta is located in the dorsal midline.
- The root of the cranial mesenteric artery can be palpated in the dorsal midline, running ventrally.
- Palpation in the left part of the caudoventral abdomen will often identify the pelvic flexure as a soft viscus of doughlike consistency and possibly some of the associated colonic taenia.

Abnormal Findings

Principles Involved in the Interpretation of Rectal Findings Associated with Intestinal Obstruction. Although there are findings that regularly accompany a particular type of obstruction, the variation between cases makes it impossible to provide a set of characteristic findings for each condition that will allow a precise diagnosis to be made. In many cases it is impossible to specify the lesion any more accurately than to localize it to the small or large intestine. Knowledge of the sequence of events that occurs with gastrointestinal obstruction makes it easier to interpret the findings, some of which are listed:

- Mechanical (foreign body, twist) or functional (ileus) obstruction of any section of the gut causes an accumulation of gas, ingesta, and fluid proximal to the site of obstruction.
- Incomplete obstruction, by reducing rather than eliminating onward passage of ingesta, tends at first to cause pain without the dramatic signs of fluid and gas accumulation.
- Loops of small intestine become palpable, as ingesta and intestinal secretions accumulate in the small intestine (Fig. 11–17A).
- The cause of a small intestinal obstruction, such as an intussusception, foreign body, ileal hypertrophy, ileal impaction, are sometimes identifiable before becoming obscured by the distended intestine.
- When the obstruction is mechanical, the loops of small intestine are likely to be tightly distended eventually, but when the obstruction is functional, the distension is not so marked.
- Edema of the intestinal wall occurs with inflammation and venous obstruction. The thickness of the intestinal wall can be gauged by pressing a section between the fingers and the abdominal wall or pelvis.
- When the obstruction is high in the tract, or when it has been present for sufficient time to allow the retrograde accumulation of fluid, the distended duodenum can be palpated as a transverse loop in the dorsal abdomen caudal to the base of the cecum (Fig. 11–17A).
- Obstruction of the small intestine leads eventually to dilation of the stomach, which is detected rectally by caudal displacement of the spleen.

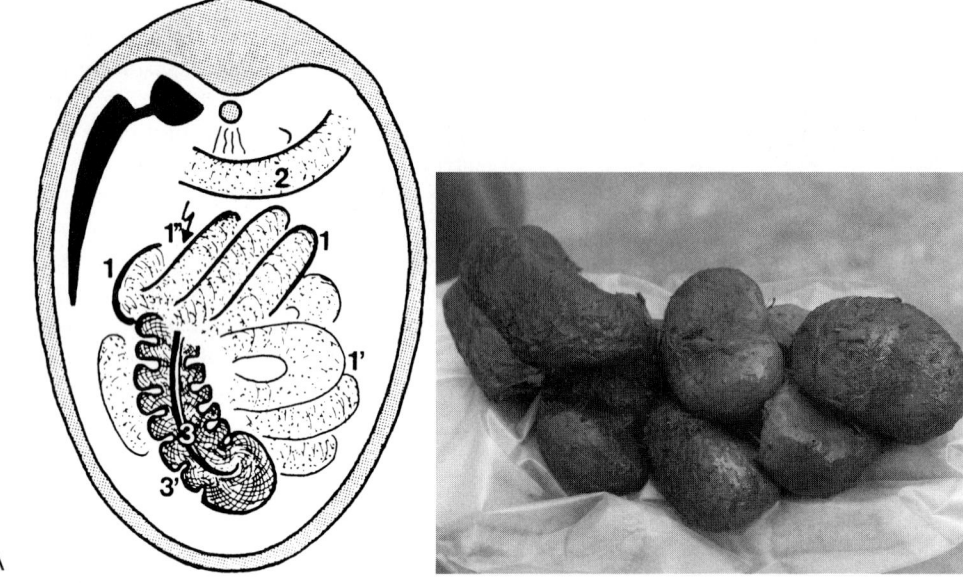

A   B

▶ **FIGURE 11-17**

Rectal examination, abnormal findings. **A.** Rectal findings in small intestinal obstruction. Strangulated portion of small intestine with thickened wall (1). Distended small intestine proximal to the site of strangulation without thickening of the wall (1'), painful region (1''), flexure of distended duodenum (2), large colon containing inspissated content (3), palpable sacculations (haustrae) of the large colon (3'). (From Kopf N: Rectal examination of the colic patient. *In* Robinson NE (ed), Current Therapy in Equine Medicine, ed 3. Philadelphia, Saunders Company, 1992, p 198. Reprinted with permission.) **B.** Inspissated feces covered with shreds of mucus. These are often found in cases of obstruction when the transit time of ingesta is prolonged.

- Obstruction of the large or small colon can place tension on the duodenocolic mesentery and so obstruct gastric outflow and produce gastric dilation.
- Reduction or failure of the onward passage of fluid from the small intestine results in the inspissation of cecal and colonic content (11–17A). Likewise, obstruction in the cecum or colons also results in inspissation of content distal to the obstruction. Inspissation of the content of these organs causes a reduction in their size, and their increasingly firmer content becomes more easily palpated (not to be confused with primary impaction when the content is similar but the organ is enlarged).
- Obstruction causes a reduction or cessation of the transport of ingesta, resulting eventually in an empty or nearly empty rectum. If any feces are present, they are usually inspissated, smaller than normal, and have a covering of shreds and sheets of mucus (Fig. 11–17B).
- Displacement of the large colon occurs in a variety of directions. A common form is its displacement first to between the spleen and left body wall and then to the nephrosplenic space (Fig. 11–17C). The condition is de-

tected by palpating intestine lateral to the spleen or in the normally empty nephrosplenic space. Initially the organ is relatively flaccid, and only a small portion is involved, but, as the duration of displacement increases, gas and ingesta accumulate, especially in the dorsal colon, and a greater length of colon is drawn caudally through the space until almost its full length is involved. The large colon can also be displaced in clockwise or anticlockwise (viewed from above) directions around the cecum. With clockwise displacement the colon is flexed laterally to the right side (dorsal displacement with lateral flexion) and passes caudally between the cecum and the right abdominal wall. When the displacement is anticlockwise, the pelvic flexure passes cranially between the cecum and the right abdominal wall (dorsal displacement with medial flexion). The direction of displacement around the cecum is often impossible to detect with a rectal exam, but the condition can be detected by noting that the large colon extends across the pelvic inlet to obscure the cecum and passes between the cecum and right abdominal wall. These conditions are often complicated by torsion of the colon.

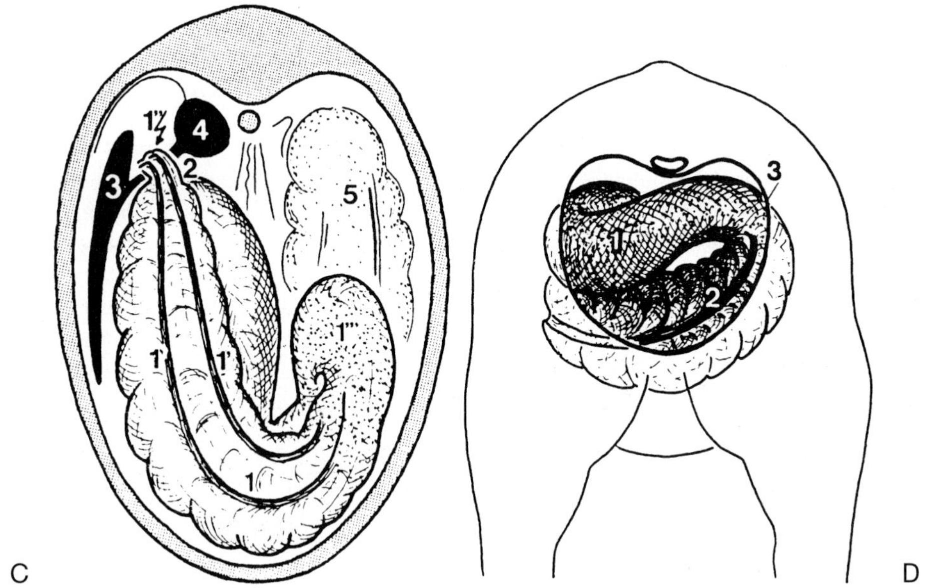

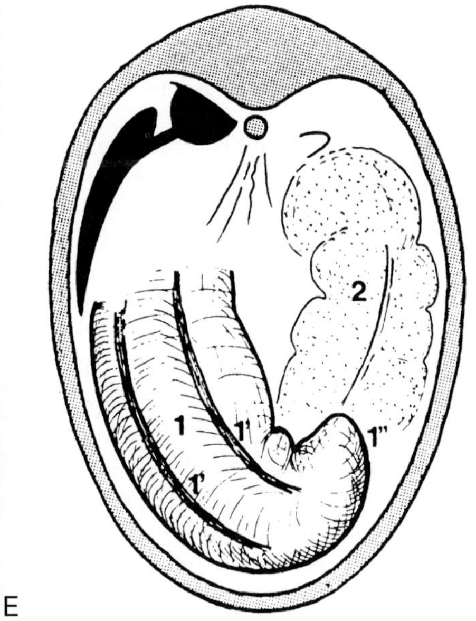

▶ **FIGURE 11–17** *Continued*
C. Rectal findings with left dorsal displacement of the large colon (nephrosplenic entrapment). Enlarged colon containing gas and ingesta (1), tense colonic teniae (1'), site where a pain response can usually be elicited (1''), displaced pelvic flexure (1'''), suspensory ligament of the spleen (2), spleen (3), left kidney (4), tympanitic cecum (5). (From Kopf N: Rectal examination of the colic patient. *In* Robinson NE (ed), Current Therapy in Equine Medicine, ed 3. Philadelphia, Saunders, 1992, p 199. Reprinted with permission.) **D.** Rectal findings with torsion of the large colon. The dorsal colon is enlarged and usually contains gas (1), the ventral colon is identified by its sacculations, and is usually edematous and also gas-filled (2), the mass of viscera obstructs the pelvis and prevents a deep examination of the abdomen (3). (From Kopf N: Rectal examination of the colic patient. *In* Robinson NE (ed), Current Therapy in Equine Medicine, ed 3. Philadelphia, Saunders, 1992, p 199. Reprinted with permission.) **E.** Rectal findings in impaction on the pelvic flexure and left ventral colon. The left ventral colon is enlarged and contains doughy ingesta that indents on digital pressure. (1), Palpable taeniae (1'), the cone-shaped end of the impacted mass in the pelvic flexure (1''), cecum is often distended with gas (2). (From Kopf N: Rectal examination of the colic patient. *In* Robinson NE (ed), Current Therapy in Equine Medicine, ed 3. Philadelphia, Saunders, 1992, p 198. Reprinted with permission.)

• Torsion of the large colon causes the organ to be grossly enlarged with gas and to extend caudally to block the pelvic inlet and prevent deeper rectal exploration of the abdomen (Fig. 11–17D). The pelvic flexure is often displaced across the inlet toward the right side. If the condition persists, it is possible to detect the developing edema of the gut wall, mesentery, vessels, and taenia. The extent of rotation can frequently be ascertained by using the taenia and haustrae, if palpable, to determine whether the dorsal or ventral colon lies dorsally. In the later stages, especially when distension prevents a thorough exam, the condition can be confused with a colonic displacement. As a general rule torsion is more acute and is characterized by dramatic gaseous distension.

• Impaction of the left ventral colon is a common condition and is characterized by an accumulation of doughy ingesta in the left ventral colon. As the condition persists, the organ enlarges and the colon and its pelvic flexure are displaced caudally toward, into, or across the pelvic inlet (Fig. 11–17E). The pelvic flexure with its content of impacted ingesta is typically cone shaped.

The ingesta pits on digital pressure, contrary to gas.

- Impaction of the ampulla of the right dorsal colon is characterized by a firm swelling, approximately 30 cm in diameter lying to the right side of the root of the cranial mesenteric artery. As with the artery, it is palpable only in medium-size horses or by examiners with very long arms. Obstruction by an enterolith can also occur at this site, and, occasionally, the stone can be palpated.
- Impaction and dilation of the cecum. The cecum can be enlarged by gas or by ingesta. Gaseous distension produces an acute condition, whereby impaction is chronic. The enlarged viscus is easily identified as being the cecum by its location to the right of the abdomen and its attachments to the roof of the abdomen. Digital indentation can differentiate between gas and ingesta, with inspissated ingesta remaining indented, as described.
- An obstructing mass in the small colon, such as a fecolith or foreign body, can be located cranial to the pelvic brim and can be moved about. The dilated loops of small colon, proximal to the obstruction, can also be palpated. With volvulus of the small colon the distended loops are located directly in front of the pelvic inlet and can prevent deeper examination.
- After rupture or perforation of a part of the gut, the normally smooth serosal surfaces of the abdomen and its viscera become coated with ingesta that imparts a roughness to the serosal surfaces when palpated. In addition, when the ingesta has a significant fluid content, the viscera tend to float and to be separated by the fluid.
- Confirmation of a rectal tear is best carried out under epidural anesthesia in order to allow a thorough examination while reducing the chances of enlarging the lesion. Rectal perforations vary in severity and are classified in the box.[12]

It is often better to explore rectal injuries without a rectal glove, thus making it easier to detect the fine details of a wound. A fresh rectal perforation is characterized by free blood and blood clots on the glove, with even a small mucosal tear sometimes associated with a surprisingly large volume of blood. Although large

---

CLASSIFICATION OF RECTAL TEARS

- *Grade 1.* Mucosal layer is disrupted.
- *Grade 2.* Muscular layer is disrupted.
- *Grade 3.* All layers (mucosa, submucosa, muscularis) except serosa are disrupted. The serosa prevents contamination of the abdominal cavity. They are subclassified according to location of the perforation:

    Grade 3A. Perforation is located in the ventral or lateral aspects of the rectum.

    Grade 3B. Perforation is located in the dorsal midline and extends between the two serosal layers of the mesocolon.
- *Grade 4.* Penetrates all layers and extends into the abdominal cavity.

---

wounds are easily detected, small lesions often require a thorough search. The wound must be accurately defined because management will vary with the extent of the lesion.

COMPLICATIONS

Blood Found on the Rectal Sleeve. This is a frequent finding and, in most cases, is not related to any detectable lesion. Small smears of blood rarely indicate significant injury. If larger volumes of blood are seen, a reexamination of the rectum should be conducted. Sedation or epidural anesthesia should be carried out if necessary. The indications for reexamination cannot be defined precisely, and, although the examination will vary between clinicians, it is better to explore the rectum and fail to find an injury than to risk leaving an injury undetected. Initial management of rectal injury is described in the following section.

Rectal Tears. Rectal palpation is always associated with the possibility of accidental rectal injury, sometimes related to improper technique. The condition, depending on degree, is potentially fatal. Because successful management depends on prompt and correct treatment, the clinician must always be prepared to institute immediate first aid. After establishing that an injury is present, the objective of the first phase of management is to prevent fecal contamination of the injury and the abdominal cavity. The owner of the horse should be informed immediately that a perforation is suspected or has occurred. Failure to notify constitutes negligence. The immediate management of different grades of perforation is as follows:[13]

- *Grade 1.* Although suturing is not usually necessary, antibiotic prophylaxis against peritonitis and a fecal softener are indicated.
- *Grade 2.* These are rare and do not require suture.
- *Grade 3 (A & B).* Under epidural anesthesia, all feces within reach should be removed carefully. To keep feces away from the injury, a rectal pack can be inserted to fill the rectum from the anus to cranial to the lesion. The pack is constructed from dampened cotton wool and stockinette, which is soaked in an antiseptic (Betadine or Hibiclens) and coated with a lubricant jelly (obstetrical lubricant, lubricating jelly) (Fig. 11–18). Additional cotton can be added to fill the pack until it is level with the anus. To retain the pack, epidural anesthesia must be maintained and a purse-string suture or towel clamps should be placed in the anus. The anesthesia should be repeated as necessary. Optimum supportive treatment consists of a broad-spectrum antibiotic (e.g., penicillin and gentamicin), tetanus prophylaxis (antitoxin, toxoid booster, or antitoxin and toxoid), and a fecal softener (mineral oil, or dioctyl sodium sulfosuccinate, 10–20 mg/kg of 5% solution) given per os via nasogastric tube.

- *Grade 4.* A grade 4 injury is catastrophic. The management is identical with that described for Grade 3 tears. Even though the abdomen is invariably contaminated, prevention of further contamination can be the difference between the horse having no chance of survival and having some chance.

Feces

Feces are examined in a number of different ways. Most examinations will be carried out in a laboratory, but the clinician will often perform some of the tests in the field.

Gross Examination

Gross examination involves checking for consistency, color, mucus shreds, blood, foreign bodies, and parasites. This can be done on feces already excreted or on fresh feces obtained from the rectum. Fresh feces are likely to provide more information because they have not had time for drying, being disturbed, or discolored. A sample of fresh feces is easily collected from the rectum with a rectal sleeve. After the sample is retrieved in the palm of the gloved hand, it should be examined and, if required, placed in a container for transport to the laboratory. The simplest form of container is obtained by turning the glove inside out, the feces remaining on the inside at the hand end of the glove. The glove is not always secure and, therefore, to prevent spillage during transport it is necessary to place the glove and feces, or feces alone, in a plastic beaker. Sand is a special form of foreign material, present in the

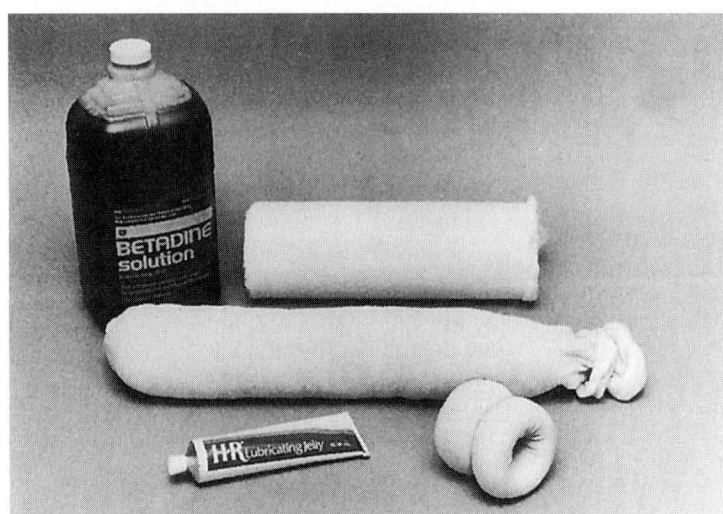

▶ **FIGURE 11–18**

Rectal pack. Materials used for packing the rectum after a rectal tear has been diagnosed. (From Baird AN: Rectal tears. *In* Robinson NE (ed), Current Therapy in Equine Medicine, ed 3. Philadelphia, Saunders, 1992, p 234. Reprinted with permission.)

feces of many horses living in a sandy environment, and is occasionally responsible for colic. Although sand imparts a gritty feel to feces, if it is rubbed between the fingers, it is distributed uniformly and is often not easily seen. A reliable way to see exactly how much sand is present is to take a quantity of feces, place it in a container of water, mix it well with the water, and then allow the sand to settle to the bottom of the container. This can be done quickly, and it often shows that a surprisingly large proportion of sand is present.

Diagnosis of Internal Parasites

DIRECT FECAL SMEAR. A sample of feces is placed on a glass slide, mixed with a drop of water, and covered with a cover slip.[14] It is important to use only a very small volume of feces. The extremely small sample renders the simple smear a relatively inaccurate method.

CONCENTRATION OF EGGS AND OOCYSTS BY FLOTATION. A greater number of eggs and oocysts, in a clear fluid medium, can be obtained by a flotation technique. Flotation is based on the fact that eggs and oocysts will float in a solution that has a specific gravity greater than their own. Examples of hypertonic solutions include saturated salt, saturated sodium nitrate, and Sheather's solution. Zinc sulphate solution has been used to isolate *Giardia* cysts and Sheather's solution for *Cryptosporidium* oocysts.

Measurement is made using a McMaster slide, or some variation of it. To prepare the sample a specified amount of feces is weighed and mixed with a known volume of the flotation solution. A sample of the mixture is transferred by pipette and placed under the counting grid of the slide. The eggs and oocysts will rise to the surface of the medium where they will be found in the same focal plane as the air bubbles, which also rise to the surface. They are counted under a magnification of 100, and then, taking into account the dilution factor, the number of eggs per gram of feces are calculated. The main use of an egg count is to gain an appreciation of the pasture contamination. The following factors should be considered when interpreting the results:

- There is little correlation between the actual number of worms and the fecal egg count.
- Immature, migrating, or hypobiotic worms do not produce eggs.
- Different worm species lay eggs at different rates.

- Not all female worms produce eggs at the same time.
- Strongyle eggs in feces of foals less than 6 weeks old are the result of coprophagia.
- Egg production can be suppressed by increased host immunity.

COLLECTION OF EGGS OF *Oxyuris equi*. The female of this species deposits most of her eggs around the anus. These are collected by applying a strip of adhesive cellophane paper to the perianal region and then sticking it to a glass slide.

LARVAL CULTURE. Differentiation between large strongyles and cyathostomes is made by examining their larvae, rather than by examination of their eggs, which are similar. Infective third-stage larvae are obtained by incubating feces for 7 days. The larvae are collected by using either of the two following methods:

- *Method 1.* A 16-oz jar is one third filled with well-mixed feces, loosely sealed, and left for 7 days at 26°C–29°C. Daily stirring will prevent fungal growth. The feces should be kept moist by adding water or, if too wet, an absorbent material such as charcoal or sterilized feces, as necessary. After 7 days the jar is filled with water and inverted over a petri dish, which is in turn half filled with water. The larvae then migrate into the petri dish from where they are collected by pipette, killed by adding a few drops of Lugol's iodine, and examined.
- *Method 2 (Baermann Method).* Larvae can be collected from fresh and incubated feces, pasture, soil, and tissues. This apparatus consists of a funnel with a stem connected to a test tube by a piece of rubber tubing. The tubing is clamped closed, and the funnel is filled with warm water. The sample, held in a sieve or wrapped in cloth, is then placed in the water, which is deep enough to cover it. The warmth and moisture stimulate the larvae to emerge from the sample and enter the water from where they descend into the neck of the funnel. After a few hours the clamp is released and the larvae pass into the test tube, from where they can be collected with a pipette. The diagnostic features of the larvae are listed in the box.

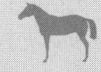

Characteristics of Larvae Cultured From Feces[14]

- *Strongylus vulgaris.* Large, broad, length 1,010 µm, 28–32 gut cells
- *Strongylus edentatus.* Thin, length 790 µm, 18–20 gut cells.
- *Cyathostomes.* Length 830 µm, 8 gut cells.
- *Trichostrongylus axei.* Short tail, length 650 µm, 16 gut cells.
- *Dictyocaulus arnfeldi.* Small spike at tail tip, length 420–480 µm.

Cytological Examination

Cytological examination is carried out mainly to detect evidence of internal parasites or sometimes leukocytes, which often indicate bacterial enteritis and compromise of the distal intestinal tract. Ova of large and small strongyles, tapeworms, round worms, and *Strongyloides westeri,* as well as coccidia, are often seen. A fresh sample of feces is required.

Fecal Culture

Fecal examination is frequently carried out to identify causative bacteria and viruses in cases of diarrhea. A sample of approximately 10 g of feces is required. In the case of *Salmonella* spp., at least five samples, collected at 12- to 24-hour intervals, are required before a case can be declared negative. Organisms can also be isolated from a rectal biopsy (see later). Feces contain a large number of organisms, and fecal culture is directed toward the identification of a specific organism rather than the usual method of identifying all organisms. This is done by using various selective culture media to allow growth and identification of specific organisms, including selenite broth, tetrathionate broth, and brilliant green agar for *Salmonella* spp; McConkey's agar and eosin methylene blue agar for other gram-negative organisms such as *Escherichia coli;* aerobic agar for *Clostridium* spp.; and cycloserine-cefoxitin-fructose agar for *Clostridium difficile.* Other bacteria include *Actinobacillus* spp.; *Bacteroides fragilis, Rhodococcus equi, Campylobacter* spp, and *Klebsiella pneumoniae.* Demonstration of the mere presence of an organism does not prove that it is responsible for the clinical signs. This applies especially to *Clostridium* spp. and *Escherichia* spp., where tests to identify the presence of toxin are required.

Viruses are also responsible for diarrhea and enteritis in foals. Rotavirus is the most common cause, although other agents such as coronavirus and adenovirus are also isolated. Rotavirus can be identified by electron microscopy and by use of ELISA (Rotazyme II ELIZA, Abbott Labs, Chicago, IL) and latex agglutination tests.(Virogen Rotatest, Wampole Labs, Cranberry, NJ).

Endoscopy of the Alimentary Tract

Endoscopy has become a useful tool in the investigation of the esophagus (esophagoscopy), stomach (gastroscopy), and duodenum (duodenoscopy). The procedures are relatively simple but do require an endoscope of appropriate length.

Esophagus

Esophagoscopy can usually be performed in the standing patient. Physical restraint with a twitch is recommended, and, occasionally, chemical restraint is also required. Evaluation of motility or assessment of the size of the lumen should be conducted without chemical restraint.

PROCEDURE. The procedure for esophagoscopy is similar to that for upper respiratory tract endoscopy.[15] The horse should be suitably restrained, as suggested, with a holder to control the horse, and a second person to insert the endoscope, leaving the clinician free to operate the endoscope while viewing the image in the eyepiece or on a monitor. Under direct vision, the endoscope is passed up one nasal passage and

Materials for Esophagoscopy

- Flexible endoscope (150 cm, with irrigation and insufflation facilities)
- Physical restraint (twitch, stocks according to temperament)
- Chemical restraint (xylazine, 0.5 mg/kg IV)

directed toward the esophageal opening, located in the midline, dorsal, and caudal to the corniculate processes of the arytenoid cartilages. As the tip of the endoscope arrives in the vicinity of the esophagus, and especially when it is gently advanced so as to contact the caudal pharynx, swallowing usually occurs. Just as when passing a stomach tube, the endoscope should be advanced once the swallowing reflex is activated, which will take it into the first part of the esophagus. There is a momentary loss of vision as swallowing occurs. Failure to stimulate the swallowing reflex can often be rectified by squirting water through the endoscope.

After insertion of the endoscope, and provided that rupture or perforation is not suspected, the esophagus is distended with air and the endoscope passed down the esophagus until it reaches the cardia of the stomach. Esophageal contractions can make insertion difficult, and, to avoid injury, the endoscope should not be inserted when a contraction is occurring. During insertion the esophagus is carefully examined. A full examination usually requires that the endoscope

be inserted and withdrawn a number of times. Saliva or food will hinder examination and should be removed by suction or lavage.

RESULTS. The tubular esophagus is normally collapsed and requires insufflation before a good examination can be conducted. When collapsed, the esophageal mucosa lies in longitudinal folds. When distension is omitted or is incomplete, the friction between the endoscope and the mucosa tends to push the mucosa ahead of the endoscope during insertion, causing the mucosa to pucker into a series of transverse folds. The mucosa is examined for lesions such as wounds, ulcers, or scars, and the lumen is evaluated for size, shape, foreign bodies, strictures, fistulae, and diverticuli. Failure to dilate during insufflation indicates stricture or stiffness. The cardia is seen as a transverse slit in the distal esophagus. The proximal part of the cranial esophagus can be difficult to examine because of repeated swallowing motions, stimulated by the presence of the endoscope. Some examples of esophagoscopy are shown in Figure 11-19.

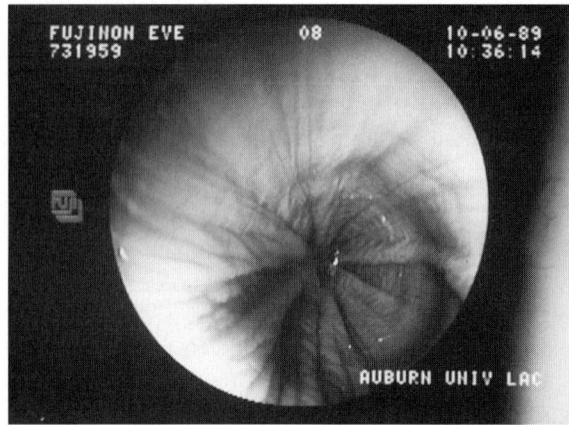

A

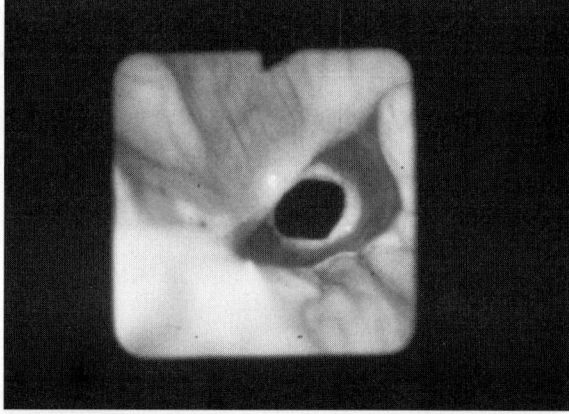

B

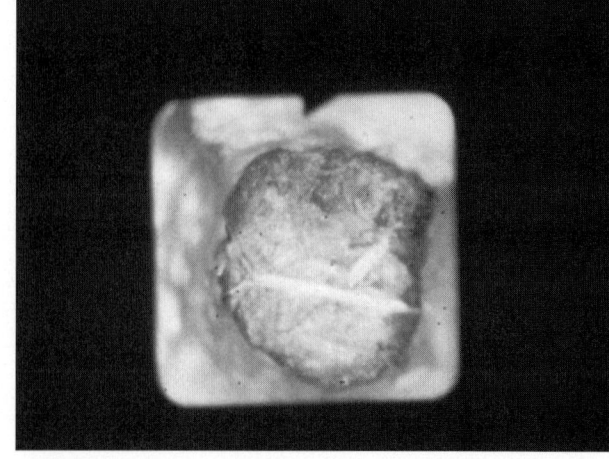

C

▶ **FIGURE 11-19**

Endoscopy of the esophagus. **A.** Normal. The proximal esophagus has been distended with air, which facilitates the examination and obliterates the normal longitudinal folds. The more distal region is not distended and, therefore, cannot be examined and also retains the longitudinal folds. **B.** Healing laceration and stricture. Note the narrow esophageal lumen at the site of a partially healed lesion. **C.** Obstruction with a bolus of food. Note the distended esophagus and the obstructing mass of food material.

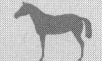

Materials for Gastroscopy

▸ Flexible endoscope (2–3 m for adults, 1–2 m for foals, with insufflation, suction, and biopsy facilities)

▸ Physical restraint (twitch, stocks)

▸ Chemical restraint (xylazine, 0.5 mg/ kg IV)

Stomach

The availability of long flexible endoscopes has allowed gastroscopy to be developed as a routine diagnostic technique.[16] The main indication for its use is gastric ulceration in foals, although other lesions, such as gastric neoplasia, in adults can also be diagnosed.

PROCEDURE. The procedure is almost identical to that described for esophagoscopy. The length of the endoscope is such that it cannot be removed quickly in case of an emergency, meaning that the horse should be restrained in stocks to prevent it from moving away from the endoscope. Foals are best controlled by using an extra handler. Most patients require sedation (e.g.,

xylazine, 0.5 mg/kg IV), although young foals can often be examined without. With the exception of young foals that ingest mainly milk, all patients should be fasted for about 12 hours to ensure that the stomach is empty. When there is a problem with gastric emptying, a longer period is often necessary.

The endoscope is inserted into the esophagus and passed to the level of the cardia, as described. The caudal esophagus and cardia should be examined for signs of ulceration, stricture, gastroesophageal reflux, and inflammation. The endoscope is then pushed through the cardia and into the stomach, resulting in momentary loss of vision. Once in the stomach, certain structures come into view and a systematic examination should follow. Whenever the objective of the endoscope contacts the wall of the stomach the image is lost momentarily. Room air is insufflated until the resulting distension will allow a thorough examination. Distension reduces some of the rugal folding, which improves visualization. If necessary, water is used to rinse food material from the surface of the stomach. The endoscope is directed dorsally and to the right side of the horse, which brings the saccus cecus (the dorsal outpouching of the stomach) and squamous mucosa into view (Fig. 11–20A). To investigate further, the endoscope is directed ventrally, to

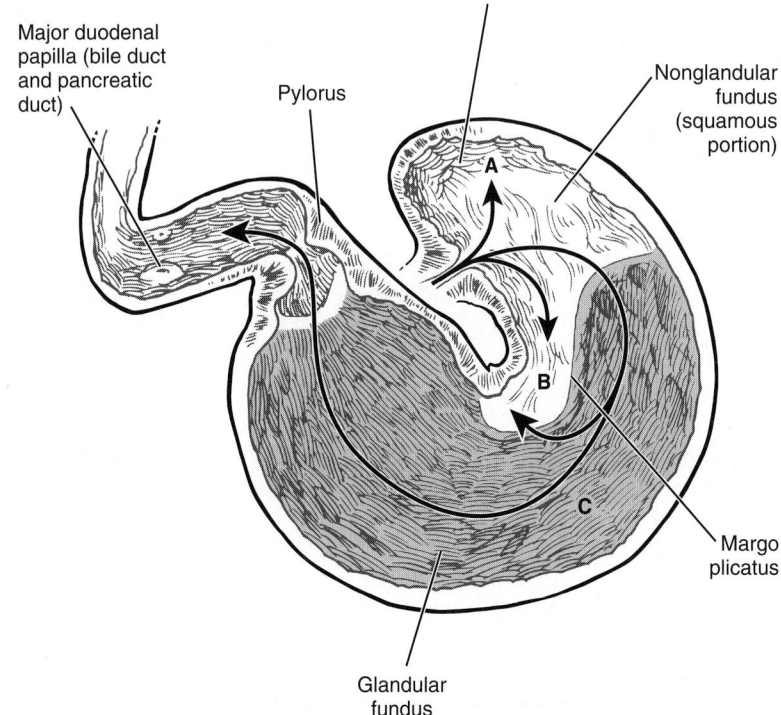

▸ **FIGURE 11–20**

Endoscopy of the stomach. Relevant gastric anatomy and how the endoscope must be moved to view the different regions.

examine the squamous fundus, margo plicatus (junction between squamous and glandular mucosa), and glandular fundus (Fig. 11–20B). The left and caudal aspects are examined by directing the endoscope toward the left side of the horse. The lesser curvature can be examined by inserting the endoscope deeper into the stomach and then directing it sharply ventrally and to the left side of the horse, which also brings the caudal pyloric antrum into view (Fig. 11–20C). Further advancement of the endoscope along the greater curvature, combined with deflection, allows the gastric pillar, and cardiac orifice containing the endoscope, to be seen. By directing the endoscope toward the pyloric antrum, the antrum and pyloris can be seen. The extent of the examination in this region is limited by the volume of fluid and ingesta present, which accumulates despite fasting. When necessary, gastric lavage can help to remove some of the ingesta. When the antral and pyloric regions are visible, their contraction can often be seen.

Complete examination of the antral region, usually indicated in foals, requires anesthesia or heavy sedation, so that the examination can be carried out with the patient recumbent. The patient should be placed in right lateral recumbency so that any fluid or ingesta tend to pool away from the antral and pyloric regions. The examination is similar to that just described. Ingesta and fluid pooled in the region of the cardia will tend to obscure the view as the endoscope enters the stomach. This can be ameliorated to some extent with aspiration and lavage. After conducting the initial examination, as described, the endoscope is inserted further and directed around the greater curvature to allow the pyloric antrum to be seen. The endoscope can often be directed into the antrum and the pylorus (examination of the pyloris and duodenum is described in the next section). If food or fluid obscure the view, improvement can usually be achieved by placing the foal in dorsal and sometimes left lateral recumbency.

RESULTS. The squamous mucosa is white, contrasting with the pink glandular mucosa. The margo plicatus is irregular and represents the junction between the glandular and nonglandular mucosa. Desquamation, erosion, and ulceration of the squamous mucosa in the region of the margo plicatus, are common findings in young foals, although most are asymptomatic and heal spontaneously.[17] Desquamation occurs in the majority of foals, and erosion and ulceration occur in approximately 50%. Lesions in the glandular region are very much less common. Clinically significant ulcers cause acute inflammation and sometimes perforation and, when chronic, can lead to stricture and obstruction. In older horses there is a much reduced incidence of ulceration, and other findings include neoplasia, *Draschia megastoma*, and *Gasterophilus nasalis* larvae.

Duodenum

Duodenoscopy can also be accomplished with the long endoscopes used today.[18]

PROCEDURE. As described for gastroscopy, the procedure can be carried out in the standing patient with appropriate restraint or in recumbency, as dictated by temperament and the presence of gastric ingesta and fluid. Access to the region of the pyloric antrum is by passing the endoscope around the greater curvature, as described. Sometimes, when gastric tone is minimal, the endoscope cannot be advanced to the desired region, and it will become coiled. The presence of gastric contraction will often assist the onward passage of the endoscope toward and through the pyloris.

RESULTS. The duodenum often contains a green-yellow fluid, a mixture of bile and pancreatic fluids. About six inches from the pyloris is the duodenal diverticulum, through which the bile and pancreatic ducts emerge, and also the minor papilla, which lies opposite and contains the duct of the accessory pancreatic duct. The mucosa is usually gray to red in color. Biopsy and aspiration of bile from the bile duct can be performed with

Materials for Duodenoscopy

▸ Flexible endoscope (with insufflation, suction, and biopsy facilities).
  Foals: 200 cm long and 9–11 mm diameter
  Larger foals and adults: Up to 300 cm long and 13.5 mm diameter

▸ Physical restraint (twitch, stocks)

▸ Chemical restraint (xylazine, 0.5 mg/ kg IV)

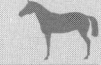

**Materials for
Rectal Biopsy**

▶ Uterine biopsy forceps

▶ Rectal examination sleeve

▶ Obstetrical lubricant

▶ Sample containers
   10% neutral formalin for histological
   examination
   Transport media (See Appendix C) for
   microbiological examination

biopsy forceps and an aspiration catheter, respectively, passed down the endoscope.

RESULTS. Findings in the duodenum include ulcers, strictures, and *Gasterophilus nasalis* larvae.

Rectal Biopsy

Biopsy of the rectum is usually done blindly with biopsy forceps. Although it is possible to carry out a rectal biopsy under direct vision through an endoscope, the small sample that is obtained has limited use.

PROCEDURE. The procedure is carried out with the horse restrained in stocks. A preliminary examination will usually have been carried out already and a site for biopsy selected. Lubricant is applied to the anus and the gloved hand. The hand with fingers coned is inserted partially through the anus, and the instrument, held in the other hand, is then guided into the palm of the hand. The hand and instrument are then inserted as one to the level of the selected biopsy site, while holding the jaws against the palm of the hand to avoid injury to the rectum. A piece of mucosa is picked up between the thumb and first finger and guided into the jaws of the biopsy forceps, which are then closed to cut the sample free. The biopsy includes only mucosa, but is suitable for histological and microbiological examinations. For histology the specimen is placed in formalin, and for microbiology, it is taken directly to the laboratory or placed in transport medium.

Radiography of the Head and Alimentary Tract

The head and alimentary tract are considered together because of the interrelationship between the conditions of the teeth and the paranasal sinuses. Although radiography of the equine alimentary tract is not as useful as it is in smaller animals, diagnostic radiographs of certain regions can be obtained. The limitation to diagnostic radiography comes as a result of the size of the equine. In adult horses radiography of the intraabdominal alimentary tract requires high-output fixed machines, which are useful for investigating conditions such as enterolithiasis, diaphragmatic hernia, and presence of sand in the large intestine. Foals and ponies are much smaller, and good radiographs can be obtained, even with portable machines. The head and cervical esophagus of any horse can be radiographed with a portable machine.

Most radiographs are taken when the animal is standing. Occasionally in adults, and more often in foals, the animal is made recumbent. In adults this requires general anesthesia, but in foals physical restraint is usually satisfactory, with or without sedation. An advantage of recumbency is that ventrodorsal and other radiographic projections are possible. A disadvantage of recumbent radiography is that gas caps and fluid levels cannot be adequately evaluated. The reader is directed to the literature for a more detailed description of techniques.[19]

Head

A portable X-ray machine can be used to produce diagnostic radiographs. The quality of the radiographs is improved by using a grid, rare earth screens, and a device to hold the cassette. The latter also is necessary to reduce radiation exposure of personnel. Whenever possible the X-ray cassette should be placed against the side of interest. A rope halter should be used to avoid the presence of metal buckles and rings in the radiographs, which invariably seem to obscure the region of interest. Lateral and slightly oblique views are usually obtained easily, and sometimes so is a ventrodorsal exposure of the rostral section of the head. More complicated oblique views and the ventrodorsal view require recumbency, usually under general anesthesia. Care is required to obtain the correct views because of the distortion produced by variations in the angle of exposure.

Although it is wise to use large cassettes, which allow most of the head to be seen on the one radiograph, it is usual to center the X-ray beam on a specific anatomical region. Regions often targeted are the cranium and base of the skull, teeth and mandible, premaxilla and rostral mandible, paranasal sinuses and maxilla, and the caudal soft tissues that compromise the pharynx, larynx, and guttural pouch.

Some conditions that can be detected include:

- *Bone.* Fractures, infection, neoplasia, developmental lesions (cysts)
- *Teeth.* Abnormality of number and shape, fracture, periapical infection, developmental lesions (cysts, heteroptopia), neoplasia
- *Paranasal sinuses and nasal passages.* Infection, neoplasia, cysts, ethmoidal hematomata (Fig. 11–21).
- *Guttural pouch.* Empyema (infection with accumulation of exudate), inspissation of exudate (chondrosis), tympany, mycosis
- *Larynx.* Ossification of cartilage, epiglottic entrapment, subepiglottic cysts, epiglottic hypoplasia, chondritis
- *Pharynx.* Soft-palate displacement, cysts
- *Temporomandibular joints.* Osteoarthritis, luxation

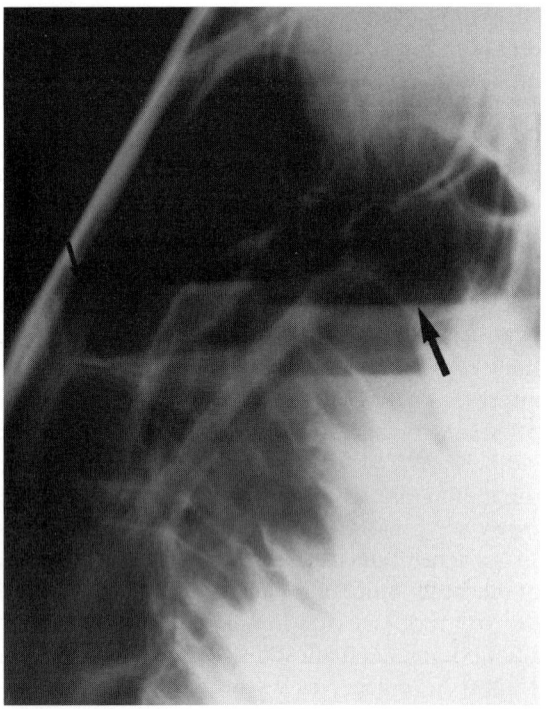

▶ **FIGURE 11–21**

Bilateral Sinusitis. The horizontal lines represent the upper border of an accumulation of fluid in the frontoconchal (*small arrow*) and caudal maxillary (*large arrow*) sinuses. The exposure has been taken at a slightly oblique angle, thus allowing the fluid–gas interfaces (fluid levels) of both the left and right sinus systems to be seen.

More specific details on some of the more important regions and conditions are available elsewhere.[20-26]

Esophagus

Radiography of the cervical and intrathoracic parts of the esophagus requires different exposures because of the different thicknesses of the neck and the thorax. A portable X-ray machine can be used under most circumstances to radiograph the cervical esophagus of all patients, small or large. Although stationary, high-output machines are most often used to radiograph the intrathoracic esophagus, the use of rare earth screens, high-speed film, and the air gap technique allow diagnostic radiographs of this region to be obtained with mobile machines (100–800 mA) and, for foals, even low-output machines (<30 mA).

The esophagus is usually radiographed with the patient standing with the cassette against the left side. If recumbency is necessary, the patient is placed in the left lateral recumbency with the cassette underneath. Plain or contrast studies can be used. Contrast can be either positive (barium or iodine-containing compounds), negative (air), or double contrast (mixture of positive and negative). Barium sulfate, in the form of a paste, is most commonly used. The paste is placed in the mouth, from where it is swallowed. Occasionally, when only a specific region must be imaged, or a larger volume of contrast is required to outline a diverticulum or megaesophagus, the barium can be given in the form of a suspension through a nasogastric tube. The volume required varies from approximately 50 to 200 mL, depending on the size of the patient. If perforation is suspected, use of an iodine-containing contrast is indicated. If necessary, a little of the contrast can be mixed with some food to study the passage of a more physiological material. More sophisticated evaluation can be achieved with fluoroscopy or image intensification, which allow a dynamic study of the movement of the bolus, or contrast, as it moves down the esophagus.

The normal esophagus is empty and is impossible to image unless it contains a little air or ingesta. After swallowing, barium paste coats the mucosa and tends to outline the normal longitudinal esophageal folds for a few minutes. A little contrast may normally be seen, momentarily, at the thoracic inlet, heart base, and cardia. Depending on how soon after swallowing the exposure is made, a bolus of barium may still be present, but should not be seen in the same site in subsequent radiographs. Liquid barium does not coat the mucosa as efficiently as does the paste. Abnormality of pharyngeal function may be associated with residues of contrast material in the larynx, nasopharynx, and nasal passages.

Plain radiography is most useful in identifying foreign bodies, although obstruction in the region of the cardia is characterized by esophageal dilation and fluid accumulation. Contrast radiography is indicated for outlining diverticuli and megaesophagus, and for identifying strictures, the sites of obstruction that hinder onward passage of contrast, space-occupying lesions, perforation, and functional abnormalities such as grass sickness. Care must be taken in evaluating motility after tranquilization or passage of a nasogastric tube, as these may slow esophageal emptying. Sometimes, a normal esophageal contraction can look like the site of stricture. However, this can be confirmed by taking a second radiograph, in which a stricture should still be present, whereas a normal contraction would have disappeared. Furthermore, xylazine, given a few minutes before examination, tends to reduce the normal esophageal activity and can therefore help avoid a false-positive diagnosis of stricture.

The reader is referred to the literature for more details on esophageal radiography.[27,28]

Gastrointestinal Tract

Radiography of the adult gastrointestinal tract is strictly limited by size to relatively easily imaged conditions such as diaphragmatic hernia, presence of sand in the large intestine, and enterolithiasis. Imaging adults is often impossible and always requires high-output machines plus rare earth screens and grids. Plain and contrast studies in foals, even with portable machines, are more rewarding, and the more extensive studies, common in dogs and cats, can often be carried out. Radiography in adults is usually done with the patient standing and the cassette positioned against the side of interest. A system of four overlapping exposures has been described for the adult abdomen, in which the first exposure covers the cranioventral region and each of the others a more caudal and dorsal region.[29] The exposure factors from this reference are listed in the box.

Foals can be imaged while standing or in lateral recumbency. Frequently, the complete abdomen can be imaged on a single exposure. Using similar screens, grids, and focal film distance to those just described for the adult abdomen, exposure factors of 14 mAs and 80 kVp were used for lateral views in foals with abdomens up to 20 cm wide (kVp was increased by 10% if required).[30] The stomach is best imaged when the cassette is against the left side of the patient. When recumbent, dorsoventral and lateral exposures can be made. The ability to see and interpret gas caps and fluid levels is lost when the foal is made recumbent. A barium enema is useful in confirming colonic atresia.

When contrast studies are to be done in adults, the patient should fast for at least 12 hours if possible (2 hours for foals). In contrast to the esophagus, where barium paste is favored, micropulverized barium sulfate solution (30% weight per volume) is preferred for gastrointestinal studies. Approximate doses are 5 mL/kg for foals and about half this for adults. The contrast is delivered to the caudal esophagus through a nasogastric tube. After administration of contrast, exposures are taken immediately, and then at one half-hour, one hour and then hourly until the contrast reaches the small colon. If a more detailed study

---

RADIOGRAPHIC EXPOSURE FACTORS FOR THE ADULT ABDOMEN: LATERAL VIEWS[29]

- 14 × 17″ (35 × 43 cm) cassettes, rare earth screens, grid (8:1, 80 lines per inch), focal film distance of 48″ (122 cm)

Site 1: Diaphragmatic and sternal flexures	180 mAs	90 kVp
Site 2: Part of LDC and LVC, RVC, part of RDC	240 mAs	110 kVp
Site 3: RDC, part of small colon	600–800 mAs	120 kVp
Site 4: small colon	240–400 mAs	110 kVp

(LDC and LVC, left dorsal and left ventral colons; RVC and RDC, right ventral and dorsal colons.)

of the stomach and duodenal region is required to evaluate ulceration, exposures can be made more frequently (e.g., immediately, and then at 10, 20, 30, and 60 minutes). To evaluate foals, a full series of left lateral, right lateral, and ventrodorsal projections should be made at each time interval. More extensive descriptions are available elsewhere.[31-33]

FOAL ABDOMEN. The foal abdomen, in addition to being smaller than that of adult horses, does not have their well-developed large intestine. The normal abdomen, seen in a standing lateral exposure, is characterized by a mixture of gas, fluid, and ingesta, with the occasional presence of intestinal loops containing fluid and gas caps. Gas is rarely observed in the cranial ventral abdomen, but it is often seen in the rectum. The stomach is located caudal to the liver, aligned with the slope of the diaphragm, has a vertical height about twice that of the width, has a dorsal gas cap in the fundus, and has fluid or ingesta located ventrally in the antral region. The haustral folds of the ventral colon may be seen lying on the abdominal floor. Change from right to left projections varies the clarity and size of some organs. The ventrodorsal position allows a better appreciation of the pylorus and duodenum and another perspective of all organs. Presence of contrast helps to identify the different regions of all the gastrointestinal tract.

The normal transit time of contrast for foals is about 6 to 8 hours. Contrast begins to leave the stomach within a few minutes, and emptying takes longer depending on the content of ingesta. Contrast reaches the cecum within 3 to 5 hours, by which time the stomach should be empty. The passage of contrast from the cecum to the colon occurs quickly.

In plain radiographs the presence of obstruction is inferred from organ distension and the accumulation of gas and fluid proximal to the site of obstruction. In contrast studies obstructive lesions may be outlined directly, seen as space-occupying lesions or inferred from delayed emptying and transit times. In foals with chronic obstruction from ulceration there may be evidence of gastroesophageal reflex and filling defects indicating the presence of ulcers. Retention of meconium causes distension of the rectum and colon with gas, which may also outline the mass of meconium. A meconium mass can also be diagnosed using a barium enema, as can colonic

atresia. Presence of contrast-filled parts of the gastrointestinal tract within the thorax indicates a diaphragmatic hernia.

ADULT ABDOMEN. The adult abdomen cannot be adequately imaged. On top of the obvious difference in size, the stomach is relatively smaller, and the cecum and colons larger than their counterparts in the foal. Useful diagnoses are limited generally to easily seen lesions such as diaphragmatic hernia (using contrast radiography), enterolithiasis, and sand impaction. The mere presence of the two latter findings does not necessarily indicate clinical disease.

Ultrasonography of the Alimentary Tract

Ultrasonography has limited application for percutaneous investigation of the adult gastrointestinal tract, and, as with radiography, the limitation is posed by the size of the abdomen. Hence, ultrasonography is most useful for investigating organs that lie relatively close to the abdominal wall, and for smaller breeds and foals. Evaluation of conditions such as abscessation, accumulation of peritoneal fluid, adhesions, and neoplasia is sometimes improved by using ultrasonography. Occasionally, transrectal ultrasonography will improve the ability to image a particular part of the gastrointestinal tract or a specific lesion by allowing the transducer to be brought closer to the object of interest. The esophagus is close to the skin surface and is therefore much easier to image. Descriptions of ultrasonography of the liver and urogenital tract are located in the respective chapters.

PROCEDURE. The procedure for skin preparation is described in Appendix B. The examination is made with the horse standing and restrained as necessary. Because foals are smaller, they are often examined when recumbent. Unless the structure or region of the abdomen to be imaged are known, selecting the correct transducer is usually done by trial and error. In foals, and when the site of interest is known to be close to the body wall, a transducer with a higher frequency will be selected, whereas for deeper structures and in adults, a lower frequency is likely to be more useful. The methods for examining some specific regions and condition are described in the paragraphs that follow.

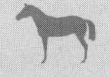

Materials for Abdominal Ultrasonography

▶ Ultrasound machine
▶ Sector transducer (frequency depends on structure imaged)
    Adult abdomen: 2.0–5.0 MHz
    Foal and pony abdomen: 5.0–7.5 MHz
    Esophagus: 5.0–7.5 MHz
▶ Ultrasound coupling gel
▶ Hair clippers (#40 head)

The Esophagus

There is little indication for ultrasonographic examination of the esophagus because it can be so easily and thoroughly examined by other means, such as radiography and endoscopy. Occasionally, useful information concerning conditions such as diverticuli, periesophageal abscessation, and foreign body can be gained by percutaneous examination.

Percutaneous Examination of the Nephrosplenic Space

As demonstrated in Fig. 11–17C, the left ventral and dorsal colons can become displaced over the nephrosplenic ligament, thereby causing colic. Ultrasonographic examination through the left paralumbar fossa, using the technique described for ultrasonography of the left kidney (see Ultrasonography of Bladder, Kidneys, and Ureter) can be useful to identify the condition when the usual diagnostic method of palpation per rectum cannot be used or is unrewarding. The normal nephrosplenic space does not contain any intestine.[34]

The Abdomen of Foals with Colic

Examination of the foal's abdomen can be very rewarding, especially because the small intestine is the site of most causes of colic. The examiner must know the appearance and motility of normal intestine in order to recognize the abnormal. Specific conditions that can be identified include intussusception, and meconium and ascarid impaction. The double-walled structure, produced by the telescoping action of an intussusception, has a typical appearance; that of a circular structure with a central core surrounded by one thick wall or by two thinner walls.[35] The single wall is seen when the segments of intestine are edematous and the two layers cannot be resolved into separate structures. Ascarids can often be imaged, either individually or as a mass. Nonspecific signs indicative of intestinal obstruction include dilation of intestine with gas and fluid and, under certain circumstances, thickening of the gut wall. Presence or absence of peristalsis can be ascertained, with increased activity often indicating enteritis and decreased activity often indicating loss of viability. Peritonitis is indicated by the accumulation of variably echogenic fluid that often contains echogenic material representing fibrin strands. Free intraabdominal gas indicates rupture of a viscus or peritonitis caused by gas-producing organisms.

The Adult Gastrointestinal Tract

The size of the adult abdomen precludes a very useful role for ultrasonography in evaluating the gastrointestinal tract. In general, considerable luck is required to be able to identify a specific lesion such as an intussusception, although the degree of distension and wall thickness of the small intestine can be determined. The presence of a much more developed large intestine introduces extra difficulties, but, here too, the thickness of the wall can be determined. The presence of large gas-filled organs prevents the transmission of ultrasound. On occasions, when a lesion can be palpated per rectum, extra information can be obtained by passing the probe into the rectum and then directly onto the lesion to carry out transrectal ultrasonography. Diagnosis of nephrosplenic displacement was described in a preceding section.

Intraabdominal Masses

Ultrasonography is very useful for examining intraabdominal masses, thereby assisting in diagnosing and selecting of sites for biopsy or drainage. Abscesses, cysts, hematomata, and soft-tissue masses can often be distinguished on the basis of their appearance. *Cysts* tend to be well-demarcated, hypoechoic structures with or without the presence of echoic septae. There are many different types of *soft-tissue masses,* and because of their variable structure, including regions of necrosis and collection of fluid, they have a varied ultrasonic appearance. Although abscesses and hematomata tend to be relatively easy to distinguish in their early phases, they tend to become similar as fibrosis and consolidation develop. The presence of a foreign body inside an abscess may present as an echoic mass with an acoustic shadow, often surrounded by fluid. *Abscesses* tend to be structures that contain numerous regions of variable echogenicity, ranging from being anechoic to being hyperechoic.

Inspissated exudate and necrotic tissue show up as irregular hyperechoic foci. *Hematomata* tend to be more uniform and less echoic than abscesses, although clotting and, later, organization introduce foci of echogenic material.

Examination of the Umbilical Structures in Foals

Ultrasonography of the umbilical structures is a very useful procedure for diagnosing and managing infection in the newly born foal.[36] The structures of interest are the urachus, umbilical vein, and two umbilical arteries (Fig. 11–22). The

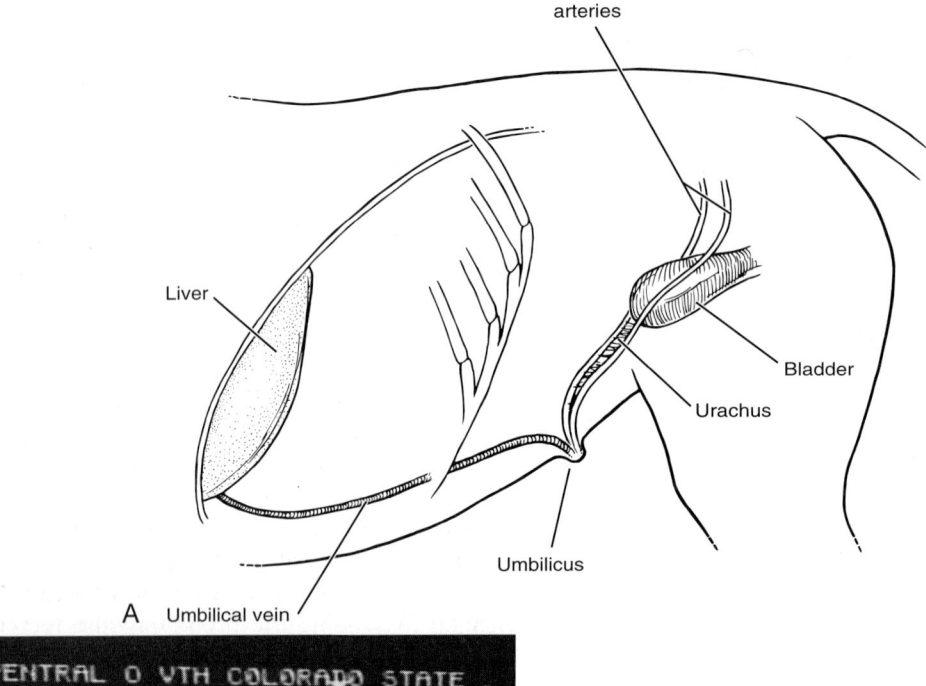

A Umbilical vein

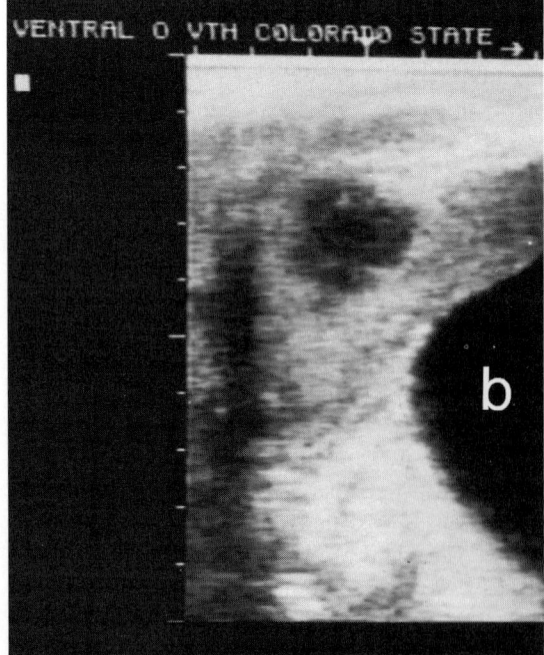

B

▶ **FIGURE 11–22**

Ultrasonography of the umbilicus and associated structures. **A.** Longitudinal diagram of the abdomen demonstrating the umbilicus and related structures. **B.** Umbilical abscess. Midline sagittal ultrasonogram of the caudal abdomen made with a 5-MHz linear transducer. There is a 2-cm-diameter fluid-filled cavity surrounded by an enlarged umbilicus cranial to the urinary bladder. ((b). (Courtesy R. H. Wrigley.)

DIMENSIONS OF UMBILICAL STRUCTURES IN FOALS (FIRST MONTH OF AGE)[36]

- Normal
  - Umbilical vein   0.52 ± 0.19 cm   (range 0.2–0.9)
  - Urachus + umbilical arteries   1.75 ± 0.37 cm   (range 1.2–2.4)
  - Umbilical arteries (single)   0.85 ± 0.21 cm   (range 0.5–1.4)
- Abnormal
  - Umbilical vein   >1.0 cm
  - Urachus + umbilical arteries   >2.5
  - Umbilical arteries (single)   >1.3 cm

---

foals can usually be imaged when standing, although lateral recumbency is satisfactory when indicated. A 2-inch (5-cm) strip of the abdomen is clipped along the midline from the xiphoid to the udder or prepuce, and also from the umbilicus to each inguinal ring. A 7.5-MHz transducer with standoff is preferred. The structures are scanned transversely to produce a cross-sectional image; the umbilical vein from just cranial to the umbilicus to where it joins the liver, and the umbilical arteries and urachus from the umbilicus to the apex of the bladder, and then each artery as it courses toward the inguinal ring. In addition to subjective examination, the structures can be measured. Measurements of the vein are made midway along its course between the umbilicus and liver (if it is oval in cross section, its vertical and horizontal dimensions are measured and then averaged). The transverse diameter of the urachus and both umbilical arteries are measured together, and then each artery is measured separately as it runs beside the bladder.

The results of measurements in foals up to 1 month old are listed in the box.

The umbilical vein is slightly larger at either end than in the middle, and it is a thin-walled structure with an echogenic wall and an anechoic center. It may contain some centrally located echogenic material. The arteries have a thick echogenic wall and an hypoechogenic center. The arterial lumen is sometimes absent. The urachus is seen as an hypoechoic tissue located between the two arteries. The bladder is seen as a fluid-filled structure caudal to the umbilicus. As the foals age, the bladder and liver cease to be in close proximity to the ventral abdominal wall, and by 2 months of age ultrasonic imaging is not always possible in normal foals. Disease may prolong the time during which imaging is possible.

The urachus is the most commonly infected structure, although all structures may be involved in varying combinations (Fig. 11–22B). In addition to an increase in size, infection is characterized by detection of exudate (echogenic) or gas (hyperechogenic).[37]

Vascular Structures in the Caudal Abdomen

Transrectal ultrasonography can be used to examine the cranial mesenteric artery and the aorta and its terminations.[38,39] Both these regions are sites of disease, and details are available concerning the investigation of cranial mesenteric arteritis and aneurysm and aortic-iliac thrombosis.[40,41] Sector or linear transducers are suitable, but it is difficult to orientate them correctly for certain sites. Although a 5-MHz transducer can produce acceptable images, a 7.5-MHz transducer is better.

Preparation consists of manual removal of feces from the rectum and terminal small colon. Sedation (xylazine, 0.5 mg/kg IV) and rectal relaxation (Propantheline, bromide, 0.014 mg/kg IV) are used as required. Ultrasound coupling gel is applied to the transducer scanning surface, which is then either inserted into the rectum unprotected or first placed inside an obstetrical sleeve and then inserted. To examine the cranial mesenteric artery (CMA), the transducer is positioned so that it scans dorsally, and it is placed against the ventral surface of the aorta. Transverse and longitudinal scans can be obtained by changing the angle of the transducer. The probe is then moved cranially until the CMA is reached, where it is repositioned against the left side of the aorta and directed dorsally and toward the right side. A little manipulation should bring the CMA into view as it branches from the aorta. The CMA can be followed by directing the transducer cranially and to the right and by then moving it ventrally to follow its branches. Transverse and longitudinal images can be obtained by repositioning the transducer. This sequence of imaging is most easily done by using the left arm for the examination. The ability to image all regions is compromised by a small colon and the presence of intestine. Changing from a linear to a sector transducer, or vice versa, is often useful when correct positioning is difficult. Renal and lumbar vertebral arteries can also be imaged. Normal arteries pulsate and have an anechoic smooth lumen. Arteritis is indicated by thickening of the walls, irregularity of the luminal surface, and presence of intraluminal masses indicative of thrombosis. Examination of the aorta and its terminal branches is simpler than examination of the CMA, although the principles of examination are identical. The transducer is passed into the rectum, directed dorsally, and placed against the ventral wall of the aorta cranial to its terminal branches. Examination consists of moving the transducer caudally along the aorta and then along its branches, the internal and external iliac arteries. Thrombosis is indicated by the presence of intraluminal masses and reduced or absent pulsation. Sometimes the pedunculated origin of a thrombus can be seen.

Laparoscopy

Abdominal laparoscopy has research and clinical applications. Although it has probably been used most frequently to examine the ovary[42,43] it is particularly suited to identify intraabdominal neoplasia. As it is carried out on the standing horse under local anesthesia, it is relatively noninvasive.[44]

PROCEDURE.   The patient must fast and have water withheld for 24 hours before the procedure. To avoid accidental puncture of any internal structures, a rectal examination should always be done to ascertain the presence of abnormal intraabdominal masses and to evaluate the size of the spleen. The site for insertion of the instrument is in the middle of the paralumbar fossa, unless otherwise dictated by the findings of the rectal examination. A 30-cm² area of skin centered on the paralumbar fossa is clipped and prepared for sterile surgery. Surgical drapes are applied as preferred. Production of a pneumoperitoneum is not required in horses. The insertion site is

---

Materials for Laparoscopy

- Sterile endoscope
    Rigid instrument, such as a Wolf 10-mm diameter, 35-cm long, direct forward viewing laparoscope (Richard Wolf Medical Instruments Corp.), with accessory instruments for biopsy or manipulation
    Flexible fiber-optic or videoendoscope (e.g., Olympus colonoscope)
- Light source and trochar-cannulae
- Hair clippers (#40 blade)
- Materials for skin preparation (antiseptic detergent [Betadine, Hibiclens], 70% alcohol, tincture of iodine)
- Local anesthetic e.g., 2% Lidocaine, 2% Mepivacaine
- Scalpel

---

anesthetized by injecting an anesthetic solution into the subcutaneous tissue and then in the muscle layers down to the peritoneum.

The manner of insertion depends on whether the rigid or the flexible instrument is used. With the rigid instrument a 2-cm skin incision is made, and the cannula with trochar inserted is pushed ventromedially through the muscle layers at an angle of approximately 45°, down to and through the peritoneum. After the abdominal cavity is entered, the trochar is removed from the cannula, through which the laparoscope is then inserted. If the flexible endoscope is used, a larger incision of approximately 5 cm is required, and the muscle layers and the peritoneum are penetrated carefully with a long forceps (e.g., Carmalt) or, alternately (preferred by the writer), if an appropriate-size trochar-cannula set is available, the endoscope can be inserted using the same procedure as described for the laparoscope. A rush of air is heard when the peritoneal cavity is opened to the atmosphere.

Examination of some organs, such as the ovary, is assisted by an accessory instrument or probe. Biopsy also requires the insertion of a suitable instrument. Operating laparoscopes have an instrument channel through which appropriate probes and instruments can be inserted. If an accessory channel is not available, a second incision must be made a few centimeters from the first. In general, a more thorough examination can be made with the flexible endoscope. Examination should be systematic and thorough, frequently necessitating approaches from both left and right sides, and the use of the accessory probes. Biopsy can be taken as indicated, but care is required to avoid perforation of an organ or production of hemorrhage.

On completion of the examination, the instruments are withdrawn and the skin incision closed. Closure of deeper tissues is required only when a more extensive access has been used.

RESULTS. The combination of pneumoperitoneum and a dorsal approach places the instrument in an air-filled space in the dorsal abdomen, from which a relatively good view is obtained. Examination is severely restricted by the presence of intraabdominal fat. A portion of most of the viscera can be examined, but a full view is impossible, except for the ovary, which can be brought into view by manipulation. Organs that can be seen in both sexes include the dorsal aspects of the colons, stomach, and spleen and part of the cecum, bladder, ureters, and left kidney. Although only the dorsally positioned small intestine can be seen, its peristaltic movement constantly brings new sections into view. In females the ovary and adjacent uterus, and in males the vaginal ring with vessels and ductus deferens, can be seen. Intraabdominal testes may also be seen in cryptorchid males.

Absorption and Digestion Tests

Intestinal absorption and digestion tests are not as useful in horses as they are in some other species. Despite this, they have some value to evaluate such conditions as chronic weight loss, small intestine inflammation and neoplasia, and malabsorptive syndromes. Some tests include:

- *Lactose tolerance test.* This test is used to evaluate the ability to digest lactose, especially in foals with enteric lesions affecting the mucosal brush border and compromising disaccharidase activity. The test consists of the oral administration of 20% D-lactose (0.5–1.0 g/kg), which, under normal conditions, results in a doubling of serum glucose within 60 minutes.

- D-glucose absorption test. An oral dose of 10% D-glucose (0.5–1.0 g/kg) is given by nasogastric tube after a 24-hour fast. Blood samples are collected in sodium fluoride tubes 0, 30, 60, 90, 120, 150, 180, 210, and 240 minutes after the glucose has been given. Sodium fluoride is used so that metabolism of the glucose is inhibited. A normal result is seen as a doubling of glucose values within 120 minutes, followed by a return to baseline levels by 6 hours. In addition to lesions that affect enzyme production, other factors, such as gastric emptying and intestinal transit time, can also affect the results.

- *D-xylose absorption test.* The D-xylose is administered by nasogastric tube as a 10% solution (0.5–1.0 g/kg). The samples are collected in heparinized tubes at the same intervals as for the D-glucose test. A normal result produces a value for D-xylose of 20–25 mg/dL 60–120 minutes after administration. The test suffers similar limitations to those of the D-glucose absorption test.

- *Fat absorption.* The ability to absorb fat can be assessed by measuring the plasma content of ^3H following administration of ^3H-oleic acid by nasogastric tube.

- *Test for protein-losing enteropathy.* Loss of protein into the intestinal tract can be evaluated by measuring the fecal content of labeled chromium, ^{51}Cr, after intravenous administration of chromium chloride, $^{51}CrCl$.

R E F E R E N C E S

1. Huntington PJ: Condition Scoring and Weight Estimation of Horses. Ag Note 2816-85. Melbourne, Department of Natural Resources and Environment, 1985.
2. Schumacher J, Schumacher J: Diseases of the salivary glands and ducts of the horse. Equine Vet Educ 1995; 7:313.
3. Schmotzer WB, Hultgren BD, Huber MJ, et al: Chemical involution of the equine parotid salivary gland. Vet Surg 1991; 20:128.
4. Sellers AF, Lowe JE: Visualization of auscultation sounds of the large intestine. Proceedings of the 29th Annual Convention of the American Association of Equine Practitioners 1984: p 359.
5. Ehrhardt EE, Lowe JE: Observer variation in equine abdominal auscultation. Equine Vet J 1990; 22:182.
6. Malark JA, Peyton LC, Galvin MJ: Effects of blood contamination on equine peritoneal fluid analysis. J Am Vet Med Assoc 1992; 201:1545.
7. Blackford JT, Schneiter HL, vanSteenhouse JL, et al: Equine peritoneal fluid analysis following celiotomy. Proceedings of the 2nd Equine Colic Res Symposium, 1985: p 130.

8. Santschi EM, Grindem CB, Tate LP, et al: Peritoneal fluid analysis in ponies after abdominal surgery. Vet Surg 1988; 17:6.

9. Hanson RR, Nixon AJ, Gronwell R, et al: Evaluation of peritoneal fluid following intestinal resection and anastomosis in horses. Am J Vet Res 1992; 53:216.

10. Tulleners EP: Complications of abdominocentesis in the horse. J Am Vet Med Assoc 1988; 182:232.

11. Kopf N: Rectal examination of the colic patient. *In* Robinson NE (ed), Current Therapy in Equine Medicine, 3rd ed. Philadelphia, Saunders, 1992, p 196.

12. Arnold JS, Meagher DM: Management of rectal tears in the horse. J Equine Med Surg 1978; 2:64.

13. Baird AN: Rectal tears. *In* Robinson NE (ed), Current Therapy in Equine Medicine, 3rd ed. Philadelphia, Saunders, 1992, p 232.

14. Herd RP: Diagnosis of internal parasites. *In* Robinson NE (ed), Current Therapy in Equine Medicine, 2nd ed. Philadelphia, Saunders, 1987, p 323.

15. Stick JA: Esophagus. *In* Traub-Dagatz JL, Brown CM (eds), Equine Endoscopy. St Louis, Mosby, 1990, ch 9, p 111.

16. Adamson P, Murray MJ: Stomach. *In* Traub-Dagatz JL, Brown CM (eds), Equine Endoscopy. St Louis, Mosby, 1990, ch 10, p 119.

17. Murray MJ, Grodinsky C, Cowles RR, et al: Endoscopic evaluation of changes in gastric lesions of Thoroughbred foals. J Am Vet Med Assoc 1990; 196:1623.

18. Darien B: Duodenum. *In* Traub-Dagatz JL, Brown CM (eds), Equine Endoscopy. St Louis, Mosby, 1990, ch 11, p 139.

19. Butler JA, Colles CM, Dyson SJ, et al: The head. *In* Clinical Radiology of the Horse. Oxford, Blackwell, 1993, ch 8, p 285.

20. Baker GJ: Some aspects of equine dental radiology. Equine Vet J 1971; 3:46.

21. Cook WR: Skeletal radiology of the equine head. J Am Vet Radiol Soc 1970; 11:35.

22. Cook WR: The auditory tube diverticulum (guttural pouch) in the horse. Its radiographic examination. J Am Vet Radiol Soc 1973; 14:51.

23. Gibbs C: The equine skull: Its radiological investigation. J Am Vet Radiol Soc 1974; 15:70.

24. Gibbs C, Lane JG: Radiographic examinations of the facial, nasal, and paranasal sinus regions of the horse. II. Radiological findings. Equine Vet J 1987; 19:474.

25. Gibbs C, Lane JG, Meynink SE, et al: Radiographic examinations of the facial, nasal, and paranasal sinus regions of the horse. I. Indications and procedures in 235 cases. Equine Vet J 1987; 19:455.

26. Stilson AE, Hening DS, Robertson JT: Contributions of the nasal septum to the radiographic anatomy of the equine nasal cavity. J Am Vet Med Assoc 1985; 186:590.

27. Butler JA, Colles CM, Dyson SJ, et al: The Alimentary and Urinary Systems. *In* Clinical Radiology of the Horse. Oxford, Blackwell, 1993, ch 12, p 471.

28. Greet TRC: Observations on the potential role of esophageal radiography in the horse. Equine Vet J 1982; 14:73.

29. Rose JA, Rose EM, Sande RD: Radiography in the diagnosis of equine enterolithiasis. Proceedings of the 26th Annual Convention of the American Association of Equine Practitioners, 1980, p 211.

30. Campbell ML, Ackerman N, Peyton LC: Radiographic gastrointestinal anatomy of the foal. Vet Radiol 1984; 25:194.

31. Dik KJ, Kalsbeek HC: Radiography of the equine stomach. Vet Radiol 1985; 26:48.

32. Fischer AT, Kerr LY, O'Brien TR: Radiographic diagnosis of gastrointestinal disorders in the foal. Vet Radiol 1987; 28:42.

33. Butler JA, Colles CM, Dyson SJ, et al: The Alimentary and Urinary Systems. *In* Clinical Radiology of the Horse. Oxford, Blackwell, 1993, ch 12, p 483.

34. McGladdery AJ: Ultrasonography as an aid to the diagnosis of equine colic. Equine Vet Educ 1992; 4:248.

35. Bernard WV, Reef VB, Reimer JM, et al: Ultrasonographic diagnosis of small intestinal intussusception in three foals. J Am Vet Med Assoc 1989; 194:395.

36. Reef VB, Collatos C: Ultrasonography of umbilical structures in clinically normal foals. Am J Vet Res 1988; 49:2143.

37. Reef VB, Collatos C, Spencer PA, et al: Clinical, ultrasonographic, and surgical findings in foals with umbilical remnant infection. J Am Vet Med Assoc 1989; 195:69.

38. Wallace KD, Selcer BA, Becht JC: Techniques for transrectal ultrasonography of the CMA of the horse. Am J Vet Res 1989; 50:1695.

39. Schmidt AR: Transrectal ultrasonography of the caudal portion of the abdominal and pelvic cavities in horses. J Am Vet Med Assoc 1989; 194:365.

40. Wallace KD, Selcer BA, Tyler DE, et al: Transrectal ultrasonography of the CMA of the horse. Am J Vet Res 1989; 50:1699.

41. Reef VB, Roby KA, Richardson DW, et al: Use of ultrasonography for the detection of aortic-iliac thrombosis in horses. J Am Vet Med Assoc 1987; 190:286.

42. Heinze VH, Klug E, von Lepel JD: Optische Darstellumg der inneren Geschlechsorgane beim Equiden zur Diagnostik und Therapie. Deutsche Tierärzt Wochenschrift 1972; 79:49.

43. Witherspoon DM, Talbot RB: Ovulation site in the mare. J Amer Vet Med Assoc 1970; 157:1452.

44. Witherspoon DM, Kraemer DC, Seager SWJ: Laparoscopy in the Horse. *In* Harrison RM, Wildt DE (eds), Animal Laparoscopy. Baltimore, Williams & Wilkins, 1980, ch 9, p 157.

45. Brownlow MA, Hutchins DR, Johnston KG: Reference values for equine peritoneal fluid. Equine Vet J 1981; 13:124.

46. Nelson AW: Analysis of equine peritoneal fluid. Vet Clin North Amer: Large Anim Pract 1979; 1:267.

47. Swanick RA, Wilkinson JS: A clinical evaluation of abdominal paracentesis in the horse. Aust Vet J 1976; 52:109.

48. McGrath JP: Exfoliative cytology of equine peritoneal fluid—an adjunct to hematologic examination. Proceedings of the 1st International Symposium on Equine Hematology, 1975; p 408.

49. Bach LG, Ricketts SW: Paracentesis as an aid to the diagnosis of abdominal disease in the horse. Equine Vet J 1985; 6:116

50. Grindem CB, Fairley NM, Uhlinger CA, et al: Peritoneal fluid values from healthy foals. Equine Vet J 1990; 22:359.

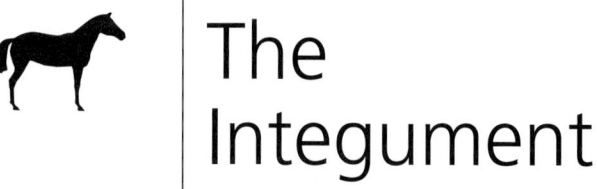

The Integument

12

COMPONENTS

The skin, or integument, consists of outer (epidermis) and deeper (dermis) layers. There is considerable variation in thickness and certain components between different regions of the body. Skin structures, such as sweat and sebaceous glands, hair bulbs, nerves, and blood vessels, are located within the dermis. Some nerves extend up into the epidermis. The epidermis is composed of a series of cell layers extending from a basal membrane to a superficial, keratinized layer, the stratum corneum. The epidermis is penetrated by the hair follicles into which sweat and sebaceous glands open.

MANIFESTATIONS OF DISEASE

Skin disease has numerous causes, including infection (bacterial, viral, parasitic), trauma (physical, chemical), immune system abnormalities (vasculitis, hypersensitivity), nutritional abnormalities (zinc deficiency), neoplasia, and functional abnormalities (anhidrosis). Depending on the type, extent, and location of the insult, the signs are localized or extensive and deep or superficial. Necrosis of skin (burns, infection, thrombosis) is manifested by presence of dead plaques of skin that eventually slough to expose a healthy base of granulation tissue. Granulation tissue is composed mainly of new capillary buds. Horses are prone to produce excessive amounts of granulation tissue, especially in regions where there is movement, such as over a joint. Infection of hair follicles produces local (folliculitis) or extensive abscessation (furunculosis). Inability to sweat (anhidrosis) is dominated by systemic signs, but absence of sweating is apparent as a local sign. Dermatophytosis (ringworm) is characterized by itching (pruritis) and localized loss of hair (alopecia), and a careful examination will reveal that many broken hair shafts remain. Lesions resulting from hypersensitivity include pruritis and thickening (*Culicoides* spp.), and bulla formation (drug allergy). Other immune-based diseases include pemphigus which produces blisters and cutaneous vasculitis, which causes focal cutaneous swellings. Signs resulting from nutritional problems tend to be generalized and include alopecia and flaking of epidermis (zinc deficiency), and rough hair coat (iodine deficiency, vitamin A deficiency or excess).

GENERAL PHYSICAL EXAMINATION

Cutaneous lesions have many different causes, including infectious agents (bacteria, fungi, parasites, viruses), neoplasms (sarcoid, squamous cell carcinoma), physical (wire and rope trauma, solar dermatitis), chemical agents (contact dermatitis), immune-mediated (drug allergy, pemphigus), spider and insect bites, and a variety of miscellaneous causes. Lesions can be characterized according to pathological description, location, extent, and tendency to be pruritic. Terms such as nodule, pustule, abscess, wheal, plaque, alopecia, papule, vitiligo, and leukoderma (deficiency of pigment in skin), leukotrichia (deficiency of pigment in hair), folliculitis and furunculosis are used to describe the type of lesion. Lesions can be widely distributed (urticaria), localized to specific anatomical regions (limbs with chorioptic mange), or localized to certain regions of skin according to pigmentation (squamous cell carcinoma and photosensitization in regions with white hair and unpigmented skin). Special attention should be given to the mucocutaneous junctions and the mucosae. Palpation helps identify the presence of crusts of dried exudate beneath or at the base of the hair and subcutaneous nodules. Ease of epilation should be evaluated.

Although many of the organisms responsible for skin disease require special diagnostic techniques, careful observation will allow the identification of biting insects such as horse flies (*Tabanus* spp.), deer flies (*Chrysops* spp.), horn flies (*Haematobia irritans*), stable flies (*Stomoxys calcitrans*), and black flies (*Simulium* spp.). *Culicoides* species and mosquitoes tend to bite outside daylight hours when visibility is poor. Lice (*Damalinia equi* and *Hematopinus ascini*) and ticks (*Dermacentor amblyomma, Ixodes holocyclus, Boophilus microplus*) can be seen with the naked eye.

SPECIAL EXAMINATION TECHNIQUES

Skin Scraping

Skin scrapings are very simple procedures, used most commonly to demonstrate microscopic ectoparasites.[1]

PROCEDURE. Most horses do not object to the procedure, although some will require sedation. Any long hair should be removed by

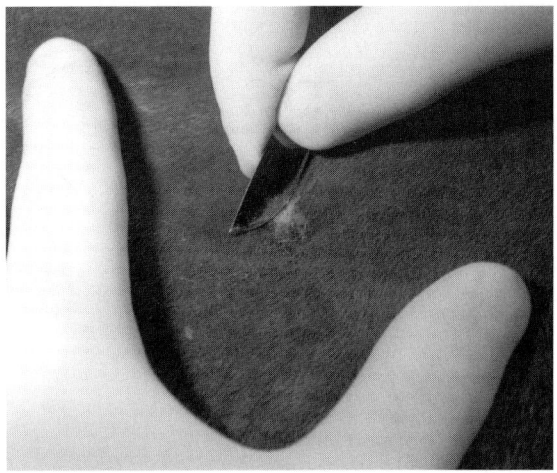

▶ FIGURE 12–1

Skin scraping. A blade is used to scrape the skin surface, ensuring penetration into the dermis.

clipping. The mineral oil can either be placed directly on the skin to be scraped or added to the sample on the glass slide after collection. The sample is collected by scraping the scalpel blade across the selected site, a sufficient number of times and with sufficient force, to ensure that a sample of adequate depth is obtained (Fig. 12-1). To obtain *Demodex,* the depth of the scraping is such that tissue fluid and blood should appear in the site. Squeezing also improves the chances. Samples should be taken from a number of sites in order to increase the chances of a positive result. Each scraping is placed in a container for later examination or on a slide for immediate examination. Mineral oil is added to the sample, as necessary, to ensure that no air bubbles are present beneath a coverslip. Microscopic examination is made under low (×10) and then higher magnification (×40).

A variation of the technique is required to obtain a sample for verification of ear mites (*Psoroptes cuniculi*). As this mite exists in and around the ear, a sample is best obtained by inserting a finger into the ear and scraping the finger nail along the inner surface of the canal in order to obtain some of the secretion. Alternately, a wooden tongue depressor or metal curette can be used carefully.

RESULTS. The organism most likely to be found is *Chorioptes equi,* located in the superficial layers of scrapings obtained from the limbs. Lice and their nits can also be seen, but these would usually have been detected during the visual examination. Larval forms of the nematodes *Strongyloides*

Materials for Skin Scraping

▶ Scalpel blade (#10)

▶ Mineral oil

▶ Glass slide

▶ Coverslip

▶ Hair clippers–#40 clipper head

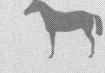
westeri and *Pelodera strongyloides* can also be found on occasions. Rarely, other findings, include *Trombicula* spp. (scrub itch mites of Australia, harvest mites of Europe, and chiggers of North America), *Psoroptes equi, Sarcoptes scabeii* var. *equi, Demodex folliculorum* var. *equi,* and *Psoroptes cuniculi* (found in exudate from the ear.

Identification of *Onchocerca microfiliariae*

The adult form of the filarid parasite *Onchocerca cervicalis* resides in the ligamentum nuchae, and the microfilariae are found in the dermis where they are often the cause of dermatitis characterized by multifocal and coalescent lesions, pruritis, alopecia, ulceration, and crusting of exudate. The microfilariae are widespread and their presence is often asymptomatic. The ventral midline is most commonly affected, also the middle of the forehead and, in severer cases, lesions are found over much of the body.

PROCEDURE. The site for biopsy often is hairless and therefore does not require clipping. Analgesia can be obtained by infiltration of local anesthetic solution or deep sedation. After preparation of the skin a full-thickness sample is obtained with the biopsy punch (see Biopsy for Histological Examination). The wound is usually left to heal by secondary intention, although closure by simple interrupted suture or skin staple is preferred by some. The sample is cut in half and one piece placed in formalin for routine histologi-

cal examination. The other piece is placed on the slide, sliced finely with the blade, covered with a few drops of saline, and allowed to stand at room temperature for about 30 minutes. The slide is then scanned under ×4 magnification, noting especially the regions adjacent to the tissue for signs of emerging microfilariae. When signs of movement are detected, the higher-power objective is used to examine the microfilariae in detail. If microfilariae are not found, the sample should be allowed to incubate for up to 24 hours.

RESULTS. The microfilariae are slender ($\approx$8 µm × 240–270 µm). They often are present without being associated with any lesions.

Identification of Fungi

Potassium Hydroxide (KOH) Preparations

A KOH preparation is a useful method for quickly verifying dermatophytosis. The KOH is used as a clearing agent to dissolve the keratin and to bleach the hair so that the fungal elements can be more easily seen.

PROCEDURE. Hairs and skin debris should be collected from the periphery of a number of different lesions.[1] The forceps are used to pluck hairs and the blade is used to scrape and collect debris. The sample can be examined immediately or stored in a sterile container for later processing. A drop of the clearing agent is placed on the slide, the hair and skin scales are added, and a coverslip is placed over the sample. The slide is warmed for about 30 seconds or allowed to stand for half an hour, to facilitate clearing, and the examination is started with a ×10 objective. The initial search is for hairs that appear to have an irregular inner region. When suspicious hairs are found, they are examined under higher magnification.

To improve identification of fungi, a more rapid method of clearing, with a mixture of KOH and dimethylsulfoxide (DMSO) solution (Dermassay Clearing Solution, Pitman Moore), which requires immediate examination, or an alternate stain, consisting of a mixture of 100 mg Chlorazol Black E stain (Sigma Chemical), 10 ml DMSO, 90 ml water, and 5 g KOH, can be used. To produce the latter stain, which stains the fungal elements green, the Chlorazol is dissolved in the DMSO and then added to the water in which the KOH has been dissolved.

RESULTS. A positive result demonstrates the presence of uniform septate fungal hyphae and arthroconidia on the hair shaft. Care must be taken to make a good preparation and to examine it carefully to avoid false-positive or false-negative results. To avoid false negative results, the sample should be cultured.

Fungal Culture

SUPERFICIAL FUNGI. Ringworm, also known as dermatophytosis, is the main form of superficial fungal infection and is a common occurrence.

Procedure. The lesions are washed gently with nonantiseptic soap and rinsed with water to remove most of the nonpathogenic and saprophytic bacteria and fungi.[1,2] The samples are taken from the periphery of a number of different lesions. Hairs are collected with the forceps and scales, debris and crusts are scraped with the scalpel. Materials can be plated directly or stored in the sterile containers for later processing. Sterile forceps are used to press the samples on to the surface of the culture medium. The samples are

---

Materials for Culture of Superficial Fungi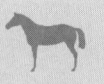

▸ Culture medium: Dermatophyte Test Medium, or Sabouraud's agar with added pH indicator, and antibacterial and antifungal agents

▸ Nonantiseptic soap

▸ Forceps

▸ Scalpel blade (#10)

▸ Sterile containers

---

left to incubate at room temperature for up to 4 weeks. A duplicate set of plates incubated at 37° is recommended because *Trichophyton verrucosum* grows better at this temperature.

Results. A positive result is indicated by a powdery or fluffy, cream-colored growth, associated with a simultaneous change from amber to red in the medium. (The color is due to the pH indicator, phenol red, which changes to red in the alkaline environment created by the alkaline metabolites of dermatophytes. Most bacteria and saprophytic fungi produce acid metabolites but can cause a color change eventually.) The most commonly isolated dermatophytes are *Trichophyton equinum,* and *Trichophyton mentagrophytes.* Other forms are *Trichophyton verrucosum, Microsporum canis,* and *M. gypseum.* (The use of the Wood's lamp is of little use in horses because, in the above list, only *M. canis,* which is uncommon, fluoresces). All horses carry a population of saprophytic fungi (most commonly *Cladosporium* spp, *Penicillium* spp. and *Rhizopus* spp.), and a small proportion also carry some potentially pathogenic fungi in the ascomycetous state (*Microsporum* and *Trichophyton*).[3] In addition, it can be expected that similar fungi will be isolated from hair and underlying skin.

DEEP FUNGI. Diagnosing fungi that cause deep infections is a little more complicated than for superficial fungal infections.[2] There are several groups of fungi in this category, producing most commonly phycomycosis and less commonly maduromycosis and sporotrichosis. *Pythium insidiosum,* the cause of pythiosis, is the commonest organism in the phycomycosis group that causes a pyogranulomatous reaction. Case reports also rarely identify several other fungi. The appropriate form of sample collection depends on the type of lesion, which includes closed and open subcutaneous nodules, ulcers, and large granulating lesions with single or multiple necrotic cores. Identification depends on finding the agent in the sample or by culture and, therefore, samples are collected to provide the laboratory with the appropriate options. Depending on the lesion, the laboratory should be presented with all or some of the following: an impression smear, an aspirate, or an excision biopsy.

Identification of Bacteria

Skin houses a population of nonpathogenic bacteria that are always potential contaminants in any attempt to culture pathogenic organisms.[1,4]

Contamination is minimized by suitable pretreatment of the surface of the lesion.[1] The skin overlying subcutaneous nodules can be given a full sterile preparation. The contents of the nodule can then be collected by needle aspirate or by incision or total excision. Ulcerated lesions are likely to be contaminated, and isolates are unlikely to be significant. If the ulcer is covered with scabs or crusts, the latter can be removed with forceps or scalpel and a sample taken from the underlying tissues.

A specific form of bacterial infection, that caused by *Dermatophilus congolensis,* is the cause of "rain scald." The infection is characterized by crusting of exudate and matting together of the hair. When moist exudate is present beneath the crusts, it can be sampled by impression smear or transferred on a swab or scalpel blade to a glass slide. When the crusts are dry, they should be collected, trimmed of hair, cut into small pieces with scissors or scalpel, and placed on a glass slide and mixed with a few drops of water. When the crusts are soft, excess debris is removed and the crusts are crushed, allowed to dry, and then stained (Gram's, Giemsa, Wright's). The bacteria are gram-positive and have a branching filamentous structure. Material can also be submitted to a laboratory for culture. Bacterial infection takes several different forms including granulomata and nodular lesions often termed botryomycosis *(Staphylococcus aureus),* abscessation with edema and localized emphysema *(Clostridium perfringens),* and abscessation with or without lymphangitis and ulceration (e.g., *Corynebacterium pseudotuberculosis, Staphylococcus aureus*), and folliculitis and furunculosis caused by a variety of organisms.

Biopsy for Histological Examination

A skin biopsy is indicated for most lesions in which a superficial scraping or culture is not indicated or has proven negative, for suspected neoplasia, and for any persistent lesion not responding to therapy.[1,5] Depending on the temperament of the patient, biopsy usually is carried out under sedation and local anesthesia in the form of a subcutaneous infiltration, or ring block. The type of surface preparation varies with the type and extent of the lesion, but, as a rule, it is contraindicated to carry out a rigorous surface preparation because of the high probability of disturbing or removing surface features of the

---

Materials for Biopsy for Histological Examination

- Biopsy punch (e.g., Baker's Cutaneous Punch, Chester A Baker Labs, Miami, FL) 4 mm, 6 mm, 10 mm
- Fine forceps (e.g., Adson)
- 70% alcohol
- #10 or #22 scalpel blade
- Scissors
- Needle holder and suture material (e.g., ⅔ polypropylene or skin staples)
- 2% lidocaine hydrochloride
- 5-cc syringe, 22–25-gauge needle
- Tongue depressor or piece of cardboard
- 10% neutral buffered formalin (volume = ×10 volume of specimen)

---

lesion. To ensure fixation, samples should be limited to about 1 cm. Larger pieces should be sliced to this thickness. When possible, samples should be pinned to a tongue depressor or allowed to adhere, dermal side down, to a piece of cardboard, before fixation, in order to preserve normal architecture. Biopsy types include needle, shave, elliptical, and excision biopsies.

Needle Biopsy

Needle biopsy is useful to obtain samples from subcutaneous nodules (e.g., mastocytoma, abscess). The overlying skin can be clipped free of hair and lightly covered with 70% alcohol. Local anesthesia is usually unnecessary. A needle with syringe attached is inserted into the nodule and the sample aspirated by applying negative pressure with the syringe. The sample is smeared on to a microscope slide and then stained for histological examination.

Shave Biopsy

A shave biopsy is useful for superficial lesions, especially those involving delicate regions such as the ear or eyelid. A few milliliters of local anesthetic is injected beneath the lesion, with the 25-gauge needle, taking care to avoid the lesion itself, dermis, and epidermis. The skin is squeezed up into a fold and the biopsy made by removing a slice of epidermis and dermis, with the plane of incision parallel with the skin surface (Fig. 12–2). Suture of the wound is not indicated. The sample is attached to the cardboard or tongue depressor, placed in the 10% buffered formalin, and submitted for histology.

Punch Biopsy

A punch biopsy is useful for obtaining a full-thickness section of a lesion in a relatively atraumatic fashion. Punch biopsies are less useful when the skin surface is disrupted by lesions such as vesicles or ulcers. A cutaneous biopsy punch is used to collect a sample that extends through the epidermis, dermis, and subcutaneous fat layer to include the panniculus (Fig. 12–3). The 6-mm instrument is adequate for most occasions. After injection of local anesthetic solution beneath the lesion, the punch is placed and the biopsy cut by simultaneously rotating and applying pressure to the punch. The sample usually remains attached to the subcutaneous tissue or the panniculus, from which it must be severed with scissors. Care must be taken to avoid squashing or distorting the sample with the forceps. The wound is usually left unsutured to heal by secondary intention. When required, closure can be made with suture or skin staples. The sample is placed in formalin for later histological examination.

Excision and Elliptical (Wedge) Biopsy

Excision and elliptical (wedge) biopsies allow a large full-thickness piece of skin and deeper tissue to be sampled. They differ only in the proportion of the lesion that is removed. An excision biopsy is indicated when the lesion is small or nodular and the procedure, by removing the complete lesion, provides treatment as well as diagnosis. An elliptical biopsy is used when complete removal of the lesion is not possible or indicated. After injection of local anesthetic beneath the lesion, or as a ring block for large lesions, the biopsy is made by making two opposing elliptical incisions with a scalpel. The incisions extend into the panniculus. When making an elliptical biopsy it is important that the sample includes normal tissue, the advancing edge of the lesion, and abnormal tissue. Deliberate selection of the central part of a lesion will often yield necrotic tissue that is not representative of the pathological process and from which a diagnosis cannot be made. Excision and elliptical biopsy wounds should be closed by suture. The sample is placed in formalin for later histological examination.

Biopsy for Immunofluorescence Testing

Immunofluorescence testing is done when immune mediated diseases such as the various forms of pemphigus, lupus erythematosus, and vasculitis are suspected.[1] The method of sample collection is identical to that described for punch or excisional biopsies, with the exception that a special fixative, Michel's fixative (Zeuss Scientific, Raritan, NJ), is required by most laboratories. (Identification of immunoglobulins can also be done using immunoperoxidase procedures, which can often be carried out on formalin-fixed samples).

Intradermal Testing

Intradermal testing is a useful method for helping to determine the antigens responsible for certain allergic conditions not necessarily restricted to the integument. The test involves the intradermal injection of a series of different allergens and evaluation of the tissue response to each over a period of up to 24 hours.[6,7]

PROCEDURE. The hair is clipped from an area 20×30 cm on the lateral cervical region. For some horses a nose twitch or sedation is required. Each antigen is diluted to a concentration of 1,000 protein nitrogen units (PNU) per milliliter, and then 0.1 mL of each is injected intradermally. Saline and histamine are injected to act as negative and positive controls, respectively. Each injection site is identified by using a marker pen to make a

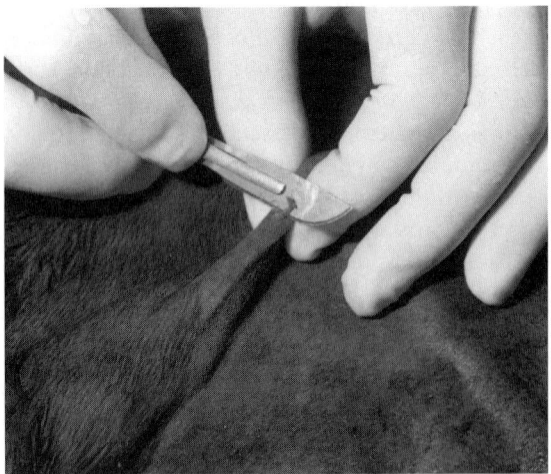

▶ FIGURE 12–2

Shave biopsy. A blade is used to take a thin superficial slice from a fold of skin.

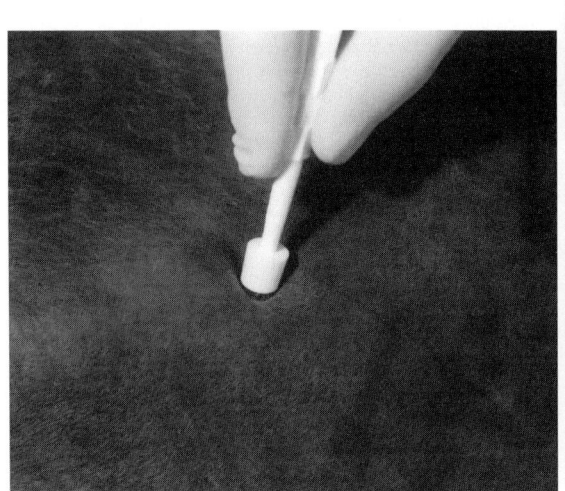

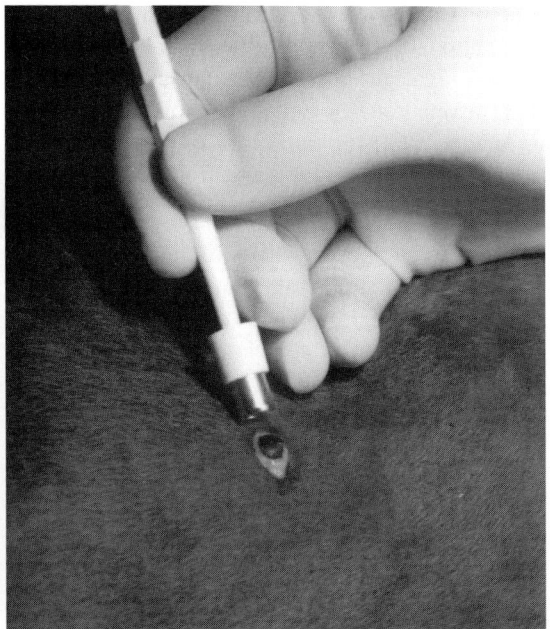

A

B

▶ FIGURE 12–3

Punch biopsy. **A.** The biopsy is cut by placing the punch on the skin and then rotating it while downward pressure is exerted. **B.** Biopsy has been cut but is still attached by the subcutaneous tissues. **C.** Extracting biopsy by cutting the deeper attachments.

C

Materials for Intradermal Testing

▶ Allergens, including inhalents, pollens, grasses, weeds, dusts, and molds
▶ Controls
   Saline
   Histamine (1 : 100,000)
▶ Tuberculin syringe, 25-gauge needle

line or dot below each site. Care must be taken to ensure that the injection is intradermal and not subcutaneous. The reactions are evaluated after 30 minutes, 4 hours, and 24 hours. The diameter of any reactions is measured, and each is assessed by noting whether it is raised, firm or soft, or painful. Lesions are compared with the controls, with saline being 0+ and histamine 4+.

RESULTS. Each reaction is compared with the controls. A positive reaction does not always indicate the presence of clinical allergy to the allergen. False-positive reactions can occur in response to factors such as nonspecific irritation, excess antigen, physical trauma, contaminants, or preservatives. False-negative reactions can result from inadequate preparation of antigens and the effects of agents that inhibit a response. Reactions are classed as follows:

- Type I or immediate (mediated by IgE and certain IgG). These antibodies are antigen-induced and bind to tissue mast cells and circulating basophils, which undergo de-granulation with release of a number of mediators, including histamine, in the presence of the specific antigen.
- Type II or late (mediated by IgG). These antibodies bind to cell membranes, and, in the presence of the specific antigen, induce activation of complement with subsequent cell lysis and cell phagocytosis.
- Type IV or delayed (mediated by lymphokines). These are produced by sensitized T-lymphocytes in response to antigen, and are chemotactic for lymphocytes and macrophages. This response is cell-mediated and does not depend on antibody formation.

R E F E R E N C E S

1. Evans AG, Stannard AA: Diagnostic approach to equine skin disease. Compend Contin Educ Pract Vet 1986; 8:652.
2. Mullowney PC, Fadok VA: Dermatologic diseases of horses. Part III. Fungal skin diseases. Compend Contin Educ Pract Vet 1984; 6:S324.
3. Ihrke PJ, Wong A, Stannard AA, et al: Cutaneous fungal flora in twenty horses free of skin or ocular disease. Am J Vet Res 1988; 49:770.
4. Mullowney PC, Fadok VA: Dermatologic diseases of horses. Part II. Bacterial and viral skin diseases. Compend Contin Educ Pract Vet 1984, 6; S16.
5. Pascoe RR: Equine nodular and erosive skin conditions: The common and not so common. Equine Vet Ed 1991; 3:153.
6. Beech J: Testing for allergies. *In* Beech J (ed), Equine Respiratory Disorders. Philadelphia, Lea & Febiger, 1991, p 36.
7. Evans AG: Recurrent urticaria due to inhaled allergens. *In* Robinson NE (ed), Current Therapy in Equine Medicine, 2nd ed. Philadelphia, Saunders, 1987, p 619.

A D D I T I O N A L   R E A D I N G S

Foil LD, Foil CS: Arthropod pests of the horse. Compend Contin Ed Pract Vet 1990; 12:723.
Mullowney PC: Dermalogic diseases of horses. Part IV. Environmental, congenital, and neoplastic diseases. Compend Contin Ed Pract Vet 1985, 7:S22.
Pascoe RR: A Color Atlas of Equine Dermatology. London, Wolfe publications, 1990.
Scott DW: Large Animal Dermatology. Philadelphia, Saunders, 1988.
Scott DW, Manning TO: Equine folliculitis and furunculosis. Equine Pract. 1980; 2:11.
The Veterinary Clinics of North America, Equine Pract, Dermatology April 1995 vol 2.

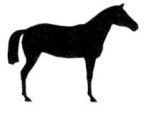

The Hemolymphatic System

13

COMPONENTS

This chapter discusses the fluid and cellular components of the lymphatic and hempoietic systems, the vascular and lymphatic network of vessels, and the sites of production and storage of the various cellular components.

MANIFESTATIONS OF DISEASE

Although the hemolymphatic system is involved in a secondary capacity in many disease states, it is far less often affected by primary disease. The manifestations of disease vary greatly in their location and extent. The widespread nature of the system dictates that the search for signs of disease be conducted in many of the other organ systems. Furthermore, nonspecific signs such as inappetance, depression, weight loss, and fever are common presenting signs in all forms of disease of the system. In the lymphatic system the most obvious specific clinical signs of disease are enlargement of lymph nodes (lymphadenopathy), distension of lymphatic vessels, and sometimes fistulous tracts in the case of infection. The clinical signs of disease of the hemopoietic system depend on the underlying abnormality, including:

- Anemia due to loss, destruction, or reduced formation of red cells: Produces mucosal pallor and reduced exercise tolerance.

- Red cell hemolysis due to blood parasites, immune-mediated disease, infections, oxidant-induced disease, and miscellaneous causes, such as heavy metal toxicosis, and snake envenomation: produces icterus, hemoglobinuria.
- Vasculitis due to immune-mediated disease and infection: Produces mucosal petechiation, ecchymosis, and ulceration, edema, and skin infarction and necrosis.
- Neutropenia due to aplastic anemia: Produces susceptibility to infection.
- Coagulopathy due to interference with function of the clotting mechanism or production of its components (hemophilia A, warfarin toxicosis, disseminated intrasvascular coagulation, thrombocytopenia): Produces a tendency to bleed and contributing to organ failure, particularly in the kidneys.

GENERAL PHYSICAL EXAMINATION

There are a myriad signs of disease in this system, and, because of the location of the organs involved, they often are invisible to an external examination. Subsequently, internal examination, especially the extensive use of clinicopathologic tests are often required.

Mucous Membranes

Examination of the mucosae has been described in the cardiovascular system. Oral and conjunctival mucosae are the usual sites for examination. In females, the vaginal mucosa is also useful, especially when the former locations have been rendered less useful by head trauma or swelling. The oral mucosa is exposed by lifting the upper lip, opening the eyelids, or by separating the vulvae (Fig. 13-1). With respect to the hemolymphatic system mucosal color and presence of petechiation are the main abnormalities. When there is a deficiency of hemoglobin, the mucosae lose their pink color, becoming paler and in extreme cases, white. Hemolysis may result in jaundice, resulting from accumulation of bilirubin. The presence of small foci of bleeding (petechiation) may indicate vasculitis or disseminated intravascular coagulation.

Veins

Palpation

The large veins should be examined and palpated for pain, swelling, thickening, and occlusion, which indicate thrombosis. The jugular veins are most accessible, and are examined by firm digital palpation (Fig. 13-2). Thrombosis

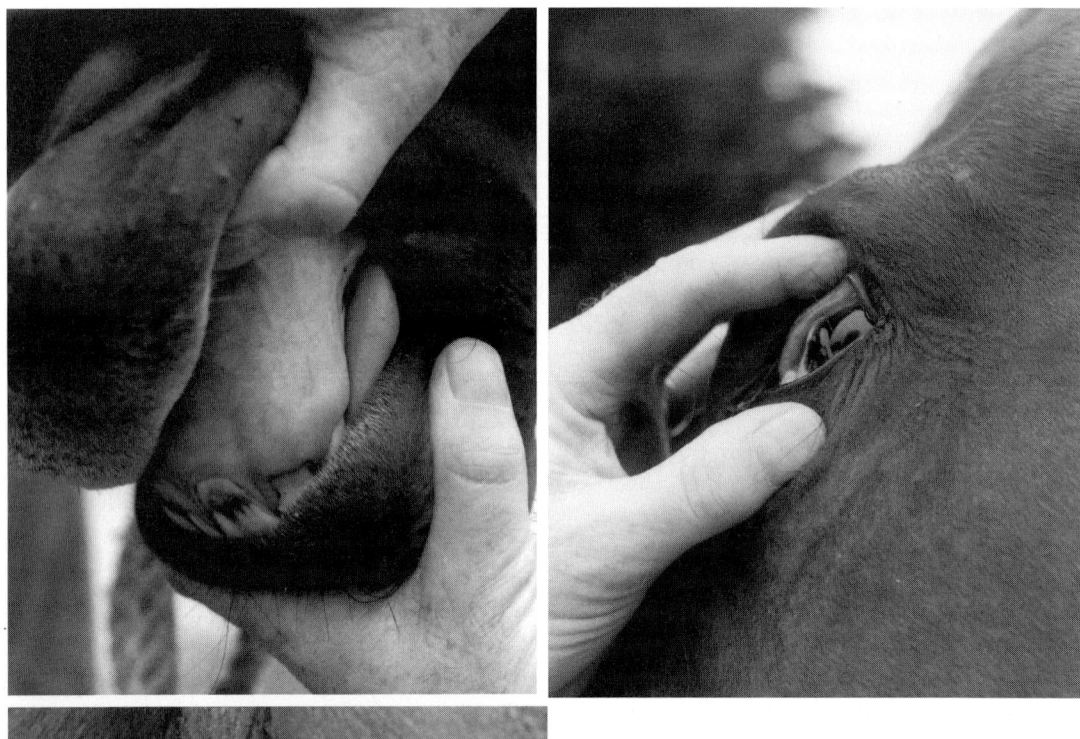

A

B

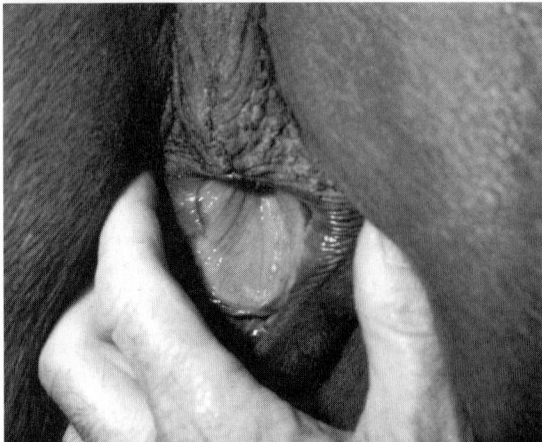

C

▶ FIGURE 13-1

Sites for examination of the mucous membranes. Oral **A,** conjunctival **B,** and vaginal **C,** mucosae.

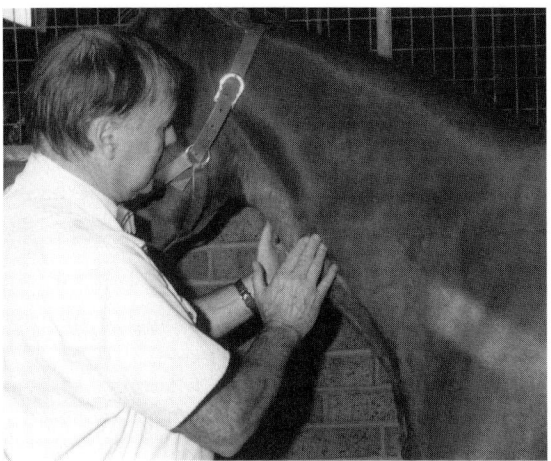

▶ FIGURE 13-2
Palpation of the jugular vein.

initially causes pain and gradual decrease in flow and, later, thickening and occlusion. Venous obstruction causes upstream edema, especially in dependent sites. Therefore, jugular obstruction tends to cause edema of the head and obstruction of limb veins causes limb edema.

Ultrasonography

The jugular veins can also be imaged by ultrasonography, to which they are rendered especially suitable by their anatomy and superficial location.

PROCEDURE. The skin overlying the vein is prepared as described in Appendix B and then scanned in longitudinal and transverse section. The vein should be scanned from below to above the suspected lesion. When sepsis is present, a sample of fluid can be obtained from within the thrombus, using the ultrasound image to guide the needle into the correct location. The sample should be collected after clipping the hair and preparing the skin for a sterile aspiration. It should then be stained for cytological examina-

tion and submitted for aerobic and anaerobic culture and antibiotic sensitivity testing as described in Appendix C.

RESULTS. The normal vein appears as an anechoic tubular structure whose diameter decreases when the transducer is pushed firmly against it and increases during a Valsalva maneuver. This deformability is diminished and eventually abolished as a thrombus develops. A thrombus is seen as a regular, echoic mass within the vein to which a point of attachment is often seen. When sepsis is present, the mass is less regular and contains hypo- or anechoic foci indicating regions of granulation tissue and fluid (Fig. 13-3). Pockets of gas are seen as hyperechoic foci within the thrombus.

Lymph Nodes and Vessels

The lymphatic system consists of the vessels, tissue, and lymphatic fluid (lymph). The lymph drains from the intertitial tissues into thin-walled capillaries and then into successively larger lymphatic vessels, ducts, and trunks, and eventually into the venous system. Lymph nodes, which are distributed throughout the lymphatic system, consist of a tissue meshwork that contains lymphocytes. Lymph flows into the nodes, passing through the cortical and medullary regions to exit from the hilus. Lymph nodes tend to be located in the same regions in different individuals, where they consist of a single node, or group of nodes, termed a lymphocenter, and

Materials for Jugular Vein Ultrasonography

▶ Ultrasound machine
  Sector or linear technology
  7.5-MHz transducer
▶ Ultrasound coupling gel

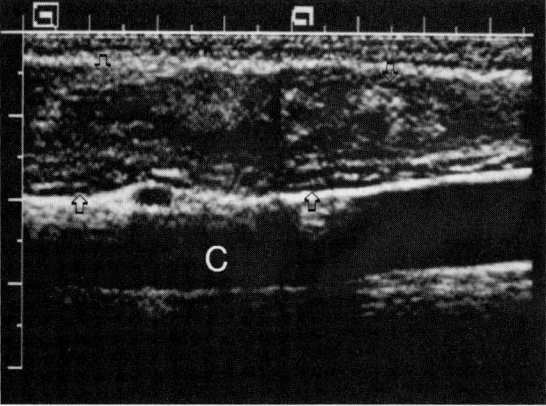

▶ FIGURE 13-3
Septic jugular thrombophlebitis. Longitudinal ultrasonogram acquired with a 7-MHz transducer. The superficial jugular vein (arrows) is distended with patchy echogenic material, which represents the thrombus. The carotid artery (C) is normal. (Courtesy R. H. Wrigley.)

drain a specific region. The main regions and their lymphocenters are:

- Head: Mandibular, parotid, and retropharyngeal lymphocenters
- Neck: Superficial and deep cervical lymphocenters
- Thoracic limbs: Axillary lymphocenter
- Thorax: Dorsal and ventral thoracic and mediastinal and bronchial lymphocenters
- Abdomen
    Abdominal and pelvic walls. Lumbar, iliosacral, inguinofemoral (superficial inguinal), and ischiatic lymphocenters
    Abdominal viscera. Celiac, cranial and caudal mesenteric lymphocenters
- Pelvic limb. Iliofemoral (deep inguinal) and popliteal lymphocenters

The major drainage from the abdomen and hind limbs is eventually into the cysterna chyli, located to the right of the aorta and extending from the second or third lumbar to the last thoracic vertebrae. It extends into the thorax as the thoracic duct and thence flows into the cranial vena cava.

Palpation

In the normal state the only superficial nodes that are easily palpable are the mandibular nodes. The others can be palpated if they are sufficiently enlarged (lymphadenopathy). The intrathoracic nodes are not accessible for palpation. The intraabdominal nodes in the caudal abdomen can be palpated, per rectum, when enlarged (see Palpation of the Abdomen per Rectum). When involved in inflammatory processes, the nodes are likely to be painful on palpation, whereas lymphadenopathy because of neoplasia often produces a painless enlargement.

Lymph vessels become visible when obstructed or infected. When infection is present, they are also very painful if palpated. The most common location is the limbs where lymphangitis is a relatively frequent clinical occurence.

Lymph Node Biopsy

The lymph node can be biopsied by aspiration, needle, or excision. Collection by aspiration is useful for bacteriological evaluation, but when tissue architecture must be preserved, needle biopsy (see Appendix F) or, better still, excision biopsy are preferred (see Excision and Elliptical Biopsy, Examination of the Integument).

Collection of Venous Blood Samples

Venous blood is used for most clinicopathological measurements, the exception being the need for arterial blood for pH and blood gas analysis when pulmonary function is tested. Venous blood is usually collected from the jugular veins, although any suitable vein can be used when necessary. The need to use other veins arises when the jugular veins are unavailable, usually because of thrombosis or occlusion.

The technique of collection is simple, varying slightly according to whether a needle and syringe or needle and vacuum tube are used. The collection tubes are either plain or contain different additives in accordance with the type of test to be conducted. When blood culture is required, the collection must be conducted under sterile conditions, using one of several commercially available blood culture systems, as described in Appendix C.

PROCEDURE. To avoid artificial elevation of red cell parameters, the collection must be made with the horse in a relaxed state. Most routine

Materials for Collecting Venous Blood

- Collection device: Vacuum tube (e.g., Vacutainer, Becton Dickinson, Rutherford, NJ) or Syringe of appropriate size and 20-gauge 1-inch needle)
- Types of additives
    Potassium EDTA (purple-top Vacutainer) for routine cytology
    Sodium citrate (3.8%) (blue-top Vacutainer) for coagulation tests and fibrinogen (Clauss method)
    Sodium citrate (3.1%); black-top Vacutainer) for erythrocyte sedimentation rate
    Sodium fluoride, potassium oxalate (gray-top Vacutainer) for glucose
    Lithium heparin (green-top Vacutainer) for plasma measurements and fibrinogen (heat precipitation method)
    Plain tube (red-top Vacutainer) for serum biochemical assays

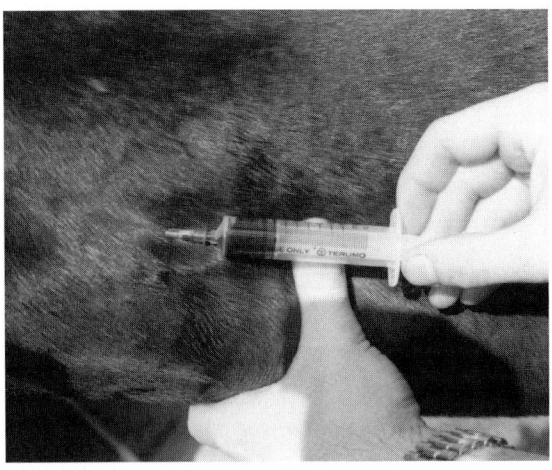
A
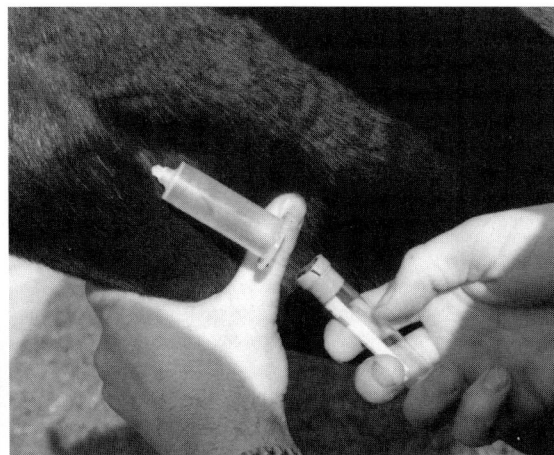
B

▶ FIGURE 13-4
Collection of a venous blood sample from the jugular. **A.** Venipuncture with a hypodermic needle and syringe. **B.** Venipuncture with an evacuated system (Vacutainer).

collection is conducted without sterilizing the hair and skin over the puncture site, although, as a token gesture, it is usual to wipe the site with 70% alcohol. Although adequate antisepsis is impossible without removing hair, many clinicians will use an alcohol rub so that they are seen to be making an effort to avoid iatrogenic infection. The use of an alcohol swab does have the advantage of flattening the hair, which makes the vein easier to see, which is of value in horses with a long hair coat and for the inexperienced collector. Under no circumstances should a dirty or obviously contaminated site be used.

The vein is occluded distal to the site of collection by digital pressure. The resultant backup of blood distends the vein, thus making it more visible and a bigger target into which to insert the needle. The technique of collecting a sample from the left jugular is shown in Figure 13-4. The left thumb is used to occlude the vein, and the right hand holds the collection tube or syringe and needle. The needle is inserted through the skin and into the vein at an angle of about 30°, and then, after entering the vein, the angle is changed so that the needle is directed almost parallel to the vein. The reasons for stressing the angle of insertion are to ensure that the needle does not pass right through the vessel and that as much as possible of the needle is within the vein, rather than lying subcutaneously. After the needle has been inserted, the finger occluding the vein is removed and the sample collected from the flowing blood. If a syringe and needle are being used, the vacuum is created by withdrawing the plunger of the sy-

ringe. When using a vacuum tube, the needle and tube are placed in the holder and the needle is directed into the vein as described, after which the vacuum is activated by forcing the collection tube into the holder.

Samples should be processed as soon as possible. Routine cytology should be carried out within a few hours, during which time the sample must not be exposed to hot conditions. Between collection and processing optimum handling of the sample consists of storing in a refrigerator or on ice. If processing is expected to be delayed, cytology can be preserved by preparing a smear.

RESULTS. Reference values for the hemogram are presented in Table 13-1. There is considerable variation in the erythron with age and type of horse.

Bone Marrow Biopsy and Aspiration

Bone marrow biopsy is used when blood values suggest that bone marrow function is abnormal. A sample of marrow can be obtained from the tuber coxae, sternum, or rib. In foals, the tuber coxae is preferred, but in adults the sternum is the most reliable.[1]

PROCEDURE.

Adults. The procedure is carried out in the standing horse, with sedation and analgesia as required (see Chapter 1, Chemical Restraint of the Adult Horse). The site for sternal collection is in

▶ **TABLE 13–1**

REFERENCE VALUES FOR HEMATOLOGY

Parameter	Reference Range (mean ± 2 SD)
Erythrocytes (×10^{12}/L)	6.5–12.5
Hemoglobin (g/L)	110–190
Packed cell volume (L/L)	0.32–0.52
Mean corpuscular volume (fL)	34–58
Mean corpuscular hemoglobin (pg)	12–18
Mean corpuscular hemoglobin content (g/L)	310–370
Reticulocytes (%)	0
Total protein (g/L)	60–80
White blood cells (×10^9/L)	5.50–12.50
Segmented neutrophils	2.50–6.50
Band neutrophils	0–0.10
Metamyelocytes	0
Myelocytes	0
Lymphocytes	1.50–5.50
Monocytes	0–0.80
Eosinophils	0–0.60
Basophils	0–0.20
Platelets (×10^9/L)	100–500
Fibrinogen (g/L)	1–4
Prothrombin time (s)	7–19
Activated partial thromboplastin time (s)	37–54
Total clotting time (s)	5–21
Fibrin degradation products (μg/mL)	<10

Source: Data are reference values used in the Central Veterinary Diagnostic Laboratory, Mt. Waverley, Melbourne, Australia. (Courtesy Dr. P. M. Lording.)

the ventral midline slightly caudal to the olecranon. The site is clipped and prepared for sterile collection. A few milliliters of anesthetic is infiltrated in the midline, subcutaneously and down on to the sternum. The spinal needle is inserted through the bleb of anesthetic solution in a vertical direction and pushed until the sternum is reached. To facilitate the insertion of the biopsy instrument, a small stab incision can be made first. The needle is inserted until contact with the sternum is made, at which stage firm upward pressure is maintained and combined with forward and backward rotation of the needle to force it through the rather soft cortex of the sternabrae. Once the needle is firmly embedded, the stylet is removed and the 20-mL syringe attached. The plunger of the syringe is quickly withdrawn to the 10-mL mark and released. This procedure is repeated two or three times or until blood is seen in the syringe. Do not continue aspiration once an adequate sample has been collected, as this tends to increase the chances of collecting blood rather than bone marrow. When a sample cannot be

obtained, the stylet should be reinserted and the assembly pushed a little deeper. If this is unsuccessful, it may indicate that the needle is located between the cavities of two adjacent sternabrae, in which case the biopsy site must be changed cranially or caudally and the procedure repeated.

Foals. Foals are restrained in lateral recumbency, with assistance of sedation and analgesia as necessary (see Chemical Restraint of the Foal). The extremity of the tuber coxae, which is rectangular in shape is clipped and prepared as described above for sternal collection from the adult. The needle is inserted in the middle of the rectangle, and directed ventromedially and slightly caudally into the wing of the ilium. Collection is as described above for adults.

Although the sample can be placed in anticoagulant, it is often advised to make thin, pull smears directly. This is done by placing a drop of the sample near the edge of a slide, placing a second slide on top of the first, allowing the sample to spread, and then sliding the slides apart. They are then air-dried, fixed in ethanol, and stained. Different stains are used for different purposes (e.g., Wright's stain for morphology, methylene blue for reticulocytes, and Prussian blue for identification of iron granules). If the original sample is to be submitted to the laboratory, clotting should be prevented by aspirating a few drops of an anticoagulant into the needle before carrying out the collection.

Materials for Bone Marrow Biopsy

▶ Biopsy needle: Spinal needle (14–18 gauge 3.5″ [8.75 cm]) or biopsy needle (14–18 gauge)

▶ Clippers (#40 head)

▶ 70% alcohol

▶ Skin antiseptic (e.g., Betadine)

▶ 2% lidocaine hydrochloride, 2% mepivacaine hydrochloride, 5-mL syringe, and 20-gauge needle

▶ 20-mL syringe

▶ Microscope slides

RESULTS. The slide should be scanned at low power (×20 or ×40 objective) to assess cell density and the presence of excess blood contamination. Detailed cell counts are made with a ×100 objective. The sample is evaluated for the presence of abnormal cell types, the ratio of myeloid to erythroid cells (M:E) based on a count of 500 cells, and the number of reticulocytes per 1,000 erythrocytes. The normal M:E ratio ranges from 0.5 to 1.5. Active erythropoiesis is indicated by the number of reticulocytes per 1,000 erythrocytes, exceeding 2%.

R E F E R E N C E

1. Mayhew IG, Rossdale PD: A technique for bone marrow aspiration in foals and adult horses. Equine Vet Ed 1992; 4:96.

A D D I T I O N A L   R E A D I N G S

Jain NC: The horse: Normal hematology with comments on response to disease. In Schalm's Veterinary Hematology, 4th ed., Philadelphia, Lea & Febiger, 1986, p 140.
The Veterinary Clinics of North America, Equine Pract, Clinical Pathology, December, 1995; vol 11.

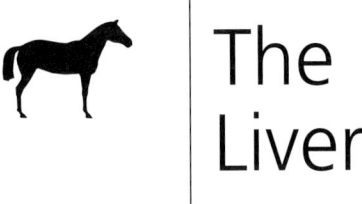

The Liver

14

The liver is difficult to examine because of its location in the cranial abdomen and because obvious malfunction occurs only after the liver has lost approximately two thirds of its functional capacity. Therefore, hepatic failure is seen only when there is extensive damage to the hepatic parenchyma or there is obstruction to biliary drainage. Nevertheless, careful clinical examination and clinicopathological testing with assistance of ultrasonography, laparoscopy, and biopsy allow many, possibly most, lesions to be diagnosed.

MANIFESTATIONS OF DISEASE

The liver has a multitude of functions, including gluconeogenesis; metabolism of ammonia to urea; protein synthesis; metabolism of amino acids, fats, and carbohydrates; production and excretion of bile; conjugation of bilirubin; synthesis of clotting factors; and metabolism of various drugs and toxins. Interference with these processes produces a corresponding variety of clinical signs. Signs related to liver failure involve the central nervous system and result primarily from increased levels of blood ammonia, hypoglycemia, and imbalance of aromatic to branched-chain amino acids. The signs of yawning, circling, head pressing, depression, seizure, and coma are typical of hepatoencephalopathy. Mild liver injury or malfunction occurs in association with some generalized systemic states, such as shock, where the only manifestation of liver disease is the elevation in serum of intrahepatic enzymes and the main clinical signs are related to the primary problem. Other signs include icterus and discoloration of urine (interference with biliary excretion), spontaneous bleeding (interference with production of clotting factors) photosensitization (interference with excretion of phylloerythrin), and weight loss (interference with intermediary metabolism, especially albumin production). Clinical signs will not be evident with mild diffuse injury or with severe but localized lesions, in which cases detection depends on clinicopathological testing.

GENERAL PHYSICAL EXAMINATION

Unless the liver is greatly enlarged or very painful, physical examination of the liver is impossible because of its protected position deep in the cranial abdomen. On rare occasions, an enlarged liver may be detected by percussion caudal to the margins of the rib cage or the sternum. Deep palpation may also, occasionally, elicit a pain response when a lesion such as an abscess is present. As described in the preceding section, liver disease can result in many signs involving other organs, and, accordingly, liver disease is most often diagnosed by inference after noting these signs. Therefore, a thorough examination of the other organ systems is indicated.

SPECIAL DIAGNOSTIC TESTS

Liver Biopsy

A liver biopsy allows microscopic examination of a sample of liver, which is useful to establish the type of lesion that, depending on the lesion and its cause, may or may not have diagnostic or prognostic value. An exact diagnosis is possible where the histological features are typical (e.g., neolasia, pyrrolizidine alkaloid toxicosis), but in other cases a diagnosis is not possible. If the sample is collected as an aspirate, it is suitable only for cytology, but if the architecture is preserved, routine histology is possible.

PROCEDURE. The possibility of an abnormality of coagulation as a result of liver disease, although uncommon, dictates that a coagulation profile be conducted before biopsy. If any coagulation abnormality is detected, a prebiopsy transfusion of fresh serum can be given to supply the missing factors. The usual site for biopsy is in the right 12th intercostal space, just above a line drawn from the tuber coxae to the point of the olecranon (Fig. 14-1).[1] When liver atrophy is present, blind biopsy often is unsuccessful. The accuracy of location can be improved by using ultrasonography, either to localize the liver or to allow biopsy

---

Materials for Liver Biopsy
▸ Biopsy instrument: Tru-Cut Biopsy Needle, Automatic Disposable Temno Needle (Products Group International, Inc., Boulder, CO), or 4″ × 18-gauge needle
▸ Sterile gloves
▸ Hair clippers (#40 clipper head)
▸ Scalpel blade (#15)
▸ Antiseptic detergent (e.g., Betadine, Hibiclens)
▸ 70% alcohol
▸ Local anesthetic solution - 2% Lidocaine hydrochloride, 2% mepivacaine hydrochloride
▸ 10-mL syringe and 20-Gauge × 1.5″ needle
▸ 10% neutral buffered formalin

---

under direct ultrasonographic guidance. Liver biopsy can also be carried out from the left side in the cranial abdomen, but this always requires the use of ultrasound.

Needle Biopsy

For routine biopsy an area about 10 × 10 cm square, centered over the site, is clipped and prepared for sterile biopsy. Local anesthetic is injected subcutaneously and deeper into the muscle layers and the parietal pleura. A small stab incision is made with the scalpel blade, adjacent to the cranial border of the rib to avoid intercostal nerves and vessels. The biopsy needle is inserted slowly through the stab incision until it touches the diaphragm, at which stage it will move as the diaphragm moves during breathing. The needle is then inserted a further 4 cm, which takes it through the diaphragm and into the liver. The sample is collected and placed in 10% buffered formalin. Use of the Tru-Cut and Temno needles is described in Appendix F. If unsuccessful, subsequent attempts can be made at sites dorsal to the originally selected site, but not higher than a line from the tuber coxae to the point of the shoulder. Repeated, blind attempts are contraindicated.

An aspirate is made in an identical fashion, except that a needle and syringe are used. When the needle has been positioned in the liver, negative pressure is applied by withdrawing the plunger of the syringe. The negative pressure should be released before the needle is withdrawn to avoid aspiration of other tissues or air, which will disrupt the liver sample. A smear should be prepared from the sample.

Ultrasonographic-Assisted, or Guided, Biopsy

With ultrasonographic-assisted biopsy the liver is first localized by ultrasonography and its depth determined by using the freeze-frame facility and measuring calipers. Then, after preparing the skin for sterile biopsy and injecting an anesthetic, the sample is collected with the biopsy needle, as described. For ultrasonically guided biopsy the probe must be sterile, and after localization of the liver the biopsy needle is inserted through the biopsy guide on the ultrasound probe to the appropriate depth, under direct vision, and the sample collected as described.[2]

RESULTS. As stated, a specific diagnosis can often be made from the biopsy when it exhibits

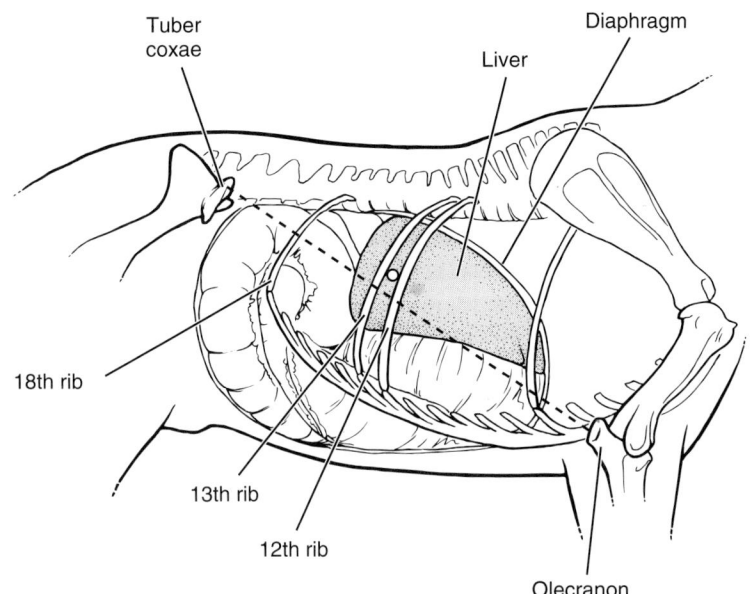

Tuber coxae

Liver

Diaphragm

18th rib

13th rib

12th rib

Olecranon

▶ **FIGURE 14–1**
Site for percutaneous liver biopsy.

changes pathognomonic for a specific condition. Most often, this is not possible, and the pathology report is limited to a description of the findings.

COMPLICATIONS. Although lung, or a section of the gastrointestinal tract, are frequently penetrated by the biopsy needle, there is rarely any significant sequelae. If it is known that the bowel has been entered, prophylactic antibiotics can be given, although the need for this has not been established definitely. Postbiopsy bleeding is a potential, but relatively, uncommon hazard. Prebiopsy testing of coagulation can detect horses in which bleeding is likely, and prophylactic serum transfusion can be used if indicated.

Ultrasonography

Ultrasonography of the liver is useful for selecting a biopsy site and evaluating parenchyma and liver size.

PROCEDURE. The liver can be imaged from the left and right sides.[1] In young horses imaging is carried out from the right side in the 6th to 15th intercostal spaces and ventral to the lung. Older horses tend to have atrophy of the right lobe of the liver, and imaging from the right is difficult or impossible. From the left side imaging is usually possible in the 7th to 9th intercostal space in horses of all ages. The skin is prepared by clipping the hair and applying coupling gel to the skin and the probe.

RESULTS. The liver is of a uniform density and contains anechoic regions representing the hepatic and portal vessels, with the walls of the latter being more echogenic (Fig. 14-2). The normal biliary system is usually invisible. Focal lesions with increased echogenicity suggest chronic abscessation or primary neoplasia, whereas those that are hypoechoic to anechoic are likely to be cysts, hematomata, or new abscesses. A diffuse increase in echogenicity suggests inflammation, fibrosis, or fatty infiltration (Fig. 14-3A). Cholelithiasis is characterized, typically, by distension of bile ducts, hepatomegaly, and hyperechoic regions within the ducts, often with an acoustic shadow (Figure 14-3B). Distension of bile ducts indicates cholestasis, but not necessarily cholelithiasis. It is difficult to differentiate between blood vessel and distended bile ducts, although use of the Doppler technique can help differentiation by detecting flow in the blood vessels.[3]

Materials for Ultrasonography

▶ Ultrasound machine
▶ Transducer: Sector (preferred) or linear (3.0 or 5.0 MHz)
▶ Clippers #40 clipper head
▶ Ultrasound coupling gel

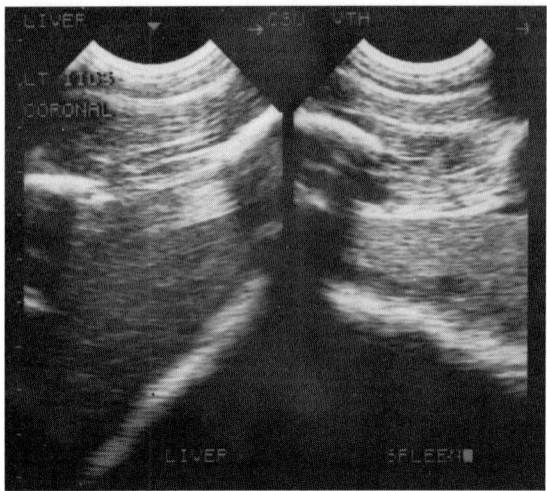

▶ **FIGURE 14–2**

Dual stored ultrasonograms, made with a 3-MHz transducer, to compare the relative echogenicities of the left liver and spleen in a normal horse. The liver parenchyma is usually less echogenic than the spleen. (Courtesy R. H. Wrigley.)

Clinicopathological Examination

Clinicopathological examination is an integral component of liver diagnosis and consists of liver function tests, and serum levels of hepatic enzymes, bile salts, ammonia, glucose, bilirubin, and clotting factors.[1] Elevations in white blood cells may be seen in association with biliary sepsis or abscessation.

The various enzymes can be used to differentiate between active and chronic disease, as well as between biliary and hepatocellular disease. Numerous enzymes can be measured, including gamma glutamyl transferase (GGT), aspartate amino transferase (AST), sorbitol dehydrogenase (SDH), ornithine carbamyl transferase (OCT), and alkaline phosphatase (AP). Gamma glutamyl transferase is the most useful screening enzyme because, although it is produced by biliary epithelium and is elevated in cases of biliary disease, it also rises with heptocellular injury. In addition to GGT, AP is elevated by cholestasis. Enzymes elevated by active hepatocellular injury include AST, OCT and SDH, although only SDH and OCT are specific for liver. Because of technical difficulties measuring SDH, and the short serum half-life of SDH and OCT, these two enzymes are not used routinely, although the short half-lives render them useful for monitoring the ongoing state of liver injury. Isoenzyme 5 of lactic dehydrogenase (LDH$_5$), is a useful alternative to SDH as it has a similar half life and is easier to measure. As the enzymes AST and LDH$_5$ also occur in muscle, the muscle-specific enzyme creatine kinase is often used to help differentiate between hepatic and muscle disease. Normal values are presented in Table 14–1.

Bile salts are sensitive indicators of biliary obstruction as well as hepatic disease. Failure to

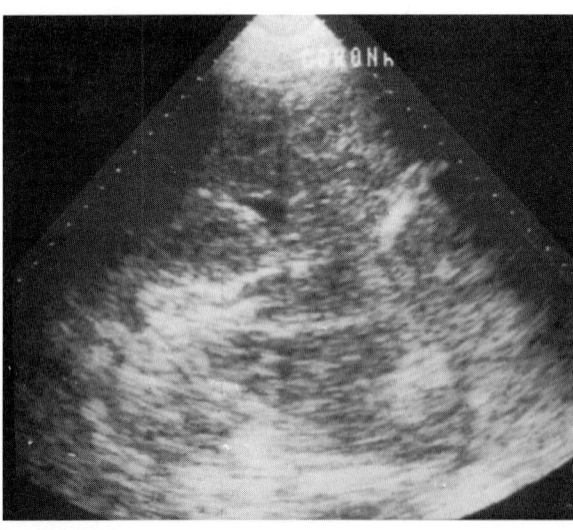

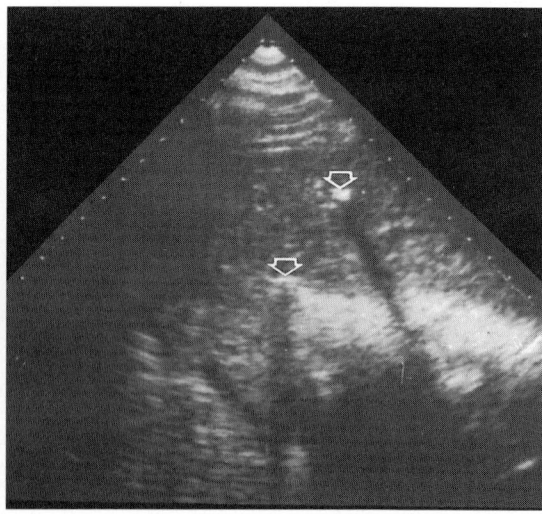

A   B

▶ **FIGURE 14–3**

Ultrasonograms of some liver lesions. **A.** Liver fibrosis and necrosis. Dorsal intercostal ultrasonogram of the right liver made with a 3-MHz sector transducer. The liver is enlarged and shows variable hyperechoic parenchyma. (Courtesy R. H. Wrigley.) **B.** Cholelithiasis and cholangiohepatitis. Dorsal intercostal ultrasonogram of the right liver made with a 3-MHz sector transducer. There are multiple hyperechoic foci *(arrows)* with far field shadowing in a variably echogenic liver parenchyma. (Courtesy R. H. Wrigley.)

TABLE 14-1

REFERENCE VALUES FOR SOME PARAMETERS USED
FOR EVALUATING LIVER FUNCTION AND DISEASE

Parameter	Reference Range (mean ± 2 SD)
Bilirubin, total (μmol/L)	4–100
Bilirubin, unconjugated (μmol/L)	4–90
Bilirubin, conjugated (μmol/L)	0–10
Protein (g/L)	58–76
Albumin (g/L)	28–38
Globulins (g/L)	26–40
Urea (mmol/L)	3.6–8.9
Aspartate aminotransferase (IU/L)	150–400
Alkaline phosphatase (IU/L)	50–250
Creatine phosphokinase (IU/L)	50–400
Lactate dehydrogenase (IU/L)	50–400
Triglycerides (mmol/L)	0.1–0.9
Gamma glutamyl transferase (IU/L)	<30
Sorbitol dehydrogenase (IU/L)	0.5–2.0
Bile salts (μmol/L)	<20

Source: Data are reference values used in the Central Veterinary Diagnostic Laboratory, Mt. Waverley, Melbourne, Australia. (Courtesy Dr. P. M. Lording.)

convert ammonia to urea causes an elevation in blood ammonia and often a decrease in blood urea nitrogen. The hyperlipemia syndrome is associated with elevation of triglycerides and a milky opalescent plasma. Hepatic disease, especially cholestasis, produces an elevation in plasma bilirubin, especially the unconjugated (indirect) fraction. A reduction in synthesis of protein produces low values for plasma fibrinogen and prolongation of indicators of coagulation.

The sulfobromophthalein (BSP) and indocyanine clearance tests are useful for assessing the functional capacity of the liver. The BSP clearance test is based on measuring the ability of the liver to excrete, or clear, a dose of BSP, measured against time. The test consists of taking a pretest blood sample before administering 1 g of BSP into a jugular vein, and then taking subsequent blood samples from the opposite jugular vein at 3-, 5-, 7-, and 9-minute intervals after the test dose. The concentration of BSP in each sample is measured and the result graphed against time. The half life, or time taken to clear half of the drug, should be approximately 4.5 minutes, with a longer half-life indicating a reduction in function.

REFERENCES

1. Divers TJ: Hepatic disease. *In* Robinson NE (ed), Current Therapy in Equine Medicine, 3rd ed. Philadelphia, Saunders, 1990, p 253.
2. Modransky PD: Ultrasound-guided renal and hepatic biopsy technique. Vet Clin North Am Equine Pract 1986; 2:115.
3. Traub-Dargatz JL: Biliary disorders. *In* Robinson NE (ed), Current Therapy in Equine Medicine, 3rd ed. Philadelphia, Saunders, 1990, p 259.

ADDITIONAL READINGS

Johnston JK, Divers TJ, Reef VB, et al: Cholelithiasis in horses: Ten cases (1982–1986). J Am Vet Med Assoc 1989; 194:405.
Rantanen NW: Diseases of the liver. Vet Clin North Am Equine Pract 1986; 2:105.

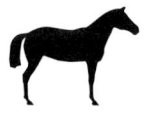

The Mammary Gland

15

The mammary gland is not very often affected by disease, and its relatively protected location often leads to its being omitted from the clinical examination. It should be remembered that the gland consists of left and right halves with a teat for each side and, further, that each side is also divided into two lobes, each with a separate teat cistern and openings onto the teat. There are, therefore, two and occasionally more openings in the teat (Fig. 15-1).

GENERAL PHYSICAL EXAMINATION

Visual Examination

The normal gland is always symmetrical, being small in mares that have not had a foal, and enlarging after the first lactation. Reasons for abnormal enlargement include infection (mastitis, abscess), trauma, and neoplasia. Physiological enlargement occurs prior to parturition and is maintained during lactation. The gland begins to enlarge approximately 3 to 4 weeks before parturition, although the teats tend to remain empty until the last few hours. Many mares, especially when having their first foal, will exhibit edema of the gland and surrounding tissues. The preparturient secretion is at first thick, sticky, and has an amber color, becoming less viscid and more like milk as parturition approaches. When parturition is iminent, the sticky amber fluid tends to hang in strands from the teat orifices, a process known as "waxing."

Palpation

To palpate the mammary gland the clinician should stand adjacent to the horse's side, an arm's length from the gland. This will reduce the possibility of being kicked. If the mare is fractious, chemical and physical restraint are indicated. In addition to sedation and a twitch, a simple procedure is to hold the ipsilateral foreleg off the ground in order to make kicking difficult. When examining from the left side, the usual technique, the left hand is placed over the horse's back and the right hand is placed on the flank and then moved carefully and slowly down and on to the mammary gland. Resentment is shown by crouching, moving away, or by kicking. If resentment is detected, the procedure should be stopped and the mare reassured before further attempts are made. Most mares will allow an examination to be conducted. The gland is palpated to detect localized swelling, pain, temperature elevation, and firmness. When pain is present, there is often an ipsilateral hindlimb lameness.

Collection of Mammary Gland Secretions

Although mares are often milked to obtain milk or colostrum for foals, mammary secretions are also required for bacteriological evaluation and electrolyte status.

PROCEDURE. Although milk is often seen running freely from the gland just before parturition or when milk "let down" has been stimulated by the foal, collection of a sample usually requires

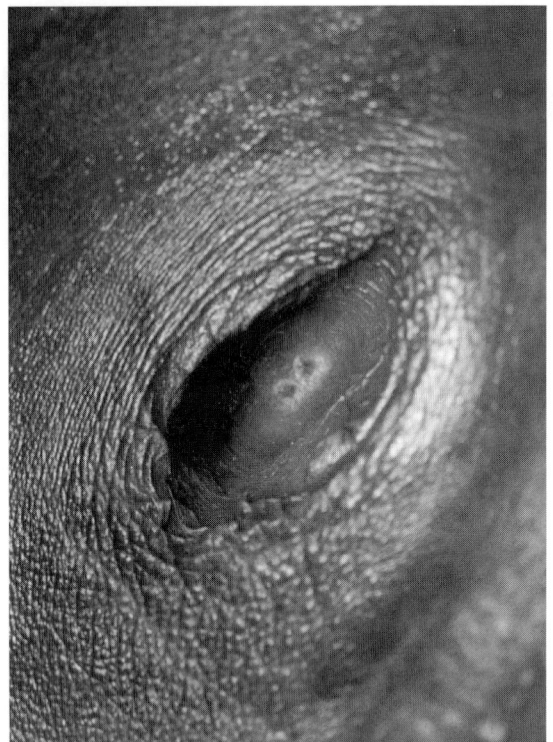

▶ FIGURE 15-1

Teat showing the two openings.

active participation by the clinician (Fig. 15-2). This is done by using the thumb and first finger to strip the fluid out of the teat and into a container. When there is thick purulent material present, the stripping action must often be commenced above the teat and it may even be necessary to gently squeeze the gland as well. When the gland is infected or inflamed, the process may be painful, thus requiring gentle and careful technique.

If the sample is to be submitted for culture and sensitivity testing, the end of the teat should be cleaned and rubbed with a swab containing an antiseptic (e.g., Betadine) and a sterile container used to collect it. The sample is submitted as described in Appendix C. For cytological examination of milk or other discharge, a few drops of the sample are placed on a slide, smeared, fixed in alcohol, and stained (e.g., Quik-diff, trichrome[1]). A Gram stain can be used to identify Gram-positive or -negative organisms and thereby help select an antibiotic. If electrolytes are to be evaluated, there is no need for sterility, and a clean container is suitable. Although electrolytes can be measured in the laboratory, a number of simple commercial tests will provide rapid approximate results. Cal-

cium content can be assessed by color change (Predict-A-Foal, Animal Healthcare Products, Vernon, CA). Calcium and magnesium content can be evaluated with water hardness test strips (Merchoquant Water Hardness Test Strip No. 10 025; E. Merck, Postfach 4119, 6100 Darmstadt, West Germany). Immunoglobulin G content can be estimated by measuring specific gravity with a modified hydrometer.

RESULTS

Cytology. The cytology of the normal gland depends on the physiological condition at the time of collection and the type of stain. Findings based on the Pollack trichrome, Sano modification are as follows:[2]

- *Colostrum* (collected within 12 hours of parturition). Granular or homogenous protein background with karyorrhectic debris and red-purple spheres and, occasionally, clear lipid vacuoles and secretory cells
- *Lactational milk.* Acellular, except for an occasional neutrophil, with greenish-brown protein background
- *Postweaning milk.* The involuting gland is characterized by vacuolated macrophages, which may contain yellow or brown vacuoles or granular material. As involution continues, the macrophages diminish in number, possibly to be replaced by a variable collection of single or grouped irregular macrophages, lymphocytelike cells, a few neutrophils, and casts of secretions

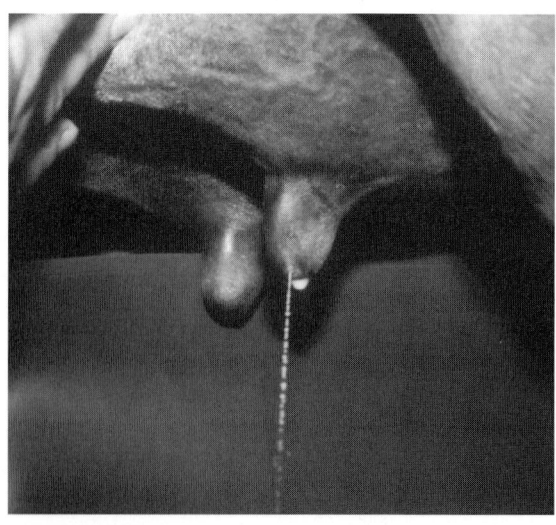

▶ FIGURE 15-2

Milk running freely from the mammary gland of a lactating mare.

- *Mastitis.* When mastitis is present, there are increased number of neutrophils, degenerated and nondegenerated, debris, and other unidentifiable cells. Bacteria are not always present, but those likely to be identified include beta-hemolytic *Streptoccocus* spp., *Strep. zooepidemicus, Escherichia coli,* or *Klebsiella* spp.[3,4] Anaerobic bacteria appear to have little significance in equine mastitis.[4]

Chemistry: Electrolyte Content. The electrolyte content of colostrum changes significantly in the last days of pregnancy and, as a result, can be used to help predict when parturition will occur. This may be of interest for management reasons, but it is mainly used when parturition is to be induced. In the weeks prior to foaling, electrolyte values are as follows: sodium (125–135 mEq/L [mmol/L]); potassium (7–12 mEq/L [mmol/L]); calcium (2 mmol/L [8mg/dl]). Specific gravity is 1.06. Within 48 hours of parturition sodium decreases to <30 mmol/L, potassium increases to >30 mmol/L, and calcium increases to 10 mg/dl (40 mmol/dl).

Chemistry: Immunoglobulin Content. There is a breed difference in colostral immunoglobin G (IgG) content, as well as a considerable difference among individuals of the same breed. The levels of colostral IgG decline precipitously in the first few hours after parturition, for example, in one study, from $9{,}691 \pm$ SEM 1.639 to 1,000 mg/dl in 19.1 hours for Arabians, and from $4{,}608 \pm$ SEM 2,138 to 1,000 mg/dl in 8.9 hours for Thoroughbreds.[5] The contribution of different immunoglobulins in a population of Standardbreds is as follows (mean $\pm$ SD):[6] IgG($8{,}911.9 \pm 6{,}282.2$ mg/dl), IgM (122.9 ± 77.3 mg/dl), IgA ($957 \pm 1{,}088.1$ mg/dl), for a total of $10{,}022.4 \pm 6{,}957.9$ mg/dl.

R E F E R E N C E S

1. Freeman KP, Carroll B: Use of wet-fixed, trichrome-stained cytologic specimens in private equine practice. Compend Contin Ed 1989; 11:485.
2. Freeman KP, Roszel JF, Slusher SH, et al: Cytologic features of equine mammary fluids: Normal and abnormal. Compend Contin Ed 1988; 10:1090.
3. McCue P, Wilson W: Equine mastitis–A review of 28 cases. Equine Vet J 1989; 21:351.
4. Perkins NR, Threlfall WR: Mastitis in the mare. Equine Vet Ed 1993; 5:192.
5. Pearson RC, Hallowell AL, Bayly WM, et al: Times of disappearance of colostral IgG in the mare. Am J Vet Res 1984; 45:186.
6. Kohn CW, Knight D, Hueston W, et al: Colostral and serum IgG, IgA, and IgM concentrations in Standardbred mares and their foals at parturition. J Am Vet Med Assoc 1989; 195:64.

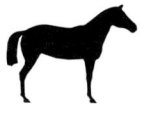 # Endoscopic Instrumentation

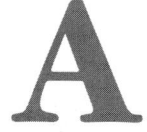

Endoscopy has become an indispensable part of the clinician's armamentarium. As the instruments are expensive and easily damaged by improper use and improper methods of disinfection, it is important that the people who use and prepare them be familiar with their correct management. Endoscopes can be divided into rigid and flexible types. Rigid endoscopes are used commonly for a variety of tasks, including arthroscopy and laparoscopy, and the flexible instruments are used primarily in the respiratory, gastrointestinal, and urinary tracts.

RIGID ENDOSCOPES

The older type of rigid instrument, used predominantly for examination of the upper respiratory tract and uterus, consists of a stiff tubular section with an eye piece at one end and a light source, a bulb, at the other (Fig. A-1). The image is conducted by prisms located in the instrument. Power for the bulb is supplied by a battery pack connected through a flexible lead. The newer rigid endoscopes, used for laparoscopy and arthroscopy, have a similar construction, but the light source (known as a cold light) is located in a separate apparatus, from which light is conducted to the endoscope with optical fibers (Fig. A-2). The main disadvantage of this system is that its rigidity means it is limited to use in regions where the object to be examined is in direct line with the viewer. Rigidity is an advantage for arthroscopy. The image is usually of very high quality.

FLEXIBLE ENDOSCOPES

Fiber-optic Endoscopes

The flexible fiber-optic endoscope overcomes most of the disadvantages of the rigid instrument in that its flexibility allows it to be inserted through almost any suitable orifice and into a number of internal organs. Additional properties are that the endoscopes come in a large number of different lengths, have a distal tip that can be manually deflected, and contains biopsy and air and flushing channels (Fig. A-3). Although only one person at a time can view the image with the basic fiber-optic instrument, this can be remedied by using a second, flexible extension cable for a second viewer, or, alternatively, a video camera can be attached to allow the image to be displayed on a monitor. The modern endoscope has image guide (IG) and light guide (LG) fiber bundles. The LG bundle transmits light from the cold light source to the distal end of the endoscope where it illuminates the object in view. The IG bundle transmits the image back to the viewer, through fibers that must occupy the same relative positions at the distal and proximal ends of the instrument, in order to avoid image distortion. Larger endoscopes have more fibers in the IG bundle, which produces a better image. Because an image is formed by adding many fibers, a broken fiber shows up as a pinhead-size black spot in the picture (i.e., there is no image at the site occupied by the broken fiber). In addition to the fibers, there is a lens system that produces wide-angle illumination from the LG bundle, an

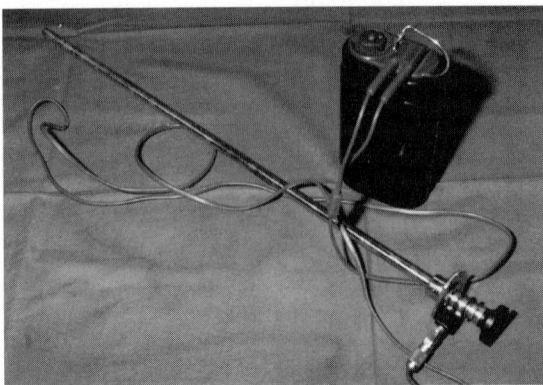

▶ **FIGURE A-1**

A rigid endoscope.

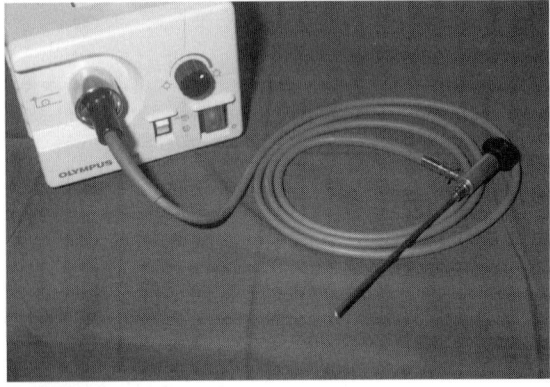

▶ **FIGURE A-2**

Arthroscope and cold light source.

objective lens that focuses the image on to the IG bundle, and the ocular lens, located in the head, for final magnification of the image.

The cold light source is a halogen or xenon lamp that comes in a unit with an air and water pump, although not all units offer a choice of either lamp. The xenon lamp is brighter than the halogen lamp.

Hard copy images can be obtained with endoscope-specific cameras, 35-mm single-lens reflex (SLR), or Polaroid cameras, as well as by using a video camera. Most veterinary pictures are probably taken with a 35-mm SLR camera using an adapter for attachment to the endoscope. The adapter usually has contacts that allow communication between camera and light source to control flash and exposure. When using a xenon lamp daylight film is required, and for the halogen light it should be tungsten film.

Videoendoscope

The second form of flexible endoscope is the videoendoscope, in which the image is seen on a video monitor and illumination, imaging, and processing are under electronic control (Fig. A–4). The light comes from a separately housed 300-W xenon lamp. Light is passed through a rotating color wheel to produce pulses of red, green, and blue that are transmitted down optical fibers to illuminate the object. The illuminated image is transmitted through an objective lens and focused onto a charge-coupled device (CCD) that transmits a black-and-white image back to the central processor, which then reconstitutes a color image on the video monitor. The image can

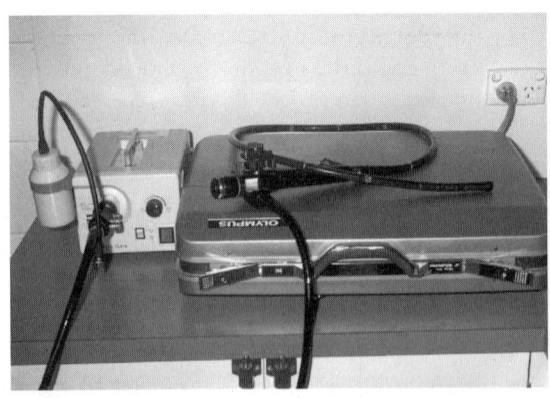

A

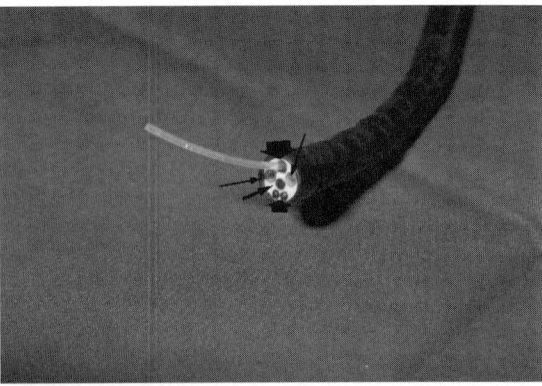

B

▶ **FIGURE A-3**

A. Flexible fiber-optic endoscope with cold light source. **B.** Distal end of a flexible endoscope showing the illumination lenses of the light guide bundles *(long thin arrows)*, the objective lens of the image guide bundle *(long thick arrow)*, the air/water nozzle *(small fat arrow)*, and biopsy channel *(large thick arrow)*.

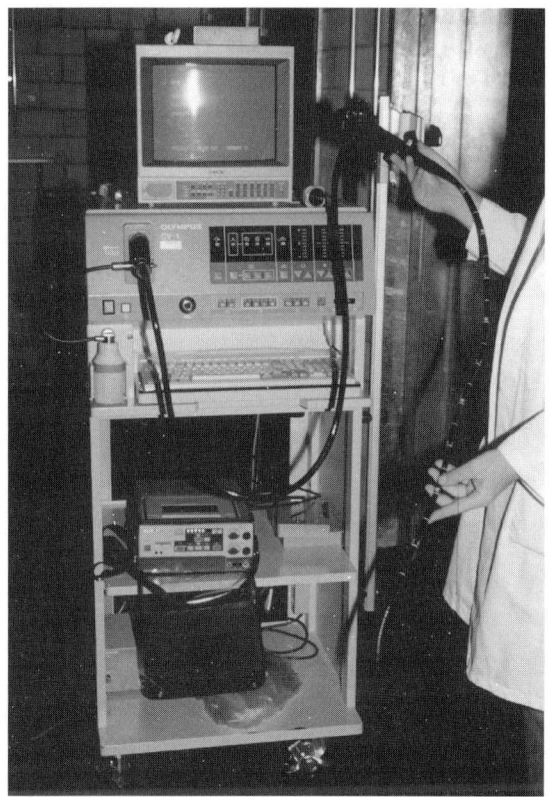

▶ **FIGURE A–4**

Videoendoscope with central video processor, keyboard, and video recorder. (Courtesy, Austvet Pty. Ltd., Melbourne, Australia.)

be stored on tape, disc, and in still format. A color CCD also exists, in which an intermediate black-and-white image is bypassed. The main advantage of the videoendoscope is its superior image quality. Its main disadvantages are its relative lack of portability and its significantly higher cost.

Endoscopic Accessories

Numerous biopsy instruments are available, although their small size renders them unsuitable for the majority of veterinary work. Cytology brushes also are available for obtaining material for cytological and microbiological evaluation. Other accessories include facilities for electrosurgery, as well as forceps and baskets for removing foreign bodies and calculi.

Care and Use of Flexible Endoscopes

The value of the instrument dictates that great care be taken during use. Damage to the endo-

scope takes several forms, including breakage of the optical fibers, disruption of the watertight seal of the casing, and damage to or breakage of the cables controlling movement of the distal tip. Under normal circumstances, loss of fibers usually is a gradual process that can be monitored by regularly counting the number of black spots in the image. Disruption of the casing allows water to enter, which causes fogging of the image that cannot be removed by adjusting the focus ring. Manipulation of the controls should always produce immediate and appropriate deflection of the distal tip. Failure to do this indicates damage or breakage of the cables. To avoid cable damage, the tip should never be manually deflected, and full deflection should be used only when indicated. General protection is afforded by always transporting the endoscope in its padded case and ensuring that the patient is adequately restrained when it is in use.

Although the instruments can be sterilized, this is not often required. The following is a simple, and feasible, system of cleaning between horses:

- Wipe the casing with a cloth dampened with a dilute solution of surgical soap (e.g., 20% Hibiclens).
- Clean the distal end with the same solution if mucus, blood, or other debris have become lodged there.
- Aspirate some of the solution through the instrument by using the suction device, or flush it through manually by syringe.
- Repeat the above with a solution of alcohol
- Ensure that all fluid is expelled from the air/water channel by disconnecting the flushing bottle and then activating the flush control while holding a finger over the connector from which the flushing bottle was disconnected.
- Dry the channel by aspirating air through it.
- Ideally, the instrument should be stored by hanging it in a cupboard.

Obviously, it is not feasible to use this procedure between every patient when a number of horses must be examined in quick succession. In this circumstance, it is recommended that the first three steps be carried out and the more complete procedure carried out before the instrument is stored. The manufacturers' brochures contain instructions for regular maintenance that should be performed from time to time.

Sterilization is possible, but the manufacturers' brochures must be read for specific details. Disinfectants include ethylene oxide gas and glutaraldehyde solution, the former being a slow method and the latter requiring only a few minutes. Some endoscopes can be fully immersed in the disinfecting solution, but others cannot and disinfection must be achieved by a combination of partial immersion and wiping with a cloth.

R E A D I N G

1. Lamar AM: Standard fiberoptic equipment and its care. *In* Traub-Dargatz JL, Brown CM (eds), Equine Endoscopy. St Louis, Mosby, 1990, ch 1, p 1.

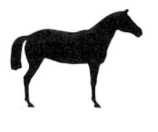

Ultrasonography

Dr. Robert H. Wrigley

B

Sound waves are present when a material experiences alternately compression and rarefaction, with a sequence of compression and rarefaction being equal to one cycle. The frequency of an ultrasound wave is measured in hertz, with 1 hertz (Hz) equalling one cycle per second, and the distance between identical points in successive cycles is equal to the wavelength:

Wavelength = Velocity (m/s)/Frequency (Hz)

When the sound frequency exceeds the audible human range, it is regarded as *ultrasound.* Frequencies between 2 and 10,000,000 Hz (2–10 MHz) are used for medical imaging. The pulses of ultrasound are produced by applying intermittent electrical pulses to crystals (piezoelectric material) that convert the electrical energy into a series of corresponding mechanical pulses. The crystals are mounted onto a transducer to provide mechanical rigidity and an efficient method to transmit the ultrasound to and from tissues.

The velocity of sound in tissues is very similar for the various organs and fluid cavities. The average velocity for soft tissue is 1,540 m/s. In compact bone the velocity increases. In air and gas the velocity decreases very significantly. As the ultrasound wave passes through a medium, the intensity is rapidly attenuated. The energy is converted to heat. High-output ultrasound therapy machines are used to generate tissue heating for physical therapy of injured tissues.

Small clusters of cells with diameters less than the wavelength cause scattering in all directions. Absorption and scatter contribute to most of the energy loss. As a result of the foregoing, ultrasound is attenuated to different degrees by different tissues, some examples being 1.05, 1.8, 0.18, and 0.63 dB/cm/MHz for liver, muscle, blood, and fat, respectively. Higher-frequency sound is more rapidly attenuated than lower-frequency sound. Also, the output power of diagnostic ultrasound machines is strictly controlled to prevent the likelihood of injury to the patient. This, combined with the attenuation of the ultrasound beam, sets practical limits to the depth of displayed tissues. Low-frequency transducers (2–3 MHz) can image about 25 cm deep. High-frequency transducers (7 MHz) will image only 3 to 5 cm deep.

When a pulse of ultrasound traverses a boundary where there is a change in tissue density or interface between different tissues, sound reflection occurs, resulting in an echo. If the reflected echo is detected by the transducer, then reconversion into electrical pulses occurs and is processed to produce a gray-scale image. The strength of the reflection is proportional to the square of the difference in acoustic impedance across the tissues. If the surface is large with respect to the wavelength, then reflection is mirrorlike, or specular. Such echoes are reflected in an equal and opposite angle to the acoustic interface. So it is important for the ultrasonographer to direct the sound beam perpendicular to specular reflecting boundaries to obtain consistent echo patterns. If the interface is small in relation to the wavelength, then scatter occurs in all directions. A loud echo is seen as a white image, weaker echoes as varying levels of gray, and no echo as a black region. The intensity represents the echogenicity of the interface, with bone and gas producing a hyperechoic region in the image, and, conversely, hypoechogenic tissue (e.g., granulation tissue) producing a hypoechoic image. An absence of echoes produces a black or anechoic image. Typically, modern scanners can display 64 to 128 levels of gray, and more expensive machines use 256 shades of gray.

A diagnostic ultrasound machine consists of multiple electronic components to control the transducer, detect and amplify returning echoes, calculate the location of the position of the echo source, and display the information on a video monitor. Plugs are usually provided to allow for exchange of transducers. Accessories include a mobile cart or carry pack and various recording devices (Polaroid camera, videotape recorder, multiformat camera, video printer). Additional specialized components include simultaneous display of an electrocardiographic trace, biopsy guide, and other displays including motion (M) mode and Doppler displays.

The ultrasound image consists of a cross-sectional view (i.e., slice of the tissue), which is continually reinforced as each echo is collected and processed. The image can be displayed with tissue depth on the x axis and the intensity of the echo on the y axis modulated with respect to echo amplitude represented as brightness ("B" mode) spots (Fig. B-1). Calculation of depth position is based on the time delay of returning echoes. A further variation, "M" (movement) mode, is obtained by placing the "B" mode tracing on the y axis and sweeping it across the display so that time is recorded on the x axis as another dimension. The introduction of time allows motion of tissue to be recorded, which is extremely useful to evaluate cardiac movement.

The resolution of the image depends on a multitude of factors. Small and increasing numbers of crystals under higher levels of computer control often lead to higher-resolution images. The ultrasound beam is focused to enhance resolution, and the best resolution is in the focal zone. The structure of interest should be in this zone. Less expensive machines may have only one focus depth. The connection of additional transducers would enable the election of an alternate focal depth. Multiple crystal transducers with higher-level computer control can allow the ultrasonographer to vary the focal depth and best optimize the resolution for each patient. Improved resolution also occurs with increasing transducer frequency. So higher-frequency transducers (7 MHz) are needed to obtain diagnostic information on small parts such as tendons.

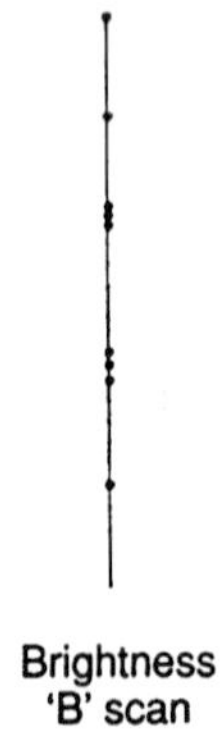

TYPES OF TRANSDUCERS

Sector Transducers

The sector transducer consists of one or more crystals mounted on a rotating wheel or rocking pivot with each pulsing at a set time to produce divergent series of pulses and a pie-shaped image (Fig. B-2A). Crystals of different frequencies can be mounted to allow a choice of frequency and focal depth within the one head. Alternately, a single crystal can be installed and made to oscillate through the sector angle at various speeds to vary the frame rate (Fig. B-2B). The transducer contains fluid to transfer the sound wave through the window in contact with the patient. The main advantages of sector transducers include a small region of contact ("footprint") with tissue, good image quality in the focal zone, ability to image dynamic structures, and good portrayal of deeper structures. Disadvantages include poor near-field resolution, near-field artifacts, mechanical failure, and fragility.

Linear Array Transducers

A linear array transducer is a rectangular structure that contains a series of thin strips of piezoelectric material arranged transversely. The number of elements varies from 64 to 256, and each element participates individually in transmission and reception. The pulse emitted from each element is parallel with all the others (Fig. B-3A). If the complement of elements is divided into sections consisting of an adjacent group of elements that are interconnected, an image can be obtained by activating each group separately in a chosen sequence (Fig. B-3B). As each group is activated, the active beam moves along the probe to form a rectangular image. The manner in which the switching of elements is achieved is complex,

▶ **FIGURE B-1**

A brightness "B" scan. (From Bentley A, Dyson S: Practical ultrasound physics. How to make optimal use of your machine. Equine Vet Educat 1991; 3:228. Reprinted with permission.)

Brightness 'B' scan

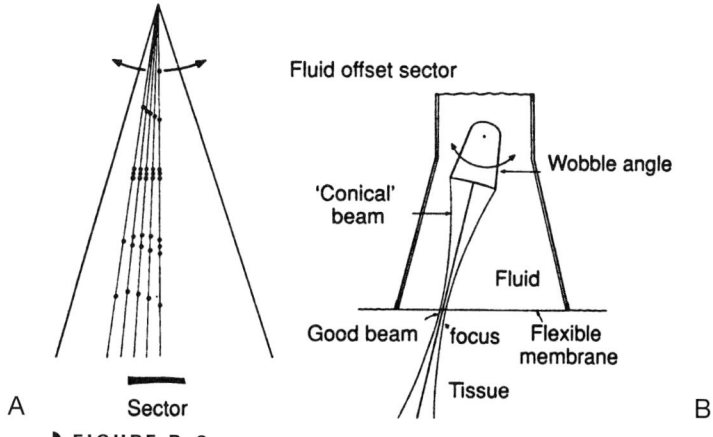

▶ FIGURE B-2

Sector scanner. **A.** Formation of a sector image. **B.** Sector transducer using a single crystal element that is made to oscillate or "wobble" through a specified sector angle. (From Bentley A, Dyson S: Practical ultrasound physics. How to make optimal use of your machine. Equine Vet Educat 1991; 3:228. Reprinted with permission.)

and in more expensive machines, with electronic switching, there is better depth of field and focal length control. Simultaneous multiple frequency images can also be performed to obtain the highest overall resolution. The main disadvantage of linear array transducers is that they require a large area of tissue contact. Excellent images of tendons, uterus, and adjacent organs can be achieved.

Convex Transducers

Convex transducers are linear array transducers modified by arranging the elements so that they lie in a curved path along the length of the probe, thus producing a divergent series of pulses similar to a sector transducer (Fig. B-4). Their advantage over a linear array system is that a larger area can be imaged in deeper regions because of the diverging emissions. Convex transducers

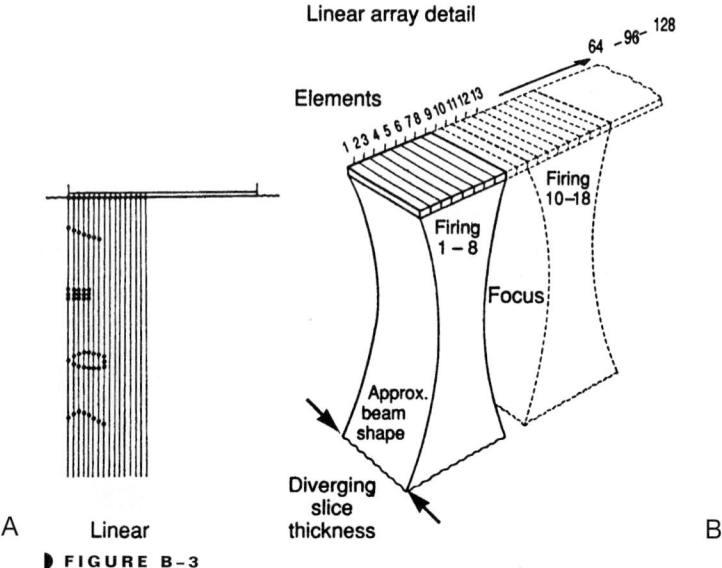

▶ FIGURE B-3

Linear array transducer. **A.** Formation of a linear image. **B.** Linear array detail. (From Bentley A, Dyson S: Practical ultrasound physics. How to make optimal use of your machine. Equine Vet Educat 1991; 3:228. Reprinted with permission.)

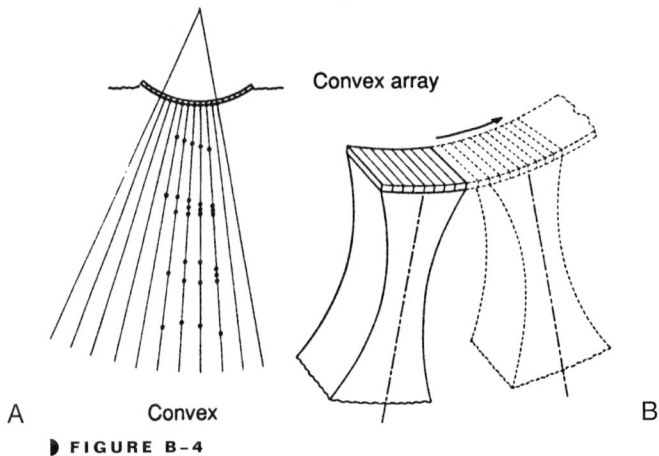

▶ **FIGURE B-4**

Convex transducer. **A.** Formation of a convex image. **B.** Convex array detail. (From Bentley A, Dyson S: Practical ultrasound physics. How to make optimal use of your machine. Equine Vet Educat 1991; 3:228. Reprinted with permission.)

require a larger contact area than sector transducers. Focal zone adjustment and simultaneous multiple frequency image can enable high-resolution imaging.

Phased Array Transducers

A phased array transducer is another form of short linear array with a complex pulsing sequence for 64 or 128 elements. The system produces a sector display by varying the angle of the ultrasound beam. It has special application for cardiac imaging.

STANDOFF MATERIALS

Many sector transducers have a focal zone set at a distance from the transducer. This, combined with the small superficial image display, results in poor near-field resolution. To circumvent this problem, the focal zone can be brought closer to the skin surface by inserting a sound-conducting spacer between the skin and the transducer. The spacer, or "standoff" includes materials such as silicon pads, saline-filled bags, and a variety of proprietary products. The standoff is placed between the transducer head and the skin or, alternately, can be an integral part of the transducer head (fluid offset) and contained by a membrane on the surface used for tissue contact. Depending on its design, standoff materials can be attached manually to the limb, the transducer, or held in place. In addition to improving near-field

resolution, the standoff, because of its flexible surface, improves contact between skin and transducer, especially when the surface is curved or irregular. A selection of standoffs and transducers is shown in Figure B-5.

SETTING THE SCANNER'S CONTROLS

Monitor Brightness

The brightness should be adjusted so that the background lines on the monitor are just visible in normal light. This setting adjusts the black level of

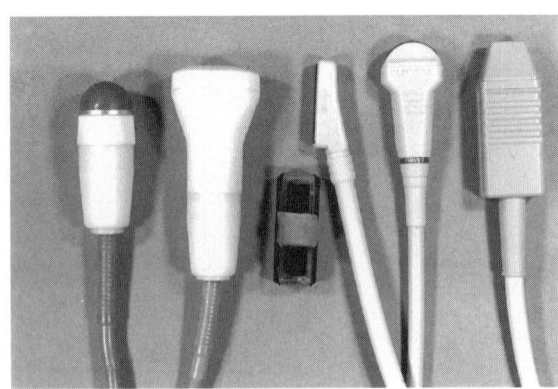

▶ **FIGURE B-5**

Comparative shapes and sizes of commonly used transducers. From left to right: Mechanical sector; mechanical sector with built-in fluid offset (standoff) suitable for tendon scanning; linear array transducer and detachable silicone standoff pad; convex transducer; and phased array transducer.

the image, which ensures that low-level echoes are not lost. If the monitor is too bright, low-level echoes are lost in the bright background and stronger echoes are unfocused and coalesce to full white. Readjustment will be necessary when the machine is moved into bright sunlight or a darkened room.

Monitor Contrast

The contrast should be adjusted so that the brightest echoes are white and in sharp focus.

Gain or Sensitivity

The control adjusts the overall sensitivity of the system. This needs to be continually fine-tuned during each examination. If too high, the image is compromised by the background "noise" that masks low-level echoes and makes the image too white. If too low, specular echoes will be more obvious and nonspecular echoes will disappear.

Slope/Time Gain Compensation or Far and Near Gain

These controls are used to balance the brightness of the top and bottom of the image by compensating for the absorption of ultrasound as tissue depth increases. The individual gain controls should be adjusted to lower the sensitivity for superficial regions and to increase it for echoes from deeper tissues. The relationship between gain levels for different tissue depths is known as the slope or time gain compensation (TGC). The TGC alters the amplitude of the returning echoes depending on the delay time of their arrival, with later arriving echoes from deeper objects being amplified to a greater degree.

Output/Power

This control adjusts the power output from the transducer and helps determine the brightness of the image. Power should be kept as low as possible consistent with ability to recognize low-level echoes. Not all machines allow output power levels to be adjusted.

Display Range/Depth of Field

This control allows the image to be magnified or reduced along with a measurement scale. Magnification produces a grainier image, that, when excessive, makes interpretation more difficult.

Alteration in magnification also alters the extent of the imaged organ that can fit on the screen, being reduced by magnification, and vice versa.

Frame Rate

This control allows the frame rate, or frequency of image updating, to be altered. In general, better resolution is associated with lower rates, and higher rates are necessary to image moving structures. Not all machines allow the frame rate to be adjusted.

Pre- and Postprocessing

In addition to the initial setting up of the machine, the postadjustment controls may allow a frozen image to be altered. Care is necessary because image details can be lost as well as enhanced. The machine settings should be recorded, so the setup can be duplicated at follow-up ultrasound examinations.

Freeze

The freeze control allows an image to be held in memory for documentation, viewing, and measurement.

Image Scrolling

When a reduced image is displayed or when a standoff is used, deeper structures may be off-screen. Scrolling, which can be done on some machines, enables such regions to be viewed.

Split Screen

A split screen allows two images to be displayed simultaneously, thus allowing comparison or abutting images of an object longer than the field of view to be displayed.

M Mode

M mode is used to view moving structures. The range, or depth, is displayed on the y axis and time on the x axis.

Measurements

Electronic calipers can be activated to measure the curved or straight line distance between points, area, and circumference. Measurements are made on the assumption that velocity of sound through soft tissues is approximately 1,540 m/s. To make a measurement, one cursor is placed at a chosen reference point, and the other is moved to the second point, with the parameter measured depending on which has been selected.

Video

The video output is used for recording or monitoring.

SELECTION OF A MACHINE

The first consideration when choosing an ultrasound machine is the expected use to which the machine will be put. The four principal regions of interest in horses, the reproductive tract, appendicular soft tissues, abdomen, and heart, are, because of tissue depth and surface anatomy, best imaged with differently shaped transducers of a particular frequency(ies). In most cases, with the exception of the heart and deeper regions of the thorax and abdomen, a linear transducer can be used. The small access window between ribs dictates that a sector transducer be used on most occasions for imaging deeper intrathoracic and abdominal structures. Comprehensive cardiac imaging requires M-mode, Doppler, and ECG facilities. Image quality often depends on price, and more expensive machines produce higher-resolution images. A standoff is necessary for imaging superficial tendons and ligaments in the distal limb.

The optimum selection of transducer frequency depends on the distance between the contact surface and the region of interest. Structures immediately below the contact surface, such as tendons and ligaments in the distal limb, which are imaged percutaneously, or the bladder, which can be imaged percutaneously or transrectally, are best imaged with higher-frequency sound (i.e., 7-MHz transducer). Structures at a distance, such as the heart, require a transducer with a frequency as low as 2.5 MHz. There are structures that are midway between these extremes, either by virtue of their location or size, that require more than one frequency for adequate imaging. These include the uterus and ovaries (7 or 5 MHz) viewed transrectally, intraabdominal structures such as spleen, liver, and kidney (3 or 5 MHz) viewed percutaneously,

and miscellaneous structures such as abscesses and hematomata (5 MHz).

FACILITIES AND RESTRAINT

In addition to the usual need for operator safety, the value of the equipment dictates that it be protected from damage. The degree of restraint usually employed varies greatly with the procedure, the temperament of the horse, and the circumstances. The main concern with unrestrained horses is that equipment is at risk from sudden movement that will not be detected in time by the clinician who is usually observing a monitor while controlling the transducer. Optimum conditions are provided by use of stocks, chemical restraint as indicated, and an enclosed darkened room.

PATIENT PREPARATION

Good-quality images cannot be obtained unless there is good contact between the transducer and the skin. This is most reliably achieved as follows:

- Clip hair from area of contact.
- Shave hair stubble if necessary and when standoffs are used.
- Apply acoustic coupling gel to transducer.

The gel should be thick and sticky to ensure that it sticks to the skin and does not run off easily, and it should not contain air bubbles. Adequate images can often be obtained with other acoustic couplers, such as alcohol, methylcellulose, and paraffin oil as long as they are approved by the transducer manufacturer, and by massaging these into the hair. The gel should be removed from the skin after the procedure to avoid infection or a hypersensitivity reaction.

READINGS

Bentley H, Dyson S: Practical ultrasound physics—How to make optimal use of your machine. Equine Vet Educ 1991; 3: 227.

Dyson S: Selecting a machine for diagnostic ultrasound examinations in horses. Equine Vet Educ 1991; 3:161.

Powis RL: Ultrasound science for the veterinarian. In Diagnostic Ultrasound. Vet Clin North Am: Equine Pract 1986; 3:32.

Clinical Bacteriology

As part of the diagnostic process the clinician collects samples that will be subjected to microbiological examination. This may simply be an examination of a sample to determine whether organisms are present or involve the culturing of organisms. In either case the sample must be appropriate for the type of lesion and the suspected organisms, and it must not be allowed to deteriorate between the time of collection and its evaluation. Failure to observe basic precautions is a significant waste of time and expense, and diminishes the effectiveness of diagnosis. Guidelines for the collection, transport, and handling of clinical samples have been described and are summarized in the following.[1]

COLLECTION OF SAMPLES

The manner in which the sample should be collected depends on the type of bacteria expected and also on the site from which it will be collected. For example, internal fluids are collected by needle aspiration, but cutaneous or mucosal lesions are usually collected by scraping or swabbing.

Sterile Collection of Internal Fluids (Blood, Cerebrospinal Fluid, Subcutaneous Tissue Fluid, and Synovial Fluid from Joints, Tendon Sheaths, and Bursae)

These sites are normally sterile and samples should be collected using sterile technique, not only to ensure an optimum sample but also to avoid contamination and iatrogenic infection in the cavities.

Procedure

Clip hair from the site, and prepare it for sterile puncture by scrubbing with the detergent antiseptic, washing with 70% alcohol which is allowed to dry, and finally by painting or spraying with the tincture, which is also allowed to dry. The clinician should wear a sterile cap, mask, and gloves to avoid contaminating the site. A needle is then inserted into the appropriate location and the sample is collected by aspiration into the syringe.

Collection of Samples from Sites with Resident Flora (Skin, Mucosae)

Some body regions carry a resident population of organisms that can interfere with evaluation of a sample. There are a number of ways to reduce the number of normal flora in the sample:

- Swab the surface of the lesion with alcohol and then take the sample from deeper tissue (e.g., swab the surface of a pustule and then sample by aspiration or after opening it with a scalpel).
- Swab the surface of a lesion and then remove crusts and scabs, and sample from the exposed region.
- Remove secretions from mucosae with a dry swab, and then sample with a moistened swab.

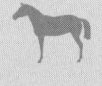

Materials for Sterile Collection of Samples of Internal Fluids for Bacteriological Examination

‣ Hair clippers #40 clipper head
‣ Materials for skin preparation
    detergent antiseptic (povidone-iodine, Hibiclens)
    70% alcohol
    Tincture Iodine (2% in 70% alcohol) or hibitane
‣ Gloves, caps, masks
‣ Syringe
‣ Needle: Spinal needle for CSF, 20-gauge 1″ hypodermic needle for the other sites
‣ Sample containers

Handling of Samples after Collection

The objective after collection is to ensure that the causative organism(s) can be identified. This is done by keeping the organisms viable, by ensuring that the sample does not dry out, and that multiplication is limited. The procedures that ensure this are as follows:

• Preparation of a smear. The availability of a smear ensures that some idea of the organisms present at the time of collection can be gained by the clinical pathologist. For fluid samples, a drop is placed on a microscope slide and a smear made. For tissue samples an impression smear is made.
• Process sample as soon as possible.
• Keep sample cool but not frozen.
• Use transport media whenever the sample cannot be processed immediately.

The methods for handling different types of material vary, as described in the sections that follow.

Swabs

AEROBES, FACULTATIVE ANAEROBES. Dry swabs must be moistened either before collection (e.g., BBL Transport Systems, BBL Division of Bec-

ton Dickinson and Co., Cockeysville, MD) or afterward by placing directly on a transport medium (e.g., Stuart's Medium, which is used in the Marion Scientific Culturette transport system, Marion Scientific, Kansas City, MO). Amies medium is required for *Taylorella equigenitalis,* the cause of contagious equine metritis.

ANAEROBES. Swabs are not suitable for collecting samples suspected to contain anaerobes. If there is no alternative, a suitable transport medium should be used (e.g., Port-A-Cul Tube, BBL Division of Becton-Dickinson and Co., Cockeysville, MD; BD Vacutainer Anaerobic Specimen Collector, BB Division of Becton-Dickinson and Co., Rutherford, NJ, or The Scott Two-Tube System, Scott Laboratories, Inc., Fiskeville, RI).

Fluids

AEROBES, FACULTATIVE ANAEROBES. These are best transported in a syringe with all air expelled. Alternately, if processing will be delayed, the material should be innoculated into a transport culture medium (e.g., Culture Collection and Transport System, Curtain Matheson Scientific, Inc., Precision Dynamic Corporation, Burbank, CA).

ANAEROBES. These should be transported in a syringe that has had all air expelled and with the needle sealed with a rubber stopper. Transport media can be used (e.g., BD Vacutainer Anaerobic Specimen Collector, BB Division of Becton-Dickinson and Co., Rutherford, NJ, for anaerobic bacteria only, or Port-A Cul Vials, BBL Microbiology Systems, PO Box 243, Cockeysville, MD).

Solid Tissue

AEROBES, FACULTATIVE ANAEROBES. The sample can be placed in a sterile screw-topped container with minimal air space. The sample can also be placed in a syringe into which a little saline is aspirated to prevent drying and then the air expelled. A transport medium can also be used (e.g., Port-A-Cul Transport System Vial, BBL Division of Becton-Dickinson and Co., Cockeysville, MD).

ANAEROBES. Place tissue in sterile container with minimal airspace, or use a transport medium (e.g., Port-A-Cul Vial, BBL Division of Becton-

Dickinson and Co., Cockeysville, MD). Do not refrigerate.

Urine

Collect into sterile, screw-top containers. These samples must be processed very rapidly. They should be kept at 5°C if they cannot be processed within 20 minutes. Storage at this temperature for up to 24 hours is acceptable, although some deterioration of leukocytes and bacterial viability will occur. Horse urine is usually cloudy, and it is therefore recommended that a smear be made immediately so that a Gram stain can be carried out to check for microorganisms and inflammatory cells. Infection is indicated if there are more than 10 white blood cells and more than 20 bacteria per microscopic field (oil immersion, ×1,000). Quantitative bacteriology can also be carried out using a disposable chamber (e.g., Kova Glasstic Slide 10 with grids, Hycor Biomedical, Inc., USA). With this method, infection is indicated if the count of white blood cells is greater than 10^4/mL of urine.

Blood

Blood should be collected under sterile conditions, as described. Vacutainer tubes should not be used so as to avoid possible aspiration of organisms into the sample.

AEROBES, FACULTATIVE ANAEROBES. If samples cannot be processed immediately, they should be inoculated into a blood culture medium (e.g., Signal Blood Culturing System, Oxoid USA, Columbia, MD) or laboratory-prepared broth (e.g., Brain Heart Infusion Broth [BHIF], Oxoid USA, Columbia, MD).

ANAEROBES. Samples should be placed in transport medium (e.g., Signal Blood Culture Bottles, Oxoid USA, Columbia, MD).

R E F E R E N C E

Love DN: Clinical Bacteriology. *In* Rose RJ, Hodgson DR (eds), Manual of Equine Practice, Philadelphia, WB Saunders Company, 1993, ch 15, p 396.

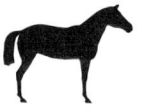

Evaluation of Pleural and Peritoneal Samples

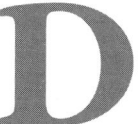

SAMPLES

Samples are collected so that examination can be carried out on clotted and unclotted fluids and under aerobic and anaerobic conditions. Accordingly, fluid should be collected into a tube containing EDTA (to ensure an unclotted sample), a plain tube with no additives (for a clotted sample), and also in a sealed syringe or transport medium for microbiological evaluation. Glucose and lactate estimations require a tube containing sodium fluoride and potassium oxalate, to inhibit further cell metabolism.

SLIDE PREPARATION AND STAINING

Although a clinician may be able to submit a sample directly to the laboratory without carrying out any further preparation, this is not always possible, especially for practitioners. For this reason a clinician should know how to prepare a sample that will be satisfactory for evaluation. The understanding of the preparation process also facilitates cooperation between clinician and laboratory, as well as improves a clinician's ability to understand some of the difficulties involved in interpreting presented material. Cytological evaluation depends on the presence of a sufficient number of suitably preserved cells. When the fluid is obviously turbid, and therefore probably contains many cells, a simple direct smear may be satisfactory. These smears can be made using "pull" or "squash" techniques on well-mixed fluid without the need for centrifugation. When the cell concentration is low, concentration by centrifugation is necessary. Smears prepared using a cytospin centrifuge are ideal, but the equipment is expensive. Luckily, sediment smears can be made using a standard centrifuge if the necessary equipment is not available. The sample is centrifuged for 5 minutes at 1,000 to 1,500 rpm, removing the supernatant until there is just sufficient left in which to resuspend the pellet of cells forming the centrifugate. After resuspension by gentle agitation, a drop of fluid is placed on a glass slide, and a "pull" or "squash" smear is made. If centrifugation is impossible, a portion of the sample can be concentrated by making a line smear by pushing the slide into, but not through, the droplet of fluid and then lifting it directly upward, leaving behind a transverse line of cell-rich fluid. As a precaution, in case of breakage during transport, some premade smears can also be submitted.

A number of different stains are suitable (Diff-Quik is easy to use). Other stains, such as Wright's Stain, methylene blue, or trichrome, are also useful. Identification of bacteria is best done with one of these stains before attempting classification with a Gram or acid-fast stain.

CYTOLOGY

Total and differential cell counts are carried out by automated or manual techniques, although the former may also count debris if the sample is not clear. Erythrocytes are not usually counted. However, their presence is noted to indicate contamination of the sample with blood during collection, frank hemorrhage, or lesions of thoracic or abdominal viscera involving vascular injury.

TOTAL PROTEIN

Total protein is measured by refractometry or biochemically, the former method being simple and requiring only a refractometer. To avoid interference from particulate matter, it is best to carry out refractometry after centrifugation, but, provided the sample is clear, this is not absolutely necessary. Refractometry is not as accurate as the chemical tests, especially when the value is below 2.5 gm/dL.

SPECIFIC GRAVITY

This parameter compares the density of the sample with that of distilled water, the difference being related to the dissolved solids.

CHEMICAL ANALYSIS

The worth of the various chemical analyses has been questioned. However the importance of comparing measurements on serum with those in peritoneal fluid are of proven value in diagnosing uroperitoneum where peritoneal fluid is contaminated with urine followed by equilibrium between blood and peritoneal fluid across the peritoneum.

CULTURE OF MICROORGANISMS

The simplest method of collecting samples for culture is to collect them into a syringe, carefully exclude air by depressing the plunger, cap the syringe by bending the needle or by using a plastic cap, and then submit it immediately to the laboratory. If this is not possible, preservation in a transport medium that will support both aerobic and anaerobic bacteria is necessary (see Appendix C, Clinical Bacteriology).

CLASSIFICATION OF EFFUSIONS

Effusions can be classified as transudates, modified transudates, or exudates, using values for total protein and total nucleated cell count:

Transudates

Transudates have low values for total protein (<2.5 gm/dL) and total nucleated cell counts (<1,500 cells/µL). Normal fluid is in this category. Accumulation of an abnormal volume of a transudate will occur if there is a disturbance in osmotic pressure usually related to hypoalbuminemia. Nondegenerate neutrophils and mesothelial/macrophagelike cells usually predominate in this group of effusions.

Modified Transudates

These are transudates modified by adding cells (1,500–10,000 cells/µL) and/or protein (2.5–6.5 gm/dL), and they generally occur in response to generalized or localized hemodynamic abnormalities, such as when there is obstruction to venous or lymphatic flow. They vary in color from amber to red to white. This is a difficult category to interpret because values for normal horses and horses with nonspecific diseases often fall here. Nondegenerate neutrophils will usually predominate.

Exudates

Effusions with high cell counts (>10,000 cells/µL) and high protein concentrations (>3.0 gm/dL) fall in this category and usually reflect significant pleuritis or peritonitis. A classification as an exudate does not provide a diagnosis, as the vascular changes can be the result of any of the myriad causes of inflammation such as sepsis, immune-mediated problems, or devitalized tissue. The predominant cell type often reflects the underlying pathological process; for example, neutrophils usually predominate in purulent effusions, appropriate neoplastic cells in cases of neoplasia, and lymphocytes in chylous or pseudochylous effusions. To account for bacteria, the exudate is subdivided into septic and nonseptic. Septic exudates contain bacteria (intra- or extracellular), degenerate neutrophils, and yield a positive culture, whereas nonseptic exudates do not contain bacteria, contain healthy neutrophils, and yield a negative culture. Interpretation is not always simple because bacteria are not always easy to find or culture, and the effect of their toxins on neutrophils varies with their virulence. Furthermore, as the broad classification is based on the concentrations of protein and cells classification may vary if the volume of fluid changes independently of protein or cells, or if there is a tendency for cells to concentrate by gravitating to the lower levels of the fluid load accumulating in the body cavity. As a result, it can be seen that the protein concentration for an exudate overlaps that of a modified transudate.

R E A D I N G

Cowell RL, Tyler RD, Clinkenbeard KD, et al: Collection and evaluation of equine peritoneal and pleural effusions. Vet Clin North Am: Equine Pract 1987; 3:543.

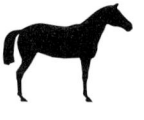

Sample Contamination with Blood

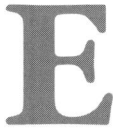

The clinician is often faced with the dilemma of deciding whether the blood in a sample is associated with the collection procedure (i.e., iatrogenic) or is related to the disease process. Sometimes the answer can be obtained quickly by examining the sample with the naked eye, but often a microscopic examination is necessary.

CHARACTERISTICS OF A SAMPLE CONTAMINATED WITH BLOOD

- Swirling of red cells during collection or agitation of the sample.
- Presence of blood platelets.
- No erythrophagocytosis.
- Tendency for sample to clot.
- Fluid only faintly pinkish.

CHARACTERISTICS OF A SAMPLE CONTAINING BLOOD ASSOCIATED WITH THE DISEASE PROCESS

- Acute-peracute
  May clot.
  Platelets may be present.
  Gross appearance and cell morphology are similar to peripheral blood, but cell numbers and protein values are less.
  Erythrophagocytosis may be present.
- Chronic
  Neutrophils often are hypersegmented and pycnotic.
  Platelets are absent.
  Blood will not clot.
  Phagocytosis of erythrocytes and their breakdown products, as well as aged neutrophils, is present.

Needle Biopsy

Percutaneous needle biopsy is used to obtain tissue samples from organs, such as the lung, liver, kidney, and from various tumors. The biopsy is usually carried out as a sterile procedure, which requires that the hair be removed by clipping or shaving, and that the skin surface be prepared with, in turn, a detergent antiseptic (povidone-iodine or chlorhexidine gluconate), 70% ethanol, and a tincture of the antiseptic used first. Subcutaneous injection of a bleb of local anesthetic, at the precise site where the needle will be inserted, is necessary. Prior to inserting the needle, a small stab incision should be made through the skin with a #15 scalpel blade to allow relatively friction-free insertion of the needle.

The most frequently used biopsy instrument is the Tru-Cut needle, demonstrated in Figure E–1A with the needle extended and the biopsy knotch exposed. The technique for using it is shown in Figure E–1B: The instrument, with the needle within the outer cannula, is inserted through the stab incision in the skin and then into the organ or mass to be biopsied. The needle is then pushed out from the cannula and deeper into the target, which allows the tissue to protrude into the knotch. Then, with the needle supported, the cannula is advanced quickly over the needle, to cut off the piece of tissue in the knotch. The instrument is then removed and the needle again extended to expose the knotch containing the tissue sample, which is scraped into the fixative, 10% neutral buffered formalin (Fig. E–1C). The technique requires practice, as controlling the needle and the cannula is a little awkward.

An alternate instrument, the Temno Automatic needle (Fig. E–2) is spring-loaded, and automates the action of advancing the cannula. It is designed to be used single-handed. Before use, it is loaded by pulling on the rectangular end of the needle while stabilizing the rest of the instrument by holding the two finger loops. When loaded, the needle is free and can be moved in and out of the cannula. To collect the biopsy, the instrument is loaded and the first and second fingers are inserted, as shown in the diagram. It is then inserted into the tissue, causing the needle to slide back within the cannula. When the needle is inserted to the appropriate depth, the thumb is used to push gently on the rectangular base of the needle, thus advancing it into the tissue and exposing the knotch, as described for the Tru-Cut needle. The instrument is then fired by pushing firmly on the base of the needle, causing the cannula to advance very rapidly and cut the biopsy. The instrument is then withdrawn with the tissue enclosed.

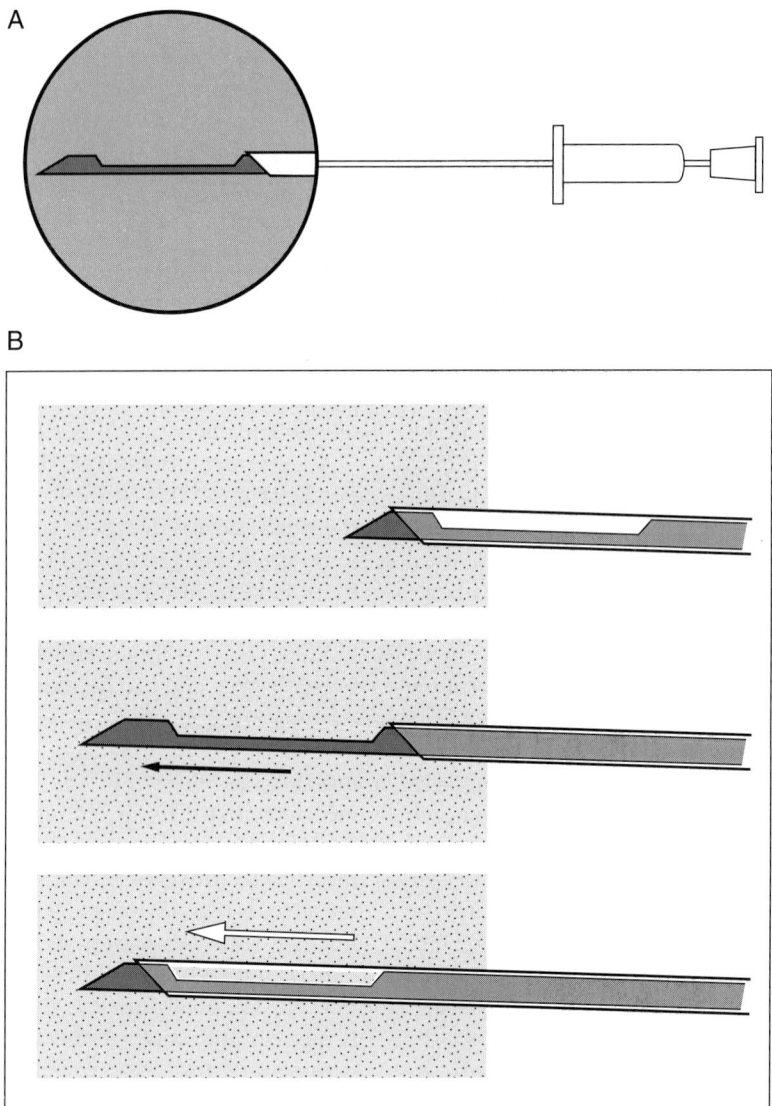

▶ **FIGURE E–1**

Technique of needle biopsy. **A.** Tru-Cut needle with needle extended and biopsy knotch exposed. **B.** Illustration demonstrating how the needle and sheath are inserted into tissue and the biopsy collected.

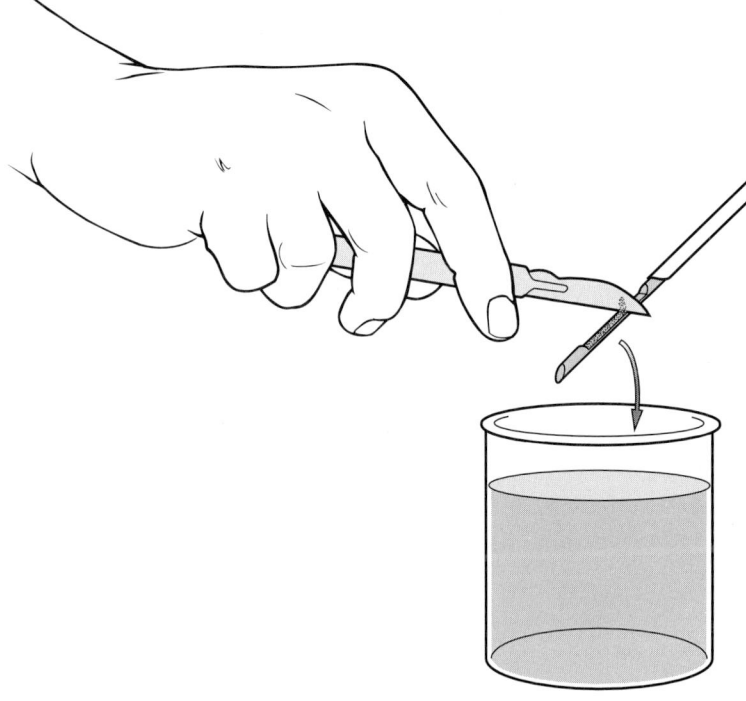

C

▶ **FIGURE E–1** *Continued*
C. Specimen is transferred to the fixative.

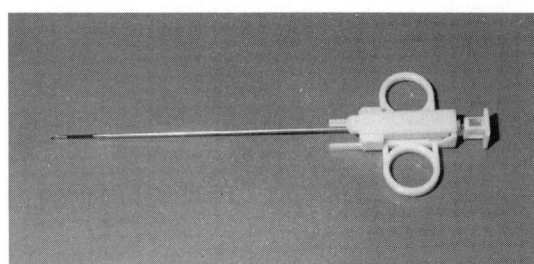

▶ **FIGURE E–2**

The Temno Automatic Disposable Guillotine Soft Tissue Needle (Products Group International, Inc). Note the finger loops that facilitate single-handed use.

Index

Note: Page numbers in *italic* refer to illustrations; those followed by t refer to tables.

ISBN 0-7216 6506-3

90038

9 780721 665061